Fundamentals of Pharmacology for Children's Nurses

Fundamentals of Pharmacology for Children's Nurses

Edited By

IAN PEATE, EN(G), RGN, DipN (Lond) RNT, Bed (Hons), MA (Lond) LLM, OBE, FRCN, JP

Principal
School of Health Studies
Gibraltar Health Authority
St Bernard's Hospital
Gibraltar, UK

PETER DRYDEN, MSc, BSc (Hons), PGCE, PGDip HE, FHEA, Dip HE Children's Nursing

Programme Lead and
Senior Lecturer
Department of Nursing
Midwifery and Health
Northumbria University
Newcastle upon Tyne, UK

WILEY Blackwell

This edition first published 2022
© 2022 by John Wiley & Sons Ltd

All rights reserved. No part of this publication may be reproduced, stored in a retrieval system, or transmitted, in any form or by any means, electronic, mechanical, photocopying, recording or otherwise, except as permitted by law. Advice on how to obtain permission to reuse material from this title is available at www.wiley.com/go/permissions.

The right of Ian Peate and Peter Dryden be identified as the authors of editorial work has been asserted in accordance with law.

Registered Offices
John Wiley & Sons, Inc., 111 River Street, Hoboken, NJ 07030, USA
John Wiley & Sons Ltd, The Atrium, Southern Gate, Chichester, West Sussex, PO19 8SQ, UK

Editorial Office
9600 Garsington Road, Oxford, OX4 2DQ, UK

For details of our global editorial offices, customer services, and more information about Wiley products visit us at www.wiley.com.

Wiley also publishes its books in a variety of electronic formats and by print-on-demand. Some content that appears in standard print versions of this book may not be available in other formats.

Limit of Liability/Disclaimer of Warranty
The contents of this work are intended to further general scientific research, understanding, and discussion only and are not intended and should not be relied upon as recommending or promoting scientific method, diagnosis, or treatment by physicians for any particular patient. In view of ongoing research, equipment modifications, changes in governmental regulations, and the constant flow of information relating to the use of medicines, equipment, and devices, the reader is urged to review and evaluate the information provided in the package insert or instructions for each medicine, equipment, or device for, among other things, any changes in the instructions or indication of usage and for added warnings and precautions. While the publisher and authors have used their best efforts in preparing this work, they make no representations or warranties with respect to the accuracy or completeness of the contents of this work and specifically disclaim all warranties, including without limitation any implied warranties of merchantability or fitness for a particular purpose. No warranty may be created or extended by sales representatives, written sales materials or promotional statements for this work. The fact that an organization, website, or product is referred to in this work as a citation and/or potential source of further information does not mean that the publisher and authors endorse the information or services the organization, website, or product may provide or recommendations it may make. This work is sold with the understanding that the publisher is not engaged in rendering professional services. The advice and strategies contained herein may not be suitable for your situation. You should consult with a specialist where appropriate. Further, readers should be aware that websites listed in this work may have changed or disappeared between when this work was written and when it is read. Neither the publisher nor authors shall be liable for any loss of profit or any other commercial damages, including but not limited to special, incidental, consequential, or other damages.

Library of Congress Cataloging-in-Publication Data

Names: Peate, Ian, editor. | Dryden, Peter, editor.
Title: Fundamentals of pharmacology for children's nurses / edited by Ian
    Peate, Peter Dryden.
Description: Hoboken, NJ, USA : Wiley-Blackwell, 2022. | Includes
    bibliographical references and index.
Identifiers: LCCN 2021010955 (print) | LCCN 2021010956 (ebook) | ISBN
    9781119633211 (paperback) | ISBN 9781119633228 (adobe pdf) | ISBN
    9781119633235 (epub)
Subjects: MESH: Pharmacological Phenomena | Pharmacokinetics | Child |
    Adolescent | Pediatric Nursing | Nurses Instruction
Classification: LCC RM301.5 (print) | LCC RM301.5 (ebook) | NLM QV 37 |
    DDC 615.7083–dc23
LC record available at https://lccn.loc.gov/2021010955
LC ebook record available at https://lccn.loc.gov/2021010956

Cover Design: Wiley
Cover Images: © sturti/Getty Images, © Karl Tapales/Getty Images

Set in 9.5/11pt Minion by Straive, Pondicherry, India
Printed and bound by CPI Group (UK) Ltd, Croydon, CR0 4YY

C9781119633211_221121

This text is dedicated to all health and social care workers who, during the COVID-19 pandemic, lost their lives whilst in the line of duty. The text is also dedicated to those students who experienced the impact of the pandemic on their education and training.

Contents

Contributors xv
Preface xxv
Acknowledgements xxvii
Prefixes and Suffixes xxix
Abbreviations xli
About the Companion Website xliii

1 Introduction to Pharmacology, Children and Young People 1

Introduction to Pharmacology 2
Professional Framework 2
The Importance and Value of Medicine Within Healthcare 3
Therapeutic Pharmacology 3
Social Prescribing 4
Safety Within Paediatric Care 5
Medicines Optimisation 5
Medicines 6
Medicine Management 6
Safety: Rights of Medication Administration 7
Specific Considerations for Babies, Children and Young People 7
Infancy 7
Adolescents 9
Tablets 10
Distraction Techniques 10
Conclusion 11
Glossary 11
References 12
Further Resources 12
Multiple Choice Questions 13
Find Out More 14

2 How to Use Pharmaceutical and Prescribing Reference Guides 17

Introduction 18
The British National Formulary and the British National Formulary for Children 19
Paper Copy BNFc 19
How to navigate the BNFc 19
Online and Mobile Application BNFc 23
Monthly Index of Medical Specialities (MIMS) 24

Electronic Medicines Compendium   26
What Can Be Prescribed on an NHS Prescription?   26
Other Guides to Prescribing   27
The Evidence Base to Prescribing: Prescribing Guidelines   28
Conclusion   30
References   30
Further Resources   30
Multiple Choice Questions   30

3   Legal and Ethical Issues   33

Introduction   34
The Law   34
The Bolam Test   35
The Children Act 2004   36
Duty of Care and Healthcare   37
Regulation of Healthcare   37
Ethical Principles and Theories   38
Research   39
Children and Young People who are under 16 years – Gillick and Fraser Guidance   42
Assessing and Promoting Competence   42
Parental Responsibility   43
Medication Adherence and Administration   43
Conclusion   44
References   45
Further Resources   47
Multiple Choice Questions   47
Find Out More   48

4   Medicines Management and the Role of the Healthcare Provider Working with Children, Young People and Families   49

Introduction   50
Being an Accountable Professional   51
Nursing and Midwifery Council   51
Employer and Colleagues   51
Promoting Health and Preventing Ill Health   52
Holistic Assessment   52
Assessing Needs and Planning Care   53
Self-Medication   55
Complementary and Alternative Medication (CAM)   58
Planning   58
Providing and Evaluating Care   58
Checking   59
Evaluation   59
Leading and Managing Nursing Care and Working in Teams   60
Improving Safety and Quality   62
Coordinating Care   63
Conclusion   65
References   65
Further Resources   66
Multiple Choice Questions   66
Find Out More   68

5 Pharmacodynamics and Pharmacokinetics 69

Introduction 70
Royal Pharmaceutical Society 70
The Nursing and Midwifery Council 70
Pharmacokinetics 70
Think Paediatrics 79
Pharmacodynamics 81
Conclusion 85
Glossary 85
References 85
Further Resources 87
Multiple Choice Questions 87

6 Drug Formulations 89

Introduction 90
Licensing of Paediatric Medicines 90
Types of Formulations 91
Excipients 96
Enteral Feeding Tubes 97
Displacement Values 100
Conclusion 101
Glossary 101
References 101
Further Resources 103
Multiple Choice Questions 103
Find Out More 105

7 Medications Used in the Cardiovascular System 107

Introduction 108
Gross Anatomy Related to Cardiovascular System (CVS) Pharmacology 108
Cardiovascular Drugs Affecting Chronic Conditions 110
Anticoagulant Medications 112
Angiotensin Converting Enzyme (ACE) Inhibitors 113
Angiotensin II Receptor Antagonists 114
Peripheral Alpha Antagonist or Alpha-Adrenergic Blockers: 'Alpha Blockers' 114
Cardiovascular Drugs for Use in Acute Clinical Scenarios 114
Electrophysiological System Recap 114
Drugs with an Inotropic Effect 117
Drugs with a Chronotropic Effect 121
Conclusion 123
Glossary 124
References 124
Further Resources 125
Multiple Choice Questions 126
Find Out More 127

8 Medications Used in the Renal System 129

Introduction 130
Anatomy and Physiology of the Renal System 130

x   Contents

Common Renal Conditions   132
Nephrotic Syndrome   132
Treatment of MCNS   134
Drugs Used to Treat Electrolyte Disorders   138
Conclusion   145
Glossary   145
References   146
Further Resources   147
Multiple Choice Questions   148
Find Out More   149

9   Medications Used in the Endocrine System   151

Introduction   152
The Endocrine System   152
Medications Used in Endocrine Disorders Affecting Growth   154
Endocrine Disorders of Puberty   157
Drugs Used to Block Puberty or the Action of Sex Steroids   160
Drugs Used to Reduce the Action of Sex Steroids   161
Medications Used in Disorders of the Adrenal Glands   162
Medications Used in the Management of Diabetes   163
Conclusion   163
Glossary   169
References   169
Further Resources   170
Multiple Choice Questions   170
Find Out More   172

10   Medications Used in the Respiratory System   173

Introduction   174
Asthma   175
Croup   177
Bronchiolitis   178
Pneumonia   178
Cystic Fibrosis   179
Respiratory Medicines   180
Antibiotics   187
Mucolytics   188
Other Respiratory Drugs   188
Conclusion   189
Glossary   190
References   190
Further Resources   191
Multiple Choice Questions   191
Find Out More   192

11   Medications Used in the Gastrointestinal System   195

Introduction   196
Overview of the Anatomy and Physiology of the Gastrointestinal System   196
The Stomach   197
Small Intestines   198
The Liver   199

The Gallbladder   199
The Pancreas   199
The Large Intestine   199
Gastro-Oesophageal Reflux Disease (GORD)   200
Enteral Feeding Tubes and Medication Administration   204
Constipation   208
Crohn's Disease   211
Conclusion   214
Glossary   214
References   215
Further Resources   216
Multiple Choice Questions   216
Find Out More   218

12   Medications Used in the Nervous System   219

Introduction   220
Epilepsy   221
Guillain–Barré Syndrome   228
Migraine   230
Status Migrainosus   234
Conclusion   234
Glossary   234
References   234
Further Resources   237
Multiple Choice Questions   237
Appendix 1: AEDs Used in Treatment of Childhood Epilepsy   239

13   The Immune System and Immunisations   241

Introduction   242
Types of Immunity   242
How Immunisations Work   243
Immunisation and Public Health   245
Immunisation Schedule   246
Vaccine Uptake   246
The 'Cold Chain'   248
Patient Specific Directions and Patient Group Directives   248
Administration of Vaccines   248
Common Reactions and Anaphylaxis   250
Communication with the Child and Family   251
The Green Book   252
Conclusion   252
Glossary   252
References   252
Further Resources   253
Multiple Choice Questions   253
Find Out More   255

14   Medications and the Integumentary System   257

Introduction   258
Anatomy and Physiology of the Integumentary System   258
The Epidermis   258

Common Skin Conditions   259
Conclusion   270
Glossary   271
References   271
Further Resources   272
Multiple Choice Questions   272
Find Out More   274

15   Medications Used in Children and Young People's Mental Health   275

Introduction   276
What Is Psychopharmacology?   276
Medications   276
Conclusion   288
Glossary   288
References   289
Further Resources   290
Multiple Choice Questions   291
Find Out More   292

16   Medications Used in Children and Young People's cancer   293

Introduction   294
Cancer   294
Cell Cycle   295
Chemotherapies   296
Immunotherapies in Treating Cancer   301
Corticosteroid Use in Cancer   308
Conclusion   312
Glossary   312
References   312
Further Resources   314
Multiple Choice Questions   314
Find Out More   316

17   Analgesics   317

Introduction   318
Pain Pathways   318
Definitions and Categories of Pain   319
Importance of Individualised Pain Assessments   320
Assessment Tools   321
Multimodal Management Strategies   323
Pharmacological Management   324
Non-opioids   325
Non-Steroidal Anti-Inflammatory Drugs (NAIDs)   327
Opioid Agonists   327
Codeine Phosphate   331
Dihydrocodeine   331
Tramadol   331
Morphine   332
Fentanyl   332
Adjuvants and Co-analgesics – Gabapentinoids   333

Inhalation Analgesics   333
Local, Regional and Topical Analgesia   334
Conclusion   337
Glossary   337
References   338
Further Resources   340
Multiple Choice Questions   341
Find Out More   342

18   Antimicrobial Medications   343

Introduction   344
Microorganisms   344
Antimicrobial Medications   345
Antibacterial Medications   345
Penicillins   347
Antiviral Medications   351
Antifungal Medications   354
Antiprotozoal Medications   357
Antimicrobial Resistance   359
Antimicrobial Stewardship   360
Prescribing Antimicrobials   362
Conclusion   362
Glossary   363
References   363
Further Resources   364
Multiple Choice Questions   365
Find Out More   366

19   Adverse Drug Reactions   367

Introduction   368
Adverse Events   369
Side Effects   369
Preventing ADRs   370
Recognising ADRs   371
ADRs and Immunisations   372
Allergic Reactions   373
Anaphylaxis   373
Medicines Safety and Reporting ADRs   376
Reporting ADRs via The Yellow Card System   377
Conclusion   379
References   379
Further Resources   380
Multiple Choice Questions   380

Answers   383
Index   387

Contributors

Jaden Allan

MSc, PG Dip, BSc (Hons), RN, SFHEA. Director of Transnational Education (TNE)
Senior Lecturer, Learning Leadership Lead (Peer support), Department of Nursing, Midwifery and Health.

Jaden joined Northumbria University having spent several years working in a partnership hospital post as a practice placement facilitator (PPF) organising a range of health professional student placements and providing support to students and mentors during their clinical rotations. Jaden's clinical nursing experience is in critical care (respiratory, neurological and plastics) at the Newcastle upon Tyne NHS Foundation Trust, and earlier in acute surgery (GI and general) at Northumbria NHS Trust. Since joining the university, Jaden has held a number of complex module lead roles and he has been instrumental in developing the use of simulation within the nursing curriculum. Having many years of senior lecturer experience in teaching and leadership gives Jaden a sound foundation for his strategic and departmental work. Over the past four years Jaden's roles have include Director of Programs and Director of Learning and Teaching (DLT) with responsibility for curricula revalidation, quality teaching and assessment monitoring, departmental development and university vision delivery. He has also led on departmental timetabling, and faculty integration of timetabling systems. Jaden is currently working as Director of International Development and Recruitment for the faculty of Health and Life Sciences, liaising with international partners and universities to develop the university's portfolio of Transnational Education (TNE) and international students both on campus and globally. Jaden has developed, and been implementation lead, for a number of complex practice modules in Northumbria University's UK BSc (Hons) Nursing program. He is a lead on the implementation for a BSc (Hons) Nursing curricula in Malta. He has led the development, and the successful implementation, of the 'Learning Leadership scheme' within Northumbria's Nursing programs. This peer support scheme prepares and develops students on nursing programs to support newer students as they make the transition into higher education and the world of nursing. Jaden's learning and teaching interests are developing clinical skills, simulation (all levels), leadership, peer support and compassion in nursing. Jaden also has a particular interest in the use of technology to enhance and share learning.

Sasha Ban

Deputy Head of Department (Nursing, Midwifery and Health), Senior Lecturer in Children's Nursing, Chair of Governors Whickham School and Sixth Form, Independent Panel member (Health) for the Fosters Carers Association.

Sasha starting her nursing career in 1990, she practised in neonatal intensive care and paediatric oncology, she moved into public health as a health visitor, working in Sure Start centres. She has worked in nurse education since 2005, Sasha's key areas of interest are adolescence, global health, social inequality and interprofessional education. She is a senior fellow of the HEA.

Janis Bloomer

Janis Bloomer started her nurse training in April 1979 at Gateshead school of nursing, she then went on to Newcastle school of Nursing to become a Registered Sick children's Nurse.

Janis worked in General Paediatrics as a staff nurse until she became a CF Nurse Specialist in October 1989, where she was instrumental in developing the Nurse Specialist role within CF and was a founder member of the National CF Nurses Group. Within this time she was part of a subcommittee who developed

Nursing standards for CF. Janis has always been passionate about the care of children with CF and has developed the service we have today, In 2015 Janis joined the NICE CF Guideline committee which developed strategies for the care of both children and adults. Throughout her career Janis has always been an advocate for children and their families, she has recently retired from Nursing after 42 years.

Jane Callum

RSCN, RGN, BSc (Hons) CCN Specialist practitioner, MSc, FHEA

Senior Lecturer at Northumbria University Jane qualified as an RGN at Leeds General Infirmary where her first staff nurse post was in gastroenterology. Following a short period in High Dependency at the Queen Elizabeth Hospital Gateshead, Jane moved to Liverpool to qualify as a children's nurse at Alder Hey Hospital and John Moores University. Within Paediatrics Jane has been a staff nurse in medicine and oncology and a research nurse before finding her true passion as a Children's Community Nurse and matron at Newcastle Hospitals Foundation Trust. Jane's keen interest in supporting children in the community started in a special school and included creating educational days on Autism and multi-disciplinary training in Tracheostomy care. Jane has also been part of a working group with the Department of Health to develop CCN services. Since moving to Northumbria University in 2012, student experience, care in the community and children with complex health needs remain a passion.

Claire Camara

Graduate Tutor in Children and Young People's Nursing at Northumbria University.

Claire began her nursing career studying at Middlesex University and working as a Therapeutic Care Worker at the Ellern Mede Centre for Eating Disorders. Since qualifying Claire has worked in paediatric oncology and as a paediatric research nurse at Newcastle Hospitals Trust before beginning in nurse education in 2018 at Northumbria University. Claire is currently studying towards her PhD and a Post Graduate Certificate in Academic Practice. Her areas of interest are paediatric chronic conditions, quality of life, research and ethics.

Louise Carr

Lead Clinical Pharmacist for Paediatric Intensive Care at the Great North Children's Hospital in Newcastle upon Tyne.

Louise achieved a Masters in Pharmacy at the University of Manchester in 2005. Following completion of a pre-registration year, she embarked on her career as a clinical pharmacist in the Newcastle upon Tyne Hospitals NHS Foundation Trust in 2006. Louise worked as a rotational pharmacist for the Trust, covering a wide range of clinical specialities, before being appointed the role of specialist pharmacist for adult critical care in 2008. In 2015 she joined the paediatric pharmacy team at the Great North Children's Hospital within the Newcastle upon Tyne Hospitals, where she has since worked as the lead clinical pharmacist for paediatric intensive care. Louise completed a postgraduate Masters in Medicines Use in Paediatrics and Neonates with Liverpool John Moores University in 2019, and is currently undertaking an independent prescribing qualification.

Sadie Diamond Fox

Advanced Critical Care Practitioner (FICM member) & Senior Lecturer in Advanced Critical Care Practice (FHEA)

Sadie qualified as an adult nurse in 2008 and has since worked in various critical care departments since. During this time, she has progressed from Registered Nurse to her current specialist roles as Advanced Critical Care Practitioner (ACCP), non-medical prescriber and Senior Lecturer. Sadie has always had a great passion for academia and has developed an extensive teaching portfolio which spans multiple disciplines within postgraduate healthcare education, making a wide range of contributions on local and international levels. Sadie has various national links and responsibilities within the field of advanced practice. Her key areas of interest are post-graduate healthcare education, acute, emergency, and critical care, physiology and pharmacology, advanced level practice and simulation and virtual reality education modalities.

Barbara Davies
RGN, RSCN, BSC(Hons), PG Dip MSc

Director of Education and Senior Lecturer in Children's Nursing at the University of Northumbria in Newcastle upon Tyne, England.

Barbara is a Senior Fellow of the Higher Education Academy. Barbara is an Adult Registered Nurse who then qualified as a Registered Sick Children's Nurse. Within clinical practice, she has 20 years' experience of working with children, young people and their families in a variety of roles. Her final clinical post was as a Paediatric Rheumatology Nurse Specialist/Clinical Co-ordinator setting up the regional rheumatology service for children and young people. Moving into academia, Barbara is involved in both teaching and research. Her research interests lie within paediatric rheumatology, family nursing, student mentor relationships and the observation of students in practice.

Following collaborative research with the Great North Children's Hospital and Newcastle University to explore the needs of nurses working with children with inflammatory arthritis. pmm.nursing, an online, free, educational resource, was launched in November 2017. Barbara has presented the research findings at national and international conferences and it was at a conference in Denmark that she became acquainted with the concept of Family Nursing and is now a member of the Executive Group of the IFNA – UK and Ireland Chapter.

Peter Dryden
MSc, BSc (Hons), PGCE, PGDip HE, FHEA, Dip HE Children's Nursing

Peter started his nursing career as a health care assistant caring for adults with learning disabilities in 1991. Peter qualified as a children's nurse in 1998 and worked in paediatric acute assessment and then as a Specialist Nurse in paediatric Inflammatory Bowel Disease (IBD). Peter has worked in Health Education since 2014 in both pre-registration nursing and Continuing Workforce Development and is currently studying for his PhD in children and young people (CYP) IBD transition, which follows on from his MSc dissertation. Peter is currently a Programme Lead and Senior Lecturer in Children's Nursing at Northumbria University.

Katherine Drape
MSc, BSc (Hons), PGCE, PGDip HE, FHEA

Senior Lecturer in Children's Nursing Northumbria University

Katherine commenced her nursing career as a registered children's nurse in Newcastle upon Tyne working in general paediatrics at Newcastle's Royal Victoria Infirmary. After 2 years Katherine specialised in paediatric renal medicine and worked with children and young people in acute and chronic renal failure. This included supporting children and their families at home requiring peritoneal dialysis. Katherine then worked in a clinical educator's role in children's services before moving into a specialist nurse role in safeguarding. Katherine joined Northumbria University in 2017 and works within the Children's nursing team teaching and supporting undergraduate nursing students.

Dr Christine English
RGN, RSCN, DPSN, BSc (Hons), MSc, PGDE, SFHEA, PhD

Visiting Scholar, Northumbria University; Senior Fellow (Higher Education Academy); Trustee Board Member and Chair of Clinical Governance and Clinical Quality Committee, St Oswald's Hospice; Executive Committee Member, International Family Nursing Association (UK and Ireland Chapter); Committee Member IFNA Education Committee; Committee Member International Child and Family Centred Care Network.

Christine initially worked in adult services before moving to children's nursing at the Royal Victoria Infirmary, Newcastle. Her career has spanned practice, education and research, where she has held strategic leadership positions. Previous roles include: Head of Subject (Nursing Midwifery and Health); Director of Student Engagement/Experience; Faculty Director of Outreach/Widening Participation; Programme Director; Senior Matron (Child and Teenage Oncology Service); Ward Sister; Staff Nurse. She continues to publish, network and collaborate within children, young people and family nursing.

Christine's main research interests are child and family perspectives on care and quality improvement in children's care.

Claire Fagan

Specialist Nurse Children and Young Peoples Cystic Fibrosis at Great North Children's Hospital, Newcastle upon Tyne.

Claire qualified as a children's nurse in 2006, having previously studied Biomedical Sciences. She started her nursing career at the Royal Victoria Infirmary in Newcastle upon Tyne. Working within the Children's services directorate her main experiences involve acute admissions and emergency care, general paediatrics and intensive care. She became a Cystic Fibrosis Nurse Specialist at the Great North Children's Hospital in 2014 and is currently the north east regional representative for the Cystic Fibrosis Nursing Association.

Dr Claire Ford

Fellow of Higher Education Academy (FHEA), PhD, PG Diploma Midwifery, BSc (Hons) Adult Nursing, Registered Nurse (RN)
Senior Lecturer Adult Nursing, Northumbria University.

Claire joined the teaching team at Northumbria University in 2013, having spent time working within perioperative care and completing a Postgraduate Diploma in Midwifery. She studied for her BSc (Hons) and PG Dip at Northumbria University, and won academic awards for both, as well as the Heath Award in 2009. As a Lecturer, she teaches on a range of modules national and international preregistration healthcare programmes. In addition to teaching, Claire is involved in several research projects ranging from the examination of pain practices in perioperative care to exploring the use of technology-enhanced learning and virtual reality to augment undergraduate students learning. Claire has a passion for pain management, clinical skills, women's health, gynaecology, perioperative care and simulation and has published many articles. She also has an interest in using other forms of media and technology to facilitate and enhance deep learning and is the co-founder of the 'Skills for Practice' website, which acts as a central repository for videos, posters, and podcasts focusing on a range of clinical nursing procedures. In 2016, the website was shortlisted for the Student Nursing Times Awards – Teaching Innovation of the Year.

Anthony Garbutt

Anthony completed his undergraduate adult nurse training at Northumbria University in 2010. Anthony subsequently worked within cardiothoracic surgery as staff nurse, surgical first assistant and senior charge nurse roles during this time. Anthony completed his MSc in 2015, investigating effectiveness of pre-operative anxiety interventions for cardiac surgery. This work was undertaken across adult and paediatric specialities, including transplantation.

Currently, Anthony is Senior Lecturer in Adult Nursing and Operating Department Practice at Northumbria University, with specialist interests in cardiovascular, respiratory and advanced clinical practice. He is currently studying for his PhD, investigating workplace socialisation, linked to education.

Alexandra Gatehouse

Alex Gatehouse graduated from Nottingham University in 2000 with a Bsc (Hons) Physiotherapy. Following Junior Rotations in the Newcastle Trust she specialised in Respiratory Physiotherapy in Adult Critical Care, also working within New Zealand. In 2012 she trained as an Advanced Critical Care Practitioner, completing a Masters in Clinical Practice in Critical Care and qualifying in 2014. Alex subsequently completed her non-medical prescribing qualification and continues to rotate within all of the Critical Care Units in Newcastle Upon Tyne, also enjoying teaching on the regional transfer course. She is a co-founder of the Advanced Critical Care Practitioner Northern Region Group and is a committee member of the North East Intensive Care Society. Alex has presented abstracts at the European Society of Intensive Care Medicine and the North East Intensive Care Society conferences.

Sophie Gilmour-Ivens

Sophie began her nursing career at Stoke Mandeville hospital in 1995 after completing her paediatric nursing degree at Oxford Brookes University.

She worked on the medical ward at Ipswich hospital before moving to Newcastle upon Tyne Hospitals NHS Trust where she worked as a staff nurse on a neurology/ neuro-oncology ward for 6 years. She was appointed as an epilepsy nurse specialist in 2006 and this role was expanded to a neurology nurse specialist role in 2014.

Sophie has always had a special interest in epilepsy and now works as a paediatric epilepsy nurse specialist at Northumbria Healthcare NHS Foundation Trust.

Liz Gormley-Fleming

RGN, RSCN, RNT, PG Cert (Herts) PG Dip HE (Herts), BSc (Hons), MA (Keele), SFHEA
Associate Director Academic Quality Assurance. University of Hertfordshire.

Liz commenced her nursing career in Ireland where she qualified as an RGN and RSCN. Initially she worked in paediatric oncology before moving to London where she held a variety of senior clinical nursing and leadership roles across a range of NHS Trusts, both in the acute care setting and community.

Educationally, Liz has worked in education since 2001, initially as a clinical facilitator before moving into full-time Higher Education in 2003. She has had held a range of leadership and management roles including being an Associate Dean for Academic Quality Assurance and Head of Department for Nursing. Liz has extensive experience in academic quality assurance and also works as an NMC quality assurance visitor. She is still actively engaged in both teaching and research. Her areas of interest are care of the acutely ill child, healthcare law and ethics, professional values, curriculum development, practice-based learning and degree apprenticeships.

Sinéad Greener

Paediatric Bone Marrow Transplantation Pharmacist at the Great North Children's Hospital in Newcastle Upon Tyne, Research Associate at Newcastle University, Newcastle Upon Tyne.

Sinéad studied biochemistry with immunology in Trinity College Dublin before training in pharmacy in Robert Gordon University, Aberdeen. She completed her pre-registration training year in St Mary's Hospital in London before moving to Newcastle upon Tyne Hospitals NHS Foundation Trust to begin training as a junior pharmacist. She has been working as a pharmacist since 2009. She became a senior pharmacist in paediatrics in 2012 and specialised as a paediatric bone marrow transplantation pharmacist in 2016. She enjoys undertaking research alongside her clinical role.

Sarah Greenshields

RN (child), BNurs, MSc Specialist Community Public Health Nursing, Post Graduate Certificate of Academic Practice, Fellow of HEA

Sarah qualified as a children's nurse from Manchester University in 2008. She worked on a ward which cared for children and young people with a variety of needs. This included neurology, neuro oncology, immunology and general paediatrics. Following this Sarah moved into community nursing. This included being responsible for immunisations and working in schools. Sarah qualified as a Specialist Public Health Practitioner in 2015. She then led a team of nurses who worked into specialist provisions, caring for children with complex needs and their families. During 2017 she completed her masters in Public Health. In late 2018 Sarah started a role as a Lecturer in the Children and Young Peoples nursing team at Northumbria University. She also has a role in teaching on the Specialist Public Health Practitioner programme and is working towards her PhD.

Dr Annette Hand
DNursing, MA, PG Dip CR, Dip HE, RGN
Nurse Consultant/Associate Professor/Clinical Lead – Nursing, Northumbria Healthcare NHS Trust/ Northumbria University/Parkinson's Excellence Network

Annette has a clinical academic position and divides her time between three roles: Nurse Consultant, Associate Professor and UK Clinical Lead for Nursing (Parkinson's).

Annette has worked in the field of Parkinson's for many years and as a Nurse Consultant has an active clinical, research and educational role within this area. She qualified as a non-medical prescriber over 15 years ago and continues to use this skill in day to day clinical practice. She was the non-medical prescribing lead for Northumbria Healthcare NHS Foundation Trust for many years, supporting and developing other non-medical prescribers. Annette, an Associate Professor with Northumbria University, has lectured on the non-medical prescribing programme (V300) for over 5 years, and supports prescribing students and the continual development of the V300 programme. Annette was appointed to the national role of Clinical Lead for Nursing within the Parkinson's UK Excellence Network, as part of the clinical leadership team. This role was developed to support service improvements through education, knowledge exchange and evidence based practice and support the role of the Parkinson's Nurse across the UK.

Barry Hill
MSc Advanced Practice, PGC Academic Practice, BSc (Hons) Intensive Care Nursing, DipHE Adult Nursing, OA Dip Counselling Skills, Registered Nurse (RN). Registered Teacher (NMC RNT/TCH). Senior Fellow (SFHEA), Programme Leader (Senior Lecturer) Adult Nursing, Northumbria University. Clinical and Commissioning Editor for the British Journal of Nursing.

Barry is an experienced leader, academic, educator, researcher, and clinical nurse. His current role is director level and as part of the senior leadership team, as 'Director of Education (Employability)' for the department of Nursing, Midwifery and Health, and Programme Leader (BSc Nursing Sciences). He has a demonstrated history of working within academia particularly in the Higher Education (HE) industry. Barry is a Senior Fellow (SFHEA) and a HEA mentor, Barry is a certified Advanced Nurse Practitioner (ANP), NMC Registered Nurse (RN), NMC Registered Teacher (TCH), and NMC Registered independent and supplementary prescriber (V300). Barry is skilled in clinical research; clinical education and is passionate about Higher Education, especially Advanced Clinical Practice (ACP), Critical Care, and Non-Medical Prescribing (NMP), and pharmacology. Barry has been a Nurse leader for more than 15 years and was trained in London's best teaching hospitals at Imperial college NHS Trust. He is a strong education focused professional, Barry has published books, book chapters and peer reviewed journal articles. Barry is the clinical editor and commissioning editor for the at a glance and advanced practice series within the British Journal of Nursing. Barry is currently a fourth year Doctor of Philosophy (PhD) candidate at Northumbria University in Newcastle upon Tyne.

Noreen Kilkenny
Noreen qualified as a adult nurse in 2008 from the University of Hertfordshire. She worked as a cardiac and respiratory staff nurse at the Royal Brompton and Harefield Hospital and completed her MSc in Cardio Respiratory Nursing at Imperial College London.

Noreen has worked as a Cardiac Rehabilitation Nurse specialist in Hertfordshire and in Ireland and Australia as an agency nurse, telephone nurse triage specialist and clinical educator.

Noreen commenced her academic career in nurse education in 2014 and works at Northumbria University, Newcastle as a Senior Lecturer. Noreen is currently studying her PhD in patient safety and human factors education.

Louise Lingwood
MBA, MA-Ed, PGDip-ANP, PGDip-Ed, APMG, BSc (Hons), RNMH, FHEA
Senior Lecturer Mental Health Nursing at Northumbria University at Newcastle.

Louise completed her undergraduate mental health nurse education and training at Northumbria University in the year 2000. She has worked extensively across children and young people's mental health services (CAMHS) since qualifying and has worked as a mental health nurse, project manager and clinical manager within specialist CAMHS across the North East and nationally. Louise has worked clinically within forensic teams, looked after children Teams, primary mental health, CAMHS, National D/deaf CAMHS, autism, eating disorder and learning disability services. She commenced her post at Northumbria University at Newcastle in 2013. She is currently the Programme Lead for Mental Health Nursing and teaches across pre-registration programmes across all fields. She has a specialist interest in enhancing nurse education, anatomy, parity of esteem, autism and disability. She is involved in a number of research projects and is currently reading for her PhD.

Harriet Minto
Senior clinical pharmacist at the Great North Children's Hospital in Newcastle upon Tyne.

Harriet began her pharmacy career at the University of Huddersfield; following that she completed her pre-registration year at the Newcastle Upon Tyne Hospitals Trust (NUTH) working between the Royal Victoria Infirmary and the Freeman Hospital. After qualifying as a pharmacist, she continued to work for NUTH as a rotational pharmacist alongside studying for a Diploma in Clinical Pharmacy at the University of Sunderland. Over the past few years she has worked in the paediatric respiratory and cystic fibrosis team at the Great North Children's Hospital and is currently working towards becoming an independent pharmacist prescriber in this area.

Jackie O'Sullivan
Specialist Nurse Children and Young Peoples Endocrinology at Great North Children's Hospital, Newcastle upon Tyne.

Jackie trained as a nurse in the QARANC nursing soldiers, civilians and their families in Germany, Aldershot, Woolwich and Hong Kong for 11 years.

After leaving the Army in 1992 Jackie worked in general paediatric wards at Gateshead and Newcastle for 10 years. She has always had an interest in endocrine and metabolic processes and became an Endocrine Nurse Specialist at the RVI in 2002, a role she continues to thrive in, speaking regularly at local and national endocrine meetings and within the university to student nurses. She has had a publication in *Archives of Disease in Childhood* and has worked on research projects in diabetes and endocrinology with local teams.

Dr Claire Pryor
MSc
Advancing Healthcare Practice, PGC Advanced Practice (Clinical), PGC Teaching and Learning in Professional Practice, NMC Teacher (NMC/TCH), V300 Independent Prescriber, Grad Cert Practice Development, Fellow Higher Education Academy (FHEA) Registered Nurse Adult (RN).

Claire Pryor is a senior lecturer in adult nursing at Northumbria University. Claire's educational interests lie predominantly in nursing care for the older person and she is module lead for non-medical prescribing. Her teaching activity spans both adult pre and post registration professional development.

Claire's specialist area of interest include delirium and delirium superimposed on dementia, which forms the basis of her PhD research, and integrating physical health and mental healthcare education and service provision.

Prior to lecturing, Claire worked in a variety of primary and secondary care settings, including acute medical assessment, critical care, intermediate care and as an older persons nurse practitioner in a mental health setting.

Matthew Robertson

BSc (Hons) Operating Department Practice. Graduate Tutor. Department of Nursing, Midwifery and Health.

Matthew is a registered Operating Department Practitioner with the HCPC. He is also a member of the College of Operating Department Practitioners. Matthew completed his BSc (Hons) at the University of Central Lancashire in Operating Department Practice, where he was able to experience a range of complex surgical specialities. Once qualified, Matthew was employed by Newcastle Hospitals within the Cardiothoracic Surgical Department where he undertook the role of the scrub practitioner, specialising in paediatric and congenital cardiac surgery.

He commenced employment at Northumbria University in November 2017 and since then he has developed a specialist interest in Human Factors within the perioperative environment and is completing a PhD on this topic, focussing on staff well-being and stress management. Recently, Matthew has had several publications regarding 'the care of the surgical patient' and has written two book chapters on the use of analgesics in practice and other related pharmacology. Matthew also sits as a registrant panel member for the Health and Care Professionals Tribunal Service and provide expertise on the disciplinary cases that are presented to him and the rest of the panel.

Elaine Robinson

Elaine qualified as a children's nurse in 1996 and worked as a staff nurse in Newcastle upon Tyne. Elaine has worked in care of children in acute and critical settings, moving to a specialist role as part of the children's immunology team.

In 2005 Elaine changed direction and trained as Specialist Public Health Nurse (Health Visitor). This role further developed into community practice teacher. She joined the academic team at Northumbria University in 2017, working across pre-registration children's nursing and the Public health community nursing and prescribing programmes. Elaine is now programme lead for the Specialist community public health programme at Northumbria University and continues to work within the children's nursing team.

Leah Rosengarten

BSc (Hons) Nursing Studies (Child), MSc Practice Development
Lecturer Children and Young People's Nursing, Northumbria University.

After qualifying as a Children's Nurse in 2012 from the University of Teesside, Leah began work as a staff nurse on the Children and Teenage Cancer Unit at the Great North Children's Hospital, Newcastle. Leah worked on this unit for 6 years whilst studying for her MSc in Practice Development, part time. In 2018, Leah commenced working as a Children and Young People's Nursing Lecturer at Northumbria University. Leah's areas of interest include Oncology, Human Factors and Continuing Professional Development and she is currently studying for her PhD.

Alison Sewell

Clinical Nurse Specialist (paediatrics) in the Regional Cystic Fibrosis unit at Great North Children's hospital, Newcastle Upon Tyne.

Alison completed RGN training alongside BSc (Hons) nursing, in Leeds and initially worked as in adult medicine for several years. Following completion of RSCN paediatric qualification, she worked as a staff nurse in paediatric medicine, before relocating to Newcastle. Whilst working in paediatric medicine and pursuing her interest in Cystic Fibrosis, she also gained BSc (Hons) community health care studies at Northumbria University. Alison has specialised in Cystic Fibrosis and the care of children and families following her appointment as Clinical Nurse Specialist.

Carol Sharpe

Nurse Specialist (CYP) Cystic Fibrosis
Carol trained and qualified as a Registered General Nurse in 1986 and as a Sick Childrens Nurse in 1988. Having initially working as a staff nurse specialising in paediatric oncology she changed focus and for the last 27 years has worked as a children's cystic fibrosis (CF) nurse specialist. She gained a BSc(Hons) degree as a paediatric nurse practitioner and is an independent nurse prescriber. Carol has contributed locally and nationally to the care of children with cystic fibrosis and has a particular interest in new born screening. She has presented work at European and American CF conferences.

Laura Stavert

MPharm, PgDip Clinical Pharmacy, PGCert Independent Prescribing, MRPharmS, Advanced Pharmacist Practitioner Cumbria, Northumberland Tyne and Wear NHS Foundation Trust.

Laura began her training in 2005 as a Pharmacy undergraduate at The Robert Gordon University (RGU) in Aberdeen before completing Pre-Registration training at the Royal Infirmary of Edinburgh in 2009 and developing a range of skills across a number of clinical specialties, including a passion for mental health and medicines of the elderly. After qualification in 2010 she completed a number of basic grade rotations at the Western General Hospital in Edinburgh before taking up a specialist role in Mental Health services with Cumbria, Northumberland Tyne and Wear NHS FT in 2012. Laura began in a specialist role in mental health of older adults in 2016 before qualifying as an independent prescriber in 2017.

Laura now has an advanced practice role working in the community with Older Adults with functional and organic mental health disorders. She currently teaches on the V300 Independent Prescribing course at the University of Sunderland and hopes to pursue a doctorate in the near future.

Edward Stephenson

Lecturer University of Sunderland School of Health and Wellbeing.

Experienced Education Manager with a demonstrated history of working in the higher education industry. Skilled in Lecturing, Research, Adult Education, Qualitative Research, and Curriculum Development. Strong healthcare services professional graduated from Northumbria University.

Carol Wills

MSc Multidisciplinary Professional Development and Education, PGDip Advanced Practice, Bsc (Hons) Specialist Community Public Health Nursing (SCPHN) (Health Visiting), DipHE Adult Nursing, Registered Nurse (RN), Enrolled Nurse (EN), Registered Health Visitor (HV), Community Practitioner Prescriber (NP), Registered Lecturer/Practice Educator (RLP), Senior Fellow (SFHEA), Subject and Programme Leader Non Medical Prescribing at Northumbria University.

Carol began her nursing career in Northumberland and enjoyed a range of exciting roles within neuro trauma, coronary care and intensive care in the North East of England before focussing on primary care and the prevention of ill health. This includes working as a staff nurse, practice nurse and nurse practitioner and then health visitor. During this time she undertook several leadership and teaching roles before her academic career.

Carol is a Senior Lecturer at Northumbria University and has led a range of post-graduate professional programmes. She has also undertaken a range of national roles as subject expert. Her key areas of interest and research are around developing learning and teaching, non medical prescribing and advanced level practice.

Preface

This text aims to provide you with an understanding of the fundamentals that are associated with pharmacology, children and young people (CYP) so as to improve patient safety and outcomes. This book can help the reader to develop their skills and confidence within the scope of pharmacology related a number of care settings, allowing them to recognise and respond in a compassionate way to the needs of CYP and their families.

The idea of studying pharmacology related to the health and well-being of CYP may appear overwhelming – indeed, the contents list of this text may also seem overwhelming. You could be thinking: how you will ever be able remember and recall so much information and apply it all to the safe and effective care of CYP and their families? *The Fundamentals of Pharmacology for Children's Nursing and Healthcare Students* has been written for you, for those nursing and other healthcare students who need to have a fundamental understanding of pharmacology as applied to care. This text has been written by clinicians and academics who are experienced in the care of CYP and their families, and they bring with them a wealth of experience that they share, helping you to come to terms with the fascinating subject of applied pharmacology.

The chapters begin by providing an overall aim along with a number of learning outcomes. At the end of the chapters, so as to promote supplementary learning, a further reading list has been provided. *The Fundamentals of Pharmacology for Children's Nursing and Healthcare Students* uses a number of strategies to help you learn about pharmacology and how to apply the knowledge acquired. Episodes of care are included in most chapters – this brings, as near as possible, the clinical environment to the theory being discussed. The clinical consideration features boxes and the skills in practice features are there to encourage you to link the theory with practice. Test your knowledge questions are provided at the beginning and end of the chapters and a suite of additional learning in the form of multiple choice questions and other types of quiz are provided.

The Nursing and Midwifery Council (NMC) (2018a; 2018b and 2018c) require all of those seeking entry to the professional register to be able to demonstrate the knowledge and skills required in order to offer safe and effective care to people of all ages and across all care settings. Upon entry to the register the nurse must be able to demonstrate knowledge of pharmacology and the ability to recognise the effects of medicines, allergies, drug sensitivities, side effects, contraindications, incompatibilities, adverse reactions, prescribing errors and the impact of polypharmacy, including over the counter medication usage. There is also a requirement to understand how prescriptions can be generated and the role of generic, unlicensed and off-label prescribing. As well as this, the nurse has to demonstrate how they relate their understanding (knowledge) of pharmacology to those people and their families whom they have the privilege to care for. Within the NMC proficiencies (NMC, 2018a; 2018b) it is noted that at the point of registration the registered nurse must apply knowledge of pharmacology to the care of people, demonstrating the ability to progress to a prescribing qualification following registration.

True, meaningful learning is not just about remembering endless facts and recalling them – whilst this is important, the application of that learning then completes the circle. Adapting your learning to respond to the people you offer care and support to as well adding to it as you progress in your career: this is the crux of lifelong learning. Pharmacological interventions are always developing and new drugs being introduced to the market, and therefore as new discoveries are made and as new information emerges the nurse is required to ensure that they are on top of this.

The 19 chapters within this introductory text will go some way to helping prepare future nurses and other healthcare workers as they work towards registration with statutory professional bodies such as the NMC and the Health and Care Professions Council.

Terminology

In this text we are using the term 'children' to refer collectively to 'children and young people' and 'family' relates to the significant adults who are involved in the child's life, such as parents, carers or guardians.

The term 'registered nurse' includes those on the NMC register who are Nursing Associates. Nursing Associate is a role introduced within the England nursing team, working with healthcare support workers and registered nurses to deliver care for patients and the public working across the four fields of nursing.

When we refer to 'students', these include students of nursing from all fields of nursing. We also include other students who are learning to become members of a regulated health and social care profession who may be engaged with medications and medicines management.

We sincerely hope you enjoy using this text as you strive to improve care for children, young people and their families across a variety of care settings. The responsibilities of becoming a registered practitioner bring with them many obligations, but they also brings with them your opportunity to make a difference and to contribute to the health and well-being of individuals, communities and nations.

References

Nursing and Midwifery Council (2018a). Future Nurse: Standards of Proficiency for Registered Nurses. www.nmc.org.uk/globalassets/sitedocuments/education-standards/future-nurse-proficiencies.pdf (accessed August 2020).

Nursing and Midwifery Council (2018b). Standards of Proficiency for Nursing Associates. www.nmc.org.uk/globalassets/sitedocuments/education-standards/nursing-associates-proficiency-standards.pdf (accessed August 2020).

Nursing and Midwifery Council (2018c). The Code. Professional Standards of Practice and Behaviour for Nurses, Midwives and Nursing Associates. www.nmc.org.uk/globalassets/sitedocuments/nmc-publications/nmc-code.pdf (accessed August 2020).

Acknowledgements

We would like to thank the contributors who, during a COVID-19 pandemic, remained steadfast in their commitment to providing chapters for this text.

Ian would like to thank his partner Jussi Lahtinen for his support, and his friend Mrs Frances Cohen who, for many, many years, has encouraged and supported him.

Peter would like to thank Louise, Emme and Elliot, his Mam and Dad and colleagues past and present for their priceless support.

Prefixes and Suffixes

Prefix: A prefix is positioned at the beginning of a word to modify or change its meaning. 'Pre' means 'before'. Prefixes may also indicate a location, number or time.

Suffix: The ending part of a word that changes the meaning of the word.

PREFIX OR SUFFIX	MEANING	EXAMPLE(S)
a-, an-	not, without	analgesic, apathy
ab-	from; away from	abduction
abdomin(o)-	of or relating to the abdomen	abdomen
a.c.	ante cibum	before food
acous(io)-	of or relating to hearing	acoumeter, acoustician
acr(o)-	extremity, topmost	acrocrany, acromegaly, acroosteolysis, acroposthia
ad-	at, increase, on, toward	adduction
aden(o)-, aden(i)-	of or relating to a gland	adenocarcinoma, adenology, adenotome, adenotyphus
adip(o)-	of or relating to fat or fatty tissue	adipocyte
ad lib.	ad libitum	to the desired amount
adren(o)-	of or relating to adrenal glands	adrenal artery
-aemia	blood condition	anaemia
aer(o)-	air, gas	aerosinusitis
-aesthesi(o)-	sensation	anaesthesia
alb-	denoting a white or pale colour	albino
-alge(si)-	pain	analgesic
-algia, -alg(i)o-	pain	myalgia
all(o-)	denoting something as different, or as an addition	alloantigen, allopathy
ambi-	denoting something as positioned on both sides	ambidextrous
amni-	pertaining to the membranous fetus sac (amnion)	amniocentesis
ana-	back, again, up	anaplasia
andr(o)-	pertaining to a man	android, andrology

xxix

PREFIX OR SUFFIX	MEANING	EXAMPLE(S)
angi(o)-	blood vessel	angiogram
ankyl(o)-, ancyl(o)-	denoting something as crooked or bent	ankylosis
ante-	describing something as positioned in front of another thing	antepartum
anti-	describing something as 'against' or 'opposed to' another	antibody, antipsychotic
arteri(o)-	of or pertaining to an artery	arteriole, arterial
arthr(o)-	of or pertaining to the joints, limbs	arthritis
articul(o)-	joint	articulation
-ase	enzyme	lactase
-asthenia	weakness	myasthenia gravis
ather(o)-	fatty deposit, soft gruel-like deposit	atherosclerosis
atri(o)-	an atrium (especially heart atrium)	atrioventricular
aur(i)-	of or pertaining to the ear	aural
aut(o)-	self	autoimmune
axill-	of or pertaining to the armpit (uncommon as a prefix)	axilla
b.d. or b.i.d.	bis in die	twice a day
bi-	twice, double	binary
bio-	life	biology
blephar(o)-	of or pertaining to the eyelid	blepharoplast
brachi(o)-	of or relating to the arm	brachium of inferior colliculus
brady-	slow	bradycardia
bronch(i)-	bronchus	bronchiolitis obliterans
bucc(o)-	of or pertaining to the cheek	buccolabial
burs(o)-	bursa (fluid sac between the bones)	bursitis
c.	cum	with
carcin(o)-	cancer	carcinoma
cardi(o)-	of or pertaining to the heart	cardiology
carp(o)-	of or pertaining to the wrist	carpopedal
-cele	pouching, hernia	hydrocele, varicocele
-centesis	surgical puncture for aspiration	amniocentesis
cephal(o)-	of or pertaining to the head (as a whole)	cephalalgy
cerebell(o)-	of or pertaining to the cerebellum	cerebellum
cerebr(o)-	of or pertaining to the brain	cerebrology
chem(o)-	chemistry, drug	chemotherapy
chol(e)-	of or pertaining to bile	cholecystitis
cholecyst(o)-	of or pertaining to the gallbladder	cholecystectomy
chondr(i)o-	cartilage, gristle, granule, granular	chondrocalcinosis
chrom(ato)-	colour	haemochromatosis
-cidal, -cide	killing, destroying	bacteriocidal

Prefixes and Suffixes xxxi

PREFIX OR SUFFIX	MEANING	EXAMPLE(S)
cili-	of or pertaining to the cilia, the eyelashes	ciliary
circum-	denoting something as 'around' another	circumcision
col(o)-, colono-	colon	colonoscopy
colp(o)-	of or pertaining to the vagina	colposcopy
contra-	against	contraindicate
coron(o)-	crown	coronary
cost(o)-	of or pertaining to the ribs	costochondral
crani(o)-	belonging or relating to the cranium	craniology
-crine, -crin(o)-	to secrete	endocrine
cry(o)-	cold	cryoablation
cutane-	skin	subcutaneous
cyan(o)-	denotes a blue colour	cyanosis
cyst(o)-, cyst(i)-	of or pertaining to the urinary bladder	cystotomy
cyt(o)-	cell	cytokine
-cyte	cell	leukocyte
-dactyl(o)-	of or pertaining to a finger, toe	dactylology, polydactyly
dent-	of or pertaining to teeth	dentist
dermat(o)-, derm(o)-	of or pertaining to the skin	dermatology
-desis	binding	arthrodesis
dextr(o)-	right, on the right side	dextrocardia
di-	two	diplopia
dia-	through, during, across	dialysis
dif-	apart, separation	different
digit-	of or pertaining to the finger (rare as a root)	digit
-dipsia	suffix meaning '(condition of) thirst'	polydipsia, hydroadipsia, oligodipsia
dors(o)-, dors(i)-	of or pertaining to the back	dorsal, dorsocephalad
duodeno-	duodenum	duodenal atresia
dynam(o)-	force, energy, power	hand strength dynamometer
-dynia	pain	vulvodynia
dys-	bad, difficult, defective, abnormal	dysphagia, dysphasia
ec-	out, away	ectopia, ectopic pregnancy
-ectasia, -ectasis	expansion, dilation	bronchiectasis, telangiectasia
ect(o)-	outer, outside	ectoblast, ectoderm
-ectomy	denotes a surgical operation or removal of a body part; resection, excision	mastectomy
-emesis	vomiting condition	haematemesis
encephal(o)-	of or pertaining to the brain; also see **cerebr(o)-**	encephalogram
endo-	denotes something as 'inside' or 'within'	endocrinology, endospore

xxxii Prefixes and Suffixes

PREFIX OR SUFFIX	MEANING	EXAMPLE(S)
enter(o)-	of or pertaining to the intestine	gastroenterology
eosin(o)-	red	eosinophil granulocyte
epi-	on, upon	epicardium, epidermis, epidural, episclera, epistaxis
erythr(o)-	denotes a red colour	erythrocyte
ex-	out of, away from	excision, exophthalmos
exo-	denotes something as 'outside' another	exoskeleton
extra-	outside	extradural haematoma
faci(o)-	of or pertaining to the face	facioplegic
fibr(o)	fibre	fibroblast
fore-	before or ahead	forehead
fossa	a hollow or depressed area; trench or channel	fossa ovalis
front-	of or pertaining to the forehead	frontonasal
galact(o)-	milk	galactorrhea
gastr(o)-	of or pertaining to the stomach	gastric bypass
-genic	formative, pertaining to producing	cardiogenic shock
gingiv-	of or pertaining to the gums	gingivitis
glauc(o)-	denoting a grey or bluish-grey colour	glaucoma
gloss(o)-, glott(o)-	of or pertaining to the tongue	glossology
gluco-	sweet	glucocorticoid
glyc(o)-	sugar	glycolysis
-gnosis	knowledge	diagnosis, prognosis
gon(o)-	seed, semen; also, reproductive	gonorrhoea
-gram, -gramme	record or picture	angiogram
-graph	instrument used to record data or picture	electrocardiograph
-graphy	process of recording	angiography
gyn(ec)o-	woman	gynecomastia
haemangi(o)-	blood vessels	haemangioma
haemat(o)-, haem-	of or pertaining to blood	haematology
halluc-	to wander in mind	hallucinosis
hemi-	one half	cerebral hemisphere
hepat- (hepatic-)	of or pertaining to the liver	hepatology
heter(o)-	denotes something as 'the other' (of two), as an addition, or different	heterogeneous
hist(o)-, histio-	tissue	histology
home(o)-	similar	homeopathy
hom(o)-	denotes something as 'the same' as another or common	homosexuality
hydr(o)-	water	hydrophobe
hyper-	denotes something as 'extreme' or 'beyond normal'	hypertension

PREFIX OR SUFFIX	MEANING	EXAMPLE(S)
hyp(o)-	denotes something as 'below normal'	hypovolemia
hyster(o)-	of or pertaining to the womb, the uterus	hysterectomy, hysteria
iatr(o)-	of or pertaining to medicine, or a physician	iatrogenic
-iatry	denotes a field in medicine of a certain body component	podiatry, psychiatry
-ics	organised knowledge, treatment	obstetrics
ileo-	ileum	ileocecal valve
infra-	below	infrahyoid muscles
inter-	between, among	interarticular ligament
intra-	within	intramural
ipsi-	same	ipsilateral hemiparesis
ischio-	of or pertaining to the ischium, the hip joint	ischioanal fossa
-ismus	spasm, contraction	hemiballismus
iso-	denoting something as being 'equal'	isotonic
-ist	one who specialises in	pathologist
-itis	inflammation	tonsillitis
-ium	structure, tissue	pericardium
juxta- (iuxta-)	near to, alongside or next to	juxtaglomerular apparatus
karyo-	nucleus	eukaryote
kerat(o)-	cornea (eye or skin)	keratoscope
kin(ae)-, kin(o)-, kinesi(o)-	movement	kinaesthesia
kyph(o)-	humped	kyphoscoliosis
labi(o)-	of or pertaining to the lip	labiodental
lacrim(o)-	tear	lacrimal canaliculi
lact(i)-, lact(o)	milk	lactation
lapar(o)-	of or pertaining to the abdomen wall, flank	laparotomy
laryng(o)-	of or pertaining to the larynx, the lower throat cavity where the voice box is	larynx
latero-	lateral	lateral pectoral nerve
-lepsis, -lepsy	attack, seizure	epilepsy, narcolepsy
lept(o)-	light, slender	leptomeningeal
leuc(o)-, leuk(o)-	denoting a white colour	leukocyte
lingu(a)-, lingu(o)-	of or pertaining to the tongue	linguistics
lip(o)-	fat	liposuction
lith(o)-	stone, calculus	lithotripsy
-logist	denotes someone who studies a certain field	oncologist, pathologist
log(o)-	speech	logopedics

PREFIX OR SUFFIX	MEANING	EXAMPLE(S)
-logy	denotes the academic study or practice of a certain field	haematology, urology
lymph(o)-	lymph	lymphedema
lys(o)-, -lytic	dissolution	lysosome
-lysis	destruction, separation	paralysis
macr(o)-	large, long	macrophage
-malacia	softening	osteomalacia
mammill(o)-	of or pertaining to the nipple	mammillitis
mamm(o)-	of or pertaining to the breast	mammogram
manu-	of or pertaining to the hand	manufacture
mast(o)-	of or pertaining to the breast	mastectomy
meg(a)-, megal(o)-, -megaly	enlargement, million	splenomegaly, megametre
melan(o)-	black colour	melanin
mening(o)-	membrane	meningitis
meta-	after, behind	metacarpus
-meter	instrument used to measure or count	sphygmomanometer
metr(o)-	pertaining to conditions of the uterus	metrorrhagia
-metry	process of measuring	optometry
micro-	denoting something as small, or relating to smallness	microscope
milli-	thousandth	millilitre
mon(o)-	single	infectious mononucleosis
morph(o)-	form, shape	morphology
muscul(o)-	muscle	musculoskeletal system
my(o)-	of or relating to muscle	myoblast
myc(o)-	fungus	onychomycosis
myel(o)-	of or relating to bone marrow or spinal cord	myeloblast
myri-	ten thousand	myriad
myring(o)-	eardrum	myringotomy
narc(o)-	numb, sleep	narcolepsy
nas(o)-	of or pertaining to the nose	nasal
necr(o)-	death	necrosis, necrotising fasciitis
neo-	new	neoplasm
nephr(o)-	of or pertaining to the kidney	nephrology
neur(i)-, neur(o)-	of or pertaining to nerves and the nervous system	neurofibromatosis
normo-	normal	normocapnia
ocul(o)-	of or pertaining to the eye	oculist
odont(o)-	of or pertaining to teeth	orthodontist
odyn(o)-	pain	stomatodynia
-esophageal, esophag(o)-	gullet	gastroesophageal reflux

Prefixes and Suffixes xxxv

PREFIX OR SUFFIX	MEANING	EXAMPLE(S)
-oid	resemblance to	sarcoidosis
-ole	small or little	arteriole
olig(o)-	denoting something as 'having little, having few'	oliguria
o.m.	omni mane	every morning
-oma (sing.), -omata (pl.)	tumour, mass, collection	sarcoma, teratoma
o.n.	omni nocte	every night
onco-	tumour, bulk, volume	oncology
onych(o)-	of or pertaining to the nail (of a finger or toe)	onychophagy
oo-	of or pertaining to an egg, a woman's egg, the ovum	oogenesis
oophor(o)-	of or pertaining to the woman's ovary	oophorectomy
ophthalm(o)-	of or pertaining to the eye	ophthalmology
optic(o)-	of or relating to chemical properties of the eye	opticochemical
orchi(o)-,orchid(o)-,orch(o)-	testis	orchiectomy, orchidectomy
-osis	a condition, disease or increase	ichthyosis, psychosis, osteoporosis
osseo-	bony	osseous
ossi-	bone	peripheral ossifying fibroma
ost(e)-, oste(o)-	bone	osteoporosis
ot(o)-	of or pertaining to the ear	otology
ovo-, ovi-, ov-	of or pertaining to the eggs, the ovum	ovogenesis
pachy-	thick	pachyderma
paed-, paedo-	of or pertaining to the child	paediatrics
palpebr-	of or pertaining to the eyelid (uncommon as a root)	palpebra
pan-, pant(o)-	denoting something as 'complete' or containing 'everything'	panophobia, panopticon
papill-	of or pertaining to the nipple (of the chest/breast)	papillitis
papul(o)-	indicates papulosity, a small elevation or swelling in the skin, a pimple, swelling	papulation
para-	alongside of, abnormal	paracyesis
-paresis	slight paralysis	hemiparesis
parvo-	small	parvovirus
path(o)-	disease	pathology
-pathy	denotes (with a negative sense) a disease, or disorder	sociopathy, neuropathy
p.c.	post cibum	after food
pector-	breast	pectoralgia, pectoriloquy, pectorophony

PREFIX OR SUFFIX	MEANING	EXAMPLE(S)
ped-, -ped-, -pes	of or pertaining to the foot; -footed	pedoscope
pelv(i)-, pelv(o)-	hip bone	pelvis
-penia	deficiency	osteopenia
-pepsia	denotes something relating to digestion, or the digestive tract	dyspepsia
peri-	denoting something with a position 'surrounding' or 'around' another	periodontal
-pexy	fixation	nephropexy
phaco-	lens-shaped	phacolysis, phacometer, phacoscotoma
-phage, -phagia	forms terms denoting conditions relating to eating or ingestion	sarcophagia
-phago-	eating, devouring	phagocyte
-phagy	forms nouns that denote 'feeding on' the first element or part of the word	haematophagy
pharmaco-	drug, medication	pharmacology
pharyng(o)-	of or pertaining to the pharynx, the upper throat cavity	pharyngitis, pharyngoscopy
phleb(o)-	of or pertaining to the (blood) veins, a vein	phlebography, phlebotomy
-phobia	exaggerated fear, sensitivity	arachnophobia
phon(o)-	sound	phonograph, symphony
phot(o)-	of or pertaining to light	photopathy
phren(i)-, phren(o)-, phrenico	the mind	phrenic nerve, schizophrenia
-plasia	formation, development	achondroplasia
-plasty	surgical repair, reconstruction	rhinoplasty
-plegia	paralysis	paraplegia
pleio-	more, excessive, multiple	pleiomorphism
pleur(o)-, pleur(a)	of or pertaining to the ribs	pleurogenous
-plexy	stroke or seizure	cataplexy
pneumat(o)-	air, lung	pneumatocele
pneum(o)-	of or pertaining to the lungs	pneumonocyte, pneumonia
-poiesis	production	haematopoiesis
poly-	denotes a 'plurality' of something	polymyositis
post-	denotes something as 'after' or 'behind' another	post-operation, post-mortem
pre-	denotes something as 'before' another (in [physical] position or time)	premature birth
presby(o)-	old age	presbyopia
prim-	denotes something as 'first' or 'most important'	primary
p.r.n.	pro re nata	whenever necessary
proct(o)-	anus, rectum	proctology

PREFIX OR SUFFIX	MEANING	EXAMPLE(S)
prot(o)-	denotes something as 'first' or 'most important'	protoneuron
pseud(o)-	denotes something false or fake	pseudoephedrine
psor-	itching	psoriasis
psych(e)-, psych(o)	of or pertaining to the mind	psychology, psychiatry
-ptosis	falling, drooping, downward placement, prolapse	apoptosis, nephroptosis
-ptysis	(a spitting), spitting, haemoptysis, the spitting of blood derived from the lungs or bronchial tubes	haemoptysis
pulmon-, pulmo-	of or relating to the lungs	pulmonary
pyel(o)-	pelvis	pyelonephritis
py(o)-	pus	pyometra
pyr(o)-	fever	antipyretic
q.d.	quaque die	every day
q.d.s.	quaque die sumendum	four times daily
q.i.d.	quater in die	four times daily
q.q.h.	quater quaque hora	every four hours
quadr(i)-	four	quadriceps
R.	recipe	Take
radio-	radiation	radiowave
ren(o)-	of or pertaining to the kidney	renal
retro-	backward, behind	retroversion, retroverted
rhin(o)-	of or pertaining to the nose	rhinoplasty
rhod(o)-	denoting a rose-red colour	rhodophyte
-rrhage	burst forth	haemorrhage
-rrhagia	rapid flow of blood	menorrhagia
-rrhaphy	surgical suturing	nephrorrhaphy
-rrhexis	rupture	karyorrhexis
-rrhea	flowing, discharge	diarrhoea
-rupt	break or burst	erupt, interrupt
salping(o)-	of or pertaining to tubes, e.g. Fallopian tubes	salpingectomy, salpingopharyngeus muscle
sangui-, sanguine-	of or pertaining to blood	exsanguination
sarco-	muscular, flesh-like	sarcoma
scler(o)-	hard	scleroderma
-sclerosis	hardening	atherosclerosis, multiple sclerosis
scoli(o)-	twisted	scoliosis
-scope	instrument for viewing	stethoscope
-scopy	use of instrument for viewing	endoscopy
semi-	one half, partly	semiconscious
sial(o)-	saliva, salivary gland	sialagogue

PREFIX OR SUFFIX	MEANING	EXAMPLE(S)
sigmoid(o)-	sigmoid, S-shaped curvature	sigmoid colon
sinistr(o)-	left, left side	sinistrocardia
sinus-	of or pertaining to the sinus	sinusitis
somat(o)-, somatico-	body, bodily	somatic
s.o.s.	si opus sit	if necessary
-spadias	slit, fissure	hypospadias, epispadias
spasmo-	spasm	spasmodic dysphonia
sperma(to)-, spermo-	semen, spermatozoa	spermatogenesis
splen(o)-	spleen	splenectomy
spondyl(o)-	of or pertaining to the spine, the vertebra	spondylitis
squamos(o)-	denoting something as 'full of scales' or 'scaly'	squamous cell
stat.	statim	at once
-stalsis	contraction	peristalsis
-stasis	stopping, standing	cytostasis, homeostasis
-staxis	dripping, trickling	epistaxis
sten(o)-	denoting something as 'narrow in shape' or pertaining to narrowness	stenography
-stenosis	abnormal narrowing in a blood vessel or other tubular organ or structure	restenosis, stenosis
stomat(o)-	of or pertaining to the mouth	stomatogastric, stomatognathic system
-stomy	creation of an opening	colostomy
sub-	beneath	subcutaneous tissue
super-	in excess, above, superior	superior vena cava
supra-	above, excessive	supraorbital vein
tachy-	denoting something as fast, irregularly fast	tachycardia
-tension, -tensive	pressure	hypertension
t.d.s.	ter die sumendum	three times daily
tetan-	rigid, tense	tetanus
thec-	case, sheath	intrathecal
therap-	treatment	hydrotherapy, therapeutic
therm(o)-	heat	thermometer
t.i.d.	ter in die	three times daily
thorac(i)-,thorac(o)-,thoracico-	of or pertaining to the upper chest, chest; the area above the breast and under the neck	thorax
thromb(o)-	of or relating to a blood clot, clotting of blood	thrombus, thrombocytopenia
thyr(o)-	thyroid	thyrocele
thym-	emotions	dysthymia
-tome	cutting instrument	osteotome

PREFIX OR SUFFIX	MEANING	EXAMPLE(S)
-tomy	act of cutting; incising, incision	gastrotomy
tono-	tone, tension, pressure	tonometer
-tony	tension	
top(o)-	place, topical	topical anaesthetic
tort(i)-	twisted	torticollis
tox(i)-, tox(o)-, toxic(o)-	toxin, poison	toxoplasmosis
trache(a)-	trachea	tracheotomy
trachel(o)-	of or pertaining to the neck	tracheloplasty
trans-	denoting something as moving or situated 'across' or 'through'	transfusion
tri-	three	triangle
trich(i)-, trichia, trich(o)-	of or pertaining to hair, hair-like structure	trichocyst
-tripsy	crushing	lithotripsy
-trophy	nourishment, development	pseudohypertrophy
tympan(o)-	eardrum	tympanocentesis
-ula, -ule	small	nodule
ultra-	beyond, excessive	ultrasound
un(i)-	one	unilateral hearing loss
ur(o)-	of or pertaining to urine, the urinary system; (specifically) pertaining to the physiological chemistry of urine	urology
uter(o)-	of or pertaining to the uterus or womb	uterus
vagin-	of or pertaining to the vagina	vagina
varic(o)-	swollen or twisted vein	varicose
vasculo-	blood vessel	vasculotoxicity
vas(o)-	duct, blood vessel	vasoconstriction
ven-	of or pertaining to the (blood) veins, a vein (used in terms pertaining to the vascular system)	vein, venospasm
ventricul(o)-	of or pertaining to the ventricles; any hollow region inside an organ	cardiac ventriculography
ventr(o)-	of or pertaining to the belly; the stomach cavities	ventrodorsal
-version	turning	anteversion, retroversion
vesic(o)-	of or pertaining to the bladder	vesical arteries
viscer(o)-	of or pertaining to the internal organs, the viscera	viscera
xanth(o)-	denoting a yellow colour, an abnormally yellow colour	xanthopathy
xen(o)-	foreign, different	xenograft
xer(o)-	dry, desert-like	xerostomia
zo(o)-	animal, animal life	zoology
zym(o)-	fermentation	enzyme, lysozyme

Abbreviations

Some abbreviations used in prescriptions

ABBREVIATION	LATIN	ENGLISH
a.c.	ante cibum	Before food
ad lib.	ad libitum	To the desired amount
b.d. or b.i.d.	bis in die	Twice a day
c.	cum	With
o.m.	omni mane	Every morning
o.n.	omni nocte	Every night
p.c.	post cibum	After food
p.r.n.	pro re nata	Whenever necessary
q.d.	quaque die	Every day
q.d.s.	quaque die sumendum	Four times daily
q.i.d.	quater in die	Four times daily
q.q.h.	quater quaque hora	Every four hours
R.	recipe	Take
s.o.s.	si opus sit	If necessary
stat.	statim	At once
t.d.s.	ter die sumendum	Three times daily
t.i.d.	ter in die	Three times daily

About the Companion Website

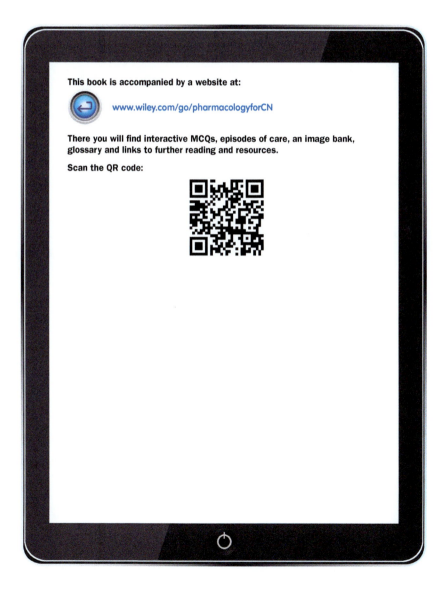

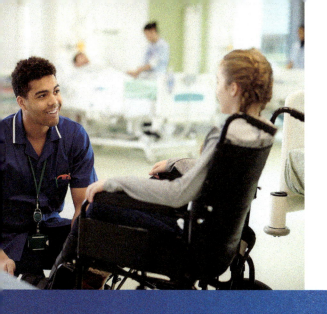

1

Introduction to Pharmacology, Children and Young People

Jane Callum

Aim
This chapter provides the reader with an introduction to pharmacology and its application to children and young people (CYP).

Learning Outcomes
After reading this chapter the reader will:
- Understand the importance of following policies and the issues associated with medicine management
- Recognise the legal frameworks and NMC code within this important aspect of care
- Increase knowledge and understanding of pharmacological principles associated with the child, young person and their family
- Appreciate the importance of the role of the family/carer and family-centred care

Test Your Knowledge
1. What is your role in medicine management?
2. What are the five principles of medication administration?
3. What is the difference between the terms 'drug' and 'medicine'?
4. Describe family-centred care and its importance in your practice?
5. What does medicine optimisation mean?

Fundamentals of Pharmacology for Children's Nurses, First Edition. Edited by Ian Peate and Peter Dryden.
© 2022 John Wiley & Sons Ltd. Published 2022 by John Wiley & Sons Ltd.
Companion website: www.wiley.com/go/pharmacologyforCN

Table 1.1 Pharmacokinetics and pharmacodynamics.

PHARMACOKINETICS	PHARMACODYNAMICS
absorption	molecular
distribution	biochemical
metabolism	physiological effects of drugs on the body
excretion of drugs in the body	

Source: Based on Haddad and Nutt, 2020.

Introduction to Pharmacology

Pharmacology is present in daily life, from medicines bought over the counter in shops such as decongestants, nappy rash cream and pain relief, to prescription-only medicines including antibiotics and inhalers. Lifestyle and what we eat and drink also have an impact on our bodies and our health, which can often be categorised as drugs. This includes drinks containing cafeine, chocolate, alcohol, vitamins and minerals as well as illegal substances. Before going further into this chapter, it is useful to define the terms 'drug' and 'medicine', which are often used interchangeably in texts. Medicine can be defined as a drug or other preparation for the treatment or prevention of disease, whereas a drug is described as a medicine or other substance that can be natural or artificially made which has a physiological effect when inhaled, ingested or inserted into the body or applied topically to the skin. The definitions link to each other except that the word 'drug' can be used for a product not necessarily designed to treat or prevent disease.

Pharmacology can be described in its most simple terms as a science or branch of medicine that looks at all aspects of medicinal drugs, including how they are used, what effect they have on the body and how they are excreted. It is important to understand how medications work and the actions they have on the systems of the body for the safety of the people you offer care and support to. You may read the term 'drug actions', which is the commonly used shortened term for this.

Pharmacology has been divided into two overarching categories, pharmacokinetics and pharmacodynamics and it is important to understand the difference (see Table 1.1). The pharmacokinetic aspect of pharmacology examines the absorption, distribution, metabolism and excretion of drugs in the body. Pharmacodynamics is a more detailed scientific aspect of the molecular, biochemical and physiological effects of drugs. As a lifelong learner you will learn about and develop your understanding of the pharmacokinetics of different medications, as well as the side effects, how to manage these and how medications interact with each other. This is an important aspect of healthcare, ensuring that you are providing safe and effective care to CYP, whilst being knowledgeable in detecting side effects or contraindications and seeking further support in managing these for the safety of individual patients.

Professional Framework

The Nursing and Midwifery Council (NMC) set the standards that all nurses must adhere to as outlined in the Code of Conduct (NMC, 2018a). As part of a nurse's role the NMC highlight that the CYP in your care, and their family, must be able to trust you with their health and well-being (NMC, 2018a). To be able to justify that trust, nurses must adhere to the following four P's:

- Prioritise people
- Practise effectively
- Preserve safety
- Promote professionalism and trust

Within Preserving Safety, section 18 of the Code specifically focuses on aspects of medicine management and the role of the nurse which includes:

Advise on, prescribe, supply, dispense or administer medicines within the limits of your training and competence, the law, our guidance and other relevant policies, guidance and regulations.

NMC, 2018a – see Table 1.2

Table 1.2 Medicine administration, preservation of safety.

To preserve safety in relation to medicine administration, you must:

18.1	Prescribe, advise on, or provide medicines or treatment, including repeat prescriptions (only if you are suitably qualified) if you have enough knowledge of that person's health and are satisfied that the medicines or treatment serve that person's health needs
18.2	Keep to appropriate guidelines when giving advice on using controlled drugs and recording the prescribing, supply, dispensing or administration of controlled drugs
18.3	Make sure that the care or treatment you advise on, prescribe, supply, dispense or administer for each person is compatible with any other care or treatment they are receiving, including (where possible) over the counter medicines
18.4	Take all steps to keep medicines stored securely
18.5	Wherever possible, avoid prescribing for yourself or for anyone with whom you have a close personal relationship

Source: NMC (2018a). This extract is reproduced and reprinted with permission with thanks to the Nursing and Midwifery Council.

It must be clarified at this point that not all registered nurses are permitted to prescribe, as further qualifications and registration with the NMC as an Independent Prescriber must be achieved first. The NMC's Future Nurse: Standards of Proficiency for Registered Nurses (2018b) are designed for newly registered nurses to be 'prescriber-ready' on admission to the register, and therefore have more knowledge of pharmacology as detailed within the previous education standards. Although the knowledge level will be in more depth, further training, practice and supervision will be required to be a registered prescriber. This is reinforced in the NMC Code, section 13.5, which states that you must complete the necessary training before carrying out a new role (NMC, 2018a). Table 1.2 outlines the NMC's (2018a) requirements regarding medicine administration.

The Importance and Value of Medicine Within Healthcare

It has been identified that medicines are the most common intervention in healthcare and are used to prevent, treat and manage conditions and illnesses for people of all ages (National Institute for Health and Care Excellence (NICE), 2015). With the increase in technology and the increase in survival rates of premature births and complex health conditions, the need for medicines has increased. As with adults, more CYP are living with several long-term conditions that are being managed with an increasing number of medicines. Medicine use can be complex and how patients can take their medicines safely and effectively can be a challenge for the health service (NICE, 2021).

The safety of administering medicines is imperative as healthcare professionals strive to 'do no harm'. Despite this, it has been estimated that there are 237 million medication errors within England each year across all ages and areas of primary and secondary care (Elliott et al., 2020). It is also estimated from the same systematic review that 72% of errors have little or no harm on the patient and they are identified before the medication reaches the patient. The National Patient Safety Agency (NPSA) monitors medication errors across all aspects of the process and reports to the multidisciplinary team involved in medication management. The NPSA (2007) reported that 1 in 10 patients experience medication-related errors somewhere in the process and that 41% of the most serious incidents that are reported are caused by errors in administration. Within the literature, it is considered that many errors are unreported and so the statistics available are not completely accurate.

Therapeutic Pharmacology

In general, when a prescription is issued it should not be issued unless a detailed clinical assessment is completed and before having explored the psychological mechanisms underlying symptoms (this especially important in the case of mental ill health).

Healthcare providers and patients should consider that mental health disorders can effectively be managed by the use of pharmacological and non-pharmacological interventions. When a decision has been made to prescribe, for example, a psychotropic drug, it should never be suggested that psychological and/or psychosocial interventions will not be indicated. Combining medicines with psychosocial interventions can be associated with better patient outcomes. Considering medications as the only therapeutic strategy is very often unacceptable (World Health Organization, 2009). Articulated, comprehensive and individualised treatment plans can very often be seen as the best therapeutic option.

Social Prescribing

Social prescribing is a key component of universal personalised care (NHS, 2020). Based on the notion that medicine alone may not always provide a solution, it can help to point patients in the right direction to seek advice or social activities that aim to encourage partnership working between health and social sectors in order to attend to the wider determinants of health. Those patients who have non-clinical needs can be referred to community activities with the intention of improving their health and well-being. Social prescribing can work for a wide range of people, including:

- Those with one or more long-term conditions
- People who need support with their mental health
- Individuals who are lonely or isolated
- People who have complex social needs which affect their well-being.

Horner (2019) discusses how social prescribing can provide social support for those young people who have been socially excluded. The key elements associated with social prescribing that need to be in place for effective social prescribing are summarised in Figure 1.1.

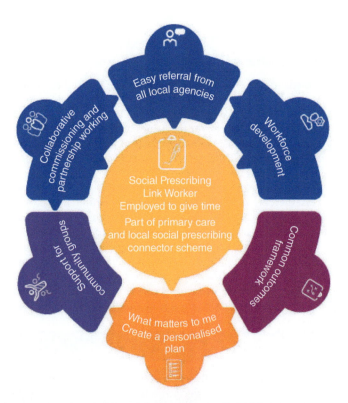

Figure 1.1 The key elements associated with social prescribing (NHS, 2020). *Source:* National Health Service/Public Domain/Open Government Licence.

Safety Within Paediatric Care

Within paediatric environments care may be provided for CYP across a wide age range, from birth (possibly premature) to 16 years or potentially older depending on the clinical environment and the needs of the young person. Calculating medicine doses can be complicated as they can be very small doses in neonates and babies, requiring accurate calculation skills. Even a small miscalculation resulting in an overdose can have a severe or life-threatening effect due to the prematurity of the infant's development and the body's ability to process the medication. Barber (2013) identified that children are three times more likely to receive a medication error than an adult due to the complexity of the calculations required, a misplaced decimal point and the complexity of calculating the individual dosage for each CYP based on weight, height or surface area. Within neonatal care this risk is higher due to the size of the neonates and the complexity of calculations.

Episode of Care

Lucy is a 3-month-old baby who presented to a Children's Emergency Assessment Department with a 36-hour history of not taking her milk, being unsettled and crying more than usual. In the last 24 hours her temperature has increased to 38.5°C, she looks flushed, but her hands and feet are cool to touch.

On examination Lucy is crying and not being comforted by being held. As the doctor examines Lucy she is concerned at Lucy's condition and temperature and is prescribing paracetamol to reduce the discomfort that Lucy appears to be in. The nurse allocated to Lucy weighs her with no clothes on, to gain an accurate weight to be able to calculate the accurate dose of paracetamol for her body weight. Lucy's weight is 12lb 4oz (5.8kg) and '12.4' is verbally passed on to the doctor writing the prescription.

As the measurement unit was passed on verbally (it was not communicated by writing it down), the doctor wrote the paracetamol dose based on a weight of 12.4kg and not 5.8kg. It was only when drawing up the amount of liquid paracetamol needed that an experienced nurse realised that this was too much for the age of the baby.

- What would you do in this situation?
- What dangers have you identified?
- How could this potential error be prevented in the future?

Medicines Optimisation

NICE guidance has identified the term 'medicines optimisation', meaning 'to make the best or most effective use of' medicines, equipment or resources. To this end the Royal Pharmaceutical Society (2013) have developed four guiding principles:

- Aim to understand the patient's experience
- Evidence-based choice of medicines
- Ensure medicines use is as safe as possible
- Make medicines optimisation part of routine practice

Medicines optimisation is a wider encompassing approach than the system approach of medicine management. Medicines optimisation is an important concept in health and social care and is relevant for CYP with chronic or long-term conditions or those who are taking more than one medication. The optimisation approach is person-centred and develops an individual patient- or professional-led self-management plan for patients. Within paediatrics, depending on the age of the CYP, the family-centred care approach maybe more appropriate, with the family being involved in the development of the self-care plan for the child. It is also important to identify any over the counter medications or complementary therapies that may interfere with the effectiveness of any prescribed medication.

Where a child is on multiple medicines or the medicines need to be administered in a different way such as via a feeding tube, additional support and follow-up might be needed. This should be identified whilst in hospital and support arranged before discharge. Within elderly care environments a screening tool is available to identify potential medicine-related patient safety incidents. Within CYP care environments there does not appear to be such a screening tool available.

Medicines

Medicines can be grouped into four types in terms of access.

- General sales list
- Pharmacy medicines
- Prescription-only medicines
- Controlled drugs.

Medicines within the general sales list are readily available in shops and there is no legal age restriction for the purchase of these medicines, although some shops have their own age limits for sales. GPs and nurses will not prescribe over the counter medications, such as paracetamol, for minor illnesses for a child or adult when they can be bought readily and at a cheaper cost to the individual and NHS, although there is a list of exemptions. The cost of prescribing over the counter medications to the NHS is approximately £136 million per year (NHS, 2018).

Pharmacy medications are also known as restricted medicines and are a small group of medicines that a pharmacist can prescribe without the patient seeing a doctor or a nurse.

Prescription-only medicines are prescribed by a GP, nurse, dentist, midwife or a doctor working in environments other than general practice. The medications on this list are considered to be needed to be used under the supervision of a licensed healthcare practitioner due to the potential to cause harm. There are also many medicines that are used but are not licensed for CYP and these can only be prescribed by a paediatrician or hospital-based doctor. In comparison to general sales and pharmacy medications, prescription-only medicines are prescribed for an individual after assessment and the dose is calculated on the child or young person's height and weight or surface area rather than a standard dose that is more often found with adults.

Controlled drugs are a group of medicines that can be abused and cause dependence and therefore they are controlled and regulated by the government. The term 'control' covers how and where the medicine is made, how it is used, the way that it is handled and stored as well as how it is distributed. In a hospital environment, GP surgery or community care environment such as a hospice or children's unit, controlled drugs are stored in a metal locked cupboard inside another locked cupboard on a wall, usually in a specific room where medicines are checked and prepared. Access to the keys to the cupboards is limited and controlled. The stock levels of controlled drugs are checked daily by two people and new supplies are also often checked by two people and everything is recorded in a specific logbook (sometimes known as the controlled drugs register) according to local policy and procedure. When preparing a controlled medication to administer to a patient the stock level is checked against the logbook and the details of the patient including the dose, date and time are recorded and signed by two members of staff. The types of controlled substances most often used include opioids (morphine, diamorphine), sedatives (diazepam, temazepam), stimulants (amphetamines used in attention deficit hyperactive disorder), central nervous system depressants (diazepam), hallucinogens and anabolic steroids (testosterone).

Medicine Management

Medicine management involves the safe storage, management and administration of medications, which includes following local and national policies and guidelines for the safe administration of medication. Monitoring the effectiveness of any medication given, as well as understanding the side effects and contraindications, and being able to explain these to CYP and their family is part of the advancing role in healthcare. The 'Professional Guidance on the Administration of Medicines in Healthcare Settings' (RPS and RCN, 2019) outlines professional accountability and covers these aspects in more detail. This document is essential reading for all healthcare staff involved in medicine management and administration. Healthcare students and healthcare professionals are involved in medicine management in a variety of settings and should refer to the Standards of Proficiency for Pre-registration Nursing Education for Guidance (NMC, 2018b) as well ensuring they are familiar with and abiding to local policy and procedure.

The Standards of Proficiency for Nursing Associates along with the Standards for Pre-registration Nursing Associate Programmes (NMC, 2018c, 2018d) provide details regarding the preparation of nursing associates and the proficiencies that have to be met prior to the nursing associate's name being entered on the professional register. The nursing associate (as is the case for the registered nurse) must be able, at the point of registration, to demonstrate and apply knowledge of pharmacology when delivering care. There is also a need to understand the principles of safe and effective administration and optimisation of medicines. Importantly, this must be done in accordance with local and national policies. Procedural competencies (very much related to local policy) must be demonstrated concerning the safe administration of medicines.

Safety: Rights of Medication Administration

Safety elements when administering medication include the 5 Rights, more commonly known as the 5 Rs (NMC, 2007):

- Right patient
- Right medication
- Right dose
- Right time
- Right route.

Working within these 5 principles whilst preparing medications and again at the bedside ensures a safe process. As more confidence is amassed in medicine management these principles can be expanded. Elliott and Liu (2010) believe that you should also include giving the medication for the 'right reason' and ensure that the 'right documentation' is completed correctly. As more understanding of the reasons for errors in medication management are understood, a further 5 rights can be added to the list, culminating in 10 rights, which include the original 5 Rs listed earlier as well as the following five (Edwards and Axe, 2015):

- The right to refuse (know what to do if the patient refuses)
- Right knowledge and understanding (of the drug and patient)
- Right questions (if there is any doubt with the process)
- Right response (monitor the effectiveness of the medication
- Right advice.

Chapter 4 of this text discusses medicines management and the role of the healthcare provider working with CYP and families in detail.

Specific Considerations for Babies, Children and Young People

When caring for CYP there are many aspects of medicine administration that need to be given special consideration, including the age of the child, gaining consent, if they have the ability to swallow tablets, the taste of medicines and what to do if a child refuses to take it. Consent will be explored in more depth in Chapter 3.

The changes in body proportions and composition in CYP change rapidly and this affects the efficacy, toxicity and dosage of medicines for children. Proportions of body fat, protein and extracellular water change over months in newborn babies, whereas at the age of 1 to 2, metabolism and elimination of medications from the liver and kidneys is at its greatest (NICE, 2021). Development of the gastrointestinal tract also affects the absorption of oral medications, and difficulties with this may indicate an intravenous route being more appropriate.

Infancy

Babies are unable to communicate their needs and feelings and assessment of a baby through body language and vital signs is important. The first 12 months of life involve rapid stages of development, from milk feeds through weaning to tolerating solid food as one example. Taste is developing and unusual tastes or textures can often be spat out or refused. It has been recommended that new foods should be introduced to babies four times before giving up, but this might not be possible with medicines. In babies and young children who cannot swallow tablets, liquid medicines or syrups are prescribed. Some liquid medicines/syrups do not have a palatable taste, antibiotics being the most common. Flucloxacillin is an example of a syrup that has a very bitter taste and is not palatable to many. Baguley et al. (2012) recommend not prescribing such medications without first allowing the child to taste it. If a child will not comply with taking the medication, this increases the stress for the parent(s)/carers in encouraging the child to take the medication. It also increases the risk of non-concordance; the infection or condition not being treated appropriately and the development of drug resistance for the child. If a child is refusing to take liquid medicine due to the taste, further discussion should be had with the prescriber and involve the parent and child (where possible) to promote concordance to treatment.

Additional negative aspects to liquid medicines or syrups are that they often have sugar added to sweeten the taste and promote concordance in taking the medication (Baguley et al., 2012). If a medicine is to be taken long-term or prescribed for a child with diabetes mellitus, a sugar-free version should be considered if a tablet is not an option. This will also aid dental health, where taking sugary medicine regularly throughout the day can result in tooth decay. In Chapter 4 drug formulations are discussed.

Clinical Consideration

In cases where there is not an alternative or a baby or young child spits out the medicine or refuses to take it, having a drink of the child's choice to take straight after the medicine will take away the taste quickly. If the medicine does not have to be given on an empty stomach, a favourite food or snack may also be an option. Putting the medicine into a drink or bottle of milk is discouraged due to the following risks.

- If some of the drink is left, it is difficult to estimate how much of the medicine has been taken.
- The medicine may react with the fluid.
- If the medicine is denser, it will sink to the bottom of the container or adhere to the inside of the container.
- If the drink takes a long time to drink, the medicine is not given at the same time.
- The medicine may alter the taste of `the drink or milk and the child then refuse to drink it.

Clinical Consideration

With babies, oral syringes are commonly used to drip liquid medicine into the buccal cavity or onto the tongue. Assessing the swallowing ability is important and awareness of tongue tie, or cleft lip and palate difficulties should be considered. Oral and nasal cavities are closely linked, and liquid medicine can come out of the nasal passages if the baby does not suck and swallow and is distressed or sneezes. Cradling babies, ensuring their arms are not flailing about, and talking to them provides comfort and reassurance. It is important for babies to feel secure and loved by those around them and cuddling a baby when giving a liquid medicine can often help. Family-centred care, where the family is treated as a unit, recognises the importance of the parent/carers in nurturing the child whilst in hospital.

Clinical Consideration

In the first year, babies learn to roll over, sit, crawl, stand and walk. With these developing skills toddlers often want to be in control where they can, and allowing them to hold and press the syringe to control the medicine is often a positive approach for concordance.

As children develop and become more independent with everyday skills, they should understand what medicine they are taking is for and why it is important.

Safety is the priority, and as is highlighted on all medicine containers, medicine must be kept out of the reach of children both in hospital and the community. It is important to watch a child taking their medication to ensure that they have taken it. If medicine is left next to the child in hospital or community, it may be taken by another child, knocked over or forgotten.

Chapter 1 Introduction to Pharmacology, Children and Young People

In younger children they may not have the ability to swallow a tablet and even in older CYP the tablet may be so large they have difficulty swallowing. In tablets that are enteric-coated it is important not to crush them so as to aid swallowing. Enteric coating is used for medicines that cause irritation to the upper gastrointestinal tract and the coating is broken down in the stomach by digestive acids, allowing the medication to be absorbed through the stomach and intestines. Crushing the tablet will increase the risk of gastric irritation. Where possible, liquid preparations should be prescribed. This is commonly seen in over the counter medicines that can be purchased in pharmacies or supermarkets, and an example of this is paracetamol, which is available in numerous formats.

Clinical Consideration

In a local store or pharmacy find out the following information:

	PARACETAMOL TABLETS	SOLUBLE TABLETS	MELTS	CALPOL INFANT SYRUP	CALPOL 6 PLUS	PARACETAMOL SUPPOSITORY
What is the recommended age range?						
What is the strength of the active ingredient?						
What is the cost of medicine?						
How many tablets or doses are in each container?						
What additional company (trade) names can you find for each of them?						

Adolescents

Teenagers develop through a complex range of emotions, physical changes and exploring identity. Through the onset of puberty hormones such as testosterone and oestrogen are produced, resulting in growth spurts and the production of secondary sexual characteristics such as body odour, body and facial hair, breast development and menstruation. During this time there is an increase in self-awareness and the need to be accepted by peers and society. There is an increase in mental health conditions developing in this age group, including eating disorders, anxiety, depression as well as lack of confidence. It has been noted that young people often rebel against strict boundaries and want to be treated and act like adults, leading to risk-taking behaviours.

Coping with ill health and being separated from friends and peers can be very isolating, especially when in hospital for long periods with a complex or long-term condition. Taking medication or carrying emergency medication, such as an epi pen in case of an allergic reaction, ventolin inhaler in case of an asthma attack or insulin and equipment to monitor and correct blood sugar levels in diabetes, can be rejected by some.

Young people should be involved in the decision-making process about their treatment and share the responsibility where appropriate. Their independence should be supported and plans developed to encourage their self-management as they move to adulthood and in the future leaving the family home. Encouraging independence supports normality in life and allows young people to stay at friends houses or go on residential trips with their peers. Promoting the self-management of treatment and medication develops responsibility, time-management and decision-making skills. One area that can be difficult with this is supporting parents to allow their child to have some independence and responsibility for their own health. When medication is vital, not taking medication can be life-threatening. This is very difficult for parents/carers, having maintained their child's safety and health for many years.

Episode of Care

Krishna aged 15 years has cystic fibrosis and has had 3 hospital admissions in the last 6 months for chest infections requiring antibiotics and increased physiotherapy. Krishna has regular medication including digestive enzyme tablets to take with food, salbutamol inhaler as a bronchodilator, dornase alfa to thin the secretions in his lungs and antibiotics for a chest infection. Due to the amount of regular medications taken at home Krishna brings his medications in to hospital to show the admitting nurse practitioner during the assessment so that the ongoing treatment can be maintained, and a review of the medication optimisation can occur effectively.

Whilst in hospital Krishna's own medication can be used if he were able to self-medicate and a lockable cupboard is at the side of his bed. This gives Krishna some independence and control over his treatment.

Prior to discharge the level of each of Krishna's medications are assessed by a pharmacist and a top up supply given on discharge preventing medication expiring whilst being in hospital and being wasted. This system is effective when CYP are on long-term medications.

Tablets

Tablets should be considered as more accurate than liquid medicines and therefore safer, they are cheaper and easier to obtain from pharmacies and more convenient to transport and administer. Non-enteric-coated tablets maybe broken into smaller pieces if scored or crushed, they can be given on a spoon, or placed on the back of the tongue and swallowed with a drink. It is advisable to teach children to swallow tablets as soon as possible and this can be done as an inpatient or outpatient using a structured process. Tse et al. (2019) published the KidzMed project findings, which focused on teaching children how to swallow tablets with a structured programme within one outpatient appointment. This project, how it was set up, and the successful outcomes will be discussed in more detail in Chapter 3, which concerns legal and ethical issues. Parents may also need support to encourage their child to take tablets and to be taught the most effective methods to swallow a tablet or capsule.

Distraction Techniques

Play and distraction have been used in healthcare for many years to relax children and reduce fear and anxiety. The use of role play with children should not be underestimated. Children's nurses need to develop a good relationship with their patients and a good place to start is to find out their favourite games, toys, characters and television programmes or films. Using a favourite soft toy or character to take their medicine first can help young children to take their own medicine. Praise and rewards are another way of encouraging children who are reluctant to take their medicine. Forcing a child to take medication is not ethical and will possibly engender a fear of taking medicine in the future. As previously discussed, allowing a child to taste a medicine before it is prescribed alongside education will help with concordance.

Inhaled medication via a face mask can also be frightening for children due to the noise, the sensation and having their face covered. Building up wearing a mask can help children if it is not an urgent situation. Staying with the child and talking to them to keep them calm and keeping their breathing regular is also good practice.

Clinical Consideration

Where CYP have a fear of taking medicine orally, via a nebuliser or as an injection, the inclusion of a play specialist should be encouraged to develop an individual programme to explore the issue and help the child overcome their fear.

Some conditions that CYP present with may require long-term medications with unpleasant side effects such as nausea, vomiting, swelling, hair loss, weight gain or loss. This text will focus on numerous conditions and medications used within systems such as cardiovascular gastroenterology, immune, integumentary, neurology, respiratory and endocrine systems. In addition to this, medications used for mental health and cancer care will be explained in detail, as well as analgesia and adverse drug reactions.

Conclusion

The use of medicine within healthcare is a growing area, with more people having a chronic condition or acute illness requiring medication treatment. Medication management is a multidisciplinary process including pharmacists, doctors, allied health professionals and nurses and one with risk of error. Under the professional bodies within healthcare we are expected to 'do no harm' and yet there are still errors happening with regard to medicine management. It is important to follow the professional guidelines and to work within local policies and procedures as well as ensuring individual capability. Reporting errors when found and learning from the factors surrounding those errors as a reflective practitioner can improve the safety of patients and improve the support for the various systems in place. Ensuring that nurses have the knowledge and skills going forward with regard to medicine storage, management and administration following the 10 Rs is essential. There is a need for healthcare students to develop knowledge as lifelong learners and apply skills so that when they are admitted to the professional register they will be fit for purpose and fit for practice.

Glossary

Adherence: The extent to which a person follows an agreed set of actions. It assumes an equal relationship between two people, it is a voluntary process.

Autonomy: A person's ability to make choices on the basis of that person's own preferences, beliefs and values

Capacity: An ability to understand, deliberate and communicate a choice in relation to a specific healthcare decision at a particular time

Competence: The achievement and application of knowledge, intellectual capacities, practice skills, integrity and professional and ethical values needed for safe, accountable, compassionate and effective practice as a registered practitioner

Compliance: Medication compliance refers to the degree or extent of conformity to the recommendations about day-to-day treatment by the healthcare provider with regard to timing, dosage and frequency. It relates to a more paternalistic or autocratic relationship, where a person is either following instructions (compliant) or disregarding them (non-compliant)

Conduct: A person's moral practices, actions, beliefs and standards of behaviour

Evidence-based practice: The conscious consideration and the application of the best available evidence along with the healthcare provider's expertise and a person's values and preferences in making healthcare decisions

Guidance: A principle or criterion that guides or directs action

Health and well-being: A state of complete physical, social and mental well-being, not just the absence of disease or infirmity

Pharmacology: A branch of science that deals with the study of drugs and their actions on living systems

Regulations: A rule or law designed to control or govern conduct

Social prescribing: Also known as community referral, a means of enabling healthcare staff to refer people to a variety of local, non-clinical services

Standards: Authoritative statements developed, monitored and enforced by, for example, healthcare regulators to describe the responsibilities and conduct expected of registrants

Therapeutic: Relating to therapeutics, the branch of healthcare concerned specifically with the treatment of disease.

References

Baguley, D., Lim, E., Bevan, A. et al. (2012). Prescribing for children – taste and palatability affect adherence to antibiotics: a review. *Archives of Disease in Childhood* 97: 293–7. 2.

Barber, P. (2013). *Medicine Management for Nurses Case Book*. Maidenhead: Open University Press.

Edwards, S. and Axe, S. (2015). The ten 'R's of safe multidisciplinary drug administration. *Nurse Prescribing* 13(8). doi: 10.12968/npre.2015.13.8.398.

Elliott, M. and Liu, Y. (2010). The nine rights of medication administration: An overview. *British Journal of Nursing* 19(5): 300–305.

Elliott, R., Camacho, E., Campbell, F. et al. (2020). Prevalence and economic burden of medication errors in the NHS in England. Policy research unit in economic evaluation of health and care interventions (EEPRU) www.eepru.org.uk/prevalence-and-economic-burden-of-medication-errors-in-the-nhs-in-england-2/ (accessed September 2020).

Haddad, P. and Nutt, D. (2020). *Seminars in Clinical Psychopharmacology*, 3e. Cambridge: Cambridge University Press, 124–140.

Horner, A. (2019). How social prescribing can help young people. *Nursing Children and Young People* 31(3): 14–15.

NHS England (2018). Prescribing of over the counter medications is changing. www.england.nhs.uk/wp-content/uploads/2018/08/1a-over-the-counter-leaflet-v1.pdf (accessed September 2020).

NHS England (2020). Social prescribing. www.england.nhs.uk/personalisedcare/social-prescribing/ (accessed September 2020).

NHS National Patient Safety Agency (NPSA) (2007). Safety in doses: Medication safety incidents in the NHS. London: NPSA.

NICE (2021). *British National Formulary for Children*. https://bnfc.nice.org.uk/guidance/medicines-optimisation.html (accessed April 2021).

NICE (2015). Medicines optimisation: The safe and effective use of medicines to enable the best possible outcomes. www.nice.org.uk/guidance/ng5/chapter/Finding-more-information-and-resources (accessed July 2020).

Nursing and Midwifery Council (2018a). The Code Professional Standards of Practice and Behaviour for Nurses, Midwives and Nursing Associates. www.nmc.org.uk/globalassets/sitedocuments/nmc-publications/nmc-code.pdf (accessed June 2020).

Nursing and Midwifery Council (2018b). Future Nurse: Standards of Proficiency for Registered Nurses www.nmc.org.uk/globalassets/sitedocuments/standards-of-proficiency/nurses/future-nurse-proficiencies.pdf (accessed July 2020).

Nursing and Midwifery Council (2018c). Standards of Proficiency for Nursing Associates. www.nmc.org.uk/globalassets/sitedocuments/education-standards/nursing-associates-proficiency-standards.pdf (accessed September 2020).

Nursing and Midwifery Council (2018d). Standards for Pre-registration Nursing Associate Programmes? www.nmc.org.uk/globalassets/sitedocuments/standards-of-proficiency/standards-for-pre-registration-nursing-associate-programmes/nursing-associates-programme-standards.pdf (accessed September 2020).

Royal College of Nursing and Royal Pharmaceutical Society (2019). *Professional Guidance on the Administration of Medicines in Healthcare Settings*. London: RCN and RPS. www.rpharms.com/Portals/0/RPS%20document%20library/Open%20access/Professional%20standards/SSHM%20and%20Admin/Admin%20of%20Meds%20prof%20guidance.pdf?ver=2019-01-23-145026-567 (accessed September 2020).

Royal Pharmaceutical Society (2013). Medicines Optimisation: Helping Patients to Make the Most of Medicines. https://www.rpharms.com/Portals/0/RPS%20document%20library/Open%20access/Policy/helping-patients-make-the-most-of-their-medicines.pdf (accessed April 2021).

Tse, Y., Vasey, N., Dua, D. et al. (2019). The KidzMed project: Teaching children to swallow tablet medication. *Archives of Disease in Childhood* 105: 1105–1107.

World Health Organization (2009). *Pharmacological Treatment of Mental Health Disorders in Primary Health Care*. Geneva: WHO.

Further Resources

- EasyHealth (www.easyhealth.org.uk): A resource with over 500 health leaflets that include pictures and very simple text. EasyHealth's information is accessible to those with low literacy levels, which may include people with learning disabilities.
- British Pharmacological Society (www.bps.ac.uk): The BPS, a charity, exists to promote and advance pharmacology in all its forms
- National Institute for Health and Care Excellence (NICE) (www.nice.org.uk): NICE provides national guidance and advice to improve health and social care. The role of NICE is to improve outcomes for people using the NHS and other public health and social care services.
- Royal College of Nursing (www.rcn.org.uk/clinical-topics/medicines-management): Medicines management. A resource providing guidance and clinical support for nurses and other healthcare professionals on medicines matters.

Chapter 1 Introduction to Pharmacology, Children and Young People 13

- Royal Pharmaceutical Society (www.rpharms.com): The RPS gives pharmacy a clear, strong voice in all healthcare discussions and decisions across Britain. They also publish the British National Formulary Child.
- Street Games (https://network.streetgames.org/our-work-changing-lives-health/youth-social-prescribing): Youth Social Prescribing. Learn more about social prescribing, the work of the Social Prescribing Youth Network and Street Games' involvement within it, by accessing the various resources.

Multiple Choice Questions

1. The Nursing and Midwifery Council's purpose is to:
   (a) Provide government with the details of those nurses and nursing associates who have been found guilty of misconduct
   (b) Inform nurse managers how they are to determine patient dependency
   (c) Promote and uphold the highest professional standards in nursing and midwifery to protect the public and inspire confidence in the professions
   (d) All of the above
2. To help patients make decisions about medicines:
   (a) Provide time for them to ask questions
   (b) Offer them relevant information which is easy to understand and avoid the use of jargon
   (c) Provide information that is structured and tailor this to the needs of the individual patient.
   (d) All of the above
3. Medicines optimisation is generally associated with:
   (a) The legal regulations in place to safely administer medicines
   (b) A more people-centred approach to the use of medicine as part of a person's care
   (c) Another phrase for capacity
   (d) Is only ever used when the patient lacks capacity
4. Pharmacokinetics is associated with:
   (a) The ability to safely calculate a drug dose
   (b) The biology of home remedies
   (c) What the body does to a drug, the movement of drugs into, through and out of the body
   (d) How enzymes are metabolised in plants
   (e) Infusion pumps and equipment used to administer drugs
5. Pharmacodynamics is associated with:
   (a) How toxins have effects on the body
   (b) How drugs have effects on the body
   (c) The prescribers prescribing skills
   (d) The nurse's competence in the administration of medicines
6. Adherence refers to:
   (a) Specific patient behaviours
   (b) The study of power differentials
   (c) The extent to which the patient's behaviour matches agreed recommendations from the prescriber
   (d) The extent to which the patient's behaviour matches the prescriber's recommendation
7. The purpose of a medicine is to:
   (a) Cause a build of toxins in the blood stream
   (b) Prevent, alleviate or cure a symptom, disorder or disease state
   (c) Cause a negative impact on a person's health and well-being
   (d) None of the above
8. A patient's/family's beliefs and preferences about medication:
   (a) May affect medication adherence
   (b) Should be moderated during medicines management
   (c) Is only appropriate in the adult patient
   (d) Will not impact on medication adherence
9. Non-adherence can result in:
   (a) Unnecessary health costs and unnecessary investigations
   (b) Changes to routines which lead to increased safety risks

(c) Enhanced care provision
(d) A better use of resources
10. The term 'compliance':
    (a) Is a term with positive connotations
    (b) Can also infer 'nurse knows best'
    (c) Is never used in the care of CYP
    (d) Is the same as concordance
11. Summaries of Product Characteristics (SPC) are:
    (a) Held at all general practices
    (b) Do not apply to CYP
    (c) Is a description of a medicinal product's properties and the conditions attached to its use
    (d) Only apply to medicines that are imported from the USA
12. Every medicine pack includes a patient information leaflet:
    (a) Providing information on using the medicine safely
    (b) The patient information leaflet is based on information in the SPC of the medicine
    (c) Provides information on using controlled drugs only
    (d) A and B
13. Independent prescribers:
    (a) Must be supervised at all times by a pharmacist
    (b) Are only allowed to prescribe in the independent and voluntary sectors
    (c) Are able to prescribe any medicine provided it is in their competency to do so.
    (d) Must also hold a pharmacy qualification
14. Pharmacology is:
    (a) The study of chemical reactions and medication
    (b) The study of how communities respond to the introduction of vaccinations
    (c) A branch of science that deals only with the effects of alcohol, nicotine and cannabis on living systems
    (d) A branch of science that deals with the study of drugs and their actions on living systems
15. A pharmacist is:
    (a) A doctor who has a special interest in drugs and medications
    (b) A licensed health professional who prepares, dispenses and advises on medicinal products
    (c) A scientist who researches new drugs
    (d) Another name for a chemist

Find Out More

The following are a list of conditions that are associated with this chapter. Take some time and write notes about each of the conditions and how they apply to chapter content. Think about the medications that may be used in order to treat these conditions and be specific about the pharmacokinetics and pharmacodynamics. Remember to include aspects of patient care. If you are making notes about people you have offered care and support to, you must ensure that you have adhered to the rules of confidentiality.

THE CONDITION	YOUR NOTES
Sarcoma	
Attention deficit hyperactive disorder	
Diabetes	

THE CONDITION	YOUR NOTES
Pneumonia	
Drug overdose on lysergic acid	

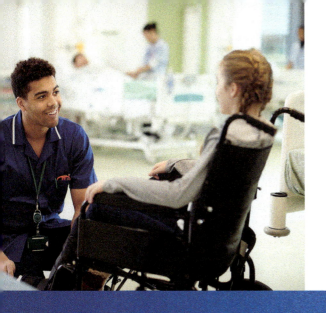

How to Use Pharmaceutical and Prescribing Reference Guides

Claire Pryor, Annette Hand and Elaine Robinson

Aim

This chapter aims to introduce the reader to commonly used pharmaceutical and prescribing reference guides and their use in practice. Specific focus is placed on the British National Formulary for children (BNFc) and other reference guides used in clinical practice.

Learning Outcomes

After reading this chapter, the reader will:

- Be aware of the different pharmaceutical and reference guides that may be used in practice
- Understand how to navigate the BNFc (in both print and electronic formats)
- Recognise the different prescribing reference guides available (local and national)
- Discuss the benefits of using pharmaceutical and prescribing reference guides in practice

Test Your Knowledge

- How many times a year is the print version of the BNFc updated?
- Is the information in the BNFc and BNF the same?
- What schedule of controlled drug is midazolam?
- What is a GSL medication?
- Where will you find national prescribing guidelines for managing constipation in children?

Fundamentals of Pharmacology for Children's Nurses, First Edition. Edited by Ian Peate and Peter Dryden.
© 2022 John Wiley & Sons Ltd. Published 2022 by John Wiley & Sons Ltd.
Companion website: www.wiley.com/go/pharmacologyforCN

Introduction

The world of medications is vast and learning about them can be daunting for all nursing and healthcare students (as well as registered professionals). The people you care for may have extensive lists of medications you need to be able to review, administer, consider interactions and monitor effects of these.

Professional bodies have specific standards of practice in relation to medicines and pharmacological knowledge and this will relate to the practitioner's role. The Nursing and Midwifery (NMC) code (NMC, 2018a) states in standard 18 that nurses and nursing associates must

> *Advise on, prescribe, supply, dispense or administer medicines within the limits of your training and competence, the law, our guidance and other relevant policies, guidance and regulations*
>
> **(Nursing and Midwifery Council, 2018a)**

Further guidance is issued for nursing associates: the NMC stipulates the requirement for nursing associates; as per section 3:16 of their standards of proficiency they must:

> *demonstrate the ability to recognise the effects of medicines, allergies, drug sensitivity, side effects, contraindications and adverse reactions*
>
> **(Nursing and Midwifery Council, 2018b)**

In order to fulfil these requirements, healthcare professionals must have a level of pharmaceutical knowledge and an awareness of how to and where to find appropriate information to support practice. In a sea of new products and complex regimens, where can you turn to for up-to-date, clear and concise information to guide your practice? There are numerous guides, websites, texts and resources that are readily available. Ensuring a robust and evidence-based selection of these is paramount, but the choice is also personal. Some are web-based, some print-based, and the recent evolution of healthcare apps for professionals means that there is a selection for all user preferences.

This chapter aims to introduce you to using pharmaceutical and prescribing reference guides with a specific focus on the British National Formulary for Children (BNFc) and other pharmaceutical reference guides. These guides are vital and valuable resources to draw upon to ensure safe, accountable and evidence-based care that is matched to the needs and wishes of the people you care for.

Skills in Practice

You are a first-year student on your first placement, with your practice supervisor you are assessing a new admission for a 12-year-old child with their parents. The parents give you a list of medication their child takes and it has lots of names on it that are new to you. You want to impress your supervisor and find out about them for your next shift. How do you do this? Where do you turn?

Your supervisor suggests you look them up and points you to a paper copy of the BNFc. Upon opening it, it appears confusing, full of sections and symbols, and you are unsure how to find the information you need.

- Open a paper copy of the BNFc and find the last drug you discussed or saw in practice
- Can you locate it in the BNFc?
- What form does it come in?
- What are the side effects?
- Are there any interactions?
- Can it be bought at the supermarket?

These are some considerations you may have to think about when supporting children, young people (CYP) and families with medication. Pharmaceutical reference guides will help you navigate this complex process and support your evidence-based practice.

The British National Formulary and the British National Formulary for Children

Produced by the Joint Formulary Committee, the BNF is one of the most commonly used and reliable sources of information for medication with distinct versions for children and adults: the BNF and the BNF for children (BNFc).The Paediatric Formulary Committee (PFC) takes responsibility for the BNFc content. Ensuring that you use the most appropriate BNF for your practice area is essential as medications, recommendations, licensing, legislation and monitoring differ for adults and children. The BNF is published in paper copy bi-annually in September and March and the BNFc is published in paper copy once a year in September. There are electronic versions (as discussed later) which are frequently updated, so it is always advisable to use the electronic version to ensure the most up-to-date information is accessed. This chapter focuses on the BNFc; the BNF follows the same layout but has additional and different information pertaining to medicines use for adults.

Practice Consideration

It is important that you use the correct version for your practice. The BNFc holds different and specific information in relation to medication and children. This is not the same as the BNF (which is for use in adults).

The BNFc is an essential tool for all practitioners working with children and young people, it is a repository of almost all drugs that are used in British health and social care settings, and offers comprehensive details on individual medications, groups of medications, uses, side effects and interactions and can assist with decision making. The information provided is sourced from summaries of product characteristics for medications, literature, consensus guidelines and peer review and employs a grading system of A–E and levels of evidence to help readers understand the strength of evidence underpinning the associated recommendations given (Joint Formulary Committee, 2019a).

Paper Copy BNFc

As a health professional you are accountable for using the most up-to-date evidence base for your practice. This means ensuring that you only use the current version of the BNFc which relates to your practice area and care of (CYP). The BNF also contains information on drugs licensed for use in children; however, the comprehensive literature relating more specifically to CYP will be found in the BNFc. A BNF will always be a good source for pharmaceutical information and can easily be used in the absence of a current BNFc, but should be used with caution.

You should consider:

- That previous paper versions may have outdated information or even sections that have been removed
- The implications of advising CYP and their families on medication regimens if the information source you have chosen is out of date. What are the potential risks to the CYP? What could this mean for your practice and accountability?

How to navigate the BNFc

At first glance the BNFc can be overwhelming; however, with a little practice it quickly becomes a fast and reliable way to gather information for yourself, patients and those you work with.

The current BNFc print versions are organised into four main sections:

- Front matter
- Chapters
- Appendices
- Back matter

Chapter 2 How to Use Pharmaceutical and Prescribing Reference Guides

Table 2.1 Text format and information purpose.

TEXT FORMAT	INFORMATION USE
Black	Information on treatment summary and therapeutic uses
Colour block	Information on drug specific information

Careful attention should be paid to the font colour (see Table 2.1), images and symbols used in the BNF as these all convey pertinent information

Front Matter

The front matter of the BNFc gives quick access to information such as how to use the BNFc, the layout of information throughout chapters and significant changes that have taken place since the previous edition. General guidance is given on prescribing and the requirements of legal prescriptions, both handwritten and computer-issued. Special attention is paid to controlled drugs, alongside adverse reactions to drugs and offers guidance on recognition and reporting.

A general overview of specific patient-centred considerations is given in relation to prescribing in hepatic (liver) and renal (kidney) failure as well considerations for pregnancy, breast-feeding and palliative care. Each section has a broad overview followed by specific considerations. For example, in prescribing for palliative care, specific information is provided on pain management, symptom control and continuous subcutaneous infusions.

Chapters

The main body of the BNFc is divided into systems chapters (i.e. gastrointestinal system) and follows the same structure.

Some drugs and chapters have a *class monograph*. A class monograph includes information that is common to all drugs within a particular class. It is important to read these in conjunction with the *drug monograph* which gives information relating to that drug in particular. Class monographs are identified by a flag in a circle ⓕ (Source: BMJ Publishing Group Ltd.). If the drug you are seeking advice on has an associated *class monograph* it will be indicated by a tab with a flag symbol and the page number where the *class monograph* can be found ⚑ 1234 (Source: BMJ Publishing Group Ltd.).

Access a copy of the current BNFc and open the gastrointestinal system chapter. It starts with a clear contents section indicating what can be found in the chapter on the gastrointestinal system and is followed by information on the associated diseases, conditions and disorders, treatment summaries and individual medication information. Focusing on constipation, find and read the description of the condition and its associated overview and management.

The *classification* of the individual drug is indicated in blue (e.g. Laxatives – Bulk-forming Laxatives) with the drug name and *drug monograph* sited below. The *drug monograph* provides comprehensive information on the drug all in one concise section. Pertinent guidance is offered relating to drug action, indications and dose, adjustments and interactions, safety information, contraindications, signposting to the correct section of interactions, side effects and medicinal forms.

Drug-class monographs have been created by the publishers of the BNF. Where there is common information relating to a class of drugs, the shared properties are contained in a drug-class monograph (Hand and Pryor, 2021). Drug-class monographs are emphasised by a circled flag symbol next to the title of the drug-class monograph The corresponding individual drug monographs generally follow the drug-class monograph, these are highlighted by a non-circled flag symbol (see Figure 2.1)

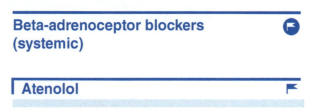

Figure 2.1 Drug-class monographs. *Source:* BMJ Publishing Group Ltd.

In the example in Figure 2.1, the monograph depicted for atenolol will display a flag; this indicates that the drug-class monograph for Beta-adrenoceptor blockers (systemic) should be consulted in tandem.

Within the drug monograph the following are also highlighted:

- Drug classification – may be based on pharmaceutical class, for example opioids, but may also be related to the use of the drug, such as cough suppressant
- Indication and dose – all the information that relates to an individual drug, for example, drug action, indication and dose, contraindications, cautions, interactions, side effects, allergies and so on
- Specific preparation name – if the dose varies with a specific preparation or formulation it appears under a heading of the preparation name
- Evidence grading – This reflects the strength of recommendations applied
- Legal categories – Applied to those preparations that are available only on a prescription issued by an appropriate practitioner and preparations that are subject to the prescription requirements of the Misuse of Drugs Act

The information found in the *medicinal forms* section of the monograph is vital for healthcare professionals to be able to understand the various routes of administration, supply, and dose schedule considerations. Alongside this, the medicinal forms section shows the legal category of the drug indicated by a specific category abbreviation or controlled drug schedule abbreviation. Table 2.2 demonstrates the abbreviations and their meanings. In practice, this information may make the difference between generating a prescription or giving health advice. The variance between categories may be determined by the drug itself, dose and amount to be dispensed (see Box 2.1).

Table 2.2 Abbreviations of medication categories.

CATEGORY	DESCRIPTION
P – pharmacy-only medicine P	A product that may only be sold in a registered pharmacy under the supervision of a registered pharmacist e.g. bisacodyl suppositories
PoM – prescription-only medicine POM	A product that may only be sold or supplied to the public on a practitioner's prescription, e.g. warfarin tablets
GSL – general sales list GSL	A product that may be sold from a retail outlet without the supervision of a registered pharmacist, e.g. NiQuitin 2mg medicated chewing gum
CD – controlled drug CD1 CD2 CD3 CD4-1 CD4-2 CD5	A product that is controlled by the Misuse of Drugs Act 1971 and is listed in the Misuse of Drugs Regulations 2001 as amended, which may be subject to specific restrictions relating to supply, prescription, storage, record-keeping, labelling and destruction, e.g. morphine sulfate (modified-release tablets) 60mg oral tablet
ACBS – Advisory Committee on Borderline Substances	A product that may be prescribed for the treatment of certain conditions. Prescriptions for these products must be endorsed 'ACBS' e.g. gluten-free bread

Chapter 2 How to Use Pharmaceutical and Prescribing Reference Guides

> ### Box 2.1 Paracetamol Sales
>
> Paracetamol 500mg tablets in 16 tablet packs are available as General Sales List (GSL) and can be purchased by an adult or young person over 16 years of age, without supervision of a pharmacist. Pharmacists may sell packs of a maximum of 32 tablets as Pharmacy only (P) drugs, requiring the supervision of a Pharmacist. Over 32 tablets per pack are Prescription-only Medication (PoM).
>
> This example shows whilst the drug itself remains the same, other factors (in this instance quantity) may impact on the classification of a medication. Other licensing considerations may change the legal status of the medication as well, even if the drug remains the same.
>
> *Source*: Medications and Healthcare products Regulatory Agency, 2009; Joint Formulary Committee, 2019b.

Skills in Practice

Using the BNFc index, locate docusate sodium.
- What is the drug classification?
- What are the cautions associated with this drug?
- Is this drug present in breast milk?

Back Matter

The back matter of the BNFc contains a number of appendices which offer detailed supplementary nformation on drug interactions, borderline substances, cautionary and advisory labels, and the specific formularies for dental practitioners and the nurse prescribers formulary (for registered community ractitioner prescribers).

Interactions

As a practitioner and professionally accountable for your actions, you must ensure that you know how to review and find out information on potential interactions. A comprehensive list of drugs with known interactions is found in appendix 1 of the BNFc (as signposted to in the drug monograph). Appendix 1 provides tables and details of specific medications, medication combinations, and their associated pharmacodynamics effects. Each drug or class listed, by name alphabetically and/or with the specific drug or group that it interacts with.

Borderline Substances

In some conditions, such as coeliac disease, food products and toilet preparations may have characteristics of drugs. These products are reviewed and determined by the ACBS, as such, may be treated as a prescribed medication. Some examples are enteral feeds, nutritional supplements, gluten-free or low-protein foods and nutritional supplements given to treat metabolic diseases (e.g. maple syrup urine disease) alongside toilet preparations for topical use (for example, E45® or Aveeno Cream® for the treatment of dermatitis).

Nutritional supplements are common in care settings. Providing support with supplement drinks and puddings, for example, may form part of your everyday practice, but these should be treated as medication and prescribed based on individual patient need as with any medication.

Clinical Consideration

You have been looking after young person for an extended period of time. It is common to offer her a feeding supplement, as she has an eating disorder. You support her to build her oral diet and the supplement is given after each attempt at eating three times a day. On discussion with your practice supervisor you realise this is not prescribed for her and she is being prepared for discharge back home with community care services.

What implications does this practice have? Jot down your initial thoughts:

1. For her? And her family? (both now and post transfer of care)
2. For you as a healthcare professional or student?
3. For discharge planning?
4. For the healthcare practitioners responsible for her medications?

Revisit these considerations and your initial thoughts when you have explored more about the legal and ethical considerations (Chapter 3 of this text) as well as pharmacokinetics and pharmacodynamics (Chapter 5 of this text).

Cautionary and Advisory Labels for Dispensed Medication

Many medications come with cautionary or advisory information that should be added by pharmacists when dispensing the requested medication. Appendix three of the BNFc is has list of approved cautionary and advisory labels each with a specific code number. The number associated with the label is found in the *drug monograph* in the *medicinal forms* section below the preparation chosen. It is important to advise the patient on the additional advice or directions given for taking their medication. A full list of the labels and wording is found in appendix three and a shorter version in the back pages of the print BNFc.

Skills in Practice

- Using the index, find ranitidine in the BNFc
- Using the drug monograph, find the medicinal form section
- Identify the cautionary and advisory label number given for effervescent tablets
- Use appendix three of the BNFc to identify what the label states
- What additional information is provided?
- How would you discuss this with the CYP and their parent/carer?
- How would you discuss this with the CYP and their parent/carer?

Emergency Care Protocols, Units, Conversions and Abbreviations

The BNFc print version acts as a reference guide for practitioners in emergency situations. The newborn life support, paediatric basic life support and paediatric advanced life support algorithms are provided along with body surface area and weight charts, and an overview of community-based medical emergency management. Additional conversion and unit tables are presented as a reference followed by the cautionary and advisory label wordings discussed previously. The inside back page lastly provides a guide to the abbreviations and symbols used which are internationally recognised.

Online and Mobile Application BNFc

In an increasingly paper-free healthcare system, you may not have access to paper copies of the BNFc. The BNFc has an online platform accessed via the National Institute for Health and Care Excellence (NICE), or via Medicines Complete (https://about.medicinescomplete.com/) as well as an offline app that can be used on smart phones and tablets. The BNF *for Children* (https://bnfc.nice.org.uk/) and BNF online (https://bnf.nice.org.uk/) are updated monthly and as such is more up-to-date than the print version and does not require a specific log in. The app is automatically updated monthly (when connected to Wi-Fi).

When you visit the home page of the BNFc online (via NICE) you are presented with clear options for navigation. All the same information is held online as in print – but navigation is different. Drugs (as drug monographs), interactions and treatment summaries can be searched for by browsing an alphabetised list or the search bar at the top of the web page. The home page also has a 'type' organisation where quick access to areas such as wound management, borderline substances and nurse prescribers' formularies can be found.

Searching for atenolol (for example) and opening its page displays information under the atenolol drug monograph. A table of contents is provided for rapid navigation of the subsections available. On scrolling down the opening page, indications and dose are clearly presented alongside routes of administration. Next, licensing information, safety information and contraindications are displayed.

Cautionary and advisory labels are indicated when medicinal form is selected both by label number and the associated text. In addition, the schedule of any controlled drug is clearly documented in its medicinal form information.

Associated class monograph information are integrated throughout the chosen drug monograph and are indicated by the phrasing 'for all . . .'. An example of this can be seen in the contraindications for atenolol (Figure 2.2)

Searching for interactions is managed within a dedicated interactions section by an initial drug search and then matching to a subsequent alphabetical list. The associated interaction is discussed in terms of potential effects of the interaction, signposting to relevant additional sections of the BNFc such as 'safety in the home' in 'Guidance on prescribing' and have associated hyperlinks for ease. Severity of interactions are defined

Chapter 2 How to Use Pharmaceutical and Prescribing Reference Guides

Contra-indications

> For all BETA-ADRENOCEPTOR BLOCKERS (SYSTEMIC)

Figure 2.2 Contraindication and class monograph.

using terms of severe, moderate, mild and unknown to support decision making alongside the type of evidence underpinning the interaction information.

Key to safe and accountable practice is the recognition and reporting of suspected adverse reactions or effects of medication. The BNF and BNFc support active reporting of adverse reactions by both healthcare professionals and patients themselves or their carers. Using the *Yellow Card Scheme*, the MHRA collects information on medications, vaccines, herbal treatments, medical devices, defective medications and from 2016 counterfeit or fake healthcare products. The print copy of the BNF and BNFc have a small supply of yellow cards in the back matter. Alternatively, concerns can be raised using the UK Medicines and Healthcare Products Regulatory Agency (MHRA) Yellow card webpage (https://yellowcard.mhra.gov.uk/). Chapter 19 provides more details of this.

Monthly Index of Medical Specialities (MIMS)

Within a primary care setting you may also come across the MIMS prescribing guide. This is an up-to-date prescribing reference for healthcare professionals and it is available both in print and online. MIMS is updated constantly online, to reflect the latest approved prescribing information, along with the addition of new drugs and formulations, and also removes products that are no longer available. The printed version of MIMS is produced quarterly and includes all the updates from the corresponding three months of the online updates. MIMS is primarily intended for use by nurses and GPs working within primary care. A subscription is required for nurses who wish to receive the print version. All other prescribing healthcare professionals, such as paramedics, dietitians and physiotherapists, need to subscribe to MIMS to access either the online or print versions. MIMS is a helpful prescribing resource and provides:

- News on changes that affect medicines and prescribing
- Drug information for branded and generic products, updated daily
- At-a-glance drug comparison tables including dosing and monitoring regimens, available presentations, prices, potential sensitisers and compatible devices
- Quick-reference summaries of key clinical guidance from authoritative national bodies including NICE and the Scottish Intercollegiate Guidelines Network (SIGN)
- Online drugs shortages tracker showing branded and generic medicines that are out of stock
- Online visual guides to help you identify, compare and recommend diabetes and respiratory devices

MIMS provides concise summaries of prescribing information for branded and generic products that can be prescribed in the UK, including devices listed in the section on permitted appliances within the Drug Tariff. Drugs that are blacklisted (i.e. not on the Drug Tariff and therefore not available on prescription within the NHS) are not listed and no information is given on the unlicensed or off-label use of drugs.

The print edition of MIMS also includes a selection of the most popular drug reference tables. The full range of tables and drug listings are available online, together with at-a-glance summaries of national treatment guidance, helpful visual guides to diabetes and respiratory devices, there is also a prescribing resource centre for specific disease areas. The legal class categories in MIMS are the same as those within the BNF and listed in Table 2.2.

How to Use MIMS Online

When you visit the home page of the MIMS online (see Figure 2.3) you are able to search for drugs (by drug name or drug class), browse news and resources by disease areas (from an A to Z list) or search for news, tables or guidance on any condition or drug. You are also able to search for drugs by manufacturer. Searching for a drug only returns a list if there is more than one hit (i.e. multiple drugs matching the search term and/or drugs matching the search term appearing in multiple sections) – otherwise you are taken to the drug entry. Clicking onto a drug will display all the different preparations, legal class, indications and dose recommendations for adults and children (where appropriate). The drug listing page will also display helpful links to any related guidelines or related conditions.

Chapter 2 How to Use Pharmaceutical and Prescribing Reference Guides

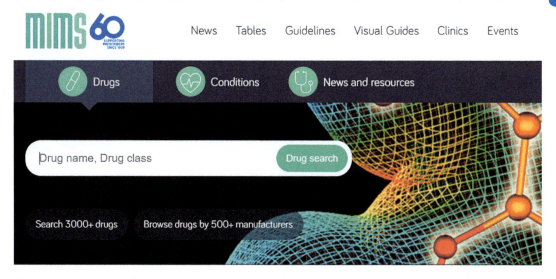

Figure 2.3 Home page of MIMS online (www.mims.co.uk/). *Source:* Haymarket Media Group Ltd.

Skills in Practice

1. Search for paracetamol using the drug search box

(Source: Haymarket Media Group Ltd.)
2. You will see that paracetamol-containing products can be used for a number of different clinical conditions (migraine, pain and fever), with different strengths, formulations and combinations.
3. When paracetamol is combined with another product it is still important to understand the strengths of the individual compounds. Clink onto co-codamol. You can see there is always 500mg of paracetamol within one co-codamol capsule, but the dose of codeine phosphate could be 8, 15 or 30mg
4. Each form of paracetamol is only licensed for specific indications. Clink onto paracetamol infusion. You can see this would only be used as a short-term treatment for moderate pain and fever when other routes are inappropriate.
5. For each paracetamol preparation there may be different contraindications. Click onto paracetamol/ibuprofen (combogesic). You will see the contraindications are alcoholism, aspirin/anti-inflammatory allergy, active or history of gastrointestinal bleeding or peptic ulcer, severe cardiac, hepatic or renal failure, cerebrovascular or other active bleeding, blood formation disturbances and pregnancy (3rd trimester)

Searching within news and resources you will find links to relevant tables and summaries of national guidelines, as well as any information about the condition that has been in the news. You can use the filters on the right-hand side to find the results of a particular type (for example, news) or from a particular year.

Many abbreviations are used in healthcare and it is important that you familiarise yourself with these to ensure you understand what they mean. Abbreviations are used within prescribing guides and in practice and it is always best to check what an abbreviation means if you are unsure what it means. A list of the abbreviations used in MIMS can be found at the front of every print issue and online.

Clinical Consideration

- You are asked to administer a medication in 'S/C' or 'S-C' form
- Do you get a glass of water for your patient, or an injection/infusion set?
- What would the implications be of not understanding the correct abbreviation?

Be aware that sometimes the same abbreviation is used to mean different things. For some healthcare practitioners the abbreviation 's/c' or 's-c' could be colloquially used to mean subcutaneous, but within MIMS ('S-C') and the BNF (S/C) the abbreviation represents 'sugar-coated' and not the route of administration. It is paramount that you are aware of the formal abbreviations in use and not colloquial, historical interpretations or slang. This is explored further in Chapter 4 of this text, Medicines Management and the Role of the Healthcare Provider.

Electronic Medicines Compendium

The electronic medicines compendium (emc) contains up-to-date, easily accessible information about medicines licensed for use in the UK and can be found at (www.medicines.org.uk/emc). The emc has more than 14,000 documents, all of which have been checked and approved by either the UK or European government agencies which license medicines. These agencies are the UK Medicines and Healthcare products Regulatory Agency (MHRA) and the European Medicines Agency (EMA). The emc is updated continually and you are able to browse for medicines, or active ingredients using the A – Z buttons. The emc contains regulated and approved information on medicines available in the UK including:

1. **Summaries of Product Characteristics (known as SPCs or SmPCs):** A SmPC informs healthcare professionals how to prescribe and use a medicine correctly. A SmPC is based on clinical trials that a pharmaceutical company has carried out and gives information about dose, use and possible side effects. A SmPC is always written in a standard format.
2. **Patient Information Leaflets (PILs, Package Leaflets or PLs):** A PIL is the leaflet that is included in the pack with any medicine. The PIL is a summary of the SmPC and is written for patients.
3. **Risk Minimisation Materials (RMMs):** Risk Minimisation Materials are resources for healthcare professionals that aim to optimise the safe and effective use of a medicine. RMMs can come in a number of forms, such as educational programmes, prescribing or dispensing guides, patient brochures or alert cards.
4. **Safety Alerts:** Safety alerts are issued by the medicine healthcare regulatory agency and/or marketing authorisation holder and contain important public health messages or safety critical information about a medicine.
5. **Product Information:** This is any additional information about a product. It may include important information such change of packaging or issues related to stock levels. (Electronic Medicines Compendium/ Datapharm Ltd.)

Within the emc there are also audio and video resources that provide additional information in a *user-friendly way*, promoting the safe and effective use of a medicine. For example, a video clip may demonstrate how to administer a certain medicine correctly.

What Can Be Prescribed on an NHS Prescription?

There are hundreds of medicinal products and devices (or appliances) available to treat and manage illnesses, conditions and diseases. A medicinal product is defined as an item which is not considered to be appliance and could be a drug, food, toiletry or type of cosmetic (Pharmaceutical Services Negotiating Committee https://psnc.org.uk/dispensing-supply/dispensing-a-prescription/medicinal-products/). An approved medical device will carry the CE mark (Conformité Européenne) which signifies that it conforms to the appropriate regulatory standards. Not all of these medical products, devices or appliances are available from the NHS. On receiving a prescription, pharmacy staff will check whether or not an item is allowed to be prescribed on the NHS prior to dispensing using the Drug Tariff.

The Drug Tariff

The Drug Tariff is produced monthly by the Pharmaceutical Directorate of the NHS Business Services Authority and the NHS Prescription Services for the Secretary of State. It is supplied primarily to pharmacists and doctors' surgeries and is available in print and online, any healthcare professional can view the most up-to-date online version. Only fully licensed and approved medications and devices, found on the Drug Tariff, can be prescribed within the NHS (unless for research purposes). Information on the Drug Tariff can be found on either the Pharmaceutical Services Negotiating Committee (PSNC) or the NHS Prescription Services Websites. Within each of these sites you will find information on how to use the Drug Tariff, the Drug Tariff Preface and the information within the different Parts of the Drug Tariff. The Drug Tariff preface is an important section as each month as it contains valuable information on additions, deletions and any other alterations to the Drug Tariff.

What the Drug Tariff Does
The Drug Tariff outlines information such as:
- What will be paid to pharmacies for the NHS services provided (for example the cost of drugs and appliances supplied against an NHS Prescription)
- Rules that need to be followed when dispensing items
- Drug and appliance prices

How to Tell if a Medicinal Product is Allowed on Prescription
The 'blacklist' can be found in Schedule 1 to the NHS Regulations 2004 and is found in the Drug Tariff (part XVIIIA). It is a list of medicinal products which cannot be prescribed on the NHS. Any medicinal product not in the 'blacklist' can be prescribed on the NHS. The prescriber may, however, be questioned during the auditing process about the appropriateness of prescribing this item at the NHS's expense. As a general rule, if a branded (proprietary) product is listed in the 'blacklist' it cannot be prescribed on the NHS. Many of the medicinal products on the 'blacklist' are available over the counter for people to buy, whilst some do not have enough evidence to show their efficacy.

The PSCN flow chart (Figure 2.4) can be used to help identify whether an item is allowed to be dispensed on an NHS prescription form. Different practitioners may use different prescription pads or resources (seen below as FP10, FP10SS, FP10SP*).

If a medicinal product or device is prescribed that is not on the Drug Tariff, it cannot be dispensed.

Skills in Practice

Go to the Drug Tariff (www.nhsbsa.nhs.uk/pharmacies-gp-practices-and-appliance-contractors/drug-tariff) and see which of the following products are blacklisted and should not be prescribed on the NHS:
- Ferrous sulfate compound tablets BP
- Gaviscon granules
- Lemsip flu strength
- Lactulose syrup

Other Guides to Prescribing

The Joint Royal Colleges Ambulance Liaison Committee (JRCALC) Clinical Guidelines
The Joint Royal Colleges Ambulance Liaison Committee Clinical (JRCALC) Guidelines is a helpful resource for paramedics and other healthcare professionals, in emergency care, on the road and in the community. JRCALC combines expert advice with practical guidance to ensure uniformity in the delivery of high-quality patient care. The book, available as either a comprehensive reference edition or a pocket guide, covers a wide range of topics, from resuscitation, medical emergencies, trauma, obstetrics and medicines to major incidents and staff well-being. It includes an extensive UK drugs formulary and Page for Age drugs tables to assist in making medicines administration simple. A digital version, via an app, of the official JRCALC guidelines is also available for prehospital clinicians to download.

Chapter 2 How to Use Pharmaceutical and Prescribing Reference Guides

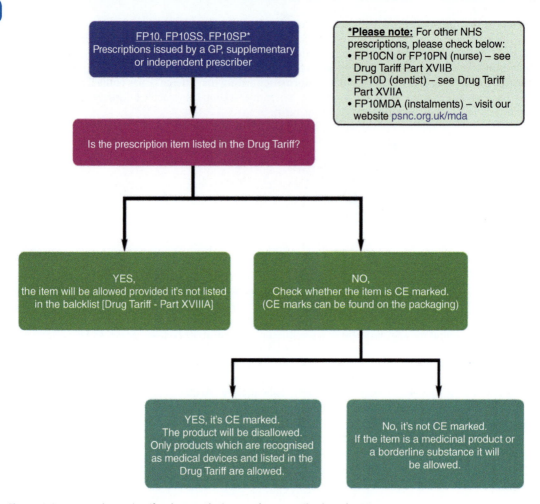

Figure 2.4 How to determine if a drug or device can be prescribed on the NHS.

Clinical Consideration

- There are also numerous prescribing and drug handbooks available, predominantly developed and produced for healthcare staff within the United States (US).
- They can be a useful resource but be aware the recommended medicines within these guides will not be based on UK NICE/SIGN guidelines and/or the medicinal products may not even have a licence to be used within the UK.

The Evidence Base to Prescribing: Prescribing Guidelines

There are many medications that can be used to treat the same condition, it is important to know which drug to use and when. To assist with choosing the most appropriate medication, in terms of efficacy, safety and cost-effectiveness, clinical guidelines (where available) must be adhered to. Clinical guidelines are systematically developed statements to assist practitioners and patients make decisions about the most appropriate healthcare for specific clinical circumstances. Guidelines provide recommendations for effective practice in the management of clinical conditions where variations in practice are known to occur and where effective care may not be delivered in uniform way. There are many guidelines available, but most are based on a consensus of 'expert opinion' or a non-systematic review of the scientific literature. Prescribing clinical guidelines can be local or national (Table 2.3 provides some examples).

Table 2.3 Examples of local and national prescribing guidelines.

LOCAL GUIDANCE	NATIONAL GUIDANCE
• The team, service or condition you are working within • NHS organisation/employer • Geographical region	• NICE or SIGN guidance • National networks • Clinical groups or • Charities

NICE Prescribing Guidance

The National Institute for Health and Care Excellence (NICE) is a non-departmental public body that provides national guidance and advice to improve health and social care in England.

NICE guidelines make evidence-based recommendations on a wide range of topics including:

- Preventing and managing specific conditions
- Improving health
- Managing medicines in different settings
- Providing social care and support to adults and children
- Planning broader services and interventions to improve the health of communities

Within each NICE guideline there are recommendations regarding the care (including medications) and services that are suitable for most people with a specific condition or need. NICE guidelines are used by NHS England and NHS clinical commissioners to develop services and are a reference guide for healthcare professionals, with recommendations about medications that should and should not be prescribed. The guidelines also cover areas that patients should be able to manage themselves and obtain, if necessary, appropriate over the counter medications.

Clinical Consideration

- In your area of practice chose a medical condition that you are familiar with.
- Check to see if there is a local (to your trust/employer) and/or national guideline for this condition
- Is the guidance the same as within the BNFc?
- Are there are any differences in recommendations? If so, think why this may be

Scottish Intercollegiate Guidelines Network (SIGN)

The Scottish Intercollegiate Guidelines Network (SIGN) was formed to improve the quality of healthcare for patients in Scotland by reducing variation in practice and outcome. SIGN collaborate with a network of clinicians, other health and social care professionals, patient organisations and individuals to develop evidence-based guidelines. SIGN guidelines are based on a systematic review of the scientific literature and are aimed at aiding the translation of new knowledge into action. The guidelines are intended to:

- Help health and social care professionals and patients understand medical evidence and use it to make decisions about healthcare
- Reduce unwarranted variations in practice and make sure patients get the best care available, no matter where they live
- Improve healthcare across Scotland by focusing on patient-important outcomes (SIGN Guidelines/Scottish Intercollegiate Guidelines Network)

NICE and SIGN both produce patient booklets that are a lay translation of the clinical guidelines. These booklets explain the recommendations in the clinical guideline and help to make patients aware of the treatment they should expect to receive. They are intended to:

- Help patients and carers understand the latest evidence about diagnosis, treatment and self-care
- Empower patients to participate fully in decisions about the management of their condition in discussion with healthcare professionals
- Highlight where there are areas of uncertainty in the management of their condition. (SIGN Guidelines/ Scottish Intercollegiate Guidelines Network)

Conclusion

This chapter has provided an overview of the main pharmaceutical and prescribing reference guides used within clinical practice. Guidance has been given to encourage you to start to navigate the BNFc in particular, to ensure you know where to find all the information needed about any medicinal product or device to ensure safe and effective practice. The differences between paper-based and online versions have been highlighted to ensure you are aware where to access the most up-to-date and accurate drug information.

References

Pryor, C. and Hand, A. (2021) How to use pharmaceutical and prescribing reference guides. In: *Fundamentals of Pharmacology: For Nursing and Healthcare Students* (ed. Peate, I. and Hill, B.), 15–32. Oxford: Wiley.

Joint Formulary Committee (2019a). *How BNF Publications are Constructed: Assessing the Evidence*. Joint Formulary Committee. https://bnf.nice.org.uk/about/how-bnf-publications-are-constructed.html (accessed 17 September 2019).

Joint Formulary Committee (2019b). *British National Formulary: How to Use BNF Publications Online*. London: Joint Formulary Committee. https://bnf.nice.org.uk/about/how-to-use-bnf-publications-online.html (accessed 17 September 2019).

Medications and Healthcare products Regulatory Agency (2009). *Paracetamol 500mg tablets (paracetamol) PL31308/0007-9 UK Public Assessment Report*. Medications and Healthcare products Regulatory Agency. Available: www.mhra.gov.uk/home/groups/par/documents/websiteresources/con071056.pdf (accessed 17 September 2019).

Nursing and Midwifery Council (2018a). *The Code: Professional Standards of Practice and Behaviour for Nurses, Midwives and Nursing Associates*. The Nursing and Midwifery Council. www.nmc.org.uk/standards/code/ (accessed 20 September 2019).

Nursing and Midwifery Council (2018b). *Standards of Proficiency for Nursing Associates*. Nursing and Midwifery Council. www.nmc.org.uk/standards/code/ (accessed 20 September 2019).

Further Resources

Electronic Medicines Compendium: www.medicines.org.uk/emc

National Institute for Health and Care Excellence (NICE) Information on medicines and Prescribing: www.nice.org.uk/about/nice-communities/medicines-and-prescribing

Joint Royal Colleges of Ambulance and Liaison Committee (JRCALC): www.jrcalc.org.uk/

Scottish Intercollegiate Guidelines Network (SIGN): www.sign.ac.uk

UK Drug Tariff: www.nhsbsa.nhs.uk/pharmacies-gp-practices-and-appliance-contractors/drug-tariff

Multiple Choice Questions

1. Which of the following are all pharmaceutical reference guides?
   (a) MIMS, NICE and emc
   (b) SIGN, BNFc and MIMS
   (c) BNFc, MIMS and emc
2. What does the BNF stand for?
   (a) British National Formulary
   (b) British National Formulations
   (c) Branded National Formulary
3. How many times a year is the BNFc published?
   (a) Once

(b) Twice

(c) Three times

4. Does the BNF/BNFc detail all the information necessary for prescribing and dispensing?

   (a) Yes always

   (b) Not always

   (c) No

5. What does PoM stand for?

   (a) Pharmacy-only medicine

   (b) Prescribed oral medicine

   (c) Prescription-only medicine

6. MIMS is primarily intended for use in which healthcare setting?

   (a) All healthcare settings

   (b) Primary care

   (c) Secondary care

7. Within MIMS how are you able to search for a drug?

   (a) By drug name

   (b) By condition

   (c) By manufacturer

   (d) All of the above

8. What does the abbreviation p.c. mean?

   (a) Before food

   (b) With food

   (c) After food

9. Where will you find the 'blacklist'?

   (a) Within the BNF

   (b) Within the Drug Tariff

   (c) Within NICE

10. On a device what does the CE mark signify?

    (a) That the device has been tried and tested and is safe to use

    (b) That the device can be prescribed

    (c) That the device has a copyright protection

11. How often is the Drug Tariff updated?

    (a) Continually

    (b) Weekly

    (c) Monthly

12. Which document informs healthcare professionals on how to prescribe and use a medicine correctly?

    (a) A clinical trial paper

    (b) Product Information

    (c) Summaries of Product Characteristics

13. A PIL is a medicine leaflet written for whom?

    (a) Healthcare Professionals

    (b) Pharmacy staff

    (c) Patients and their carers

14. Where will you find the most up-to-date information about the use of medicines?

    (a) BNFc/MIMS paper copy

    (b) BNFc/MIMS online

    (c) NICE guidance

15. You find an outdated BNFc being used within a clinical area, what should you do?

    (a) Nothing, it is still safe to use an outdated BNFc

    (b) Nothing, as it is not your place to say anything

    (c) Speak to a senior member of staff to get it replaced with an up-to-date version

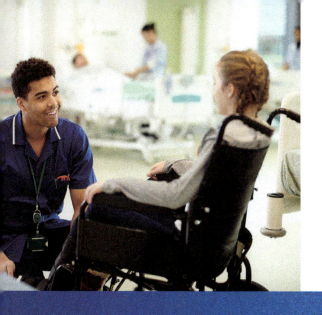

3

Legal and Ethical Issues

Sasha Ban and Peter Dryden

Aim
The aim of this chapter is to examine the legal and ethical considerations that are related to pharmacology and medicines management in contemporary healthcare settings in association with children and young people (CYP).

Learning Outcomes
By the end of this chapter the reader will be able to:

- Define commonly used legal and ethical concepts
- Identify situations where legal and ethical considerations are required to make decisions
- Explain how legal and ethical considerations influence the decision-making process
- Apply legal and ethical considerations to a variety of scenarios likely to be encountered in modern healthcare settings

Test Your Knowledge
1. According to UK law, what must be established in order to prove a case of negligence?
2. Can a grandparent consent to treatment for their grandchild?
3. What is the meaning of beneficence in relation to the child health immunisation programme?
4. At what age can a young person give consent for their own treatment?
5. What is a professional body's primary function?

Fundamentals of Pharmacology for Children's Nurses, First Edition. Edited by Ian Peate and Peter Dryden.
© 2022 John Wiley & Sons Ltd. Published 2022 by John Wiley & Sons Ltd.
Companion website: www.wiley.com/go/pharmacologyforCN

Introduction

The health and welfare of children and young people is a primary concern in paediatrics and especially in paediatric pharmacology decision making. Healthcare professionals can be faced with complex situations with regard to CYP, for example the right to refuse vaccinations, access to sexual health services and the understanding of these decisions by the CYP and/or their carers. Healthcare providers need to know when or if the CYP is competent to make their own decisions, what this means in terms of consent to treatment, refusal of healthcare including medications and how these decisions may be affected by parental responsibility. This section will introduce readers to fundamental ethical principles relating to CYP nursing and healthcare and discuss some of the key legal concepts with which healthcare professionals should become familiar in order to ensure that decisions around pharmacology have a legal and ethical basis. When caring for CYP, independent prescribers have a number of ethical and legal obligations with which they should be familiar and are outlined in best practice guidance, statute and case law.

Any pharmacology decisions made about the CYP requires careful consideration of:

- What is in the best interests of the CYP within the situation
- What you are legally obliged to do
- What you are professionally guided to do

In practice, the three usually exist together, but this chapter will consider the three components separately that underpin high-quality decision making in pharmacology:

- The law
- Ethical principles and theories
- Regulatory bodies

The Law

Laws in the UK and around the world exist to protect the public and in clinical situations, patients and their families. Clinical negligence claims in the UK quadrupled between 2007 and 2017 (National Health Service Improvement (NHSI), 2019). In general, laws can be applied in two ways.

Statute Law

Also known as an Act of Parliament or primary legislation, this is the way in which the main laws are passed in the United Kingdom Parliament, Scottish Parliament, Welsh Parliament and the Northern Ireland Assembly. In the UK, usually these acts begin as bills in the House of Commons and then pass to the House of Lords before receiving Royal Assent by the reigning monarch before becoming Law. The bills and Acts can be either public or private. Public Acts affect the whole of the UK usually and private acts are there to grant powers to public bodies such as local authorities.

Common Law

Also known as Case Law, this is the way in which judges sitting in a Court of Law make legal precedents based on the outcome of court cases, similar in nature and delivering judgements about the cases they preside over. This Common Law ensures that the law remains 'common' throughout the country of origin. Common Law can change over time since some judges interpret the law differently. Common Law can be divided into criminal and civil law.

Criminal Law

This aims to protect the public from behaviour that is deemed unacceptable and which can affect society. It may come in the form of an offence or breach of a law. If a criminal act occurs, then the person is subject to criminal prosecution by the state. In the UK, criminal proceedings are usually brought by the Crown Prosecution Service (CPS) for England and Wales, the Crown Office and Procurator Fiscal Service in Scotland and the Public Prosecution Service (PPS) in Northern Ireland. The trial will take place in a courtroom deemed appropriate to the severity of the alleged misdemeanour.

Civil Law

This is different from criminal law, it is usually concerned with the property and rights of individuals or, indeed, organisations which may not always be protected by Criminal Law. Civil Law usually involves the awarding of compensation between individuals and organisations. Examples of civil cases may include:

- Family disagreements – divorce, parental responsibility, child and safeguarding issues
- Employment law – discrimination in the workplace, unfair dismissal
- Breach of contract – whereby the contract is not honoured, or monies are unpaid
- Personal injury – medical and clinical negligence, trips and falls

Whether Civil Law cases are successful or not, often depends on whether the accused person or organisation, legally known as the defendant, had a duty of care towards the claimant and did not fulfil that duty.

Tort Law

In healthcare, Torts are Civil Laws that address the legal rights of patients and the responsibilities of the nurse in the nurse–patient relationship. Some torts specific to nursing and healthcare practice may include things like malpractice and negligence, which may be classed as unintentional torts and can occur when the wrongdoer does not intend to cause harm, but rather harm is caused by negligence or failure to act as a reasonable person or professional would normally act in the same circumstances. Intentional torts are acts done deliberately and could include assault, false imprisonment or intended emotional distress. The perpetrator in this sense acts with a purpose to intentionally cause wrongdoing.

The Medical Protection Society (MPS) produced a report in 2017 that quotes figures from NHS Resolution, formally known as the NHS Litigation Authority (NHS LA), which estimates that the provision for future clinical negligence costs, relating to claims arising from incidents that have already occurred, stands at £56.1 billion (MPS, 2017).

The Bolam Test

When considering cases of clinical negligence, courts will assess whether the health professional or organisation in question acted in line with the practice accepted as proper by a body of health professionals specialising in the specific field under scrutiny. This is known as the 'Bolam' test. The case (Bolam vs Friern Hospital Management Committee 1957), involved a patient who had suffered a fractured hip during electroconvulsive therapy (ECT). No relaxant or other restraint had been given to the patient in preparation for the treatment. The case explored this, along with the information the patient had been offered. The question was asked of a group of similar professionals and it was assessed that the practitioner had not been negligent as he had acted in accordance with accepted practice at that time. This set the standard and the Bolam test is now utilised in cases of negligence as a benchmark for whether the professional concerned, acted in a reasonable manner. However, a judge can still make the assessment that the body of opinion is not reasonable. Such was the case in Montgomery v Lanarkshire (Box 3.1), which has since impacted on the content of information when obtaining informed consent from a patient regarding the inclusion of material risk.

After the Montgomery case, the so-called Bolam test, which asks whether a doctor's conduct would be supported by a responsible body of medical opinion, no longer applies to the issue of consent. The law now requires a clinician to take 'reasonable care to ensure that the patient is aware of any material risks involved in any recommended treatment, and of any reasonable alternative or variant treatments.'

Box 3.1 The Bolam Test Tested

Case Law: Montgomery v Lanarkshire Health Board [2015]
Nadine Montgomery was a woman with Type 1 diabetes who gave birth by vaginal delivery. Her baby, Sam, was born with cerebral palsy after shoulder dystocia during delivery. The doctor, Dina McLellan, did not tell Montgomery of the 9–10% risk of shoulder dystocia. McLellan said that she did not routinely discuss the risk of shoulder dystocia with women with diabetes for fear that, if told, such women would opt for a Caesarean section. The court held that McLellan should have informed Montgomery of the risk and discussed with her the option of a Caesarean section.

Source: Modified from Medical Defence Union, 2018.

Clinicians must now ask themselves: does the patient know about the material risks? The Montgomery family were awarded over £5 million in damages, after an appeal went to the Supreme Court.

The Children Act 2004

The Children Act 2004 is a development from the 1989 Act which brought together private and public law in one framework. The Act dictates what local authorities, courts, parents and other agencies in the UK do to ensure that children are safeguarded. The guidelines set out in this Act allow for anyone working in an educational or non-educational setting and working with children to know how a child must be looked after in the eyes of the law in addition to promoting their well-being. The Act focuses on the idea that children are best cared for within their own families; however, importantly, it also deals with cases when parents and families are not the best option too.

This Act's ultimate purpose is to make the UK a safer place for children and charges each local authority to appoint a director of children's services.

Principles of the Children Act 2004

- To allow children to be healthy
- Allowing children to remain safe in their environments
- Helping children to enjoy life
- Assisting children in their quest to succeed
- Helping make a positive contribution to the lives of children
- Helping achieve economic stability for our children's futures

The main part of the Act is concerned with the maltreatment of a child. This particular element of the Act ensures that any agency that is aware of the maltreatment of a child – or the misconduct of a child's legal guardian – should make their findings known to other agencies that might have a hand in the protection of a child who would normally go unmonitored. This can include schools, nurseries, youth groups and other places and organisations that care for children or run children's events. The aim is to have a coordinated, joined up approach to child protection and the sharing of vital information which could help prevent child deaths such as Daniel Pelka (Box 3.2).

Box 3.2 Daniel Pelka

Just after 0300h on Saturday 3 March 2013 a telephone call was made by Daniel Pelka's mother to the ambulance service in respect of Daniel, who was then aged 4 years and 8 months old. The ambulance service attended the home and Daniel was subsequently admitted to hospital after having suffered a cardiac arrest. He was pronounced dead at 0350h. At the time of his death Daniel weighed just 10.7kg. He was found to be malnourished and had an acute subdural haematoma to the right side of his head, as well as other bruises on his body. Subsequent pathological examination also identified an older mild subdural haematoma of several months' or years' duration. Daniel was the middle child of a family who had migrated to this country in 2005 from Poland and who lived in Coventry for most of the time that they resided in the UK. Daniel lived with his mother and her fourth partner along with his older sibling, known as Anna, aged 7 years, and a younger sibling known as Adam, aged 1 year. On 31 July 2013, his mother and her partner were found guilty of the murder of Daniel and sentenced to a minimum of 30 years each.

Throughout Daniel's short life, several appointments were made with health visitors, GPs, community paediatricians and the school nurse. Most of these resulted in non-attendance, with some cancelled then rearranged. Concerns within the serious case review were raised around the way in which agencies lacked the ability to share information, either through lack of communication, inadequate IT systems, poor record-keeping or through assumptions around culture and language. A number of missed opportunities by professionals and agencies enabled the abuse to continue and were contributing factors identified as lessons that needed to be learned from the review into Daniel's death.

Source: Lessons To Be Learned Briefing No. 16: In Respect Of The Death Of Daniel Pelka- Coventry, 2013 / Stafford Borough Council.

Duty of Care and Healthcare

Healthcare and the law in the UK are strongly linked. The laws that are created to protect the health of an individual can be seen in the healthcare setting in the form of public health and the legal requirements of health and safety. Across the UK, the laws that exist have been created to ensure that the rights and health interests of the service user are protected throughout the duration of their care. Healthcare professionals have a legal duty to act with reasonable care when providing services. The duty of care refers to the obligations placed on people to act towards others in a certain way, in accordance with certain standards (Royal College of Nursing (RCN), 2020). This can include prescribing drug therapy and drug administration as well as consent, negligence and confidentiality and data protection. Failure to act with reasonable care could result in healthcare staff being held responsible in both criminal and civil courts.

Regulation of Healthcare

The Health and Safety Executive (HSE) is the national independent regulator for health and safety in the workplace. This includes both private or publicly owned health and social care settings in Great Britain. This regulatory body, works in partnership with co-regulators in local authorities to inspect, investigate and where necessary take enforcement action (HSE, 2020). The various regulators across the UK have a range of powers to secure improvement and/or justice. As mentioned earlier, private acts are there to grant powers to public bodies such as local authorities and other regulatory bodies who have patient/service user safety within their remit and have powers to secure justice. The HSE will not in general investigate or take action on issues that come under the jurisdiction of these bodies.

To mitigate against breaches of reasonable care, civil or even criminal law and to ensure that the public are protected, organisations such as the Nursing and Midwifery Council (NMC), General Medical Council (GMC) and the Health and Care Professions Council (HCPC) have important roles to play in ensuring that professional standards are maintained and may be better placed than HSE to improve standards or prevent a recurrence and to produce expected standards to achieve registration.

Within healthcare, regulatory bodies have a duty to protect, promote and maintain the health and safety of the public. They do this by ensuring that proper standards are in place in order to practise. The professional standards of practice and behaviour for nurses, midwives and nursing associates, 'The Code', (NMC, 2018) is structured around four themes – prioritise people, practise effectively, preserve safety and promote professionalism and trust. Such standards define the overarching goals and the expected role and duties of their practitioners through listing the obligations associated with their individual responsibilities and skill set. The overarching goals are aspirational and represent an optimal position ethically, thus encouraging the individual to strive towards the optimal position. Healthcare professionals, like the general public, possess their own values, ethical codes and beliefs which in turn influence their practice, but this should not have a detrimental effect on patient care.

There are a number of guidelines set out by various professional bodies in relation to pharmacology. The General Medical Council (GMC) have outlined expectations of doctors' ethical prescribing practices which aim to provide more detailed advice on how to apply ethical principles when prescribing and managing medicines (2020). Additionally, largely in response to the withdrawal of the Medicines Management Standards by the Nursing Midwifery Council, the Royal Pharmaceutical Society and the Royal College of Nursing collaborated in developing the 'Professional Guidance on the Administration of Medicines in Healthcare Settings' (2019). These standards seek to promote patient safety in relation to the administration of medicines by acknowledging the importance of guidance for health professionals that is enabling and supportive while being clear and concise. The document recognises the importance of a commitment to ethics, values and principles which put patients first. It is incumbent upon the individual healthcare professional to ensure that they are familiar with the most current guidance related to their own sphere of practice to ensure that ethical and legal considerations are applied.

Chapter 3 Legal and Ethical Issues

Ethical Principles and Theories

Making ethical decisions is about deciding on the right way to act in a given situation, and this is under-pinned by the moral values held by an individual or group. In 1979 Beauchamp and Childress (2009) developed a four-point theoretical framework to be used as a method of analysing ethical dilemmas in clinical medicine. The framework included beneficence, non-maleficence, autonomy and justice. These principles remain in healthcare, along with the addition of a further two principles. Today the following ethical principles apply:

- Beneficence
- Non-maleficence
- Autonomy
- Justice
- Veracity
- Fidelity

The principles outlined here are commonly felt to underpin judgements health professionals believe to be right. Firstly, *beneficence* whereby we should endeavour to do good. This extends to protecting others and defending their rights, preventing harm and helping others. It is argued by some such as Pellegrino (1988) that beneficence is the only fundamental principle within healthcare ethics and that the sole purpose of medicine should be to heal. Contraception, fertility treatment and plastic surgery support health and well-being in a myriad of direct and indirect ways, physically as well as psychologically, which is why the endeavour of beneficence is not as straightforward as it would first appear.

Utilitarian or consequentialism theory considers the rightness of an act as that which, when considering the costs and benefits, creates the greatest good for the greatest number. For example, the issue of immunisation is a controversial one, with a minority of parents deciding to opt out of immunisation programmes for their children (Box 3.3). This puts children and other vulnerable members of society at risk of developing some diseases that were previously eradicated in the UK, e.g. measles (Public Health England, 2019), with the associated implications to the individuals, wider society and to the health service. The utilitarian perspective would be that all eligible children should be immunised irrespective of the views/wishes of their parents.

Box 3.3 Immunisations and the Law

The case concerned a 5-year-old girl, B, whose parents were separated and unable to agree as to her immunisation. Before the parents separated, B had received all the recommended vaccinations. Under the recommendations of Public Health England, she was now due (or overdue) three further vaccinations.

The case was determined by His Honour Judge Clifford Bellamy, sitting as a Deputy Judge of the High Court.

The court heard evidence from Dr Elliman, a jointly instructed medical expert witness. B's guardian supported the mother's position. The parents filed written statements but did not give oral evidence. The father, though lacking relevant medical expertise, had carried out extensive research and exhibited over 300 pages of material in support of his position. The judge extrapolated the father's seven key points and Dr Elliman addressed the medical issues. The court dismissed the father's proposition that where parents disagree on a child being vaccinated, then the status quo should be preserved as wrong in law (*Re Z* [1996] 1 FLR 191; *Re B (A Child)* [2003] EWCA Civ 1148).

Dr Elliman acknowledged that no vaccination is 100% risk-free, but that vaccination has greatly reduced the burden of infectious disease. The judge noted the paramountcy principle and the principle that delay in determining the matter may be prejudicial to B's welfare. In respect to the no order principle, the judge recorded that the court should decide the matter as the parents' views were polarised. With regard to Article 8 of the European Convention, His Honour Judge Bellamy stated that any order made by the court must be proportionate and in B's best welfare interests.

Having considered the case law, the judge then determined that Dr Elliman's opinions were 'mainstream' whilst the father's views were biased and unreliable. In conclusion, the judge granted the specific issue order and made a declaration that it was in B's best welfare interests to receive the vaccinations.

Source: Judge Bellamy (2018) *'B' A Child; immunisations,* www.familylawweek.co.uk/site.aspx?i=ed191684 Judge Bellamy 2018/Law Week Limited.

Utilitarianism would not be concerned with the autonomy of the individual (the right to not give consent to the vaccine) as this is arguably in conflict with the greater good.

Deontological ethics or deontology is an approach to ethics that determines goodness or rightness from examining acts rather than consequences of the act as in utilitarianism. Deontologists look at rules and duties. For example, the act may be considered the right thing to do even if it produces a bad consequence, if it follows the *rule* that 'one should do unto others as they would have done unto them'. According to deontology, we have a *duty* to act in a way that does those things that are inherently good as acts. In this approach, the duty of care to the individual takes priority over any other considerations. Going back to the example of immunisations, children are, in reality, not forced to have immunisations where parents have opted out. Health professionals have a duty to ensure that any care given is consented to (within the parameters of the MCA 2005 as outlined earlier). Without this consent the healthcare provider cannot inject a live vaccine into a child, no matter what the potential implications might be for wider society. So the act itself is good (abiding by rules of consent) but the consequence may be a negative one (the child contracting measles and passing this on to others). For deontologists, the ends or consequences of our actions are not important, nor are our intentions. Duty is the key consideration. However, it is not always clear what one's duty is. Whilst we may agree that our duty is to 'do no harm', there will be instances where health professionals will have to override this with their duty of care.

Virtue ethics focuses on how we ought to behave, and how we should think about relationships, rather than providing rules or formulas for ethical decision making. It considers the virtues a 'good' person would have: honesty, compassion, generosity and courage for example (Velasquez et al., 1988). With the common good in mind, these virtues will be applied to actions and decisions. A group of virtues can be accredited to particular roles or professions, and it could be argued that nurses are attracted to the profession because they already function according to these virtues.

The focus of nursing ethics is on developing a caring relationship and seeks a collaborative relationship with the CYP and family. Common themes of nursing ethics emphasise respect for the autonomy of the individual and maintaining the dignity of the client by promoting choice and control over their environment.

What is deemed to be right is not therefore bound by absolute rules or duty, or purely the greatest good, but also considers the virtues that individuals and society value. The ethical views held by society affect healthcare laws and how they are implemented. As society's moral values alter, legislation follows. An example of this was in 1967, when UK society's beliefs changed regarding abortions. It became largely accepted that in some cases they were necessary for saving women's lives as well as reducing the potential for suffering (psychologically as well as physically) of the woman and her pre-existing family, and so the Act was introduced (Abortion Act 1967).

In practice, in order to do good, the medical interventions and treatments can often carry a risk of harm and therefore require justification. *Non-maleficence* means that by our actions, we should do others no harm. The principle of non-maleficence therefore cannot be absolute and must be balanced against beneficence. For example, when treating patients with cytotoxic chemotherapy drugs for cancer, we balance beneficence (the potential to do good and eradicate the cancer) against non-maleficence and the risk of the chemotherapy itself to cause the patient's condition to deteriorate possibly leading to death.

Research

The legal and ethical standards which govern research into pharmacological treatments are very specific to the context of clinical drug trials. During the Second World War, prisoners in Nazi concentration camps were used as subjects in medical experiments against their will, leading to permanent disfigurement, disability, trauma and in many cases death. In response to these atrocities, the Nuremberg Code (1947) was developed as international guiding ethical principles for the conduct of research involving human participants. They include principles of informed consent, non-coercion and the right to withdraw as well as the importance of robust protocols underpinned by beneficence. These principles were later encapsulated within the Declaration of Helsinki (1964 amended in 2008) and further legislation has evolved to ensure the safety of human participants in clinical trials, including: the Data Protection Act (1998), the Human Tissue Act (2004) and the Medicines for Human Use (Clinical Trials) Regulations (2004) as well as the Human Rights Act (1998).

Research is an important mechanism for healthcare professionals to ensure that the drug treatments we offer patients are thoroughly tested for safety and efficacy. Additionally, there is strong evidence emerging that research active organisations have better patient outcomes, highlighting the importance and the responsibility healthcare providers have to offer their service users the opportunity to be involved in clinical trials (Ozdemir et al., 2015). It is essential that legislation enables clinical researchers to conduct clinical trials in the endeavour of medical advancement, while ensuring that participants are fully informed of the potential risks and benefits, are not coerced into consenting to participate and that they are aware of their right to withdraw from participating at any time. The guiding principle is that the well-being and safety of the participants is paramount and takes priority over any other consideration (Box 3.4).

Research Ethics Committees (RECs) have the remit to review any proposed research that involves human participants. Made up of a number of lay-people and professionals experienced in their own field, it is the responsibility of the REC to interrogate the research protocol and to identify any aspects of the research consent and treatment processes which may pose an unacceptable risk to participants or the public. Approval from a REC is essential before a trial can go ahead. As the trial progresses, researchers will also need to seek ethical approval to make any amendments to the protocol which may be something as minor as a change of wording within a participant information sheet, to something more substantial such as a change in the dose of medication to be administered. These changes will be implemented in line with Good Clinical Practice (GCP) principles (MHRA, 2012).

Fortunately, however, the ethical and legal frameworks which surround clinical research, limit these incidences, and provide principles and guidance for the safe conduct of research and researchers.

It is also generally believed that people should have the right to make decisions about what is right for them, provided they have sufficient capacity or understanding to do so. This principle is a respect for the *autonomy* of the individual and relates to enabling patients to make self-determined decisions regarding their care. Consent to treatment is a fundamental component of ethical patient care in addition to a legal requirement. It involves a genuine agreement (verbal or written) to receive treatment under circumstances where the patient has been assessed as competent, has been fully informed and where there is no undue pressure exerted (Herring, 2018). Beauchamp and Childress (2009) have argued that no decision can be truly autonomous, as patients rarely have the relevant knowledge to hold a full understanding of treatment options and as such are vulnerable to the coercion of health professionals who feel that they are

---

Box 3.4 Ethical Research Involving Children and Young People

Harm and Benefits
The most fundamental consideration in undertaking research involving children is deciding whether the research needs to be done, if children need to be involved in it and in what capacity. Non-maleficence is a guiding principle in all areas of child health.

Informed Consent
Obtaining informed consent from parents/carers and children is central to the research relationship and signals respect for the research participant's dignity, their capability to express their views and their right to have these heard in matters that affect them. A child's assent to research is crucial in developing trusting relationship, maintaining the child at the heart of all treatment choices. being part of the study

Privacy and Confidentiality
Respecting the privacy and confidentiality of children participating in research involves close consideration of several aspects: privacy with regard to how much information the child wants to reveal or share. Part of the process of ethical approval is to ensure that all safeguarding measures are in place to support this process.

Payment and Compensation
Fairness and justice are guiding principles, time and effort should be rewarded, whatever the age of the research participants. This may require creativity with children and young people and must be given or offered without coercion or pressure to take part in the study.

Source: ERIC, a collaborative between UNICEF's Office of Research, Innocenti and the Centre for Children and Young People at Southern Cross University, Australia.(2013)ERIC, 2013/United Nations Children's Fund

best placed to make decisions in the interests of their patients (paternalism). However, increasingly patient groups have sought to increase autonomy for patients through changes in policies and practices which decrease the potential for coercion and increase patients' freedom to act (Williamson, 2010). An example of this has been seen in recent years, as a greater emphasis has been placed on models of shared decision making between health professionals and patients. The shared decision making approach seeks a balance between paternalistic care and the informed consent approach. Paternalistic care is where decisions about care are made by health professionals and patients passively receive the care prescribed. This model does not factor in patients' own values and beliefs and can lead to patients feeling greater distress where there is a negative outcome (Stewart and Brown, 2001). The informed consent approach offers patients greater responsibility and will often involve health professionals offering patients all of the information required and then leaving them to make the decision unsupported. This can lead to patients feeling abandoned and unsure, creating anxiety and distrust (Corrigan, 2003; Deber et al., 2007). The shared decision making approach involves health professionals and patients working together to devise a plan of care that is in line with the best available evidence as well as the values and beliefs of the individual patient, aligning to the principle of true autonomy.

Health professionals also abide by the principle of *justice*, which is the belief that people should be treated fairly, equally and reasonably. At its heart, justice is about equality but how equality is determined can be ambiguous and problematic in healthcare. An example of the difficulties posed within this principle is often seen in relation to the fair and equal distribution of resources 'distributive justice'.

Health professionals should also be honest and tell the truth to enable someone to have the full information relevant to them in order to make full rational choices about their care. This is known as veracity and involves conveying accurate and objective information to the patient. Giving children and young people information regarding treatment options is the most common application of the veracity principle; the CYP's understanding needs to be assessed and it is paramount to discuss treatment with the family (Coyne et al., 2011). Disclosures of medication errors are also an obvious example of veracity and the recent introduction of the Duty of Candour guidance for health professionals (NMC, 2021) highlights the importance of the veracity principle. Informing patients when something has gone wrong, apologising and offering a remedy, were measures that were advised by Sir Robert Francis in his report on the failings of the Mid-Staffordshire Health trust (2013). Francis stated that candour and transparency were key components of a safe and effective culture for patient care.

The principle of fidelity requires the act of loyalty and trustworthiness, it involves keeping our promises, performing our duties and doing what is expected of us within our relationships with patients. The nurse may be conflicted where their loyalty or obligation may be torn between their patients, parents/carers and colleagues or the organisation for which they work.

Clinical Consideration: Consent to Treatment

Young People Who Are Over 16

The United Nations Convention on the Rights of the Child (UNICEF, 1989) advocates the right of every child to self-determination, dignity, respect, non-interference and the right to make informed decisions

When young people and adults have capacity, the authority to treat comes solely from the patient. All young people aged 16 years and over are presumed in law to be competent to give their consent to medical treatment and to the release of information in England, Scotland, Wales and Northern Ireland (British Medical Association (BMA), 2020). According to UK law, consent by proxy is not permitted for the care or treatment of adults who have the capacity to make an informed decision. When considering 16 to 17-year-olds with capacity, according to section 8(1) of the Family Law Reform Act (1969) consent can be sought from the young person for medical and dental treatment. However, those with parental responsibility may still consent on the young person's behalf.

When young people and adults lack capacity to make an informed decision regarding their care due to an impairment or disturbance to the functioning of the mind, for example, an acute confused state, brain injury, being unconscious, then under the Mental Capacity Act (MCA) 2005 the health professional can decide upon the treatment that is deemed in the best interests of the patient without the consent of the next of kin. Where treatment is felt to be in the best interests of the child, a court order may be obtained.

Section 3(1) of the MCA 2005 sets out the following benchmarks by which are seen as fundamental to assess a person's capacity to make an informed decision:

- If they are unable to understand the information given to them relating to the decision
- They are unable to retain the information
- They are unable to weigh the information as part of the decision-making process
- They are unable to communicate their decision.

Children and Young People who are under 16 years – Gillick and Fraser Guidance

In healthcare, when decisions are being formulated for YP under 16 years of age, it is common to hear the term 'Gillick-competent' or to talk about whether they meet the 'Fraser guidelines' (NSPCC, 2021). An assessment of the child relating to 'Gillick' competence (Gillick v West Norfolk and Wisbech Area Health Authority 1986) would determine whether the child has sufficient maturity and understanding of what is involved to enable them to decide to consent to treatment or not. Each young person should be assessed on a case-by-case basis and this should be reviewed throughout the treatment or medication regime. Gillick usually refers to any form of healthcare that may affect the CYP and the Fraser guidelines apply specifically to advice and treatment about contraception and sexual health. Nurses and other allied health-care professionals (AHP) should involve the CYP in the decision-making process around their treatment (see Box 3.5). Effective communication is the key to recognising if a young person can make a valid choice about their care. The multidisciplinary team should not just assume the ability to make decisions based on the age of the CYP.

Assessing and Promoting Competence

The relationship and communication skills required by the nurse or other Allied Health Professional (AHP) must address the needs of the CYP by developing good communication skills necessary to inspire trust and maintain a professional relationship (Dryden and Greenshields, 2020). The skill in paediatrics is being able to do this with CYP of all ages and levels of emotional and psychological development, in addition to recognising any learning disabilities or difficulties the CYP may have. The family/carers must also be able to understand the information around the proposed medical care including removal of treatment or medication which may affect end of life care for example. The importance of providing understandable, unbiased and timely information in a supportive way is identified as essential in enhancing Family-Centred Care (FCC) (Coyne et al., 2011). Effective communication supports and encourages positive relationships between the family and the multidisciplinary team, while poor communication can do the opposite and undo this relationship.

Box 3.5 Competence in Children and Young People

For a young person under the age of 16 years to be competent, they should have:

- The ability to understand that there is a choice and that choices have consequences
- The ability to weigh the information and arrive at a decision
- A willingness to make a choice (including the choice that someone else should make the decision)
- An understanding of the nature and purpose of the proposed intervention
- An understanding of the proposed intervention's risks and side effects
- An understanding of the alternatives to the proposed intervention, and the risks attached to this

Source: Children and young people ethics toolkit/British Medical Association.

Parental Responsibility

43

Parental responsibility is given to those who make decisions on behalf of the CYP if they lack capacity or are unable to consent due to age, provided the decisions of the best interests of the CYP. The Children Act 2004 defines parental responsibility as 'all the rights, duties, powers, responsibilities and authority which by law a parent of a child has in relation to the child and his property'. Throughout the UK, the mother of the CYP automatically acquires parental responsibility at birth. A father's acquisition of parental responsibility can vary throughout the UK depending on where the child was registered at birth.

- If the CYP was registered in Scotland, a father acquires parental responsibility if he is married to the mother at the time of the child's conception or subsequently. If the couple are unmarried, the father will acquire parental responsibility if this is recorded on the child's birth certificate (at registration or upon reregistration) from 4 May 2006.
- If the CYP was registered in England, Wales or Northern Ireland, the father acquires parental responsibility if he is married to the mother at the time of the child's birth or subsequently. If the couple are unmarried, the father will acquire parental responsibility if he is recorded on the child's birth certificate (at registration or upon reregistration) from 1 December 2003 in England and Wales and from 15 April 2002 in Northern Ireland
- If the CYP was born outside of the United Kingdom, the rules will apply in the UK country where the child resides.

Episode of Care

Kahlil is a 16-year-old who has attended the inflammatory bowel disease (IBD) clinic to receive his first dose of methotrexate to help treat his Crohn's disease. He attends with both parents. Methotrexate belongs to a group of medicines called immunosuppressants which 'dampens down' overactivity of the immune system, reducing inflammation, and can be dangerous if not monitored properly. Kahlil has been prescribed 15 mg of methotrexate to be given orally as he prefers this route of administration to the subcutaneous route via a prefilled syringe and needle.

An Information sheet had already been given to Kahlil and his parents to read prior to attending the clinic. This information identified side effects and drug interactions including nausea and vomiting and the potential to make Kahlil more prone to opportunistic infections. There is also evidence that immunosuppressants such as methotrexate may also slightly increase the risk of other blood disorders, such as lymphoma (cancer of the lymph glands). As Kahlil has been so unwell recently, he agrees to start the treatment and have bloods taken to monitor efficacy and potential problems on a weekly basis. However, his parents state that they refuse to agree to the treatment due to the increased risk of cancer. An argument starts between Kahlil and his parents. You have cared for Kahlil since he was 10 years old and deem him competent to make an informed decision, with or without his parents' consent.

While the methotrexate may be doing 'good' (beneficence), it has the potential to do harm (maleficence). It is imperative that health professionals discuss medication plans prior to treatment to ensure that patients are aware of the impact this will have on their life and the potential limitations. In Kahlil's case, he can make autonomous decisions and although his parents may be disagree, healthcare professionals, must ensure that every decision made fully involves the patient and in Kahlil's case his parents, even though the outcome may not be a satisfactory one for both parties.

Medication Adherence and Administration

Medication comes in lots of different formulations and the age and development of the CYP must be taken into consideration (see Chapter 6). Medication given in hospital may be refused when the child returns home or tablets may be refused and require liquid medicines to be prescribed.

Liquid medicines often have a short shelf-life once reconstituted, they often need refrigeration, they are sometimes difficult to obtain from local pharmacies, can cause dental decay, and many are unpalatable

Chapter 3 Legal and Ethical Issues

(Baguley et al., 2012). Many medicines used in paediatrics are either unlicensed or used off-label, which can present problems and dilemmas for the prescriber and whoever administers the medication. The cost of the medication must also be taken into account as liquid medicines usually come at an extra cost. Children and young people often remain on liquid medications due to habit, reluctance to change or lack of knowledge on the part of staff and parents/carers about switching to tablets (Tse et al., 2019).

Conclusion

Children and young people are at the centre of paediatric care, their needs, wishes and developing autonomy should always be respected. Their families are integral to their care and should therefore be part of all decision making. Where the family involvement is contraindicated either because of safeguarding concerns or contesting beliefs, ethical and legal frameworks are available for health professionals to utilise to ensure the best outcome.

Skills in Practice: KidzMed Project

The KidzMed project is example of a quality improvement project to train staff and embed a system of converting eligible CYP attending complex renal clinics to tablet medication (where there are no contraindications, i.e. swallowing or cognitive impairment).

Working with families and the clinical teams, the project team organised an interactive hour-long training session for staff. Using positive reinforcement and play the designated trainers and demonstrated pill swallowing with the child, the pills are dummy capsules filled with sweets of increasing sizes.

The capsules were then placed in the centre of the tongue, with the head in a neutral position, the CYP swallowed by drinking or sucking from a sports bottle or a straw (Figure 3.1)

Over 3 months, 90 CYP were seen in 13 multidisciplinary renal clinics and 25 CYP on liquid medication without contraindications were suitable for conversion to tablet medication. Twenty-one CYP (median age 8.4 years, range 5.1 to 15.5) were successfully converted (only one patient required two sessions). Thirty-six medicines were switched, generating £46,588 annual savings. The project has now been expanded to other clinical teams in hospitals throughout the North-East of England and beyond. It is possible to embed the system to convert CYP to tablet medication, improve families' experience of obtaining medication and realise considerable cost savings. The project has found that pill swallowing is an easy skill to learn; children as young as five can successfully swallow pills (see Figure 3.2) (Tse et al., 2019).

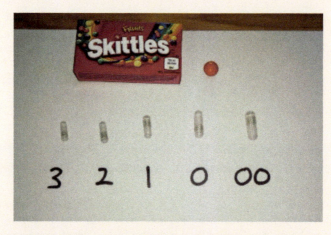

Figure 3.1 Dummy gelatine capsules in order of size compared with typical sweets.

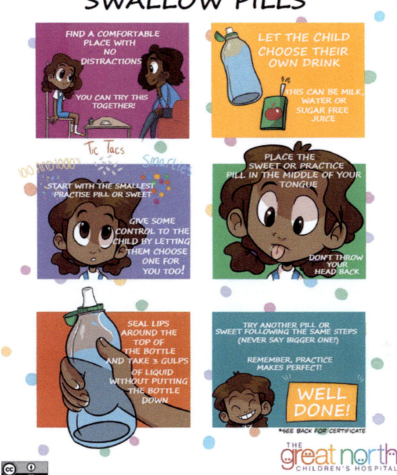

Figure 3.2 Comic poster teaching children to swallow tablets. *Source:* NHS Foundation Trust.

References

Abortion Act (1967). www.legislation.gov.uk/ukpga/1967/87/contents (accessed 26 July 2020).
Baguley, D., Lim, E., Bevan, A. et al. (2012). Prescribing for children – taste and palatability affect adherence to antibiotics: A review. *Archives of Disease in Childhood* 97(3): 293–297.
Beauchamp, T. and Childress, J. (2009). *Principles of Biomedical Ethics*, 6e. Oxford: Oxford University Press.
British Medical Association (2020). *Children and Young People Ethics Toolkit*. www.bma.org.uk/advice-and-support/ethics/children-and-young-people/children-and-young-people-ethics-toolkit (accessed 24 July 2020).
Children Act (2004). www.legislation.gov.uk/ukpga/2004/31/contents (accessed 24 July 2020).

Corrigan, O. (2003). Empty Ethics: the problem with informed consent. *Sociology of Health and Illness* 25 No.3.

Coyne, I., O'Neill, C., Murphy, M. et al. (2011). What does family-centred care mean to nurses and how do they think it could be enhanced in practice. *Journal of Advanced Nursing* 67(12), 2561–2573.

Data Protection Act (2018). www.legislation.gov.uk/ukpga/2018/12/contents/enacted (accessed 26 July 2020).

Deber, R. et al. (2007). Do people want to be autonomous patients? Preferred roles in treatment decision-making in several patient populations. *Health Expectations* 10, 248–258.

Declaration of Helsinki (2008). Ethical principles for medical research involving human subjects. www.who.int/bulletin/archives/79%284%29373.pdf (accessed 26 July 2020).

Dryden, P. and Greenshields, S. (2020). Communicating with Children and Young People. British Journal of Nursing 29(20): 1164–1166.

Family Law Reform Act (1969). www.legislation.gov.uk/ukpga/1969/46 (accessed 24 July 2020).

Francis, R. (2013). *Report of the Mid Staffordshire NHS Foundation Trust Public Enquiry*. London: Stationary Office.

Gillick v West Norfolk and Wisbech AHA (1986). A.C. 112 at 189 *per* Lord Scarman.

General Medical Council (2020). *Good Practice in Prescribing and Managing Medicines and Devices*. www.gmc-uk.org/ethical-guidance/ethical-guidance-for-doctors/prescribing-and-managing-medicines-and-devices (accessed 25 July 2020).

Health and Safety Executive (2020). Health and Safety at Work etc Act 1974. www.hse.gov.uk/legislation/hswa.htm (accessed 24 July 2020).

Herring, J. (2018). *Medical Law and Ethics*. Oxford: Oxford University Press.

Human Rights Act (1988). www.legislation.gov.uk/ukpga/1998/42/contents (accessed 24 July 2020).

Human Tissue Act (2004). www.legislation.gov.uk/ukpga/2004/30/contents (accessed 24 July 2020).

Medical Defence Union (2018). Montgomery and informed consent. www.themdu.com/guidance-and-advice/guides/montgomery-and-informed-consent (accessed 26 July 2020).

Medicines and Healthcare products Regulatory Agency (MHRA) (2012). *Good Clinical Practice Guide*. London: The Stationery Office.

Medicines for Human Use (Clinical Trials) Regulations (2004). www.legislation.gov.uk/uksi/2004/1031/contents/made (accessed 24 July 2020).

Medical Protection Society (2017). The rising cost of clinical negligence: Who pays the price? www.medicalprotection.org/docs/default-source/pdfs/policy-papers/striking-a-balance-policy-paper-65gs4rc7.pdf (accessed 24 July 2020).

Mental Capacity Act (2005). www.legislation.gov.uk/ukpga/2005/9/contents (accessed 25 July 2020).

NHS Improvement (2019). *The NHS Patient Safety Strategy*. https://improvement.nhs.uk/resources/patient-safety-strategy/ (accessed 25 July 2020).

NSPCC (2021). Gillick competence and Fraser guidelines. https://learning.nspcc.org.uk/child-protection-system/gillick-competence-fraser-guidelines (accessed 14 April 2021).

Nursing and Midwifery Council (NMC) (2021). *Guidance on the Professional Duty of Candour*. www.nmc.org.uk/standards/guidance/the-professional-duty-of-candour/ (accessed 14 April 2021).

Nuremberg Code (1947). Trials of war criminals before the Nuernberg [sic] military tribunals volume 2 'The medical case'. www.loc.gov/rr/frd/Military_Law/pdf/NT_war-criminals_Vol-II.pdf (accessed 24 July 2020).

Nursing Midwifery Council (2018). *The Code: Professional Standards Of Practice And Behaviour For Nurses, Midwives And Nursing Associates*. www.nmc.org.uk/standards/code/ (accessed 23 July 2020).

Ozdemir, B.A., Karthikesalingam, A., Sinha, S. et al. (2015). Research activity and the association with mortality. *PLoS ONE* 10(2): e0118253. doi: 10.1371/journal.pone.0118253.

Pellegrino, E.D. (1988). *For the Patient's Good: The Restoration of Beneficence in Health Care*. Oxford University Press.

Public Health England (2019). *Measles: Guidance, Data and Analysis*. www.gov.uk/government/collections/measles-guidance-data-and-analysis#epidemiology (accessed 24 July 2020).

Royal College of Nursing (2020). Duty of care. www.rcn.org.uk/get-help/rcn-advice/duty-of-care (accessed 24 July 2020).

Royal Pharmaceutical Society and Royal College of Nursing (2019). *Professional Guidance on the Administration of Medicines in Healthcare Settings*. www.rpharms.com/Portals/0/RPS%20document%20library/Open%20access/Professional%20standards/SSHM%20and%20Admin/Admin%20of%20Meds%20prof%20guidance.pdf?ver=2019-01-23-145026-567 (accessed 24 July 2020).

Stewart, M. and Brown, J. (2001). Patient-centredness in medicine. In: *Evidence-based Patient Choice* (ed. Edwards, A. and Elwyn, G.). London: Oxford University Press.

Tse, Y., Vasey, N., Damneek, D. et al. (2019). The KidzMed project: teaching children to swallow tablet medication. *Archives of Disease in Childhood*. https://adc.bmj.com/content/early/2019/10/08/archdischild-2019-317512 (accessed 23 July 2020).

UNICEF (1989). *Convention on the Rights of the Child*. www.unicef.org/child-rights-convention (accessed 23 July 2020).

UNICEF (2013). *Ethical Research Involving Children*. Florence: UNICEF Office of Research.

Velasquez et al. (1988). Ethics and virtue. www.scu.edu/ethics/ethics-resources/ethical-decision-making/ethics-and-virtue/ (accessed: 24 July 2020).

Williamson, C. (2010). *Towards the Emancipation of Patients. Patients' Experiences and the Patient Movement*. Bristol: Policy Press.

Chapter 3 Legal and Ethical Issues

Further Resources

47

Staffordshire & Stoke-on-Trent Safeguarding Children Boards: Lessons to be Learned Briefing No. 16: in respect of the death of Daniel Pelka- Coventry, 2013 www.staffordbc.gov.uk/live/Documents/PolicyAndImprovement/Serious--Case-Review---Daniel-Pelka.pdf

UNICEF Ethical Research Involving Children https://childethics.com/ethical-guidance/

Multiple Choice Questions

1. Common Law is also known as. . .
   (a) Criminal Law
   (b) Case Law
   (c) Statute Law
   (d) All of the above
2. Failure to act with reasonable care could result in healthcare staff being held responsible in which courts?
   (a) Criminal Court
   (b) Civil Court
   (c) Civil and Criminal Court
   (d) All the above
3. What year did the Medicines Act become statute?
   (a) 1966
   (b) 1967
   (c) 1968
   (d) None of the above
4. Utilitarian theory considers. . .
   (a) The greatest good for the greatest number
   (b) Your duty of care takes priority over any other considerations
   (c) How we ought to behave and seek relationships
   (d) All the above
5. When adopting principle-based ethics to guide your decision making, where do you need to gather the facts from?
   (a) From all the stakeholders involved within the scenario
   (b) From what is already known
   (c) From other facts that are relevant from other scenarios'
   (d) All the above
6. Sensitive topics such as abortion can lead to the practitioner having _____ dilemmas.
   (a) Ethical
   (b) Clinical
   (c) Legal
   (d) All the above
7. Implicit means?
   (a) Hidden
   (b) Obvious
   (c) Available
   (d) Explicit
8. Elements of implicit bias include?
   (a) Stereotypes
   (b) Prejudices
   (c) Stereotypes and prejudices
   (d) Impartialities
9. Healthcare professionals harbour the _____ level of implicit bias as the general population
   (a) Lower
   (b) Higher
   (c) Equal
   (d) None of the above

Chapter 3 Legal and Ethical Issues

10. The influences of implicit bias on the practitioner's professional behaviour include?
    (a) Making the client feel uncomfortable
    (b) Helping them access services
    (c) Correct diagnoses and treatment
    (d) Patient concordance
11. What is the Bolam test?
    (a) A test to assess patients' capacity
    (b) The opinion of a professional body as to whether the action was accepted practice
    (c) An assessment of competency of a patient under 16
    (d) All the above
12. Shared decision making. . .
    (a) Is an approach to care that increases patient engagement in treatment
    (b) Improves patient engagement with care and treatment
    (c) Reduces medico-legal claims
    (d) All the above
13. What is distributive justice in relation to healthcare?
    (a) The fair and equal distribution of health resources
    (b) The 'postcode lottery'
    (c) An assessment of patient need
    (d) All the above
14. Why is research in healthcare so important?
    (a) To test drugs for safety and efficacy
    (b) To develop better treatments for patients
    (c) To improve outcomes for patients
    (d) All the above
15. What must healthcare professionals do in order to abide by the 'Duty of Candour'
    (a) Only tell the patient when a serious incident has occurred
    (b) Inform patients and their families of everything related to the patient's care at all costs.
    (c) Apologise to patients
    (d) All the above

Find Out More

The following is a list of considerations, guiding legislation and ethical frameworks for safe and effective practice. Find out more about each of these and make notes in the section provided about what each of these involve and how these impact upon the care of patients.

THE CONSIDERATION	YOUR NOTES
Mental Capacity Act (2005)	
Children Act (1989)	
Children Act (2004)	
United Nations Convention on the Rights of the Child (1989)	
Gillick/Fraser Competence	

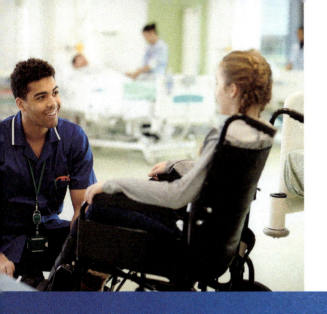

4

Medicines Management and the Role of the Healthcare Provider Working with Children, Young People and Families

Barbara Davies and Christine English

Aim

The aim of this chapter is to help the reader understand the role of the nurse in medicines management when working with children, young people and their families.

Learning Outcomes

After reading this chapter, you will be able to:

- Describe the principles of medicines management
- Discuss the responsibilities of the nurse in medicines management
- Critically discuss key aspects of partnership working with children and their families within the context of medicines management
- Outline the nurse's role in supporting children, young people (CYP) and families

Fundamentals of Pharmacology for Children's Nurses, First Edition. Edited by Ian Peate and Peter Dryden.
© 2022 John Wiley & Sons Ltd. Published 2022 by John Wiley & Sons Ltd.
Companion website: www.wiley.com/go/pharmacologyforCN

Test Your Knowledge

1. As a healthcare provider who are you accountable to?
2. What are the principles of medicines management?
3. What are your responsibilities in ensuring safe medicines administration?
4. What communication strategies may improve the medicines management experience for CYP and their families?
5. What are the benefits of partnership working in the context of medicines management?

Introduction

Public sector organisations are expected to be 'learning organisations' with a flexible workforce that has the capacity to continually develop and improve to meet changing demands across diverse care environments. The clinical governance agenda requires that organisations and individual practitioners are publicly accountable for the delivery of safe and effective evidence-based practice. All Nursing and Midwifery Council (NMC) registrants, nurses, midwives and nursing associates must possess well-developed skills for learning to enable them to function effectively in a transparent learning and working environment, this is also true for registrants from other health and social care professions.

All health and care professionals must have the requisite skills, knowledge and attitudes to interact with others in order to understand better the expressed needs of CYP and provide, lead and coordinate care that is compassionate and evidence-based to deliver high-quality person-centred care to meet their needs in a local context.

There is also greater emphasis on the development of leadership skills, the public health agenda around mental health, and high-order clinical skills, including medicine management. Practitioners must also have well-developed evaluation skills to enable reflection on practice and make an active contribution to the learning needs of employing organisations. The core aim is to enable healthcare providers to continue to develop the skills needed for effective practice in continually changing and challenging environments with the confidence and ability to think critically, apply knowledge and skills and provide expert evidenced-based care.

This chapter, exploring the role of the nurse working with CYP and families within medicines management, is based upon *Future Nurse: Standards of Proficiency for Registered Nurses* (NMC, 2018a). Proficiencies also exist for the nursing associate (NMC, 2018b). The proficiencies, divided into seven platforms, outline the 'roles, responsibilities and accountabilities of registered nurses' whilst detailing core knowledge and skills (see box 4.1.).

Focusing on medicines management, the aim is to enable you, to recognise and develop the skills required at the point of registration in readiness to complete a prescribing qualification. Medicines management covers a wide range of activities including the ordering, storage, administration, recording, monitoring and disposal of medication in adherence with legal, professional and employer requirements.

Box 4.1 The NMC's Seven Platforms

- Platform 1: Being an accountable professional
- Platform 2: Promoting health and preventing ill health
- Platform 3: Assessing needs and planning care
- Platform 4: Providing and evaluating care
- Platform 5: Leading and managing nursing care and working in teams
- Platform 6: Improving safety and quality of care
- Platform 7: Coordinating care

Source: NMC, 2018a/Nursing Midwifery Council.

Being an Accountable Professional

Registered Nurses have always held a key role in medicines administration, but the publication of the Future Nurse Standards (NMC, 2018a) raises expectations for qualifying nurses to develop competence to prescribe. In medicines management, as in all other areas of their practice, nurses are accountable for their own actions and omissions, and are required to work within the law and The Code (2018c) to provide person-centred, safe and compassionate care. These additional roles in medicines management bring with them increased autonomy along with increased levels of accountability and responsibility. In practice, nurses must ensure that they have the necessary competence and authority to perform these roles and must always work safely within the legal, ethical and professional frameworks. Key legal and ethical issues are also addressed in Chapter 3.

In medicines management, the NMC has a duty to protect the public by ensuring safe practice through the setting of standards for professional practice, providing guidance for registrants, academic education institutions and students, advising and managing misconduct or incompetence allegations against registrants including conducting fitness to practise hearings. The NMC promotes professional standards through publications and updating of The Code (NMC, 2018c), which sets out the expectations of a registrant. Academic Education Institutions (AEIs) must meet the NMC's Education standards to offer pre-registration nursing programmes (NMC, 2018d).

Locally, organisations set up their own policies and guidance for medicines management cognisant of legal and professional requirements and adherence to these procedures protects both patients and staff. In situations where errors or omissions concerning medicines occur, the employer investigates using disciplinary procedures, as necessary, if local policies and procedures are found not to have been followed. If there has been a serious breach of policy or procedure, the employer may refer the case to the NMC for consideration and this could ultimately result in the nurse concerned facing a fitness to practise panel should an investigation conclude that professional misconduct has taken place.

The nurse is accountable first and foremost to the patient and this is governed by public law, the NMC as the professional regulatory body and the employer through employment contract.

Nursing and Midwifery Council

Nurses have a duty of care to the patient to always promote their best interests and any breach of this duty could result in the nurse being called to account, for their actions or omissions, to the NMC. In clinical practice, registered nurses must acknowledge their own limitations and continue to update their knowledge and skills to enable them to make evidence-based decisions in care, including medicines management.

Employer and Colleagues

Nurses working within an organisation will have employer indemnity which means that the employer accepts liability for any acts that the nurse may commit provided that they have practised within the law and the employer's policies and procedures (vicarious liability). It should be noted that it is the professional responsibility of the nurse to notify their employer if they believe that any policy or procedure does not meet legal requirements.

Clinical Consideration

In the case of a registrant working independently, they must provide their own indemnity.

In a situation where a nurse makes a mistake, the employer has a right to investigate the incident and invoke its own disciplinary policy. However, the nurse's actions to minimise patient harm following the error and the nurse's honesty will be taken into consideration when deciding the outcome.

Nurses not only have accountability to the NMC and their employer but also with regard to other nursing colleagues. If a nurse has concerns about the behaviour of another nurse, the nurse has a legal and professional duty to report concerns to their manager and can report this more widely if the manager fails to act on the information. These duties to report have been put in place to assist in public protection.

Patients, or their relatives, do sometimes bring a case against an individual nurse for negligence, and these cases are dealt with through the civil courts. The judge will decide if the individual is liable/not liable and can award damages. In more serious cases where negligence may constitute a criminal act, prosecution through public law may be sought. Such cases are dealt with by the police, a magistrate and a jury. In these situations, the individual nurse may be found guilty/not guilty and the outcome could be a fine, community service, prison sentence or discharge.

In law, for a negligence claim to be upheld four important elements must be proven:

1. that the defendant owed a duty of care to the person harmed (duty)
2. that they breached this duty (breach)
3. that the breach caused was foreseeable (causation)
4. that harm was caused to the claimant (harm)

Promoting Health and Preventing Ill Health

It is recognised that nurses play an important role in the public health agenda and medicines education is a key aspect of health promotion. All nurses need to make every contact count (Health Education England, 2018) and use medication education as a vehicle to address health concerns, promote health and prevent further ill health. This is becoming increasingly important as more and more CYP and their families are self-managing long-term health conditions.

Holistic Assessment

The role of the nurse is to enable and empower CYP and their families, as and when appropriate, to be involved in care and care planning (Department for Education and Skills/Department of Health, 2004). The philosophy of family-centred care and partnership working is an accepted way to structure involvement (Foster and Shields, 2020) taking the needs of the CYP and family into consideration (Armitage and Knapman, 2014). A distinguishing aspect of the nursing role is to undertake holistic health assessments, building rapport with patients and discussing aspects of lifestyle that may influence medicines management. It is imperative that there is a move from compliance, lack of patient involvement and an assumption that the patients' views align with the prescriber's recommendations, to one of concordance where families are listened to and their views taken into consideration when decisions are made about their child or young person's medication (Haynes et al., 2008).

Skills for Practice

How to promote good health and well-being using brief interventions to initiate change.

A brief intervention can take as little as 30 seconds and could be as simple as opening a conversation about a health issue, relaying information, signposting for further support, raising awareness of risk or referral for further interventions.

(Health Education England, 2018)

Clinical Consideration

When working with families, healthcare providers must always consider and take seriously the CYP's views. This right is laid down in the United Nations Convention on the Rights of the Child (1989).

Nurses must support and enable CYP and their families to make informed choices as they manage healthcare challenges with a view to optimising quality of life and health outcomes (NMC, 2018a). The nurses' role is not just the giving of medications but the underlying education of the patient and their family to ensure safe administration. Children's nurses need to be creative and innovative in how they share their knowledge about medication using online, age-appropriate information from evidence-based sources. Nurses also need to consider meeting the needs of those children and families who might have trouble in understanding information, for example, those who have difficulties communicating and those whose first language is not English (Smith and Atkinson, 2012).

To engage fully in a partnership approach and be involved in medicines management decision making, all those involved must be enabled to develop knowledge. The 5 Moments of Medication Safety (World Health Organization, 2017a) is a useful tool to actively engage the child and family in conversations about their medicines (see Figure 4.1).

It is vital that both written and verbal information is made available. By providing patient-specific information, evidence-based education, reminders and reinforcement, improved adherence to medicine management can be achieved (Haynes et al., 2008). The aim is to empower and promote independence (Armitage and Knapman, 2014).

The nursing role within medicines management is one that is continually evolving and over the years nurses have taken on prescribing roles, enhancing their professional identity (Stenner et al., 2010). Most importantly there is a need to ensure that the therapeutic aspect of the nursing role is not lost and that this role expansion adds value to patient care. Nursing consultations must continue to follow a holistic nursing model involving health promotion, CYP and family-centred care (Stenner et al., 2010).

Assessing Needs and Planning Care

Assessment, in general, is a process of evaluating a patient's personal, physical, psychosocial, cultural and spiritual needs taking into consideration the patient and family's wishes. All healthcare professionals who consult with CYP should take a developmentally appropriate psychosocial history as well as enquire about generic health and disease specific issues. When assessing the medication needs of a patient, an inclusive and holistic family-centred approach is important to engage those involved and ensure accuracy of data, ensuring the patient receives the maximum benefit from the medicines they are taking whilst minimising potential harm (MHRA.gov.uk). There are different types of patient assessments that are undertaken, all of which will include, to some extent, assessment of medication use.

A mini assessment might take place in an emergency department and questions about medication may be brief to focus on immediate problems. Following this initial assessment, a move to a more focused/comprehensive assessment would be needed (see Table 4.1).

Assessment includes asking about medication usage including route of administration, times of administration, side effects, concordance and allergies. Other considerations may be whether the illness requiring the medication is acute and short term in which case it is likely that the nurse will directly prepare and administer the drugs or if long term there needs to be a plan to teach the CYP and/or the family about the drugs. Education will include ordering of medication (including emergency medication), safe storage, administration, side effects, checking expiry dates, contraindications, how to access help and the importance of follow-up. For some CYP this may mean learning to self-inject, e.g. in diabetes or severe allergies. The CYP may need to learn how to monitor their condition to enable them to decide when they should inject themselves or take a tablet, for example, a finger prick blood test for glucose level.

During assessment, some problems may not be disclosed by the patient and may only be identified when the nurse–patient relationship develops and the patient trusts the nurse. For example, it may be difficult discussing sexual health and risk-taking behaviours with young people. Ideally, these questions are asked when the young person is comfortable and able to answer openly; this often means without other family members present. Confidentiality is important and the young person may need assurance. Questions should be open-ended and aimed at building rapport with the young person.

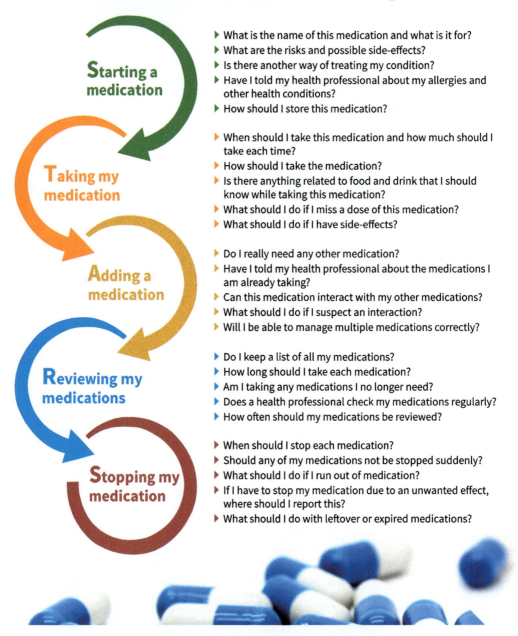

Figure 4.1 Five moments of medication safety. WHO 2017/World Health Organization

Table 4.1 Types of assessment.

Mini assessment	Snapshot of the patient. A quick visual and physical assessment. ABC approach (airway, breathing, circulation). Patient's mental status, appearance, level of consciousness and vital signs are recorded. Focus is on the patient's main problem. Where able, in these mini assessments the patient's medication use needs to be considered as it could be an indicator of the cause of the problem e.g. overwhelming infection in the case of the immunosuppressed patient.
Comprehensive assessment	In depth including physical examination, risk factors, psychological and social factors, previous health status. Usually occurs on admission. This will include medical history including medication usage. Often based upon the Activities of Living (Roper et al., 2000).
Focused assessment	Assessment of a specific condition/problem. For example, a child with juvenile idiopathic arthritis (JIA) who is experiencing a flare-up of their disease. Open-ended questions used to elicit more information; this would include in-depth discussion around medicines management.
Ongoing assessment	Assessment is cyclical and follows the giving of care; it is important to evaluate and reassess. Monitoring and observation add to the information gained from mini, comprehensive or focused assessment and changes to planned care reflect data retrieved.

Source: Ahern and Philpot, 2002; White, 2003; Holmes, 2003

Episode of Care

Charlie, a 13-year-old boy, admitted due to a 48-hour history of abdominal pain, loose stools and fatigue. Charlie was diagnosed with Crohn's disease 18 months ago. On assessment Charlie indicates his pain score to be 5 out of 10, he is pyrexial, other vital observations are within normal parameters. Charlie, following assessment by the doctor, is to start a course of prednisolone along with his other medication of azathioprine.

Charlie appears very quiet, withdrawn and does not communicate very much with the nursing staff. Both parents are present and they mention they are worried about his mental health as he has stopped socialising with friends and says he does not like school. They also mention that Charlie has a good therapeutic relationship with the gastroenterology specialist nurse.

The specialist nurse is informed of his admission and further assesses Charlie's psychological and emotional health, offering ongoing psychological and physical support.

The following day Charlie, as his pain is under control, is to be discharged home on prednisolone. Charlie will be seen again in 3 weeks in the paediatric clinic. A referral is also made to child and adolescent mental health services.

The HEADSS for Adolescents tool is often used during assessment to explore CYP adolescent issues (Cohen et al., 1991). We have adapted the tool using the headings (Home, Education and Employment, Activities, Drugs, Sexuality, Suicide and Depression) (see Table 4.2) to identify potential medication issues with CYP to ensure safe treatment and positive outcomes.

Self-Medication

An increasing number of medications can be bought over the counter (OTC) which enables self-care and can be of benefit. However, the nurse during the assessment process needs to be mindful that the CYP may have taken OTC medication in addition to prescribed medication as patients often fail to mention them. Nurses may notice side effects but may not recognise the cause if they are unaware the patient is taking OTC medication.

Equally important is to ask about medications bought from other countries. In some countries, medication such as ventolin inhalers can be purchased over the counter. If this happens on a regular basis it might,

Table 4.2 HEADSS.

HEADSS – EXAMPLES OF QUESTIONS TO ASK			REASONS
H	HOME	Who lives with the young person? What are relationships like at home? What do parents do for a living? New people in home environment?	Parents may have separated/divorced/died/left the home. It is important to identify who is supporting the CYP through diagnosis and treatment. Who can help the CYP with medication administration? Assess the medication training needs of the CYP/family. Do other people need to be involved, e.g. child minders, school teachers, workplace/employers, neighbours, friends and relatives? Do other health professionals need to be involved, e.g. specialist community public health nurses, community children's nurse, practice nurse? Consider safety including storage and disposal.
E	Education and employment	What year at school are they in? Do they like school? Favourite subjects/worst subjects What is their school attendance?	School attendance/poor school attendance may be an indicator of personal problems within their school or home life or could be an indicator of poor disease control. Further assessment needed including in-depth medicines management. How might the environment impact upon ability to access and use medications? What education is required within the school environment to ensure safe administration of medicines? Is any training required? How are medicines to be stored?
A	Activities	What do they do for fun? Where? When? Who with? What things do they do with their friends? What do they do with their free time? Are they planning to travel?	It is important to explore peer relationships as peer pressure may affect medication concordance. Some activities might impact upon medication administration, e.g. athletics, and which sites to use for insulin administration. Requirements at customs with regard to carrying some medications, syringes and needles into a different country. It may be necessary for the family to carry with them a letter from the medical staff to authorise and explain the CYP's medication needs.
D	Drugs	Smoking/alcohol/other drugs? Ask about all medicines including complementary and over the counter medicines.	Some CYP experiment with drugs and alcohol. Remember every contact is a health promotion opportunity. It is important to establish if this is a regular or an occasional activity. Try to identify what they drink or what drugs they take and frequency. Alcohol consumption may be a contraindication to medicines prescribed, e.g. methotrexate, metronidazole, nitrofurantoin.

S	Sexuality	Are you involved in a relationship? Are you using a form of contraception? Ask girls about menarche and menstrual cycle (and last menstrual period).	Do not assume that all CYP are heterosexual. Do not make assumptions about sexual orientation and gender identity. Do they know about teratogen risk with some medicines, e.g. methotrexate?
S	Suicide/ depression	Is there anything else that is worrying the young person? Do they have trouble with sleep/appetite/eating behaviour? Have they ever self-harmed? Who can they talk to if they have worries?	CYP who feel anxious or depressed have difficulty falling asleep. Tiredness may also be a sign of poor disease control. Enquiring about eating habits may lead to identification of disordered eating habits. Check the side effects of medications used, there might be contributing factors, e.g. steroids may cause mood changes and weight gain and fear of weight gain might lead to noncompliance with medication regimens.

Source: Adapted from Cohen et al., 1991

for example, appear that the patient is managing their asthma in light of reduced medication use when in fact their asthma is uncontrolled.

Complementary and Alternative Medication (CAM)

Complementary and alternative medicines refers to a diverse group of therapies and disciplines that are not part of standard medical care. Although some people may choose CAMs, believing them to be natural or risk-free, it is important to always consider the evidence base. Nurses must have an understanding of the different CAMs available and ask the patient/family about their usage.

Clinical Consideration

Interactions between herbal medicines and prescribed medicines can occur, for example St John's Wort interacting with erythromycin can potentially lead to therapeutic failure of the antibiotic.

Planning

Once an assessment is complete, interventions and outcomes are prioritised in consultation with the CYP and their family acknowledging age and stage of development. All care must be communicated and documented, the aim being to reduce risk factors, address needs, improve problems, reduce occurrence of further risk/needs/problems, utilise patient strengths and refer to other professionals as needed where an identified problem is not a nursing one. The plan needs regular review as the CYP's condition may change, medications may change and as the child matures, self-medication may be appropriate. Concordance with medication is better achieved where there is ownership and responsibility from an early age (Kaufman, 2014).

As planned care is delivered, the nurse continues to assess the ability of the CYP/parent to administer and monitor the prescribed medication. Where there are concerns that these responsibilities may not be carried out safely at home then the plan needs to be reviewed and the involvement of other health professionals considered ensuring safe medicines administration. This might be a community nurse giving the medication at home. In situations where there is a specific safeguarding concern linked to the CYP's medication, a cause for concern, additional support and advice should be put in place.

Patient safety is paramount and there is a need to have the underpinning knowledge to base care decisions upon, being aware of abilities and limitations and seeking advice and support from your practice supervisors.

Providing and Evaluating Care

The Registered Nurse is responsible for implementing the medication plan but must work in partnership with the CYP and family at each stage to ensure that medication is administered safely and effectively. Initially, partnership working may simply involve the nurse sharing with the family key information about the CYP's medicines or perhaps teaching the parents specific skills to administer the medication. Where there is a need for long-term medication, CYP and their parents will require more in-depth information and preparation to build their confidence to fully engage in future shared decision making about their medicines.

In the hospital setting it is usually the nurse who will prepare and administer medication to CYP and it is vital that these duties are carried out safely and competently. Despite continued efforts to improve safety standards, each year medication errors do occur and some of these medication errors result in fatalities. It is critical, therefore, that any nurse who is administering medicines to patients is deemed competent to do so and follows local policies and procedures, ensuring that all necessary safety checks are carried out fully.

There are a wide range of checks that the nurse is responsible for during the preparation and administration of medication. To begin with, the nurse must check the prescription itself using knowledge of pharmacology to determine if the medicine is appropriate, the dosage and route are correct, there are no contraindications or allergies to be considered. Once satisfied that the prescription is accurate, the nurse can start to calculate and prepare the dose of the medicine. Accurate calculation of medicines for CYP is of paramount importance. Most medicine dosages for CYP are calculated on the weight of the CYP so you need to be aware that what is the usual dose for one child or young person may be a dangerous dose for another.

Nurses should be aware of the normal dosage range for commonly prescribed medication and when unsure they must look up this information within a reference text such as the British National Formulary for children (BNFc) (see Chapter 2). Although the NMC (2018a) requires nurses to be numerate and students are tested on this subject (there is a requirement of student nurses to achieve a 100% success in summative numeracy assessments), many errors in paediatrics continue to occur. In CYP, calculation errors can result in a fatality, so it is imperative that calculations are checked for accuracy. It is therefore vital that all opportunities are used to practise and achieve competence in calculations of drug dosages.

There are measures in place to ensure CYP are given medication safely. Healthcare organisations embed safety checks within their local policies and procedures and although this may differ across organisations, the principles remain the same.

Checking

A first check that the nurse must undertake is that the prescription is correct. Even if the nurse is not a nurse prescriber, the nurse must have knowledge of the commonly used drugs and know the appropriate dosage, using the BNFc to check the prescription where needed. The nurse needs to understand the CYP's clinical condition to guard against the administration of any medicines which may potentially exacerbate their problems. To practise safely, nurses must also understand medication side effects, potential drug interactions and any special precautions to be taken. The nurse must check that they are administering the right drug, the right amount, to the right patient, via the right route at the right time and record on the right documentation. They must ensure that the medicine has not passed the expiry date. They should check for any contraindications and allergies to ensure that it is safe to administer the drug.

Evaluation

The nurse regularly monitors the patient, checking the effectiveness of the medicine, observing for side effects or allergic reactions that would indicate a need to stop and/or change the medication or the dosage. Similarly, if the route of administration is problematic for the patient, a change may need to be considered, e.g. if a CYP is unable to swallow a tablet, a liquid alternative may need to be used.

When evaluating the medicines management plan the nurse works in partnership with the CYP and family to determine if the medication is effective and if the CYP is experiencing any difficulties with taking the medicines. Sometimes the timing of the prescribed medication is difficult to fit in with the CYP's normal daily schedule and small adjustments to dosage timing can greatly increase the likelihood of the medication actually being taken. Remember, it is no good having a highly effective medicine available if the CYP will not or cannot take it for whatever reason.

Clinical Consideration

A side effect of long-term use of steroids can be increased appetite and weight gain. This unwanted side effect may impact upon the CYP's willingness to continue treatment. Professionals need to be alert that the CYP may stop treatment without consulting them.

CYPs who receive community care and are attending for check-ups will need to have their medicines plan regularly reviewed. Reviews need to be undertaken in partnership with the CYP and family. The WHO's (2017a) 5 Moments of Medication Safety is a useful tool to guide these conversations and assess CYP and family knowledge. Example of review questions relate to the effectiveness of the medication, dose alteration due to weight change and reports of problems and side effects of the medicines. Further points for discussion may explore whether the medication is compatible with the CYP's and family's lifestyle. To enable greater concordance, adjustments may need to be considered, e.g. changing the timing of medication so that it fits well with mealtimes, bedtimes, school. The evaluation may also encompass records of medicines taken, any emergency medicines used and possible side effects noted. In addition, some medicines need specific monitoring by the CYP/family and nurse, e.g. to measure blood levels of the drug or to identify any side effects early.

If the taste of the medicine or the size of a tablet causes difficulty for the CYP, this needs to be addressed as the medicines cannot be effective if the CYP is unable to comply with the prescription (see Chapter 6). Good practice indicates that teaching CYP to swallow a tablet can support concordance and also prove cost-effective (Tse et al., 2019).

Leading and Managing Nursing Care and Working in Teams

As you become more experienced and more knowledgeable within the role of medicines management you will be responsible for leading and managing nursing care for a small group of patients. This care delivery will include medicines management. Still under supervision from your practice supervisors and practice assessors, your role will be to work as part of the interdisciplinary team to ensure that medicines administration of the right drug, given by the right route at the right time in the right dose to the right patient occurs. You will be using your skills of assessment to monitor and evaluate patient responses to medication, evaluating care and communicating changes to the interdisciplinary team.

The giving of the medication is only a small part of medicines management. Medicines management is a team approach and that team needs to be able to work cohesively to ensure best outcomes for the patient. The team may consist of a many different professionals, with the nurse often being the facilitator of communication and collaboration (see Figure 4.2).

Developing responsibility for leading, managing and coordinating care can be difficult given the potential numbers of professional staff involved in the process. Good medicines management relies on the sharing of information in a timely way and effective communication processes are critical to success. Lapses in communication may impact upon patient care and outcomes and therefore a structured form of communication can be used to ensure information is transferred accurately.

The Situation, Background, Assessment and Recommendation (SBAR) communication tool provides clarity of information (Institute for Healthcare Improvement, 2015). SBAR is useful in a range of situations including:

- Inpatient or outpatient
- Urgent or non-urgent communications
- Conversations between clinicians, either in person or over the phone
- Conversations with peers, e.g. nurse to nurse, or between different disciplines, e.g. nurse to pharmacist
- Escalating a concern when patients move between NHS services, e.g. emergency department to ward.

This tool assists the giver and receiver of information by providing a structured and standardised approach to interactions about patients.

Using SBAR, the information giver benefits by being able to gather a standard set of information in a way that ensures that the message sent is clear. The information receiver knows the format of the message they will receive so does not need to interrupt to ask questions and can concentrate on actively listening. SBAR fits in any setting but is particularly useful to minimise communication difficulties across disciplines or where there are differences in levels of seniority. In clinical practice, the rationale for the communication is made clear by the information giver by providing a recommendation. This is a key step in the process and is especially

Chapter 4 Medicines Management and the Role of the Healthcare Provider Working with Children

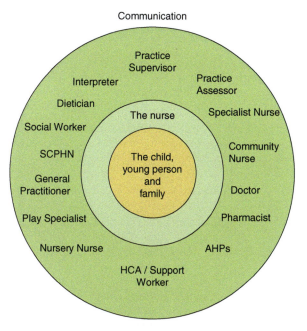

Figure 4.2 Team around the patient in clinical practice.

valuable where the person sending the message is inexperienced and has to communicate with an experienced member of staff. The clinical scenario in Table 4.3 demonstrates application of the SBAR tool in a medicines management communication.

Skills for Practice

Table 4.3 How to communicate effectively using the SBAR tool in a medicine's management situation.

S	Situation (a concise statement of the problem)	I am student nurse Smith on ward 1 calling about Raffik Ampour. I am calling because I am concerned that following the administration of intravenous antibiotics, he has developed a widespread raised itchy skin rash.
B	Background (pertinent and brief information related to the situation)	He is a five-year-old boy with no previous medical history. He was admitted today with an upper respiratory tract infection and pyrexia of 38.4°C.
A	Assessment (analysis and considerations of options – what you found/think)	I think the problem is that he is having a reaction to the antibiotics and I have stopped the infusion.
R	Recommendation (action requested/recommended – what you want)	I need you to come and see the child in the next 30 minutes, is there anything I need to do in the meantime?

Transition points in care, such as ward transfer or discharge, can be a risk factor within medicines management. Part of your role will be to ensure all those involved within the care of the patient are aware of the change in environment to prevent care becoming fragmented. For example, consideration needs to be given to the transfer of medicines from one ward to another or the planning of discharge medications.

Skills and knowledge related to medicines management takes time and practice and is something that will continue to develop following registration. Further education and training should focus on your own performance, continuation of your role as a reflective practitioner and to enhance knowledge and skills development. You will be educating the next student nurses in practice, acting as a role model and supervising their practice.

Improving Safety and Quality

This section will:

- Identify why safety and quality improvements are important in medicines management
- Outline changes in perspectives on errors and development of a safety culture in the NHS
- Discuss nurses' role in continuous quality improvement including human factors

Patient safety is a relatively new discipline within healthcare that developed in recognition that contemporary, complex care environments were witnessing a growth in adverse medical events that was widespread and preventable (www.who.int/news-room/fact-sheets/detail/patient-safety). Patient safety has been defined as:

. . . the avoidance of unintended or unexpected harm to people during the provision of healthcare.

NHS Improvement, 2019: 1

Fundamental to patient safety is the use of continuous quality improvement approaches capitalising on learning from errors and adverse events to prevent repetition of incidents. A major area of concern for patient safety currently is medicines management. Each year in the NHS in England, an estimated 237 million 'medication errors' take place, with 66 million of these being considered potentially clinically significant errors (NHS Improvement, 2019).

In 2017, the World Health Organisation launched its third Global Patient Safety Challenge – 'Medication without Harm' – with the aim of reducing the global burden of severe and avoidable medication-related harm by 50% over five years (WHO, 2017b). A Medicines Safety Improvement Programme (NHS Improvement, 2019) has been published in the UK focusing on the four domains outlined in the WHO Global Challenge: patients; medicines; healthcare professionals; systems and practices (WHO, 2017b).

Despite this, medication errors continue to occur. Traditionally, errors have been seen as merely mistakes or failings of individual nurses resulting in disciplinary action. Many organisations have now become more aware that it is unrealistic to expect that human beings will operate without error in the type of complex, high-stress environments that exist in healthcare. There is greater acceptance that where practitioners work in an environment where the systems, tasks and processes are well designed they are better protected against making mistakes (Grout, 2006). This shift in thinking about errors moves the 'blame' for such adverse incidents away from the failings of individual nurses to consider failings in the systems that allow errors to happen. The learning from these incidents is critical for development of safer practices.

Improvement strategies in medication safety now focus on improving the patient safety systems by learning from mistakes and good practice while promoting open, transparent working environments that encourage development of strong organisational safety cultures https://improvement.nhs.uk/resources/patient-safety-strategy/. Key factors for success in improving patient safety have been identified as: clear policies and procedures; effective leadership; data to underpin safety improvements; skilled healthcare professionals and patient involvement (www.who.int/news-room/fact-sheets/detail/patient-safety).

As errors in medicines management can result in serious adverse outcomes or even fatalities, nurses must continuously monitor and quality improve the systems and policies that support these aspects of care. It is important to remember that there is currently no risk-free way to manage medicines: the risks must be managed and minimised. Nurses need to actively engage in quality improvement work to problem solve, spot potential safety risks in medication processes and escalate concerns, to an appropriate senior professional in their organisation. Patient involvement is key to successful quality improvements and nurses can be pivotal in encouraging CYP and families to feedback on their experiences to improve processes.

Nurses have a key role to play both in patient safety and in continuous quality improvement related to medicines. Their position, relationship and communications with the CYP, family and other healthcare professionals places them in a unique position to be proactive in safety improvements in this area of care delivery. Nurses are well placed and also have responsibility to continually look for safety improvements (NMC, 2018a) in practice, including medicines management. They may notice recurring problems in practice with certain medicines or procedures and may offer pragmatic remedies to these issues. It is also critical that CYP and families are involved in safety and quality improvement work in medicines management as they will add a different perspective to the discussions and may suggest novel ideas for improvements.

A human factors approach is now central to analysis of patient safety problems. The term 'human factors' (or ergonomics) encompasses the study of the inter-relationships between humans, the tools and equipment they use in the workplace and the environment in which they work (Kohn et al., 1999).

The key aspects of this approach is to optimise human performance by better understanding the behaviour of individuals, their interactions with each other and their environment. The factors that support or hinder the way that people carry out the necessary tasks also need consideration. Appreciating human limitations and factors that can impact on an individual's performance within the environment and the equipment of a task enables safety improvements to be made in medicine management procedures to mitigate against human frailties, such as lack of knowledge, fatigue, stress, poor communication and inadequate skills, thus minimising errors (england.nhs.uk/wp-content/uploads2013/11/nqb-hum-fact-concordat.pdf) NHS Human factors in healthcare website).

This knowledge allows a better understanding of the potential triggers for adverse events and errors and can enable re-design of processes to include steps to minimise or eradicate the impact of human factors on task performance.

Coordinating Care

When considering coordination of care it is also equally important to explore continuity of care as both go hand in hand. The WHO (2018) provide definitions:

Continuity of care: reflects the extent to which a series of discrete healthcare events is experienced by people as coherent and interconnected over time and consistent with their health needs and preferences
and
Care coordination: a proactive approach to bringing together care professionals and providers to meet the needs of service users to ensure that they receive integrated, person-focused care across various settings.

If continuity and coordination are absent, many CYP and families will experience care which is fragmented. This has the potential to result in poorer outcomes and harm resulting from failures in communication and information giving, inadequate medicine reconciliation, repeated investigations and admission/readmission to hospital.

The focus in this section is on transitions of care, which could be in the form of:

- Transition of care to another ward
- Transition of care to another hospital
- Transition of care to home and family
- Transition of care to community services

Initially this may seem relatively straightforward; however, transition points are high risk for medication error, therefore it is important that a medication review is completed. At each stage of transition any discrepancy needs to be identified as non-identification may place the patient at risk of harm (World Health Organization, 2019).

At all transition points the empowered CYP and family, working in partnership with the MDT, can contribute to discussions. The CYP and family are the constant within care and they may be the only ones who know what medication is prescribed at each stage of transition. Not including them would increase the risk of error potentially resulting in harm.

As each CYP and family's needs will be different, a short scenario is used to help you begin to think about the aims of transition and the planning needed.

When the CYP is transitioned, it is important that new medication regimens or changes to existing prescriptions be communicated to the next healthcare provider. The aim is, through good communication, to reduce medication errors that could lead to harm/readmission to hospital. Coordination and ensuring continuity of care are essential to positive outcomes and patient safety.

Episode of Care

Alisha, 14 years old, who has Down's syndrome, has been newly diagnosed with polyarticular juvenile idiopathic arthritis (JIA). She has numerous swollen, painful joints and has been admitted to the ward for 3 days of intravenous methylprednisolone. She has been commenced on subcutaneous (S/C) methotrexate and is to be discharged home tomorrow on both S/C methotrexate and a reducing dose of prednisolone.

In this case the aims of transition planning are as follows:

AIM	ACTIONS TO CONSIDER
To prepare Alisha and her family both physically and psychologically for transfer to an agreed environment (in this case home)	Planning for transition starts on admission. Consider physical, psychological, social, cultural and economic needs. Use a family-centred care approach. Multidisciplinary team input to include pharmacist. Disease education. Ensure at appropriate level for Alisha's understanding. Discuss available support for both JIA and learning disability. Check discharge medications are ordered. Time to ask questions. Reassure. Update Alisha and her family regularly. Reassess as care is evaluated.
To provide written and verbal information to meet their needs	Patient information leaflets. Ensure at appropriate level for Alisha's understanding. Direct to appropriate websites for additional information. Give a medication list in paper or electronic format. Discuss medication: dosage including when to reduce, how to administer, side effects, contraindications, storage, safety issues such as when not to give, what to do if unwell, and adherence to regime. How to order a repeat prescription. Allow time for Alisha and her family to ask questions. Assess Alisha and family's understanding. Use 'teach back' techniques (NHS Education for Scotland, 2020).
To facilitate a smooth transfer by ensuring all necessary healthcare facilities are prepared to receive the patient	Inform those health professionals who might be involved in the care plan. This might be general practitioner (GP)/ practice nurse, children's community nurse, MDT, community physiotherapist, school nurse, specialist nurse. Hand over patient information using SBAR to enable informed plan of care to be developed. Give details and contact information of health professional involvement to Alisha and her family.
To promote the highest possible level of independence for Alisha and her family	Disease education. Consider using other formats such as pictures/video. Medicines education. Discuss teaching of injection technique, who by and when. Does Alisha want to self-administer? Consider additional support to facilitate this. Telephone helpline details if there is one so questions can be asked about medication. Discuss return to school.
To provide continuity between hospital and the agreed environment of care by facilitating effective communication	Give copy of discharge plan to Alisha and her family. Follow-up appointment arranged. Give details of who to contact if a problem arises.

Source: Adapted from Lister et al., 2020.

Conclusion

Having read this chapter, you should recognise, you have an integral role in medicines management providing safe and effective medicine delivery whilst coordinating care that is evidence-based, person and family-centred. The NMC (2018d) envisages students to be prescriber-ready at the point of registration, and with this comes increasing accountability and responsibility. To practise safely, and work within legal, ethical and professional frameworks, you must maintain competence and be authorised to prescribe and administer medications. You must be able to work autonomously, or in partnership with a range of professionals and teams responding to the demands of your role. Interprofessional team working in medicines management is recognised as important, but often the nurse is the key professional interacting face to face regularly with the patient and their family.

Within medicines management, and the wider nursing role, your contribution to health protection, health promotion and the prevention of ill health aids empowerment of the CYP and their family. By supporting them to manage their own care, where possible, you enable them to move from dependence to independence. As a student nurse, you will increasingly demonstrate leadership in the delivery of care developing confidence and demonstrating the ability to think critically, make decisions and apply your knowledge and skills of medicines management to provide evidence-based care.

References

Ahern, J. and Philpot, P. (2002). Assessing acutely ill patients on general wards. *Nursing Standard* 16(47): 47–54.

Armitage, G. and Knapman, H. (2014). *Medicine Management Toolkit, Together for Short Lives*, 2e. Bristol: Together for Short Lives.

British National Formulary for children (BNFc). https://bnfc.nice.org.uk/(accessed 1 April 2021).

Cohen, E., Mackenzie, R.G., and Yates, G.L. (1991). HEADSS, a psychosocial risk assessment instrument: Implications for designing effective intervention programs for runaway youth. *Journal of Adolescent Health*, 12: 539–544.

Department for Education and Skills/Department of Health (2004). *National Service Framework for Children, Young People and Maternity Services.* London: DH.

Lister, S., Hofland, J., and Grafton, H. (eds) (2020). *The Royal Marsden Manual of Clinical Nursing Procedures*, 10e. Oxford: Wiley-Blackwell.

Foster, M. and Shields, L. (2020). Bridging the child and family centred care gap: therapeutic conversations with children and families. *Comprehensive Child and Adolescent Nursing* 43(2): 151–158.

Grout, J.R. (2006). Mistake proofing: changing designs to reduce error. *Quality and Safety in Health Care*, 15(Suppl 1): 44–49.

Haynes, R.B., Acidoo, E., Sahoto, N. et al. (2008). Interventions for enhancing medication adherence. *Cochrane Database of Systematic Reviews.* 2.

Health Education England (2018). Making every contact count. www.makingeverycontactcount.co.uk/ (accessed 1 April 2021).

Holmes, H.N. (ed.) (2003). *3-minute Assessment.* Lippincott, Williams & Wilkins, Philadelphia: 1–19, 20–32.

Institute for Healthcare Improvement (2015). *Safer Care. SBAR. Situation, Background, Assessment and Recommendation. Information and Training Guide.* Institute for Healthcare Improvement.

Kaufman, G.G. (2014). Polypharmacy, medicines optimisation and concordance. *Nurse Prescribing* 12(4): 197–201.

Kohn, L.T., Corrigan, J.M., and Donaldson, M.S. (eds) (1999). *To Err is Human – Building a Safer Health System.* Washington, DC: Committee on Quality of Health Care in America, Institute of Medicine.

National NHS Improvement (2020) *The Medicines Safety Improvement Programme.* Updated 7 April 2020.

MHRA.gov.uk (2019). www.gov.uk/government/organisations/medicines-and-healthcare-products-regulatory-agency (accessed 27 August 2020).

NHS Education for Scotland (2020). The Health Literacy Place. www.healthliteracyplace.org.uk/tools-and-techniques/techniques/teach-back/(accessed 20 April 2021).

NHS England. www.england.nhs.uk/ (accessed 27 August 2020).

NHS Improvement (2019). https://improvement.nhs.uk/ (accessed 27 August 2020).

NHS Improvement (2020). Patient Safety Strategy. www.england.nhs.uk/patient-safety/the-nhs-patient-safety-strategy/ (accessed 27 August 2020).

Nursing Midwifery Council (2018a) *Future Nurse: Standards of Proficiency for Registered Nurses*. www.nmc.org.uk/globalassets/sitedocuments/education-standards/future-nurse-proficiencies.pdf (accessed 20 April 2021).

Nursing Midwifery Council (2018b) *Standards of Proficiency for Nursing Associates*. https://nmc.org.uk (accessed 20 April 2021).

Nursing Midwifery Council (2018c) *The Code: Professional Standards of Practice and Behaviour for Nurses and Midwives*. www.nmc.org.uk/standards/code/read-the-code-online/ (accessed 20 April 2021).

Nursing Midwifery Council (2018d) Standards for Pre-registration Nursing Programmes. Part 3 of Realising Professionalism: Standards for Education and Training. www.nmc.org.uk/standards/standards-for-nurses/standards-for-pre-registration-nursing-programmes/ (accessed 20 April 2021).

Roper, N., Logan, W., and Tierney, A. (2000). *The Roper, Logan and Tierney Model of Nursing: Based on Activities of Living*. Edinburgh: Churchill Livingstone.

Smith, J. and Atkinson, S. (2012). Children who have difficulty communicating. In: *Communication Skills for Children's Nurses* (ed. Lambert, V., Long, T., and Kelleher, D.). Berkshire: Open University Press.

Stenner, K., Carey, N., and Courtenay, M. (2010). How nurse prescribing influences the role of nursing. *Prescribing* 8(1): 29–34.

Tse, Y., Vasey, N., Dua, D. et al. (2019). The KidzMed project: teaching children to swallow tablet medication. *Archives of Disease of Childhood* 105(11): 1105–1107.

White, L. (2003). *Documentation and the Nursing Process*. Thomson Delmar Learning.

World Health Organization (2017a) 5 Moments for medication safety. www.who.int/health-topics/patient-safety#tab=tab_1 (accessed 27 August 2020).

World Health Organization (2017b) Fact sheet: patient safety. www.who.int/news-room/fact-sheets/detail/patient-safety (accessed 20 April 2021).

World Health Organization (2018). *Continuity and Co-ordination of Care: A Practice Brief to Support Implementation of the WHO Framework on Integrated People-centred Health Services*. Geneva: WHO.

World Health Organization (2019). Medication safety in transitions of care. Geneva: WHO. www.who.int/patientsafety/medication-safety/TransitionOfCare.PDF (accessed 27 August 2020).

Further Resources

Clinical Human Factors Group (Charity) www.chfg.org//

Nursing Midwifery Council www.nmc.org.uk/standards/standards-for-post-registration/standards-for-prescribers

Paediatric Musculoskeletal Matters. A free online educational resource www.pmmonline.org/nurse

Royal College of Paediatrics and Child Health www.rcpch.ac.uk/resources/qi-central-sharing-qi-experience-expertise

The third WHO Global Patient Safety Challenge: *Medication Without Harm* www.who.int/patientsafety/medication-safety/en/

Boyd, C. (2013). Student Survival Skills: Calculation Skills for Nurses. Oxford: Wiley-Blackwell.

Carter, B., Bray, L., Dickinson, A. et al. (2014). *Child-centred nursing: Promoting Critical Thinking*. Sage: London.

Griffith, R. and Dowie, I. (2019). Dimond's Legal Aspects of Nursing. A Definitive Guide to Law for Nurses, 8e. London: Pearson.

Lambert, V., Long, T., and Kelleher, D. (2012). *Communication Skills for Children's Nurses*. Berkshire: Open University Press.

Lapham, L. (2015). Drug Calculations for Nurses: A Step-by-step Approach, 4e. London: CRC Press.

Starkings, S. and Krause, L. (2018). *Passing Calculations Test in Nursing*, 4e. London: Sage.

Stewart, M., Purdy, J., Kennedy, N., and Burns, A. (2010). An interprofessional approach to improving medication safety. *BMC Medical Education* 10(19).

Multiple Choice Questions

1. The WHO have identified 5 moments of medication safety. What are they?
   (a) Starting a medication, taking a medication, adding a medication, reviewing a medication, stopping a medication.
   (b) Prescribing a medication, taking a medication, adding a medication, reviewing a medication, stopping a medication.
   (c) Starting a medication, taking a medication, adding a medication, reviewing side effects, stopping a medication.

Chapter 4 Medicines Management and the Role of the Healthcare Provider Working with Children

2. Why did WHO launch the third global patient safety challenge?
  (a) To reduce severe avoidable medication-related harm by 40%, globally in the next 5 years
  (b) To reduce severe avoidable medication-related harm by 50%, globally in the next 5 years
  (c) To reduce severe avoidable medication-related harm by 60%, globally in the next 5 years

3. How should subcutaneous methotrexate be stored?
  (a) In the fridge to keep it cool
  (b) In a cupboard at room temperature
  (c) On a windowsill
  (d) Anywhere it does not matter

4. What are the 5 rights of medication administration?
  (a) Right drug, right route, right time, right dose, right patient
  (b) Right drug, right route, right day, right dose, right patient
  (c) Right drug, right prescription, right day, right dose, right patient

5. Which of the following could transitions of care be in the form of?
  (a) Transition of care to another ward
  (b) Transition of care to another hospital
  (c) Transition of care to home and family
  (d) Transition of care to community services
  (e) All of the above

6. Who is the constant within medicines management?
  (a) The Nurse
  (b) The pharmacist
  (c) The GP
  (d) The CYP and family

7. During transition what contributes to a positive patient experience?:
  (a) Communication
  (b) Coordination of care
  (c) Continuity of care
  (d) All of the above

8. Who is the nurse accountable to first and foremost?
  (a) The NMC
  (b) The patient
  (c) The employer
  (d) Their colleagues

9. Concordance is most likely to be achieved when there is ownership and responsibility from an early age. True or false?
  (a) True
  (b) False

10. Which if the following situations is SBAR useful in?
  (a) Inpatient or outpatient
  (b) Urgent or non-urgent communications
  (c) Conversations between clinicians, either in person or over the phone
  (d) Conversations with peers e.g. nurse to nurse or between different disciplines, e.g. nurse to pharmacist
  (e) Escalating a concern when patients move between NHS services e.g. emergency department to ward.
  (f) All of the above

11. Each year in the NHS in England, approximately how many medication errors' take place?
  (a) 137 million
  (b) 237 million
  (c) 337 million
  (d) 437 million

12. Of these medication errors how many are potentially clinically significant?
  (a) 36 million
  (b) 46 million

(c) 56 million
(d) 66 million

13. Which medication may cause weight gain?
- (a) methotrexate
- (b) prednisolone
- (c) ventolin
- (d) erythromycin

14. When prescribing for children it is critical that an accurate weight is recorded.
- (a) True
- (b) False

15. Investment in patient safety can lead to better patient outcomes.
- (a) True
- (b) False

Find Out More

This further reading will supplement your learning around the role of the healthcare provider. Take some time to write notes about each example, thinking specifically about your role.

GOOD PRACTICE EXAMPLES	YOUR NOTES
Find out more about the KidzMed project – how to teach children to swallow a tablet (Tse et al., 2019).	
Find out more about the responsibilities of being a prescriber.	
Find out more about STOMP which stands for stopping over medication of people with a learning disability, autism or both with psychotropic medicines.	
Find out more about human factors in healthcare.	
Find out more about the rights of the CYP in the United Kingdom.	

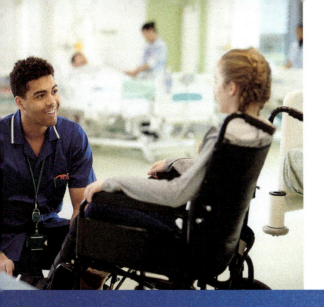

5

Pharmacodynamics and Pharmacokinetics

Barry Hill, Jaden Allan and Claire Camara

Aim

The aim of this chapter is to provide the reader with an introduction to pharmacokinetics and pharmacodynamics in paediatrics and the important issues surrounding medicines management.

Learning Outcomes

After reading this chapter the reader will:

- Acknowledge the professional responsibilities of registered nurses who administer drugs to patients.
- Define and understand the differences between pharmacodynamics and pharmacokinetics
- Understand some of the complexities of pharmacokinetics and pharmacodynamics in relation to paediatric nursing practice.
- Appreciate the complexities of how drugs work differently in every individual.

Test Your Knowledge

1. Describe the professional responsibilities of nurses who administer medications.
2. Define pharmacodynamics.
3. How many phases of pharmacokinetics are there?
4. What are the phases of pharmacokinetics?
5. Identify some of the key considerations for paediatrics.

Fundamentals of Pharmacology for Children's Nurses, First Edition. Edited by Ian Peate and Peter Dryden.
© 2022 John Wiley & Sons Ltd. Published 2022 by John Wiley & Sons Ltd.
Companion website: www.wiley.com/go/pharmacologyforCN

Introduction

This chapter explores the pharmacokinetics and pharmacodynamics of drugs.

Royal Pharmaceutical Society

As new diseases emerge, and older medicines such as antibiotics – no longer work as well as they once did, the contribution of pharmacology to finding better and safer medicines becomes even more significant in order to improve the quality of life for patients. The Royal Pharmaceutical Society (RPS) is the body responsible for the leadership and support of the pharmacy profession within England, Scotland and Wales. The RPS is the leading society within the United Kingdom (UK), and believe that 'Pharmacological knowledge improves the lives of millions of people across the world'. They also recommend all healthcare professionals have pharmacological knowledge, as it 'maximises their benefit and minimises risk and harm' (RPS, 2019). In 2019, the RPS and RCN published the Professional Guidance on the Administration of Medicines in Healthcare Settings (RPS and RCN, 2019). This guidance has replaced all previously published NMC medicines management guidance and should be the key document for all healthcare professionals.

The Nursing and Midwifery Council

The Nursing and Midwifery Council (NMC) who are the regulating body for nurses, nursing associates and midwives; require utilisation of 'critical thinking' and 'clinical judgement' when working with medicines in order to provide patient safety. Registered Nurses should be able to practise as an autonomous professional, exercising their own professional judgement, and should also be able to modify and adapt practice to meet the clinical needs of patients within the emergency and urgent care environment.

Consequently, for nurses to think critically, work within their scope of practice and most importantly improve patient safety when working with medicines, it is imperative that they understand the patients' health condition/s. This is usually in the structure of a medical model including, presenting complaint (PC), history of presenting complaint (HPC), past medical history (PMH), drug history (DH), social history (SH) and acknowledging the patient's (and their families') ideas, concerns and expectations (ICE) when providing pharmacological interventions and treatments (Bickley, 2017).

When nurses directly prepare, administer or have any input into pharmacology and medicines management, it is vital that they understand how medicines work and how they will affect the patient receiving medicinal treatment. The two most popular and well-published terms that are used to explore the effects of medications are pharmacokinetics and pharmacodynamics.

Pharmacokinetics

In its most basic form, pharmacokinetics is 'what the body does to drugs'. Pharmacokinetics can be considered as four processes: absorption, distribution, metabolism and excretion (ADME) of drugs (Young and Pitcher, 2016), and their corresponding pharmacological, therapeutic, or toxic responses in humans and animals.

Pharmacokinetic Principles (the ADME Process)

Pharmacokinetics describes the influence that the human body has on drugs foreign chemicals over time (Young and Pitcher, 2016). The key concerns of pharmacokinetics are what the body does to the drug, how drugs are absorbed by the body, how they are distributed to the tissues, how drugs are metabolised by the body (with the liver being the primary organ for metabolisation of drugs) and elimination (primarily by the kidneys and lungs) (see Box 5.1).

Pharmacokinetics is important to our understanding of why drugs are administered via different routes. For example, why is a drug administered orally (PO) via tablet or liquid suspension form, or into the tissues by subcutaneous injection (SC), intramuscularly (IM), or directly into the bloodstream by intro venous (IV) injection? See Chapter 6 for a discussion of drug formulations.

> **Box 5.1 Four Stages of Pharmacokinetics: ADME**
> 1. Absorption of drugs into the body — How does it get into the body?
> 2. Distribution of drugs to the tissues of the body — Where will it go?
> 3. Metabolism of drugs into the body — How is it broken down?
> 4. Elimination of drugs from the body — How does it leave?

Pharmacokinetics also helps us appreciate the frequency of drug administration, for example: why are some drugs are administered once a day and others administered twice a day, three times a day or four times a day, or even continuously via SC, IM or IV infusion via a mechanical pump? When thinking about the organs that work with drugs during the process of ADME, it becomes clear why absent, or diseased, or aged organs would have an effect on the metabolisation of drugs.

Figure 5.1 integrates the four main features of pharmacokinetics (ADME) and the main routes or administration of medication. Note that the IV route bypasses absorption and the topical route is used to achieve a local effect and minimise absorption.

Phase 1: Absorption

Absorption is defined as the process by which a drug proceeds from the site of administration to the site of measurement (usually blood, plasma or serum). Absorption is the process of a drug/s entering the blood circulation. Le (2017) suggests that drug absorption is determined by the drug's physicochemical properties, formulation and route of administration, i.e. enteral or parenteral. Dosage forms (e.g. tablets, capsules, solutions), consisting of the drug plus other ingredients, are formulated to be given by various routes (e.g. oral, buccal, sublingual, rectal, parenteral, topical, inhalational). Regardless of the route of administration,

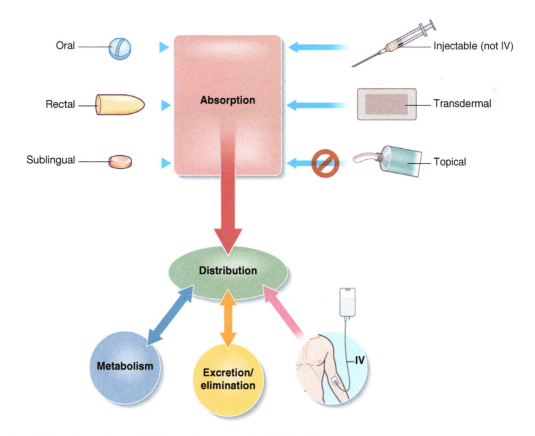

Figure 5.1 An integration of ADME and the routes of administration. Young and Pitcher, 2016/John Wiley & Sons.

drugs must be in solution to be absorbed. Thus, solid forms (e.g. tablets) must be able to disintegrate and disaggregate.

Unless given IV, a drug must cross several semipermeable cell membranes before it reaches the systemic circulation. Cell membranes are biological barriers that selectively inhibit passage of drug molecules (Figure 5.2). Being selectively semipermeable means that the cell can allow in or out the products it needs to function without allowing in or retaining the products it does not need. The membranes are composed differently, which determines membrane permeability characteristics.

How Drugs Cross the Cell Membrane

Many drugs need to pass through one or more cell membranes to reach their site of action. A common feature of all cell membranes is a phospholipid bilayer, about 10 nanometres thick. Spanning this bilayer or attached to the outer or inner leaflets are glycoproteins, which may act as ion channels, receptors, intermediate messengers (G-proteins) or enzymes.

Cells obtain molecules and ions (for example sodium or potassium) from the extracellular fluid, creating a constant in and out flow. The interesting thing about cell membranes is that relative concentrations and phospholipid bilayers prevent essential ions from entering the cell. Therefore, for drugs to move across the membrane, these problems must be addressed. In general, this is completed by facilitated diffusion or active transport. In facilitated diffusion, relative concentrations are used to transport in and out. Active transports uses energy (ATP) to transfer molecules and ions in and out of the cell.

The Concept of Drugs Crossing the Cell Membrane

Cellular signals cross the membrane through a process called signal transduction. This three-step process proceeds when a specific message encounters the outside surface of the cell and makes direct contact with a receptor.

1. A receptor is a specialised molecule that takes information from the environment and passes it throughout various parts of the cell.
2. Next, a connecting switch molecule, transducer, passes the message inward, closer to the cell.
3. Finally, the signal gets amplified, therefore causing the cell to perform a specific function. These functions can include moving, producing more proteins, or even sending out more signals.

Methods of Drug Movement Across the Cell Membrane
Passive Transport

The most common method for drugs to cross the cell membrane is by passive diffusion. Drug molecules will diffuse down its concentration gradient without expenditure of energy by the cell. A gradient simply means a lack of balance in the molecules (there are more in one place than another) moving down the gradient is the molecule being distributed more evenly. However, the membranes are selectively permeable, so the membrane has different effects on the rate of diffusion on different drug molecules. The rate of diffusion also can

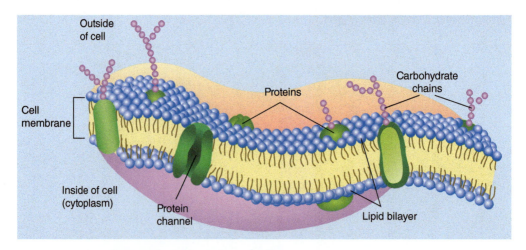

Figure 5.2 A visual representation of cell membrane layers.

Chapter 5 Pharmacodynamics and Pharmacokinetics

be enhanced by transport proteins in the membrane by facilitated diffusion. There are two types of transport proteins that carry out the facilitated diffusion: channel protein and carrier protein.

Active Transport

Active transport is an energy-requiring process. There are also two types of active transport: primary active transport and secondary active transport.

1. Primary active transport directly uses energy to transport molecules across a membrane.
2. Secondary active transport or co-transport also uses energy to transport molecules across a membrane.

Absorption depends on the administration route and can either be: *enteral*, entering the gastrointestinal (GI) tract, either by oral administration, feeding tubes, or rectal suppositories; or *parenteral*, not into the GI tract, such as via injection or topical medicine (for example creams or patches).

To be absorbed, a drug given orally must survive encounters with low pH and numerous GI secretions, including potentially degrading enzymes. Peptide drugs (e.g. insulin) are particularly susceptible to degradation and are not given orally. Absorption of oral drugs involves transport across membranes of the epithelial cells in the GI tract. Absorption is affected by:

- Differences in pH along the GI tract
- Surface area per luminal volume
- Blood perfusion
- Presence of bile and mucus
- The nature of epithelial membranes

The oral mucosa has a thin epithelium and rich vascularity (thus a thin barrier and good perfusion), which favour absorption; however, contact is usually too brief for substantial absorption. A drug placed between the gums and cheek (buccal administration) or under the tongue (sublingual administration) is retained longer, enhancing absorption.

The stomach has a relatively large epithelial surface, but its thick mucous layer and short transit time limit absorption. Because most absorption occurs in the small intestine, gastric emptying is often the rate-limiting step, differences in gastric emptying due to child development make this important in paediatric medicine (see Table 5.1). Food, especially fatty food, slows gastric emptying (and rate of drug absorption), explaining why taking some drugs on an empty stomach speeds absorption. Drugs that affect gastric emptying (e.g. parasympatholytic drugs) affect the absorption rate of other drugs. Food may enhance the extent of absorption for poorly soluble drugs (e.g. griseofulvin), reduce it for drugs degraded in the stomach (e.g. penicillin G) or have little or no effect.

The small intestine has the largest surface area for drug absorption in the GI tract and its membranes are more permeable than those in the stomach. For these reasons, most drugs are absorbed primarily in the small intestine. The intraluminal pH is 4 to 5 in the duodenum but becomes progressively more alkaline, approaching 8 in the lower ileum. GI microflora may reduce absorption. Decreased blood flow (e.g. in shock) may lower the concentration gradient across the intestinal mucosa and reduce absorption by passive diffusion. Intestinal transit time can also influence drug absorption, particularly for drugs that are absorbed by active transport (e.g. B vitamins), that dissolve slowly (e.g. griseofulvin) or that are polar (i.e. with low lipid solubility; e.g. many antibiotics). It is expected that the gastrointestinal tract of children is mature by 6 months and therefore in children and adults absorption should occur similarly; however, there are specific considerations with variable evidence (see Table 5.1)

Table 5.1 Pharmacokinetics of paracetamol.

A	Paracetamol can be given orally, via and enteral feeding device, rectally or intravenously. When taken enterally, it is absorbed in the gastrointestinal tract. Bioavailability is 70–90%. Dependent on gastric emptying.
D	It is distributed to all tissues of the body. In pregnant women, it does cross the placenta to the foetus. It is also passed through breastmilk to a nursing infant. Peak plasma concentration occurs between 30 and 120 minutes after the initial dose.
M	Approximately 90–95% is metabolised in the liver. Half-life can vary between 1 and 4 hours.
E	It is then excreted by the kidneys.

Chapter 5 Pharmacodynamics and Pharmacokinetics

To maximise adherence, clinicians should prescribe oral suspensions and chewable tablets for children less than 8 years, although innovative practice can train young children to swallow tablets whole (Tse et al., 2019). In adolescents and adults, most drugs are given orally as tablets or capsules primarily for convenience, economy, stability and patient acceptance. Because solid drug forms must dissolve before absorption can occur, dissolution rate determines availability of the drug for absorption. Dissolution, if slower than absorption, becomes the rate-limiting step. Manipulating the formulation (i.e. the drug's form as salt, crystal or hydrate) can change the dissolution rate and thus control overall absorption.

Enteral

Enteral medicines are medicines that enter the GI tract. Oral medicines, such as a tablet or liquid suspension, would normally be administered into the mouth of the patient and would pass into their GI tract. If the oral route is not an option, enteral medications may also be administered via nasogastric tube (NGT) or orogastric tube (OGT). From here, medicine would be absorbed via the GI tract wall and would enter plasma. Any substances that are absorbed via the GI wall will be transported by plasma to the liver via the hepatic portal vein (HPV); this is completed prior to being delivered to the body's tissues and organs. In pharmacology, this process is known as the first-pass metabolism.

Clinical Consideration

If a patient in is taking medications enterally and has or develops changes to their gastrointestinal functioning (for example, diarrhoea or vomiting) this may affect the absorption of their medication. If a patient has a newly fitted enteral device that bypasses part of the gastrointestinal tract (for example, a percutaneous endoscopic jejunostomy, also known as PEJ) this is also likely to affect absorption.

Two drugs given together may change the absorption of either one or both of the drugs. For example, a drug that may change the acidity for the stomach acid is likely to affect a drug that is dissolved in the stomach. Other drugs can interact and form an insoluble compound that cannot be absorbed. Sometimes an absorption interaction can be avoided by separating the administration of each drug by at least 2 hours (Scott and McGrath, 2004).

Parenteral

Drugs given IV enter the systemic circulation directly. However, drugs injected IM or SC must cross one or more biological membranes to reach the systemic circulation. If protein drugs with a molecular mass > 20,000 g/mol are injected IM or SC, movement across capillary membranes is so slow that most absorption occurs via the lymphatic system. In such cases, drug delivery to systemic circulation is slow and often incomplete because of first-pass metabolism (metabolism of a drug before it reaches systemic circulation) by proteolytic enzymes in the lymphatics.

Perfusion (blood flow/gram of tissue) greatly affects capillary absorption of small molecules injected IM or sc. Thus, injection site can affect absorption rate. Absorption after IM or SC injection may be delayed or erratic for salts of poorly soluble bases and acids (e.g., parenteral form of phenytoin) and in patients with poor peripheral perfusion (e.g., during hypotension or shock).

Topical

Applying medication to the skin or mucous membranes allows it to enter the body from there. Medication applied in this way is known as topical medication. It can also be used to treat pain or other problems in specific parts of the body.

Topical medication can also be used to nourish the skin and protect it from harm. Some topical medications are used for local treatment and some are meant to affect the whole body after being absorbed through the skin.

Additional factors that can affect how the drug is absorbed is from the drugs formation, extended release versus immediate release. Blood flow to the area of absorption and GI motility for enteral medications. A common example of enteral medication would be Ibuprofen. Common parenteral medications include insulin and heparin. Some medications, such as penicillin, have both enteral and parenteral formulations. See Table 5.2 and Figure 5.8.

Table 5.2 Factors that affect absorption of drugs.

ROUTE	FACTORS AFFECTING ABSORPTION
Intravenous (IV)	None: direct entry into the venous system
Intramuscular (IM)	Perfusion of blood flow to the muscle Fat content of the muscle Temperature of the muscle: cold causes vasoconstriction and decreases absorption; heat causes vasodilation and increases absorption
Subcutaneous (SC)	Perfusion of blood flow to the tissues Fat content of the tissue Temperature of the tissue: cold causes vasoconstriction and decreases absorption; heat causes vasodilation and increases absorption.
Oral (PO)	Acidity of the stomach Length of time in the stomach Blow flow to the gastrointestinal tract Presence of interacting foods or drugs
Rectal (PR)	Perfusion of blood flow to the rectum Lesions in the rectum Length of time retained for absorption
Mucous membranes (sublingual, buccal)	Perfusion or blood flow to the area Integrity of mucous membranes Presence of food or smoking Length of time retained in area
Topical (skin)	Perfusion or blood flow to the area Integrity of skin
Inhalation	Perfusion or blood flow to the area Integrity of lung lining Ability to administer drug properly

Source: Karch, 2017/Wolters Kluwer

Phase 2: Distribution

Distribution is the drug's dispersion through the body's fluids and tissues as it travels to its site of action (usually blood or plasma). This is dependent on blood flow, both to the area of where the drug is to be administered and how perfusion occurs to other areas of the patient's body, as well as protein binding. If a drug binds to protein, they become attached and therefore the drug cannot exert its effect on the body. The more a drug binds to protein, the less of the drug there is available for distribution.

Protein Binding

Most drugs are bound to proteins in the blood and transported around the body by venous circulation. When drugs have bound to protein, they become enlarged and cannot enter capillaries and then into tissues to react. Some drugs are tightly bound and are released slowly, meaning that they have a longer duration of action as they are not broken down or excreted by the kidneys. Some drugs are in competition with other drugs at the same protein binding site, which will change the effectiveness of the drug, or causing toxicity when two or more drugs of the same group are administer together (Karch, 2017).

Blood–Brain Barrier

The blood–brain barrier (BBB) prevents entry into the brain of most drugs from the blood, in neonates and premature infants the BBB may not yet have matured. The BBB is a protective system of cellular activity that keeps many things such as foreign invaders and poisons. Drugs that are highly lipid-soluble are more likely to pass through the BBB and reach the central nervous system (CNS). Drugs that are not lipid-soluble are not able to pass the BBB. This is clinically significant in treating brain infections. For example, antibodies are too large to cross the blood–brain barrier and only certain antibiotics can pass. The blood–brain barrier becomes more permeable during inflammation, allowing antibiotics and phagocytes to move across the BBB. However,

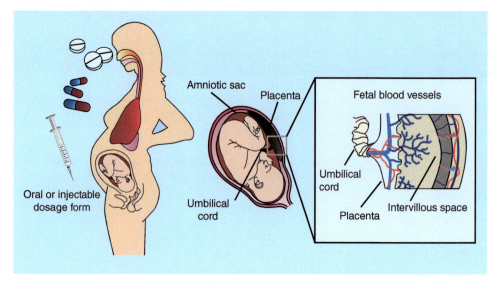

Figure 5.3 **Medication delivery to infant during gestation.**

this also allows bacteria and viruses to infiltrate the blood–brain barrier. Most antibiotics are not lipid-soluble and therefore cannot treat brain infections as they are unable to cross the BBB. IV medications such as Rifampicin would be used in such cases. The presence of the BBB makes difficult the development of new treatments of brain diseases, or new radiopharmaceuticals for neuroimaging of brain. All of the products of biotechnology are large-molecule drugs that do not cross the BBB.

Placenta and Breast Milk

The placenta is the lifeline of the developing foetus (Figure 5.3). It is a semipermeable barrier through which all nutrients and waste products must pass. Several factors affect a medication's ability to cross the placenta, although many drugs are transported by passive diffusion based on the concentration gradient. Conversely, if a medication is hydrophilic, ionised in maternal serum and highly protein-bound, little to no medication will cross. If there is little to no published safety data for a medication, the pharmacist can evaluate these details of a medication to predict the possibility of foetal exposure.

The transfer of medication into human milk shares some of the same principles as crossing the placenta, with most by passive diffusion. A medication may cross through the placenta into foetal circulation and back on the concentration gradient, just as a drug may pass into milk and diffuse back into the bloodstream as serum concentrations decrease. Certain properties of some medications may cause them to be sequestered into or actively excreted into breast milk (Hale, 2012). Drugs should only be given to pregnant women when the benefit clearly outweighs any risk. Drugs are likely to be secreted into breast milk and therefore have the potential to affect the neonate. All drugs must be checked prior to administration, this includes utilising the British National Formulary (BNF), organisation-approved guidelines and published medication guides that are up to date and based on the appropriate patient groups you are caring for, i.e. renal and liver patients have different ADME needs, paediatric patients required weight-based doses, UK-based material for the population you are caring for. By better understanding the pharmacokinetics and pharmacodynamics of medications during lactation, Nurses can assist mothers in making well-informed decisions about medication use during lactation. The most important factor in infant exposure through breast milk is the amount of medication in the mother's serum.

Phase 3: Metabolism (Biotransformation)

Metabolism, sometimes referred to as biotransformation, is the recognition by the body that the drug is present and the transformation of the drug into usable parts. Most drugs are metabolised in the liver via the cytochrome P450 family of enzymes. Other organs may include the kidneys and intestines.

Drugs can be metabolised by oxidation, reduction, hydrolysis, hydration, conjugation, condensation or isomerisation; whatever the process, the goal is to make the drug easier to excrete. The enzymes involved in metabolism are present in many tissues but generally are more concentrated in the liver. Drug metabolism rates vary among patients. Some patients metabolise a drug so rapidly that therapeutically effective blood and tissue concentrations are not reached; in others, metabolism may be so slow that usual doses have toxic effects. Individual drug metabolism rates are influenced by genetic factors, coexisting disorders (particularly chronic liver disorders and advanced heart failure) and drug interactions (especially those involving induction or inhibition of metabolism).

For many drugs, metabolism occurs in two phases.

- Phase I reactions involve formation of a new or modified functional group or cleavage (oxidation, reduction, hydrolysis); these reactions are non-synthetic.
- Phase II reactions involve conjugation with an endogenous substance (e.g. glucuronic acid, sulfate, glycine); these reactions are synthetic. Metabolites formed in synthetic reactions are more polar and thus more readily excreted by the kidneys (in urine) and the liver (in bile) than those formed in non-synthetic reactions. Some drugs undergo only phase I or phase II reactions; thus, phase numbers reflect functional rather than sequential classification.

According to Young and Pitcher (2017) certain drugs only undergo phase I metabolism, others only phase II metabolism and some drugs undergo no metabolism at all. Some drugs underdo phase II metabolism and then phase I. Certain drugs – such as levodopa, used to treat Parkinson' disease, are inactive in the body until some biotransformation takes place. These drugs are known as pro-drugs. Certain drugs, such as the antidepressant fluoxetine, are transformed into metabolites that are also active and these metabolites are partially responsible for the therapeutic activity of the drug agent.

Rate
For almost all drugs, the metabolism rate in any given pathway has an upper limit (capacity limitation). However, at the therapeutic concentrations of most drugs, usually only a small fraction of the metabolising enzyme's sites are occupied and the metabolism rate increases with drug concentration (Le, 2019). In such cases, called first-order elimination (or kinetics), the metabolism rate of the drug is a constant fraction of the drug remaining in the body (i.e., the drug has a specific half-life).

First-Pass Metabolism
The first-pass effect (also known as first-pass metabolism or pre-systemic metabolism) (Figure 5.4) was coined by Rowland (1972) to be a phenomenon of drug metabolism whereby the concentration of a drug is greatly reduced before it reaches the systemic circulation.

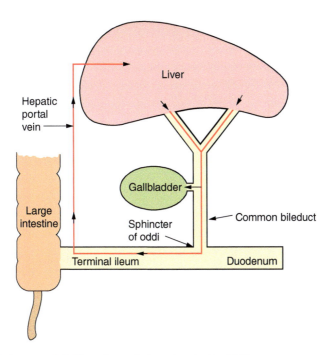

Figure 5.4 **Hepatic first pass metabolism.** *Source:* Redrawn from Rowland 1972.

The process of drug metabolism is part of the body's normal response to removal of drugs and chemicals from the system. Hepatic metabolism, or biotransformation, is the main site and method of the process of elimination. This is followed by excretion of the drug and its metabolites from the body. The liver plays an extremely important role in drug removal. When drug molecules are distributed in the blood stream, the plasma flow through the functional units of the liver present these molecules for biotransformation. This occurs after administration by any route.

The oral route of drug administration is by far the most commonly used route of giving medication to patients. It is accessible and least invasive for many patients, well tolerated and convenient. Many common drugs are available in oral formulations as well as in presentations suitable for administration by other routes. There are very few drugs in the British National Formulary (BNF) that have no oral formulation.

Hepatic First-Pass Effect

Drugs given by the oral route are absorbed from the stomach and the small intestine into the hepatic portal vein. This blood vessel goes directly to the liver. The process of biotransformation begins and the drug will start to be metabolised in preparation for excretion from the body. The drug molecules in the plasma move through the system. The drug molecules are now metabolised by the liver enzymes in the normal fashion. This 'first-pass effect' reduces the fraction of the dose administered, which then goes on to reach the systemic circulation and become available for therapeutic effect. This process occurs in the hepatic microsomal enzymes and includes the cytochrome P450 enzymes. For drugs given orally, the amount of first pass metabolism known to occur has been factored into oral dosing by the pharmaceutical companies, usually based on information found in clinical trials (see Box 5.2). This means that the bioavailability, which is a known factor, has been considered when dose and dose ranges are advised in the BNF. It is important, therefore, for the prescriber to be aware of any hepatic dysfunction when prescribing oral drugs. If there is compromised liver function or disease such as cirrhosis, then first pass metabolism will be compromised. This could lead to more active drug entering the systemic circulation due to the reduced liver enzyme functionality and may cause side effects, adverse effects or toxicity. Drug dosing may need to be reduced in patients in this situation. Some drugs are destroyed by liver enzyme systems at this first pass stage and will not enter the general systemic circulation. Not all oral drugs are destroyed by the liver at first pass, but many clinically significant drugs do undergo an extensive first pass effect. Therefore, the doses of some drugs are considerably higher when given by the oral route compared to their dosing if given intravenously.

1. The drug is absorbed by the GI tract.
2. Drug absorbed from the gastrointestinal tract travels immediately to the liver through the hepatic portal vein.
3. The first pass effect occurs at this stage. Hepatic first pass occurs when drug absorbed from the gastrointestinal tract is metabolised by enzymes within the liver to such an extent that most of the active agent does not exit the liver and, therefore, does not reach the systemic circulation.
4. The remaining drug is distributed around the body within blood cells and plasma.

Phase 4: Elimination

Elimination is the irreversible loss of drug from the site of measurement (blood, serum, plasma). Elimination of drugs occur by one or both of:

- Metabolism
- Excretion

Excretion

Excretion is the irreversible loss of a drug in a chemically unchanged or unaltered form. The two principal organs responsible for drug elimination are the kidney and the liver (see Figure 5.5). The kidney is the primary site for removal of a drug in a chemically unaltered or unchanged form (i.e. excretion) as well as for metabolites. The liver is the primary organ where drug metabolism occurs. The lungs, occasionally, may be an important route of elimination for substances of high vapour pressure (i.e. gaseous anaesthetics, alcohol, etc.). Another potential route of drug removal is via mother's milk. Although not a significant route for elimination of a drug for the mother, the drug may be consumed in enough quantity to affect the infant.

Box 5.2 Clinical Trials and Off-Label Medication Use in Paediatrics

Historically there has been a reticence to complete clinical trials with paediatric populations (Medical Research Council, 2004), thus though drugs may have a reliable scientific basis (Corny et al., 2016), paucity of robust trials leads to a lack of specific (such as pharmacokinetics and pharmacodynamics) drug information (Ginsberg et al., 2001; Anderson et al., 2006). In turn, this leads to off-label prescribing being commonplace in paediatric healthcare (Edington et al., 2006; McLay et al., 2006). Regulation in the EU (Regulation EC No 1901/2006) and America (Christensen, 2012) aimed to ensure that new medications were also trialled for paediatric populations. Yet studies continue to report varying prevalence of off-label or unlicensed prescribing for paediatrics worldwide (Khdour et al., 2011; Slažneva et al., 2012; Ribeiro et al., 2013; Czarniak at al., 2015; Jouret-Descout et al., 2015; Corny et al., 2016)

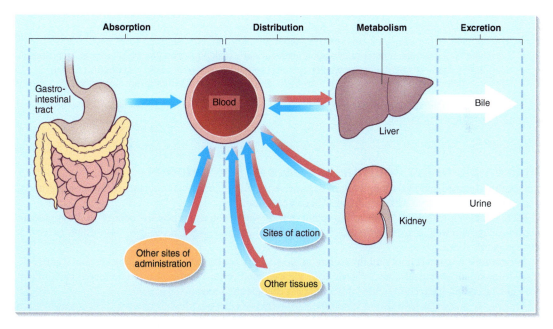

Figure 5.5 **Pharmacokinetics (ADME) and the main anatomical structures/physiological systems that are responsible for executing those processes.** *Source:* Young and Pritchard 2016/John Wiley & Sons.

Think Paediatrics

Following the overview of the ADME process there are key considerations in the following think paediatrics table contains specific differences to think about pertaining to paediatrics. It is well documented that paediatric patients are not simply small adults, due to maturational differences of infants, children and young people there are additional layers of complexity for paediatric pharmacokinetics.

A   Neonates and infants can have a less acidic gastric pH which then may change the absorption of the drug. The acidity continues into to increase in childhood until pH and transit time are similar to that of an adult around age 8 (Fallingborg et al., 1990; Nagita et al., 1996; Yu et al., 2014). Although the lability of the pH is varies across different literature (Van den Abeele et al., 2018). In addition, pH gastric fluid differences in osmolality and contents such as bile salts can also affect absorption (Van den Abeele et al., 2018). Literature varies on gastric emptying in neonates, for both preterm and term babies, with some evidence that intake has a more significant effect on gastric emptying than age or size (Anderson and Holford, 2013). Furthermore, there is a paucity of evidence relating to permeability of paediatric intestinal tract (Batchelor et al., 2014).

D	Body composition changes within the first year; until approximately 4 months (in infants born at term), water accounts for 70–80% of body weight (10–20% higher than that of an adult). In addition to body weight composition, neonates and preterm infants are unlikely to have a mature blood–brain barrier, potentially allowing filtration of molecules into the central nervous system.
M	There are two key enzymes within the 450 system, CYP1A2 and CYP3A4, these are responsible for the majority of drug breakdown. These enzymes vary in activity from very low in neonates, then higher in early and middle childhood than in adolescence and adulthood (Choonara and Sammons, 2014).
E	The majority of drugs are excreted by the kidneys. Rodieux et al. (2015) cite three primary considerations for kidney function during the elimination phase in paediatrics: • immature glomerular filtration and tubular function; • reduced kidney perfusion pressure; • inadequate osmotic load to produce full counter-current effects. As blood flow to the kidneys increases the glomerular filtration rate (GRF) also increases, the GFR also increases, reaches a peak above adult levels in early childhood and gradually reduces to normal adult levels again. Recognising the challenges of obtaining an accurate GFR or estimated GFR in neonatal patients, Muhari-Stark and Burchart (2018) discuss a range of different approaches.

N.B. As is apparent from the variability in literature, these are important considerations but always need to be viewed in context of the patient, their signs and symptoms.

An Example of the Pharmacokinetics of Paracetamol

Paracetamol is a medication frequently used in paediatrics as an antipyretic or analgesic. For consideration of the pharmacokinetics we will assume it has been given orally.

This can be seen with medication such as paracetamol, where you can repeat the dose of 1g (or appropriate dose for age and weight) every 4 to 6 hours (Figure 5.6). Greater dosages can be toxic as you have exceeded the therapeutic index.

The example of paracetamol and ibuprofen (subject to any contraindications) can be seen in Figure 5.7, where to maintain therapeutic level (black line) the two medications are used to complement each other, while not exceeding the recommended dose and thus therapeutic index.

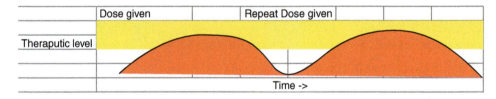

Figure 5.6 Therapeutic range.

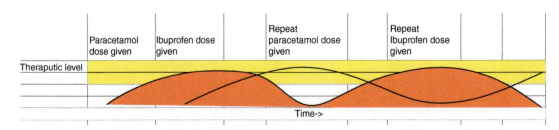

Figure 5.7 Paracetamol and ibuprofen maintain therapeutic level.

Clinical Consideration

Half-Life

The half-life of medication is how long it takes for the medication to be reduced by half of its blood concentration level. This is done through metabolisation. It can be affected by the individual's ability to metabolise, such as if the patient has renal failure and liver damage.

Clinical Consideration

Steady State

A steady state (SS) is when the amount of drug administered is equal to the amount of drug eliminated within one dose interval, resulting in a plateau or constant serum drug level. Drugs with a short half-life reach steady state rapidly, whilst drugs with long half-life can take days to weeks to reach a steady state.

Clinical Consideration

Termination of Action

A termination of action is when the medication has stopped its action at the site of requirement. This may be seen in analgesic control; when the pain returns, the medication has stopped acting.

Clinical Consideration

Therapeutic Range

A therapeutic range is similar to therapeutic index. It is the range area where the medication is effective for the individual. Linking back to analgesic control, it is the period from when pain is blocked to when it returns.

Pharmacodynamics

Pharmacodynamics explores what the drug does to the body, and specifically how the drug molecules interact within the body, what they interact with and how they cause their effects (Young and Pitcher, 2016: 21). To expand on this, a drug exerts its biological effects by interacting with the receptors located on tissues and organs throughout the body. The effects of the drug are dependent upon the drug's ability to bind to a variety of the body's receptors (Scott and McGrath, 2009). For example, if a drug's concentration is increased where many receptors are located, the intensity of the drug's effect will be improved. Therefore, the pharmacological response depends on the drugs ability to bind to its target. The concentration of the drug at the receptor site influences the drug's effect.

One of the key challenges for nurses when studying pharmacodynamics is that the drugs are affected by a patient's physiological changes, such as disease, genetic mutations, ageing and/or other drugs. These changes are likely to alter the level of binding proteins, or decrease receptor sensitivity (Campbell and Cohall, 2017). It is important that nurses recognise that some drugs acting on the same receptor (or tissue) differ in the magnitude of the biological responses that they can achieve (i.e. their 'efficacy') and the amount of the drug required to achieve a response (i.e. their 'potency'). Drug receptors can be classified based on their selective response to different drugs. Constant exposure of receptors or body systems to drugs sometimes leads to a reduced response, for example, desensitisation. There is also far less evidence of pharmacodynamics in paediatric patients (Choonara and Sammons, 2014).

All medications act in one of four ways (Karch, 2017):

1. To replace or act as a substitute for missing chemicals
2. To increase or stimulate certain cellular activities
3. To depress or slow cellular activities
4. To interfere with the functioning of foreign cells, such as invading microorganisms or neoplasms leading to cell death (drugs that act in this way are called chemotherapeutic agents).

Agonists and Antagonists

The terms 'agonist' (a molecule that binds to a receptor causing activation and resultant cellular changes) and 'antagonist' (a molecule that attenuates the action of an agonist) apply only to receptors (see Figures 5.8 and 5.9).

Agonist

An agonist is an example of a drug that interacts with receptors. Agonist drugs are attracted to receptors and stimulate them. Once stimulation has occurred, the agonist binds to the receptor and the drug effect occurs; the outcome of this activity is known as intrinsic activity. Agonists can be full, partial or inverse. Some drugs act on a variety of receptors. These are known as non-selective and can cause multiple and widespread effects (Scott and McGrath, 2004).

Pleuvry (2004) notes that a full agonist can produce the largest response that the tissue can give. The term 'efficacy' has been used to describe the way that agonists can vary in the response they produce even when occupying the same number of receptors. A high-efficacy agonist produces a maximum response even when occupying a small proportion of the available receptors. The magnitude of response to an agonist is usually proportional to the fraction of receptors that are occupied. As the concentration of an agonist at its site of action increases, so the fraction of occupied receptors rises and, in turn, the magnitude of response rises. A partial agonist cannot fully activate the receptors, irrespective of the concentration available. In contrast to a full agonist, a partial agonist cannot exert a maximal response. Finally, the simplest definition if an inverse agonist is that the compound binds to a receptor but it produces the opposite effect to an accepted agonist.

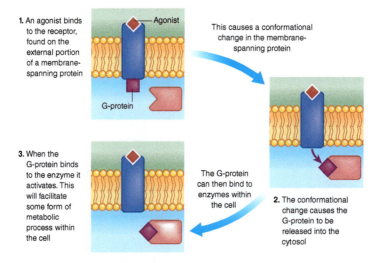

Figure 5.8 The step-by-step process of s second messenger system. *Source*: Young and Pritchard 2016/John Wiley & Sons.

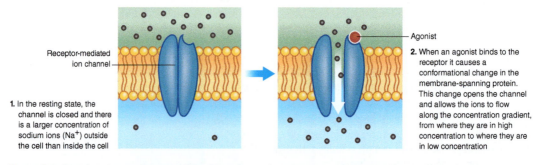

Figure 5.9 Step-by-step receptor-mediated ion channel. *Source*: Young and Pritchard 2016/John Wiley & Sons.

Chapter 5 Pharmacodynamics and Pharmacokinetics

Table 5.3 Examples of opioid by receptor binding.

FULL AGONIST	PARTIAL AGONIST	MIXED AGONIST	ANTAGONIST (ALSO KNOWN AS BLOCKERS OR REVERSALS)
Codeine	Buprenorphine	Buprenorphine	Naloxone
Fentanyl	Butorphanol	Butorphanol	Naltrexone
Heroin	Pentazocine	Nalbuphine	
Hydrocodone	Tramadol	Pentazocine	
Hydromorphone			
Levorphanol			
Meperidine			
Methadone			
Morphine			
Oxycodone			
Oxymorphone			

An example of a widely used agonist is salbutamol. Salbutamol is a beta-2 agonist. One easy way to remember the location of beta-1 and beta-2 cells simply and quickly is that humans have 1 heart and 2 lungs. Beta-1 cells are mainly based around the heart (1 heart) and beta-2 cells are mainly based around the lungs (2 lungs). Therefore, salbutamol, being a beta-2 agonist, would have its main effects on the receptors based within the lungs. Beta-1 receptors, along with beta-2, alpha-1 and alpha-2 receptors, are adrenergic receptors primarily responsible for signalling in the sympathetic nervous system. Beta agonists bind to the beta receptors on various tissues throughout the body. Beta-2 agonists are used for both asthma and COPD, although some types are only available for COPD. Beta-2 agonists work by stimulating beta-2 receptors in the muscles that line the airways, which causes them to relax and allows the airways to widen (dilate). This is why Salbutamol is known as a bronchodilator.

Using opioids as an example, Table 5.3 gives examples of opioid by receptor binding.

Antagonists

In opposition of an agonist is an antagonist. An antagonist is a type of receptor ligand or drug that blocks or dampens a biological response by binding to and blocking a receptor rather than activating it like an agonist. They are sometimes called blockers; examples include alpha blockers, beta blockers and calcium channel blockers.

Antagonists can be competitive or non-competitive:

- A competitive antagonist binds to the same site as the agonist but does not activate it, thus blocks the agonist's action.
- A non-competitive antagonist binds to an allosteric (non-agonist) site on the receptor to prevent activation of the receptor.

Episode of Care

Chris is a 15-year-old with Duchenne Muscular Dystrophy. DMD is a muscle wasting disease caused by mutation of dystrophin producing genes. There is no curative treatment currently available for DMD but corticosteroids are commonly prescribed from an early age in an attempt to prolong muscle function. Deflazecort is the preferred option but prednisolone is also still widely used (Birnkrant et al., 2018). Chris began taking prednisolone one year ago and also takes vitamin D daily. Mum is with Chris and is struggling with his weight gain and hyperactivity in the evenings.

Clinical Consideration

The side effects of medication can be wide-ranging, especially when you start a new medication. As a registrant you must understand medicines management, including side effects and monitoring the effects of medication. You should report/take action where there is a possible or actual side effect. This is often the patient's body becoming used to the medication, but it is important to ensure you keep in contact with the prescribing professional, GP or hospital staff.

Chapter 5 Pharmacodynamics and Pharmacokinetics

While there are a range of side effects associated with prednisolone such as (but not limited to) adrenal insufficiency, diarrhoea, dyslipidaemia, lipomatosis, protein catabolism, scleroderma, renal crisis, irritability, mood swings insomnia (JNF, 2020), there are also specific concerns for the paediatric practitioner. Prolonged corticosteroid use may cause impairment of the endocrine system, with compromised linear growth (height) and delayed onset puberty. Both require referral and treatment by an endocrinologist (Birnkrant et al., 2018).

To improve concordance discussion with parents and caregivers is crucial to minimise disruption to lifestyle; for example, taking steroid doses in the morning, ensuring a healthy diet to minimise weight gain or being aware of the importance of reporting vomiting.

Therapeutic Index

A therapeutic index is the range in which a medication is therapeutic to the individual. A drug with a low or narrow therapeutic index has a narrow range of safety between an effective dose and a lethal one. Alternatively, a drug with a high therapeutic index will have a wide range of safety and fewer risks of toxic effects. It should be noted that doubling a dose of a drug does not mean that the therapeutic effect will be doubled but will most likely double the toxic effect. Furthermore, administration above the dose at which the maximum effect is observed will produce no added benefit.

Therapeutic range will rise and fall depending on the medication formulation, its strength and the time it has until it is broken down and metabolised within the body. This process can be affected by the patient's health and organ condition/s, particularly the patient's liver and kidney function. Although metabolism typically inactivates drugs, some drug metabolites are pharmacologically active. An inactive or weakly active substance that has an active metabolite is called a prodrug, especially if designed to deliver the active moiety more effectively.

Some medication has what is called a Narrow Therapeutic Index (NTI), meaning the gap between effective and toxic effect is small. Some examples of drugs that are known to have an NTI can be seen in Table 5.4. Slight changes in medication dose or blood concentration level need to be carefully monitored and recorded.

Table 5.4 Narrow Therapeutic Index examples.

DRUG NAME	INDICATION	DRUG GROUP
Phenytoin	Tonic-clonic seizures, Focal seizures	Anticonvulsants
Carbamazepine	Focal and secondary generalised tonic-clonic seizures, Primary generalised tonic-clonic seizures	Anticonvulsants
Gentamicin	Infection	Aminoglycoside antibiotics
Vancomycin	Infection	Glycopeptide antibiotics
Teicoplanin	Serious infections caused by Gram-positive bacteria	Glycopeptide antibiotics
Lithium	Treatment and prophylaxis of mania, Treatment and prophylaxis of bipolar disorder, Treatment and prophylaxis of recurrent depression, Treatment and prophylaxis of aggressive or self-harming behaviour	Antimanic agents
Digoxin	Rapid digitalisation, for atrial fibrillation or flutter	Cardiac glycosides
Aminophylline and theophylline	Severe acute asthma or severe acute exacerbation of COPD in patients not previously treated with theophylline.	Xanthines

Source: Based on Joint National Formulary, 2019.

Adverse Effects

The International Union of Basic and Clinical Pharmacology (IUPHAR) (2019) suggest that the adverse effects of drugs are often dose-related in a similar way to the beneficial effects. Drugs have multiple potential adverse effects, but the concept of therapeutic index is usually reserved for those requiring dose reduction or discontinuation. Drugs with low therapeutic indices are more difficult to prescribe and hazardous for patients but they are still preferred if there are no alternative drugs with similar efficacy (e.g. anti-cancer drugs). The doses of such drugs must be titrated carefully for individual patients to maximise benefits but avoid adverse effects. This is done by monitoring drug effects, either clinically or using regular blood tests (often known as 'therapeutic drug monitoring').

Conclusion

This chapter has introduced the reader to pharmacodynamics and pharmacokinetics of medicines. The reader should now be able to acknowledge the professional responsibilities of registered healthcare professionals of whom administer drugs to patients; define and understand the differences between pharmacodynamics and pharmacokinetics and appreciate the complexities of how drugs work differently in every individual.

Glossary

Biotransformation: Also known a metabolism. The alteration of a drug within the body.

Blood brain barrier: The blood-brain barrier acts as an additional boundary between the circulating blood and the extracellular space of the brain.

Efficacy: The maximum effect that a drug can produce regardless of dose.

First pass metabolism: Whereby the concentration of a drug is greatly reduced before it reaches the systemic circulation.

Half life: The half-life of a drug is the time it takes for the amount of a drug's active substance in the body to reduce by half. This depends on how the body processes and gets rid of the drug. This can vary from a few hours to a few days or weeks.

Potency: The amount of drug that is needed to produce a given effect.

Therapeutic range: Therapeutic range is the range of drug levels in the blood of a person in which a drug has the desired effects upon the body.

Therapeutic index: A narrow therapeutic index, means that there is only a small difference between the minimum effective concentrations and the minimum toxic concentrations in the blood.

References

Anderson, B.J. and Holford, N.H.G. (2013). Understanding dosing: children are small adults, neonates are immature children. *Archives of Disease in Childhood* 98: 737–744.

Anderson, B.J., Allegaert, K., and Holford, N.H. (2006). Population clinical pharmacology of children: general principles. *European Journal of Pediatrics* 165(11): 741–746. doi: 10.1007/s00431-006-0188-y.

Batchelor, H.K., Fotaki, N. and Klien, S. (2014). Paediatric oral biopharmaceutics: Key considerations and current challenges. *Advanced Drug Delivery Reviews* 73: 102–126.

Bickley, L. (2017). *Bates' Guide to History Taking and Physical Examination*, 12e. Walters Kluwer.

Birnkrant, D.J., Bushby, K., Bann, C.M. et al. (2018). Diagnosis and management of Duchenne muscular dystrophy, part 1: diagnosis, and neuromuscular, rehabilitation, endocrine, and gastrointestinal and nutritional management. *The Lancet*, 17: 251–267.

Campbell, J.E. and Cohall, D. (2017). Pharmacodynamics – a pharmacognosy perspective. In: *Pharmacognosy: Fundamentals, Applications, and Strategies* (ed. Ba dal, S. and Delgoda, R.). Elsevier Inc.

Choonara, I. and Sammons, H. (2014). Paediatric clinical pharmacology in the UK. *British Medical Journal* 99: 1143–1146.

Christensen, M.L. (2012). Best Pharmaceuticals for Children Act and Pediatric Research Equity Act: Time for permanent status. *Journal of Pediatric Pharmacolology Therapy* 17(2): 140–141.

Corny, J., Bailey, B., Lebel, D., and Bussières, J.F. (2016). Unlicensed and off-label drug use in paediatrics in a mother-child tertiary care hospital. *Paediatric Child Health* 21(2): 83–87.

Czarniak, P., Bint, L., Favie, L. et al. (2015). Clinical setting influences off-label and unlicensed prescribing in a paediatric teaching hospital. *PLoS One*, 10(3): e0120630. doi: 10.1371/journal.pone.0120630.

Edington, A.N., Schmitt, W., and Willmann, S. (2006). Development and evaluation of a generic physiologically based pharmacokinetic model for children, *Journal of Clinical Pharmacokinetics* 45(10):.1013–1034.

Fallingborg, J., Christensen, L.A., Ingeman-Nielsen, M. et al. (1990). Measurement of gastrointestinal pH and regional transit times in normal children. *Journal of Paediatric Gastroenterology and Nutrition*. doi: 10.1097/00005176-199008000-00010.

Ginsberg, G., Hattis, D., Sonawane et al. (2001). Evaluation of child/adult pharmacokinetic differences from a database derived from the therapeutic drug literature. *Toxicological Sciences* 66: 185–200.

Hale, T.W. (2012). *Medication and Mother's Milk*, 15e. Amarillo, TX: Hale Publishing.

Health Education England (HEE) (2017). Advisory Guidance Administration of Medicines by Nursing Associates. www.hee.nhs.uk/sites/default/files/documents/Advisory%20guidance%20-%20administration%20of%20medicines%20by%20nursing%20associates.pdf (accessed 2 October 2019).

International Union of Basic and Clinical Pharmacology (IUPHAR) (2019). Pharmacodynamics. www.pharmacologyeducation.org/pharmacology/pharmacodynamics (accessed 6 February 2019).

Joint National Formulary (JNF) (2020) Prednisolone. https://bnf.nice.org.uk/drug/prednisolone.html (accessed: 19 April 2021).

Joint National Formulary (2021) BNFc. https://bnfc.nice.org.uk/ (accessed 19 April 2021).

Joret-Descout, P., Prot-Labarthe, S., Brioan, F. et al. (2015). Off-label and unlicensed utilisation of medicines in a French paediatric hospital. *International Journal of Clinical Pharmacology* 37: 1222–1227.

Karch, A. (2017). *Focus on Nursing Pharmacology*, 7e. Wolters Kluwer.

Khdour, M.R., Hallak, H.O., Alayasa, K.S. et al. (2011). Extent and nature of unlicensed and off-label medicine use in hospitalised children in Palestine. *International Journal of Clinical Pharmacology* 33(4), 650–655. doi: 10.1007/s11096-011-9520-3.

Le, J. (2017). Drug absorption. www.msdmanuals.com/en-gb/professional/clinical-pharmacology/pharmacokinetics/drug-absorption (accessed on: 11 February 2019).

Le, J. (2019). Drug metabolism. www.msdmanuals.com/en-gb/professional/clinical-pharmacology/pharmacokinetics/drug-metabolism (accessed 2 October 2019).

McLay, J.S., Tanaka, M., Ekins-Daukes, S., and Helms, P.J. (2006). A prospective questionnaire assessment of attitudes and experiences of off label prescribing among hospital based paediatricians. *Arch Dis Child* 91(7), 584–587. doi: 10.1136/adc.2005.081828.

Medical Research Council (2004). MRC Ethics Guide: Medical Research Involving Children accessed at: https://mrc.ukri.org/documents/pdf/medical-research-involving-children/ (accessed 21 August 19).

Muhari-Stark, E. and Burchart, G.J. (2018). Glomerular filtration rate estimation formulas for pediatric and neonatal use. *Journal of Paediatric Pharmacological Therapy* 23(6): 424–431.

Nagita, A., Amemoto, K., Yoden, A. et al. (1996). Diurnal variation in intragastric pH in children with and without peptic ulcers. *Paediatric Research* 40: 528–532.

NMC (2018). The Code. Available at: www.nmc.org.uk/globalassets/sitedocuments/nmc-publications/nmc-code.pdf (accessed 6 February 2019).

Pleuvry, B. (2004). Pharmacology: Receptors, agonists and antagonists. *Anaesthesia and Intensive Care Medicine* 5(10): 350–352.

Ribeiro, M., Jorge, A., and Macedo, A.F. (2013). Off-label drug prescribing in a Portuguese paediatric emergency unit. *International Journal of Clinical Pharmacology* 35(1): 30–36. doi: 10.1007/s11096-012-9699-y.

Rodieux, F., Wilbaux, M., van den Anker, J.N., and Pfister, M. (2015). Effect of Kidney 'Function on Drug Kinetics and Dosing in Neonates, Infants, and Children', Clinical Pharmacokinetics, 54: 1183–1204.

Rowland, M. (1972). Influence of route of administration on drug availability. *Journal of Pharmaceutical Sciences* 61(1): 70–74.

Royal Pharmacological Society (RPS) (2019). *What is Pharmacology?* www.bps.ac.uk/about/about-pharmacology/what-is-pharmacology (accessed on: 03.02.2019).

RPS and RCN (2019). Professional Guidance on the Administration of Medicines in Healthcare Settings. www.rpharms.com/Portals/0/RPS%20document%20library/Open%20access/Professional%20standards/SSHM%20and%20Admin/Admin%20of%20Meds%20prof%20guidance.pdf?ver=2019-01-23-14026-567 (accessed: 08 October 2019).

Rodieux, F., Wilbaux, M., van den Anker, J.N., and Pfister, M. (2015). Effect of kidney function on drug kinetics and dosing in neonates, infants, and children. *Clinical Pharmacokinetics* 54: 1183–1204.

Scott, W. and McGrath, D. (2009). *Nursing Pharmacology Made Incredibly Easy*. Wolters Kluwer Health. Lippincott Williams and Wilkins.

Slažneva, J., Kovács, L., and Kuželová, M. (2012). Off-label drug use among hospitalized children: identifying extent and nature. *Acta Facultatis Pharmaceuticae Universitatis Comenianae* 59(1): 48–54. doi: 10.2478/v10219-012-0016-6.

Tse, Y., Vasey, N., Dua, D. et al. (2019). The KidzMed project: teaching children to swallow tablet medication. *Archives of Disease of Childhood* 105(11): 1105–1107.

Van den Abeele, J., Rayyan, R., Hoffman, I. et al. (2018). Gastric fluid composition in a paediatric population: Age-dependent changes relevant for gastrointestinal drug disposition. *European Journal of Pharmaceutical Sciences* 123: 301–311.

Young, S. and Pitcher, B. (2016). *Medicine Management for Nurses at a Glance*. Oxford, Wiley.

Yu, G., Zheng, Q.S., and Li, G.F. (2014). Similarities and differences in gastrointestinal physiology between neonates and adults: a physiologically based pharmacokinetic modeling perspective. *AAPS* 16(6): 1162–1166.

Further Resources

The electronic medicines compendium: www.medicines.org.uk/emc/
The British National Formulary: https://bnf.nice.org.uk/
The British National Formulary for Children: https://bnfc.nice.org.uk/
IUPHAR Pharmacology Education Project: www.pharmacologyeducation.org/

Multiple Choice Questions

1. An accurate definition of pharmacodynamics is
  (a) The study of how a certain concentration of a drug produces a biological effect by interacting with specific targets at its site of action
  (b) The study of how the body affects the given drug
  (c) The study of how a drug affects the body

2. Pharmacodynamics is that they can be affected by physiologic changes due to disease, genetic mutations, ageing and/or other drugs.
  (a) True
  (b) False

3. Drugs usually work in which way:
  (a) To replace or act as a substitute for missing chemicals
  (b) To increase or stimulate certain cellular activities
  (c) To depress or slow cellular activities
  (d) To interfere with the functioning of foreign cells, such as invading microorganisms or neoplasms, leading to cell death (drugs that act in this way are called chemotherapeutic agents)
  (e) All of the above

4. What is meant by medications that have a Narrow Therapeutic Index?
  (a) The gap between effective and toxic effect is large
  (b) The gap between effective and toxic effect is small
  (c) The gap between effective and toxic effect is insignificant

5. Pharmacokinetics is the study of drugs and their corresponding pharmacological, therapeutic, or toxic responses in man and animals. True or false?
  (a) True
  (b) False

6. What does ADME mean?
  (a) Absorption, distribution, metabolism and elimination
  (b) Absorption, digestion, metabolism and excretion
  (c) Administration, distribution, metabolism and excretion
  (d) Absorption, distribution, metabolism and excretion

Chapter 5 Pharmacodynamics and Pharmacokinetics

7. What is ADME the process of?
   (a) Pharmacodynamics
   (b) Pharmacokinetics
   (c) Pharmacovigilance
   (d) pharmacotherapeutics
8. The two principal organs responsible for drug elimination are:
   (a) the spleen and the respiratory system
   (b) the kidneys and the bowel
   (c) the spleen and the bowel
   (d) the kidney and the liver
9. A drug that may change the acidity for the stomach acid is likely to affect a drug that is dissolved in the stomach. True or false?
   (a) True
   (b) False
10. Active transports uses energy (ATP) to transfer molecules and ions in and out of the cell. True or false?
    (a) True
    (b) False
11. Drug potency is an expression of
    (a) how much alcohol is used within the drug
    (b) the activity that judges the therapeutic effectiveness of the drug in humans.
    (c) the activity of a drug in terms of the concentration or amount of the drug required to produce a defined effect
12. Clinical efficacy. . .
    (a) judges the therapeutic effectiveness of the drug in humans.
    (b) is the activity of a drug in terms of the concentration or amount of the drug required to produce a defined effect
    (c) is how ethical it is to administer the drug
13. Another name for biotransformation is:
    (a) Administration
    (b) Distribution
    (c) Metabolism
    (d) Elimination
14. Drugs that are not lipid-soluble are
    (a) not able to pass the BBB
    (b) can pass the BBB
15. An agonist is:
    (a) A type of antidote
    (b) A molecule that binds to a receptor resulting in activation and cellular change
    (c) A molecule accentuating the action of agonist
    (d) None of the above

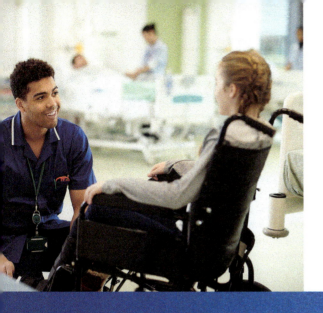

6

Drug Formulations

Sinéad Greener and Louise Carr

Aim

The aim of this chapter is to outline the many different drug formulations that providers should be aware of when they offer care and treatment to children and young people (CYP) and to highlight the key aspects that must be considered before the most appropriate formulation can be selected.

Learning Outcomes

After reading this chapter the reader will be able to:

- Describe the terms 'unlicensed' and 'off-label'
- Understand the different formulations of medications available and their advantages and disadvantages
- Understand how to administer medications via enteral feeding tubes
- Acknowledge the importance of displacement values and excipient content of medications

Test Your Knowledge

1. Explain the difference between licensed and unlicensed medications.
2. In CYP, what is the preferred route of administration? List advantages of this route.
3. Identify two formulation excipients that have potential to cause harm to CYP.
4. Explain the acronyms NG and PEG. What should be considered if administering medications via a feeding tube?
5. What does the term 'displacement value' mean?

Fundamentals of Pharmacology for Children's Nurses, First Edition. Edited by Ian Peate and Peter Dryden.
© 2022 John Wiley & Sons Ltd. Published 2022 by John Wiley & Sons Ltd.
Companion website: www.wiley.com/go/pharmacologyforCN

Chapter 6 Drug Formulations

Introduction

'Pediatrics does not deal with miniature men and women, with reduced doses and the same class of disease in smaller bodies, but....has its own independent range and horizon' (Halpern, 1988: 52). With this in mind, selection of the correct product for the right indication to treat CYP needs careful risk assessment. The European Medicines Agency (EMA) has stipulated aspects that should be considered when selecting the appropriate medicine for this population: 'the condition(s) to be treated, the treatment duration, the properties of the active substance, the necessity of particular excipients in a paediatric formulation (and their safety)...risk of dosing errors and user aspects such as the ease of administration and patient acceptability' (EMA, 2013: 6).

According to the World Health Organization (WHO), the 'guiding principle' on product selection should be based on 'the balance of risk/benefit taking into account the specific needs of this vulnerable population' (WHO, 2011: 7). Weighing up the advantages and disadvantages of available formulations leads to the use of many unlicensed and off-label medications in CYP.

Licensing of Paediatric Medicines

Most medications available on the UK market have been produced without CYP in mind. In January 2007 the paediatric regulation came into force in the EU, requiring manufacturers to complete a Paediatric Investigation Plan and submit the results of studies when applying for a medicine's marketing authorisation, its licence (EMA, 2020a, 2020b). As a result, the number of licensed paediatric medicines and indications has increased (European Commission, 2017). However, improvement is needed.

Licensed medications should be used in preference to unlicensed medications, but often there is no acceptable formulation available to deliver the right dose, via the right route. Figure 6.1 shows how pharmacists and medical staff select the most appropriate medicine for CYP.

Option 1 is the only licensed option; options 2 to 5 are unlicensed, carrying extra risk.

- 'Off-label' – licensed medication used in an alternative way to manufacturers' specifications.
- Imported – medication licensed in another country, imported and used unlicensed in UK.

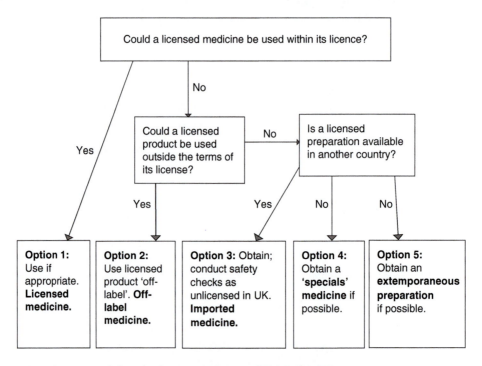

Figure 6.1 Stepwise approach for selecting appropriate medications for CYP.

Chapter 6 Drug Formulations

- 'Specials' – medicines exempt from having a licence. The Neonatal and Paediatric Pharmacists Group (NPPG) and the Royal College of Paediatrics and Child Health (RCPCH) have compiled a list of recommended strengths to be used for certain medications when a 'specials' formulation is produced (RCPCH, 2020).
- Extemporaneous – ingredients are compounded on request to fulfil a prescription for an individual patient.

The team providing an unlicensed medication and the parents/caregivers/patient must be highly vigilant for effectiveness and tolerability of the product. Using medications outside the terms of their licence increases the risk to CYP as the safety of such use has not been assessed. If no licensed preparation is available, pharmacists should be consulted for advice.

Types of Formulations

Medicines are produced by taking an active pharmaceutical ingredient (API) and combining with a suitable vehicle to develop appropriate forms for administration. The EMA provides guidance on pharmaceutical development of medicines for CYP. It states that, when choosing a medicine, advantages and disadvantages of the product and the intended route of administration should be considered (EMA, 2013). The different formulations will now be discussed and consideration given to their advantages and disadvantages.

Oral Route of Administration
Most common route of medication administration; medications provide local or systemic effects.

Advantages:
1. Self-administration is possible
2. Often easiest method of administration
3. Generally safest method of administration

Disadvantages:
1. Slow method of absorption
2. Enzymes in the gastrointestinal tract (GIT) might interfere with the medicine
3. Requires properly functioning GIT
4. Gastric emptying can be affected by food intake or disease state, potentially affecting rate of drug absorption.
5. Inappropriate route in an unconscious, vomiting or unwilling CYP (Watson et al., 2014).

Liquid Formulations for Oral Administration
Can be termed solutions or suspensions. Solutions are homogenous preparations that do not need to be shaken before use. In suspensions, the API is suspended in a liquid. Consequently, if left to stand, the API may sediment to the bottom requiring the bottle to be shaken before use. If the bottle is not shaken properly before use, the likelihood of an individual being under or over-dosed is greater.

Episode of Care

While a medication might appear appropriate for a specific CYP, in some cases, the individual may not be able or willing to take the medication as intended (EMA, 2013). Patient acceptability is an important consideration when choosing which formulation to give a CYP.

WHO recommends limiting medication volumes to less than 5ml for those under 5 years, and less than 10ml for those over 5 years (WHO, 2011). In practice, these amounts are often exceeded. For example isoniazid used as part of a tuberculosis prophylaxis regimen is dosed at 10mg/kg; a 16-month-old infant weighing 10kg would be prescribed 100mg. The recommended strength of isoniazid liquid is 50mg/5ml (RCPCH, 2020). To deliver a dose of 100mg, 10ml of isoniazid liquid is required, a volume which may prove too large for the infant.

Finn was expected to take 10ml of isoniazid liquid. He did not tolerate the medication orally due to the volume and taste, therefore a nasogastric tube was inserted for administration of this medicine. Alternative options were sought and, on pharmacist advice, isoniazid 100mg tablets were crushed and dispersed in 5ml of water. This proved acceptable to Finn, whose nasogastric tube could then be removed.

Clinical Consideration

Adding Medicines to Food

Ideally, medication should not be mixed into milk or food as this could turn the CYP off their essential nutrition. Furthermore, there is a danger of the API becoming denatured. Some exceptions to this are:

- Gaviscon infant sachets – stabilise stomach acid and reduce risk of reflux – often added to milk
- Pancreatin powder or granules – enzymes that digest food in pancreatic insufficiency – added to apple puree or milk

CYP should be encouraged to consume the full amount of food or milk if medicine has been added to it, ensuring that the whole dose is administered. Consult manufacturers' information or seek advice from a pharmacist or specialist nurse before adding medicine to food or milk.

In CYP, sugar-free preparations should be considered first. If a medicine with cariogenic sugars is taken long term, advice on dental hygiene should be provided (Paediatric Formulary Committee, 2019–2020).

Solid Dosage Formulations for Oral Administration

Solid dosage formulations are generally smaller, easier to transport and have a longer shelf-life than liquid formulations (see Table 6.1).

Table 6.1 Different types of oral solid dosage forms.

TYPE OF ORAL SOLID FORMULATIONS	DESCRIPTION
Capsules	Can be prepared as soft gelatin capsules containing liquid, or as hard-shell capsules with powder, granules or pellets inside (Watson et al., 2014).
Chewable tablets	Easier for CYP to take if they have difficulty swallowing tablets whole. Tend to be pleasant-tasting. There is often a preference for chewable tablets among school-aged children, adolescents and caregivers (Ranmal et al., 2016).
Dispersible/soluble/ effervescent tablets	Dissolved in water, hence easier to administer to CYP who have difficulty swallowing tablets. Sodium content and volume of water required to disperse tablet must be considered.
Granules and powders	Unlike tablets or capsules, which need to disintegrate to release API, powders and granules dissolve fast, releasing API quickly (Aulton and Taylor, 2018). Can be put directly into mouth, mixed with liquid – usually water – or sprinkled onto/mixed with food.
Immediate-release (IR) formulations	Shortly after administration API is released into GIT providing rapid onset of action (Aulton and Taylor, 2018). Short duration of action necessitates more frequent dosing; often three to four times a day.
Modified-release (MR) formulations; including enteric-coated (EC)/gastro-resistant and extended/ prolonged-release (XL) or sustained release (SR) formulations	Formulated to control the release of drug so that API is delivered: • At the right rate • At expected time points or • To a specific site within the GIT (Aulton and Taylor, 2018). Enteric coating prevents breakdown of the formulation within stomach, instead releasing API when it reaches intestines. EC is used to: • Deliver API to an appropriate site • Protect stomach from APIs that might cause gastric irritation or • Protect API from degradation by stomach acid or enzymes (Aulton and Taylor, 2018) API is slowly released from XL and SR formulations, offering a slower onset and longer duration of action. Dosing is less frequent; often only once or twice a day (Aulton and Taylor, 2018).
Orodispersible formulations including films, melts and tablets	Rapidly dissolving formulations for oral administration. Placed onto tongue, where they disintegrate or disperse within seconds before being swallowed. Ideal for CYP with swallowing difficulties.

Clinical Consideration

Flexible Dosing with Tablet Formulations

Tablets can be sugar-coated, film-coated or uncoated. The coating affects the palatability, how quickly the tablet will dissolve and also the ability to crush and disperse a tablet.

The solubility of a tablet's contents affects how suitable it is for crushing and dispersing in water in order to obtain a flexible dose for CYP. If a tablet does not fully dissolve in water – yet an even dispersion is assumed – there is a risk of under- or overdosing the CYP. For example, if a 20mg tablet is left to dissolve in 5ml, it cannot be guaranteed that each 1ml will contain 4mg of the API.

Another consideration is the relevance of a 'break-line' on a tablet. It is a common misconception that if a break-line is present, it means that the tablet can be halved in order to give a smaller dose. Caution is needed here if the API itself is not evenly distributed throughout the tablet, as giving half of the tablet will not necessarily mean that an individual is receiving half of the API. Occasionally, break-lines are purely present so the tablet can be broken in two, making it easier to swallow the smaller parts.

Extra care is also required when administering enteric-coated and modified-release tablets. Generally speaking, these formulations should never be manipulated due to the risk of disrupting the special properties of the product.

A pharmacist should always be consulted before crushing, dispersing or splitting any tablet which is not licensed to be administered in this way. It is also worth noting that children as young as 3 and 4 years of age have been taught to swallow tablets and capsules so that they can overcome the need to take liquid medications that are unpalatable. See 'Creating a pill school' recommendation in the Further Resources section.

Formulations for Administration Via Mucous Membranes

Products include buccal, sublingual, and rectal formulations.

Advantages:

1. Absorbed directly into bloodstream from site of placement, giving a quick onset of action
2. Avoid GIT and associated potential for degradation of API
3. Can be administered in an unconscious patient

Disadvantages:

1. Lack of formulations available
2. Eating and drinking can affect absorption of buccally and sublingually administered medicines
3. Limited range of strengths of formulations, in particular with suppositories, can lead to inflexible dosing
4. Necessary for medication to be retained in the correct site which can prove challenging in CYP

Sublingual and buccal formulations include tablets, melts and liquids. Buccal and sublingual tablets are small, porous tablets that disintegrate fast (Aulton and Taylor, 2018). Buccal tablets are placed high between upper lip and gum and left to dissolve directly into the mucous membrane, for example hydrocortisone buccal tablets used to treat aphthous ulceration of the mouth (eMC, 2020a). Sublingual tablet and melt formulations are placed under the tongue where they dissolve without the need for water, for example, DesmoMelt (desmopressin) oral lyophilisates to treat bedwetting (eMC, 2019a). Buccolam (midazolam) is a buccal liquid formulation supplied in prefilled syringes, the contents of which should be slowly inserted between gum and cheek when needed for prolonged seizures in CYP (eMC, 2019b).

Formulations for rectal administration include suppositories, creams, tablets, capsules, solutions and enemas, which can have local or systemic effects. The rich blood supply of the rectum means that medicines administered via this route can be quickly absorbed into the circulation (Waterfield and Rivers, 2012). Suppositories are solid formulations with the API incorporated into a base which is then set in a mould (Watson et al., 2014). Upon insertion into the rectum and exposure to body temperature, the preparation dissolves, melts or disperses, releasing the API. Enemas are liquids which do not require dissolution before the API is released (Aulton and Taylor, 2018). They can be made into foams, solutions, suspensions or emulsions.

Advantages of using rectal formulations:

1. Useful option in perioperative period if patient is nil by mouth
2. Alternative route of administration if patient cannot swallow is unconscious or vomiting
3. Can be used to yield local effects within the rectosigmoid region
4. Do not require taste-masking excipients

Disadvantages of using rectal formulations:

1. Limited amount of formulations available
2. Products offer fixed dosing
3. Absorption may be irregular or unpredictable
4. Patient and caregiver acceptability and tolerability may be low
5. Can be challenging encouraging CYP to maintain a certain position in order to hold the suppository or enema in place

Administration of liquid rectal formulations in CYP necessitates consideration of the length of the rectal tube, as well as the volume to be inserted (EMA, 2013). When rectal diazepam (for epileptic and febrile convulsions) is administered to CYP under 15kg, it is important that the tube nozzle is only inserted half-way into the rectum (eMC, 2019c). In all cases, specific instructions for administration in CYP must be sought from the manufacturers' information, a pharmacist, or an experienced nurse.

Formulations for Topical Administration

Topical medicines can be delivered via the skin, eye, ear or nose. This is an external route of administration usually delivering local effects although sometimes, particularly with patches, it can provide systemic effects.

Products for application via the skin include creams, ointments, gels, lotions, pastes, dusting powders and patches. They are all formulated in different ways to meet the needs of the condition they are treating. Ointments are oily preparations that usually prevent water loss, making them suitable for chronic dry skin, whereas creams are aqueous-based and often preferred by patients as they are less greasy. Patch formulations release the API through the skin into the systemic circulation. The patch aims to provide continuous absorption of the API over a period of days. As absorption through the skin can be unpredictable, patches are designed to release the API slowly, limiting the rate of absorption (Watson et al., 2014).

Key tips for using patches:

- Location and application of patch is important and should be checked in manufacturers' instructions. For example, hyoscine patches for travel sickness or excessive secretions in CYP should be applied behind the ear.
- Check patches are still in place and have not fallen off. If a patch falls off, a new patch should be applied.
- Check the patch is replaced after the required time period.
- Patches should be carefully folded over on themselves prior to disposal.
- Hands must be washed after both application and removal, ensuring no residual medicine remains on the hands.
- Heat, including hot water, may increase rate of absorption of API from a patch, increasing risk of adverse effects and toxicity.

Hyoscine hydrobromide patches are 1mg in strength. They are licensed from 10 years, but in practice are used in CYP much younger than this. The dose in the British National Formulary for Children for a 1-month-old infant is 250 micrograms, which equates to a quarter of a patch. To deliver this dose, the patch either needs to be cut to the required size, ensuring the membrane is not peeled off, or part of the patch needs to be covered so that only the required proportion is in contact with the skin (PFC, 2019–2020). Always consult the manufacturer's information or a pharmacist before manipulating patches.

Eye drops and ointments are useful for treating localised eye problems. They are sterile and particle-free. If treating an eye infection, separate containers must be used for each eye to avoid cross-contamination. They often have a reduced expiry date after first being opened; always consult the manufacturer's information and local policies to ensure that these products are used within their expiry. Eye ointments are oil-based, so they will stay in contact with the eye/eyelid for a longer period of time, and are often used at night so they remain at the site of action for longer. In addition, their oily nature may cause blurred vision if used during the day.

Ear drops are usually viscous preparations, maximising contact time with the affected area (Aulton and Taylor, 2018). Antibiotic ear drops are only recommended in cases of obvious infection and should not be continued for longer than two weeks (PFC, 2019–2020).

Formulations for nasal administration include sprays, drops, ointments and creams that can have a local or systemic effect. Drops and sprays depend on a good administration technique in order to administer the dose accurately. In 2013 a nasal flu vaccination was licensed in the UK for CYP over two years, providing a much less invasive method of administration compared with the traditional injectable flu vaccine (eMC, 2020b).

Chapter 6 Drug Formulations

Formulations for Inhalation Administration

Examples include inhalers and nebulisers where the API is either formulated as an aerosol, a dry powder or a liquid. These formulations are usually designed to provide local effects within the airways. See Chapter 10 for further details.

Advantages:

1. Medicines administered direct to the site of action, therefore lower doses of API needed, potentially reducing the incidence of systemic side effects
2. Range of inhaler devices available to suit an individual's preferred technique or ability
3. Spacer devices aid delivery of the API to the lungs. Available in different sizes to suit the individual CYP.

Disadvantages:

1. Correct technique needs to be mastered for appropriate medication delivery
2. Not easy to administer in an unwilling CYP
3. Nebuliser therapy requires specialised equipment to deliver the medication.

Formulations for Parenteral Administration

Administration of medication via the parenteral route is common within the hospital setting and may be essential for very sick CYP. Prior to giving a medication parenterally, factors such as the clinical effect, characteristics of the API, the parenteral access the CYP has, and their acceptance, need to be considered (EMA, 2013). Distraction techniques and anaesthetic creams are often needed in CYP to overcome pain, anxiety or needle-phobic feelings arising from repeated administration of parenteral medications.

The different routes available for parenteral injections are described in Table 6.2. Drugs to be administered parenterally may come as ready to use solutions or as powders that require reconstitution.

The Intravenous Route

The type of access the patient has, for example peripheral cannula versus central line, affects how the product should be diluted and at what rate it can be safely administered. Generally speaking, medications that are given peripherally must be diluted to a weaker concentration and run at a slower rate than those given via a central line.

Table 6.2 **Different routes of parenteral injection.**

TYPE OF INJECTION	DESCRIPTION
Intramuscular (IM)	Involves a small volume of drug solution being administered directly into muscle. In infants the muscle mass is lower, therefore absorption of the drug will be slower. The recommended sites of administration are the thigh for children under 1 year and the upper arm for older CYP. IM injections are painful and should be avoided where possible in CYP. The larger the volume administered, the more painful the injection. The maximum suggested IM volume to administer in CYP is 2ml, although in smaller CYP, often 1ml is the most that should be administered, especially via the deltoid muscle (Workman, 1999). If a larger volume is required, dosage should be double-checked and volume split between different sites.
Intravenous (IV)	Delivers the API into the veins and is the most used parenteral route. Depending on the individual medication, may involve bolus injections administered over 3–5 minutes, intermittent infusions administered over 20 minutes to 8 hours, or continuous infusions over 24 hours. The concentration of the prepared drug may determine the method of administration. A list of advantages and disadvantages of IV administration is discussed later.
Subcutaneous (SC)	Delivers a small amount of drug under the skin to subcutaneous tissue. Thighs, buttocks and abdomen are the most common sites for administration. SC injections are less painful than IM injections.

Advantages:

1. Fast onset of action
2. 100% bioavailability of the administered medication
3. Useful route of administration in the seriously ill or nil by mouth.

Disadvantages:

1. Lack of licensed formulations available for CYP
2. Need IV access to avoid repeated venepuncture
3. Venous cannulation can be painful and distressing
4. Risk of fluid overloading if volumes of injections are large
5. Displacement values may need to be taken into account to ensure accurate doses are delivered (see displacement values section)
6. Risk of extravasation
7. A small dosage error can have a significant impact on the CYP
8. Knowledge of appropriate diluents, final concentrations, and suitable infusion rates required. May entail complex calculations
9. Compatibility of medicines to be given via the same line must be discussed with a pharmacist if the information is not readily available

Excipients

Excipients are added to a drug formulation to perform specific functions, including aiding the manufacturing process, improving storage life, and enhancing patient acceptability. Often several different excipients are required to produce a stable medicinal product fit for purpose; however, one individual excipient may perform multiple roles within a formulation. Different brands of the same medicinal product may vary in the range and quantity of excipients included within their formulation (Graham and Turner, 2011).

The following non-exhaustive list describes some of the functions of excipients:

- Coating agent – improves palatability by masking unpleasant tastes or smells
- Preservative – improves shelf-life of formulation by stabilising API against degradation – for example, from light, oxygen or microbial contamination
- Sweetener (natural or artificial) – masks unpleasant tastes to improve palatability (Medicines for Children, 2018)

As many medications prescribed for CYP are used in an unlicensed or off-label way, it is important to ensure that these products are safe, including consideration of the full range and quantity of excipients. This data is rarely readily available; pharmacists often contact the manufacturer's medical information department to ascertain this information.

Factors Affecting Excipient-Related Toxicity

CYP are at greater risk of experiencing excipient-related toxicity than adults. Firstly, this is because their organ systems are still developing, making accumulation of excipients more likely. Secondly, CYP often require medications in a liquid formulation to allow for flexibility of dosing. Liquid formulations tend to contain a wider range of excipients than solid dosage forms, such as flavouring agents to make the liquid more palatable, and preservatives to extend shelf-life of the medicine once the bottle has been opened. Consequently, CYP are often exposed to a broad variety of excipients. Thirdly, most excipients included in medications intended for adult patients are generally considered safe for human consumption, yet the safety of such excipients in CYP has not been extensively studied (Yochana et al., 2012).

Commonly used drug formulation excipients have been found to cause CYP harm when used in certain circumstances, as described in Table 6.3.

CYP with complex medical or surgical backgrounds may require several regular medications as part of their healthcare plan. It is important to consider the cumulative excipient intake from these medications.

Chapter 6 Drug Formulations

Table 6.3 Excipients with a known potential to cause harm in CYP.

EXCIPIENT	REPORTED ADVERSE EFFECTS IN CYP
Benzoates/benzyl alcohol/benzoic acid	• Metabolic acidosis, jaundice and neurotoxicity in neonates (Graham and Turner, 2011; EMA, 2006). • Fatal toxic syndrome in premature or low-birthweight neonates (UK National Poisons Information Service, 2020). **Recommendations:** • Avoid in neonates (Medicines for Children, 2018) • Use with caution in CYP with chronic liver impairment (Yamada et al., 1992)
Ethanol (alcohol)	• CYP, especially those under 6 years, are more susceptible to the central nervous system adverse effects of ethanol, for example, poor concentration, respiratory depression and coma (EMA, 2019) • Ethanol-induced hypoglycaemia is more common in infants and young children (EMA, 2019) • Risk of dependence in adolescents following chronic consumption. • Toxic effects in neonates following absorption of ethanol through skin when topical preparations with high alcohol content have been applied (EMA, 2019) **Recommendations:** • Avoid ethanol-containing medications including topical products in CYP if possible.
Propylene glycol	• Wide range of adverse effects reported with increasing frequency in neonates and children less than 4 years, including: seizures, lactic acidosis, and cardiovascular toxicity (Ladyzhynsky, 2012) • Toxicity more likely in patients with renal or hepatic insufficiency (Ladyzhynsky, 2012) **Recommendations:** • Particular caution required in CYP with pre-existing renal and/or hepatic impairment

Enteral Feeding Tubes

These provide an important route for administering medications (see Table 6.4). Acutely unwell CYP may have a nasogastric (NG) tube inserted to temporarily facilitate feed and medication administration whilst unable to eat and drink or take medications orally. Longer-term solutions, such as a surgically inserted percutaneous endoscopic gastrostomy (PEG) tube, may be necessary for CYP with complex needs, for example those with a neurodisability or gastrointestinal condition.

The vast majority of medications are not licensed to be administered via an enteral feeding tube as manufacturers have not assessed suitability. Manipulation of a medicinal product's formulation, not expressly covered in the manufacturer's literature, constitutes an unlicensed use of the medicine. Associated risks include:

• Altered bioavailability and pharmacokinetic profile of the medication, leading to therapeutic failure
• Instability of the drug compound
• Increased side effects
• Blockage of feeding tube
• Operator exposure to compounds that could be harmful (Royal Pharmaceutical Society, 2011)

To mitigate risk when administering via an enteral feeding tube, the relevant merits and drawbacks of each formulation must be considered, see Table 6.5.

Table 6.4 Locations of the main types of enteral feeding tubes.

TYPE OF FEEDING TUBE	LOCATION
Nasogastric (NG)	Inserted into nose and fed down into stomach
Nasojejunal (NJ)	Inserted into nose and fed down into jejunum
Percutaneous endoscopic gastrostomy (PEG)	Surgically inserted through abdominal wall directly into stomach
Percutaneous endoscopic jejunostomy (PEJ)	Surgically inserted through abdominal wall directly into jejunum

Chapter 6 Drug Formulations

Table 6.5 **Merits and drawbacks of different formulations for administration via enteral feeding tubes.**

FORMULATION	CONSIDERATIONS FOR ENTERAL FEEDING TUBE ADMINISTRATION
Liquids (solutions/ suspensions/ syrups/ reconstituted sachets)	• Usually formulations of choice; predominantly drawn up and administered without the need to manipulate original product. • Viscous liquids require dilution with water for easier flushing down the tube. • Many 'sugar-free' liquids contain sweeteners, for example sorbitol, which when given in large quantities can induce diarrhoea (Wrexham Maelor Hospital Pharmacy Department, 2015). Dilution of the liquid with water may reduce this risk. • In granular suspensions, the size of the granules affects the suitability for administration via a feeding tube (White and Bradnam, 2015). • Some sachet formulations are unsuitable due to the likelihood of blocking the tube, for example ispaghula husk preparations (Wrexham Maelor Hospital Pharmacy Department, 2015). • Other sachets may contain modified-release granules which must not be crushed.
Standard tablets	• Consider if no other suitable formulation available. • Many disintegrate within 5–10 minutes when placed in water and shaken (White and Bradnam, 2015). • Non-disintegrating tablets must be crushed well, using a tablet crusher or crushing syringe, then mixed with water.
Sugar-coated/film-coated tablets	• Consider if no other suitable formulation available. • Must be crushed well, using a tablet crusher or crushing syringe, then mixed with water. • Ensure coating suitably broken down by crushing process and feeding tube well flushed after dose given, reducing chance of blocking the tube (Wrexham Maelor Hospital Pharmacy Department, 2015).
Dispersible/soluble/ effervescent tablets	• Dissolve or disperse in water; generally suitable for feeding tube administration. • Ensure tablet fully dispersed before drawing up dose. • Some dispersible tablets generate particles or granules too large to give via fine-bore tubes (White and Bradnam, 2015). • Often have high sodium contents; may be unsuitable in sodium-restricted patients (Wrexham Maelor Hospital Pharmacy Department, 2015).
EC tablets	• Not suitable for administration via feeding tubes; crushing renders the enteric coating ineffective.
MR tablets	• Not suitable for administration via feeding tubes; crushing may change modified release to immediate release.
Chewable tablets	• Not suitable for administration via feeding tubes. Some chewable tablet formulations are partially absorbed in mouth upon chewing (Wrexham Maelor Hospital Pharmacy Department, 2015). • Crushing and administering via a feeding tube, bypassing the mouth, leads to reduced absorption of API.
Buccal and sublingual tablets	• Unsuitable for administration via feeding tubes; usual site of absorption will be bypassed, leading to reduced absorption of API (White and Bradnam, 2015).

Table 6.5 (Continued)

FORMULATION	CONSIDERATIONS FOR ENTERAL FEEDING TUBE ADMINISTRATION
Capsules	Hard gelatin: • May potentially be opened and contents mixed with water (White and Bradnam, 2015). Soft gelatin: • Unsuitable for administration via feeding tubes. • No easy way of extracting entire contents as cannot be opened (White and Bradnam, 2015). • API contained within an oily solution; will not mix with water (White and Bradnam, 2015). MR capsules: • Suitability depends on size and nature of contents. If the contents will not fit down feeding tube without crushing, it is not suitable to give. • Always seek further advice from pharmacy.
Injections	• Some are suitable for short-term administration via feeding tube, only when no suitable alternative is available (White and Bradnam, 2015). • Always seek further advice from pharmacy.
Cytotoxic tablets	• Should not be crushed due to risk of operator exposure to hazardous materials, therefore not suitable for administration via feeding tubes (Wrexham Maelor Hospital Pharmacy Department, 2015).

When a medication is prescribed via a feeding tube, consider the available formulations and which would be most appropriate to administer. A multidisciplinary approach is essential to ensure the patient receives their required medication in the safest way:

- Prescribers should review the patient's medications, ensuring that the most appropriate route has been prescribed. Alternative routes to feeding tube administration, such as rectal or topical, may be suitable.
- Pharmacists can advise on:
  - Formulation choice to aid administration via feeding tube and required manipulations
  - Switching to alternative medication or route where no suitable formulation available for prescribed medication
  - Additional monitoring required due to anticipated reduced efficacy or increased toxicity of administered medications
  - Precautionary measures required by administrator to minimise risk of exposure to harmful substances.
- Nurses should regularly review route, ensuring feeding tube administration only continued while patient unable to tolerate oral medications. See 'Clinical Consideration: General Rules for Administering Medications Via Feeding Tubes'.

Clinical Consideration

General Rules for Administering Medications Via Feeding Tubes

- Always ensure medication prescribed to be given via the feeding tube. If prescription is for oral administration, discuss with prescriber and ensure prescription re-written with correct intended route prior to administration.
- Medications should be administered using enteral syringes compatible with feeding tube in situ.
- *Do not* use intravenous syringes to prepare medications for enteral administration due to risk of inadvertently giving the medication intravenously.
- Always stop any running enteral feed and flush tube with water before administration.
- Some medications interact with feeds leading to reduced absorption of API. A prolonged break in feed both pre and post dose may be required.
- Flush tube with water again after administration of medication is complete, then re-start the feed unless a prolonged break is required.

Chapter 6 Drug Formulations

Displacement Values

Some medications presented in a powder formulation require reconstitution with a solvent prior to adminis-tration. Examples include certain oral suspensions and injectables.

When a dry-powder formulation is reconstituted, the final volume of the solution may exceed the volume of solvent added; the powder itself has contributed to the volume and further diluted the solution. The difference between final product volume and original solvent volume is the displacement value of the powder. Displacement values vary between different medications and among different brands of the same medication.

The clinical significance of a powder's displacement value depends on several factors:

- therapeutic index of medication
- dose to be given
- intended recipient

Clinical Consideration

Reconstituting Oral Suspensions

When reconstituting a dry-powder oral suspension, always consult the manufacturer's guidance. The amount and type of solvent required should always be specified on the outer box or bottle label. Most dry-powder formulations will have a reduced expiry once reconstituted, and may require different storage arrangements.

The following storage and reconstitution information is provided on the bottle label of the Brown & Burk product, Amoxicillin 250mg/5ml suspension:

Dry Powder: Store powder in a dry place below 25°C.
Reconstituted suspension: Store up to 14 days at 2°C – 8°C in a refrigerator.
Discard 14 days after reconstitution.
Instructions for Pharmacists/Dispenser: Add 88ml of water to get 100ml of reconstituted oral suspension. Close the cap securely. Shake the bottle vigorously to dissolve the content.
(Brown & Burk UK Ltd., 2020).

Although the packaging directs the instructions towards pharmacy staff, nursing staff are often expected to reconstitute oral suspensions prior to use. It is important to understand directions provided. In the example above, adding 88ml of water to the powder in the bottle and shaking vigorously produces 100ml of a suspension containing 250mg of amoxicillin in every 5ml.

Remember:

1. Read packaging to check which solvent required. Drinking quality water is needed to reconstitute oral suspensions.
2. Check quantity of solvent required, then obtain appropriately-sized syringes to draw up stipulated volume. It may be necessary to use more than one size of syringe.
3. Before adding solvent, shake closed bottle to loosen powder, then remove cap.
4. Add measured-out solvent to bottle, replace cap, then shake vigorously. Visually inspect bottle to ensure all powder has mixed with the solvent.
5. Write on bottle label the date of preparation and/or date the liquid will expire (consult local policy).
6. After administering required dose, ensure product is stored appropriately. Some reconstituted suspen-sions require refrigeration, others can be kept at room temperature. Always consult product's packaging.

For oral suspensions the displacement value is taken into consideration by following the manufacturer's instructions for reconstitution, as detailed above. When dealing with injectable medications requiring recon-stitution, displacement values can prove more complex.

If the full contents of a dry-powder vial are required to deliver a dose, the powder's displacement value can generally be disregarded once reconstituted, as the full volume of liquid is simply drawn up from the vial. However, the vast majority of medications used in CYP are manufactured with adults in mind. Consequently, most inject-able products contain 'adult-sized' doses; to prepare a smaller dose for a CYP, a proportion of the contents must be used. In this situation, if the powder has a displacement value, upon reconstitution this will result in a more dilute solution. The displacement value must be taken into consideration to avoid under-dosing the CYP.

Key tips:

- Some powders do not have a displacement value, hence volume of reconstituted product is equal to volume of solvent added.
- Always check for information on displacement values and final concentrations in leaflet and packaging for dry-powder injectable products.
- Resources like the 'Injectable Medicines Guide' (Keeling and Bullock, 2020) contain paediatric-specific intravenous drug monographs detailing how to appropriately manage displacement values. Always check which relevant resources are available to use in your clinical area.

Conclusion

There are a wide variety of formulations and potential routes of administration available when dealing with medicines for CYP, all of which have their own advantages and disadvantages. A multidisciplinary team effort is often required to ensure that the most appropriate medication formulation is selected and safely delivered to an individual. Patient acceptability and parent or caregiver preference should also be considered when appropriate.

Glossary

Absorption: The passage of a medicine from the site of administration to the site of action.
Bioavailability: The proportion of API which reaches the systemic circulation following administration.
Central line: A flexible tube inserted into a large, fast-flowing central vein which can be used for fluid and medication administration.
Cytotoxic: A medication toxic to cells. An example is chemotherapy.
Enteral: Involving the gastrointestinal tract.
Extravasation: Leakage of an injectable medication from the site of administration, causing irritation and damage to surrounding tissue.
Gastrointestinal tract: The body's digestive tract from the mouth through to the anus, including several organs essential to digestion.
Homogenous preparation: Ingredients are evenly distributed throughout the whole product.
Multidisciplinary: Involving several different types of professionals.
Perioperative: The period of time around surgery, including before, during, and after the actual operation.
Peripheral cannula: A thin tube inserted into a peripheral vein which can be used for fluid and medication administration.
Rectosigmoid: The distal part of the sigmoid colon and the proximal part of the rectum.
Therapeutic index: A measure of the safety of a medication. 'Narrow therapeutic index' refers to medications with little difference between beneficial and harmful doses.
Venepuncture: Accessing a vein with a hollow needle to gain access to the bloodstream to obtain a blood sample/to give an IV.

References

Aulton, M.E. and Taylor, K. (2018). *Aulton's Pharmaceutics: The Design and Manufacture of Medicines*, 5e. Edinburgh: Elsevier.
Brown & Burk UK Ltd. (2020). Amoxicillin Sugar Free 250 mg/5 ml Powder for Oral Suspension – bottle label and outer box (accessed 23 May 2020).
Electronic Medicines Compendium (2019a). DesmoMelt 120mcg oral lysophilisate – Summary of Product Characteristics. (Last updated 16 December 2019). www.medicines.org.uk/emc/product/171/smpc (accessed 15 June 2020).
Electronic Medicines Compendium (2019b). Buccolam 5mg oromucosal solution – Summary of Product Characteristics. (Last updated 1 November 2019). www.medicines.org.uk/emc/product/7462/smpc (accessed 15 June 2020).

Chapter 6 Drug Formulations

Electronic Medicines Compendium (2019c). Diazepam Destin 5mg rectal solution – Summary of Product Characteristics. (Last updated 11 December 2019). www.medicines.org.uk/emc/product/2997/smpc (accessed 31 May 2020).

Electronic Medicines Compendium (2020a). Hydrocortisone 2.5mg muco-adhesive buccal tablets – Summary of Product Characteristics. (Last updated 9 March 2020). www.medicines.org.uk/emc/product/5037/smpc (accessed May 31 2020).

Electronic Medicines Compendium (2020b). Fluenz Tetra nasal spray suspension Influenza vaccine (live attenuated, nasal) – Summary of Product Characteristics. (Last updated 27 March 2020). www.medicines.org.uk/emc/product/3296/smpc (accessed 15 June 2020).

European Commission (2017). State of Paediatric Medicines in the EU. 10 years of the EU Paediatric Regulation. Report from the Commission to the European Parliament and the Council. https://ec.europa.eu/health/sites/health/files/files/paediatrics/docs/2017_childrensmedicines_report_en.pdf (accessed 2 June 2020).

European Medicines Agency (2006). Reflection paper: Formulations of choice for the paediatric population; EMEA/CHMP/PEG/194810/2005. (Last updated 28 July 2006). www.ema.europa.eu/en/documents/scientific-guideline/reflection-paper-formulations-choice-paediatric-population_en.pdf (accessed 15 January 2020).

European Medicines Agency (2013). Guideline on Pharmaceutical Development of Medicines for Paediatric Use; EMA/CHMP/QWP/805880/2012. www.ema.europa.eu/en/documents/scientific-guideline/guideline-pharmaceutical-development-medicines-paediatric-use_en.pdf (accessed 29 May 2020).

European Medicines Agency (2019). Information for the package leaflet regarding ethanol used as an excipient in medicinal products for human use; EMA/CHMP/43486/2018. (Last updated 22 November 2019). www.ema.europa.eu/en/documents/scientific-guideline/information-package-leaflet-regarding-ethanol-used-excipient-medicinal-products-human-use_en.pdf (accessed 10 January 2020).

European Medicines Agency (2020a). Paediatric Regulation. www.ema.europa.eu/en/human-regulatory/overview/paediatric-medicines/paediatric-regulation#:~:text=Supporting%20SMEs-,Paediatric%20Regulation,aged%200%20to%2017%20years (accessed 29 May 2020).

European Medicines Agency (2020b). Paediatric investigation plans. www.ema.europa.eu/en/human-regulatory/research-development/paediatric-medicines/paediatric-investigation-plans (accessed 29 May 2020).

Graham, S. and Turner, M. (2011). European Study of Neonatal Exposure to Excipients (ESNEE). *Infant* 7(6): 196–199. www.infantjournal.co.uk/pdf/inf_042_ien.pdf (accessed 10 January 2020).

Halpern, S.A. (1988). *American Pediatrics: The Social Dynamic of Professionalism 1880–1980*. Berkeley, CA: University of California Press.

Keeling, S. and Bullock, G. (2020). NHS Injectable Medicines Guide. https://medusa.wales.nhs.uk/Home.asp – account required (accessed 23 May 2020).

Ladyzhynsky, N.S. (2012). Propylene Glycol. In: *Handbook of Pharmaceutical Excipients*, 7e (ed. Rowe, R.C.), 672–674. London: Pharmaceutical Press.

Medicines for Children (2018). Excipients in children's medicines. (Last updated 29 November 2018). www.medicinesforchildren.org.uk/excipients-children%E2%80%99s-medicines (accessed 10 January 2020).

Paediatric Formulary Committee (2019–2020). *British National Formulary for Children*. London: BMJ Group, Pharmaceutical Press, and RCPCH Publications.

Ranmal, S.R., Cram, A., and Tuleu, C. (2016). Age-appropriate and acceptable paediatric dosage forms: Insights into end-user perceptions, preferences and practices from the Children's Acceptability of Oral Formulations (CALF) Study. *Int J Pharm* 514(1): 296–307.

Royal College of Paediatrics and Child Health and Neonatal and Paediatric Pharmacists Group (2020). Position statement 18-01 Using Standardised Strengths of Unlicensed Liquid Medicines in Children. NPPG and the Royal College of Paediatrics and Child Health (RCPCH). www.rcpch.ac.uk/sites/default/files/2020-04/position_statement_v5_april_2020.pdf (accessed 27 May 2020).

Royal Pharmaceutical Society (2011). Pharmaceutical Issues when Crushing, Opening or Splitting Oral Dosage Forms. www.rpharms.com/Portals/0/RPS%20document%20library/Open%20access/Support/toolkit/pharmaceuticalissuesdosageforms-%282%29.pdf (accessed 11 April 2020).

UK National Poisons Information Service (2020). TOXBASE®: Benzyl Alcohol monograph. (Last updated December 2018). www.toxbase.org/ – account required (accessed 10 January 2020).

Waterfield, J. and Rivers, P. (2012). *Fundamental Aspects of Medicines*. London: Quay Books Division, MA Healthcare Ltd.

Watson, J., Rees, J.A., and Smith, I. (2014). *Pharmaceutical Practice*, 5e. Edinburgh: Churchill Livingstone.

White, R. and Bradnam, V. (2015). *Handbook of Drug Administration via Enteral Feeding Tubes*, 3e. London: Pharmaceutical Press.

Workman, B. (1999). Safe injection techniques. *Nurs Stand* 13(39): 47–53.

World Health Organization (2011). Development of paediatric medicines: points to consider in pharmaceutical development. www.who.int/medicines/areas/quality_safety/quality_assurance/Rev3-PaediatricMedicinesDevelopment_QAS08-257Rev3_17082011.pdf (accessed 24 May 2020).

Wrexham Maelor Hospital Pharmacy Department (2015). General guidance on administration of medication. In: *The NEWT Guidelines for Administration of Medication to Patients with Enteral Feeding Tubes or Swallowing Difficulties*, 3e (ed. Smith, J.A.), 21–43. Wrexham: North East Wales NHS Trust.

Yamada, S., Yamamoto, T., Suou, T. et al. (1992). Clinical significance of benzoate-metabolizing capacity in patients with chronic liver disease: pharmacokinetic analysis. *Res Commun Chem Pathol Pharmacol* 76(1): 53–62. https://pubmed.ncbi.nlm.nih.gov/1518961/ (accessed 10 January 2020).

Yochana, S., Yu, M., Alvi, M. et al. (2012). Pharmaceutical excipients and pediatric formulations. *Chemistry Today* 30(5): 14–18. www.researchgate.net/publication/288599708_Pharmaceutical_excipients_and_pediatric_form ulations#:~:text=Pharmaceutical%20excipients%20used%20in%20pediatric%20formulations%20have%20 received,the%20growth%20and%20development%20process%20of%20pediatric%20population (accessed 10 January 2020).

Further Resources

The Medicines for Children website www.medicinesforchildren.org.uk/ provides useful leaflets containing advice on the use of specific medication formulations in CYP.

Creating a pill school – https://northernpaediatrics.com/kidzmed/pill-school/

Dealing with harmful excipients in medicines for CYP – www.pharmaceutical-journal.com/learning/learning-article/how-to-identify-and-manage-problem-excipients-in-medicines-for-children/20203121. fullarticle?firstPass=false

Advice on how to safely administer medicines via enteral feeding tubes – www.nursingtimes.net/clinical-archive/nutrition/administration-of-medicines-via-an-enteral-feeding-tube-17-10-2011/

Information on promoting safer use of injectable medicines –www.sps.nhs.uk/wp-content/uploads/2018/02/2007-NRLS-0434F-Promoting-safeSOP-template-2007-v1.pdf

Practical advice for performing IV drug calculations – Dixon, A. and Evans, C. (2006). Intravenous therapy: Drug calculations and medication issues. *Infant* 2(3): 110–114. www.infantjournal.co.uk/pdf/inf_009_tdc.pdf

Multiple Choice Questions

Use these questions to test your knowledge of issues surrounding drug formulations for CYP. For each question, select the correct answer from the four options given.

1. Licensed medications:
   (a) Have not undergone rigorous safety checks hence should be used with caution.
   (b) Can also be termed imported or 'off-label' medications.
   (c) Are medications that have a marketing authorisation.
   (d) Are all medications administered to CYP in the UK.
2. When administering medications in CYP:
   (a) There are always plenty of flexible dosing formulations available.
   (b) Patient acceptability does not always need to be considered.
   (c) Unlicensed medications rarely need to be obtained.
   (d) Pharmacists' advice should often be sought to provide safe and accurate dosing.
3. Oral dosage administration:
   (a) Is an appropriate method of administration in an unconscious or vomiting CYP.
   (b) Drug absorption will not be affected by food intake or disease state.
   (c) Is the most preferred and safest route of administration.
   (d) Is unaffected by enzymes in the GIT.
4. Liquid formulations:
   (a) The volume to be administered in CYP should be considered.
   (b) Palatability and patient acceptability are never a problem.
   (c) Are likely to contain less excipients as liquid formulations are always made with CYP in mind.
   (d) Shelf-life is generally longer than that of solid dosage formulations.
5. Solid dosage formulations:
   (a) Granules and powders need to disintegrate to release the API.
   (b) Enteric-coated tablets deliver the API into the intestine.
   (c) Chewable tablets tend to have a bitter taste in the mouth.
   (d) Break-lines on tablets always mean that each half contains an equal amount of API.

Chapter 6 Drug Formulations

6. Manipulating capsules and tablets:
   (a) Film-coated tablets should never be crushed.
   (b) Soft gel capsules are the only type of capsule that can be opened.
   (c) Information on crushing tablets is readily available from the manufacturers.
   (d) MR tablets should not be crushed.

7. Mucous membrane medication administration:
   (a) When sublingual tablets are used, ensure that the CYP swallows them whole.
   (b) Suppositories are ideal for administration in CYP due to the availability of flexible dosage forms.
   (c) Buccal tablets are placed on the tongue to dissolve.
   (d) The API is absorbed directly into the bloodstream from the site of placement.

8. Topical administration:
   (a) Medications administered topically will only ever have a local effect.
   (b) Patches can never be cut to allow flexible dosing.
   (c) Ointments are most suited for chronic dry skin.
   (d) Suppositories and enemas are examples of drugs used topically.

9. Parenteral administration:
   (a) The location of a child's IV access will influence the concentration that an IV infusion can be safely administered at.
   (b) IM injections are the most common route for parenteral medication administration in CYP.
   (c) Large volumes of medication can be given via IM injection.
   (d) The SC route is more painful than IM administration.

10. Excipients:
    (a) One excipient may perform multiple roles within a formulation.
    (b) Excipients are the active substances within a medication formulation.
    (c) Preservatives are added to formulations to improve their taste.
    (d) Unlicensed medication formulations do not contain excipients.

11. Safety of excipients:
    (a) CYP experience fewer excipient-related adverse effects than adults.
    (b) If an excipient is safe to give to an adult, it is safe to give to CYP.
    (c) Some excipients that are safe to give to an older child may be dangerous for a newborn baby.
    (d) If one brand of a medication is safe for CYP, then all brands of the same medication will be safe.

12. Enteral feeding tubes:
    (a) A PEG tube is inserted into the nose and fed down into the stomach.
    (b) Intravenous syringes should never be used to prepare medications for administration via a feeding tube.
    (c) Enteral feeding tubes can only be used for medication administration within a hospital.
    (d) Medications can be given via feeding tubes whilst a feed is running.

13. Least likely to be suitable for administration via an enteral feeding tube:
    (a) Hard-gelatin capsule.
    (b) Modified-release tablet.
    (c) Oral solution.
    (d) Dispersible tablet.

14. Reconstituting oral powders for suspension:
    (a) Expiry date is unaffected by the reconstitution process.
    (b) Reconstituted suspension must be stored in a refrigerator.
    (c) Pharmacy staff always perform the reconstitution process.
    (d) Powder should be loosened by shaking the bottle prior to adding the solvent.

15. If the displacement value of a powder for solution for injection is disregarded:
    (a) There is a risk of under-dosing.
    (b) It will make no difference as displacement values are only relevant to oral powders for reconstitution.
    (c) There is a risk of overdosing.
    (d) The CYP will receive the correct dose.

Chapter 6 Drug Formulations

Find Out More

Take some time to think, look up and write some notes about the following topics. Include aspects of patient care and relate this to real practice experience where possible, maintaining patient confidentiality at all times.

TOPIC	YOUR NOTES
How to use a tablet crusher	
How to administer an enema	
How to administer an eye drop	
When and how to use an anaesthetic cream	
Pill schools for CYP	

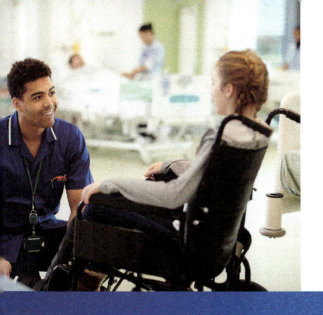

7

Medications Used in the Cardiovascular System

Anthony Garbutt and Noreen Kilkenny

Aim
Within this chapter, you will gain a broad understanding of common drugs which affect the cardiovascular system. Through discussion of drug therapy for chronic and acute conditions, this chapter will demonstrate the way these drugs act, their cardiovascular effects and some of the common side effects.

Learning Outcomes
- After completion of test questions, you will evaluate your existing knowledge and areas for development
- By the end of this chapter, you will identify physiological actions related to cardiovascular drugs
- By the end of this chapter, you will be able to distinguish between chronic and acute cardiovascular drugs
- By the end of this chapter, you will be able to clarify the uses of some less common cardiovascular drugs

Test Your Knowledge
1. The cardiovascular system is made up of the heart, major blood vessels and peripheral blood vessels. Can you name the four chambers of the heart and the two vessels which supply the lungs and body with blood?

Fundamentals of Pharmacology for Children's Nurses, First Edition. Edited by Ian Peate and Peter Dryden.
© 2022 John Wiley & Sons Ltd. Published 2022 by John Wiley & Sons Ltd.
Companion website: www.wiley.com/go/pharmacologyforCN

Chapter 7 Medications Used in the Cardiovascular System

2. What category of drugs do medications with the suffix '-pril' belong to?
3. What is the name given to an irregular heart rhythm?
4. There are three main physiological mechanisms for reducing blood pressure pharmacologically: can you name them?
5. Can you name the most common cardiovascular drug used in the treatment of cardiac arrest?

Introduction

The term 'cardiovascular' considers the heart and associated blood vessels, often segmented into atria, ventricles, great vessels and peripheral blood vessels (Ashworth, 2019). Cardiovascular disease is the most common cause of death worldwide, with 17.9 million deaths attributed to CVD, which is 31% of all deaths (World Health Organisation, 2017). An increasingly common suggestion of awareness of childhood CVD is suggested, with elevated blood pressure, abnormal lipid profiles, diabetes mellitus and smoking considered risk factors (Bloetzer et al., 2015). The British Heart Foundation (BHF, 2013) identifies similar risk factors, namely high cholesterol and obesity alongside behavioural risk factors such as diet, physical activity, alcohol and smoking. BHF (2013) also state that congenital abnormality is pertinent to childhood CVD.

Historically, Berenson et al. (1998) developed a link between childhood CVD risk factors and increased disease in adulthood. More recently, McGill et al. (2008) linked childhood CVD risks to increased severity of CVD during adulthood, supporting increased childhood and adolescent awareness, stating that effective treatment is critically important (McGill et al., 2009).

Pharmacologically, drugs to treat CVD have widely improved since the 1950s, with numerous drugs being discovered. Some examples of this are: antihypertensives, adrenergic receptor blockers, antiplatelet therapy, cholesterol-lowering medication, drugs for heart rhythm control and drugs affecting the renin-angiotensin aldosterone axis (Braunwald, 2015). Due to these complex classifications, an attempt will be made through this chapter to identify and simplify their actions where possible.

Clinical Consideration

Anxiety in clinical settings can cause 'White coat syndrome'. If there is an elevated blood pressure, it would be worthwhile taking multiple readings during the episode of care.

Gross Anatomy Related to Cardiovascular System (CVS) Pharmacology

The CVS is responsible for the supply of blood, oxygen and nutrients to the body whilst transporting waste materials for excretion. The CVS consists of the following primary structures:

- Heart
- Arteries
- Capillaries
- Veins

Please see Figure 7.1 for a visual representation of the heart.

Chapter 7 Medications Used in the Cardiovascular System

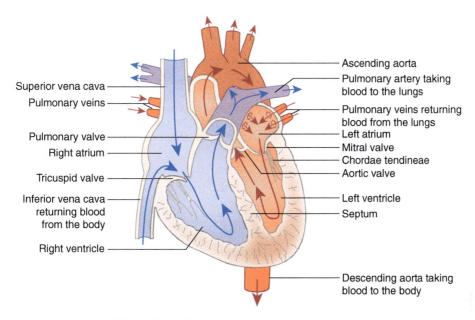

Figure 7.1 **Gross anatomy and blood flow of the heart.** *Source:* Gormley-Fleming and Peate, 2018/John Wiley & Sons.

Structure
The heart is cone-shaped and located in the mediastinum, or middle of the chest cavity. The upper part of the heart is known as the base and the lower, more pointed section is known as the apex.

There are four main chambers: the left and right atrium and the left and right ventricles. A fibromuscular septum divides the two atria, called the interatrial septum and the ventricles are divided by the intraventricular septum. During neonatal development, a connection between the two atria should close (patent foramen ovale) while remaining atrial and ventricular septal defects (ASD and VSD) can be relatively common.

Heart Valves
There are four valves, called the aortic, pulmonary, tricuspid and mitral valves. The mitral and tricuspid valves allow blood flow from the atria to the ventricles, while the aortic and pulmonary valves allow blood flow from the ventricles to the systemic and pulmonary circulation. Working heart valves should be one-way or occlusive when closed. If they are not fully occlusive, this leak is termed regurgitation but can also be valve 'stiffening', called stenosis.

Layers of the Heart
The heart is made up of three layers: epicardium (outer), myocardium (middle) and endocardium (inner). See Table 7.1 for more details.

Function
The heart contains two circulation routes, the pulmonary and systemic.
1. Pulmonary – the right side of the heart pumps deoxygenated blood to the lungs for gas exchange (under low pressure)
2. Systemic – the left side of the heart pumps oxygenated blood to the body's organs and tissues (under high pressure)

The cardiovascular system aids homeostasis via:
- Rapid transport of nutrients such as oxygen, amino acids, glucose, fatty acids, water
- Excretion of waste products such as carbon dioxide, urea and creatinine

Chapter 7 Medications Used in the Cardiovascular System

Table 7.1 The layers of the heart.

LAYER	DESCRIPTION
Epicardium	This thin outer layer of the heart contains the nerves, adipose tissue, coronary arteries and veins.
Myocardium	This is the thickest layer, it consists of cardiac muscle cells. It is thickest over the left ventricle and thinnest in the atria. Two hormones can be produced with heart distension: Atrial Natriuretic Peptide (ANP) and Brain Natriuretic Peptide (BNP). When the atrial chambers are stretched, ANP is released, while BNP will identify ventricular distension.
Endocardium	The endocardium outer layer contains Purkinje fibres, veins and nerves, a middle layer contains connective tissue, with an inner layer of flat endothelial cells

- Transportation of immune cells, antigens and other mediators acting as host defence
- Body temperature is regulated by controlling heat distribution between body core and skin
- Transport of endocrine hormones occurs via the circulation

Right Side of the Heart

Deoxygenated blood enters the heart from the superior and inferior vena cava into the right atrium (causing preload pressure). As the right atrium contracts, the pressure increases within this chamber. Blood then passes through the tricuspid valve and into the right ventricle.

The tricuspid valve closes and the right ventricle ejects blood through the pulmonary valve and into the main pulmonary artery, which bifurcates to the right and left lung. The pulmonary valve closes due to backpressure of blood and prevents backflow.

Left Side of the Heart

Oxygenated blood returns to the heart via four pulmonary veins (left and right superior and inferior) and into the left atrium. The left atrium fills and the atrial myocardium contracts forcing the blood through the mitral valve and into the left ventricle. The left ventricle now ejects blood into the aorta through the aortic valve which then closes due to backpressure (afterload pressure).

Cardiovascular Drugs Affecting Chronic Conditions

Statins

With familial hypercholesterolaemia, drug therapy may be considered by the age of 10 years but the clinical decision will be made upon the child's age, onset and age of familial coronary heart disease and other cardiac risk factors (National Health Lung and Blood Institute (NHLBI), 2012). Those who do not tolerate statins may be offered ezetimibe, bile acid sequestrants or fibrates (National Institute of Health and Care Excellence (NICE), 2020).

A full lipid profile should be established prior to commencing statins. Creatinine concentration and liver function profile should be monitored when commencing lipid-lowering therapy. Liver function tests should be repeated 3-monthly and then 12-monthly to monitor for hepatotoxicity.

Clinical Consideration

A full lipid profile will consist of the following:

1. High-density Lipoprotein (HDL) 'good'
2. Low-density Lipoprotein (LDL) 'bad' >190ml/dL may require pharmacological treatment
3. Triglycerides (certain type of fat)

NHLBI (2012) provided guidance on screening for patients under 21 years. However, recommendation acceptance is clinically limited due to reduced evidence to support utility of paediatric screening for dyslipidaemia and hypertension. Notably, obesity screening is more widely accepted. As previously noted, hypercholesterolaemia, hypertension and obesity can be predictors of further adult disease, with potential familial connections (McGill et al., 2009).

Experience around lipid-regulating drugs in children is limited and therefore should be commenced under specialist guidance. This said, a recent study found short- and intermediate-term statin use to be safe in children and adolescents with hypercholesterolaemia (Kavey et al., 2020). It is also noted that statins should be combined with health promotion, increased exercise and effective diet if possible.

The two statins of choice are atorvastatin and simvastatin; however, other statins such as fluvastatin may be considered, although fluvastatin is the least potent to LDL cholesterol levels (Joint Formulary Committee (JFC), 2021). Statin therapy may be considered in children aged 10 years and upwards for hypercholesterolaemia where cholesterol concentration is unaffected by lifestyle and diet changes (JFC, 2021).

Dyslipidaemias such as mixed hyperlipidaemia, hypoalphalipoproteinemia and hypercholesterolaemia contribute as a chief cause of atherosclerosis and are often caused by genetic lipoprotein disorders (Li, 2014). Also, conditions such as coronary heart disease, ischaemic cerebrovascular disease and peripheral vascular disease are associated.

Physiologically, three main pathways are involved in lipoprotein metabolism: the exogenous pathway which transports dietary lipids, the endogenous pathway transporting hepatic lipids and reverse cholesterol transport. When these pathways are dysregulated by genetic disorders or dietary factors, dyslipidemia presents. Table 7.2 gives useful information regarding pharmacokinetics of statins.

Statins have revolutionised the management of dyslipidaemias. Some cautions and considerations in relation to statins are shown in in Table 7.3.

Table 7.2 Pharmacokinetics of statins.

Absorption	Statins are ingested orally via the mouth. 40–75% of the drug is absorbed in the intestine apart from fluvastatin, which is absorbed completely by the intestine.
Distribution	Over 98% of the dose is bound to plasma proteins in the blood within 2–4 hours.
Metabolism	Cytochrome P450 in the liver and intestine. Bioavailability varies between 5–30% of administered doses.
Excretion	70% of statin metabolises into bile and subsequently in faeces. The excess is excreted through the renal system.

Source: Based on Drugbank, 2020.

Table 7.3 Cautions or considerations for all statins.

Liver function
High alcohol intake; history of liver disease; hypothyroidism; known genetic polymorphism

Muscle effects
Muscle toxicity can occur with all statins; risk is increased with higher doses and in patients with muscle toxicity, including those with a personal or family history of muscular disorders, previous history of muscular toxicity, a high alcohol intake, renal impairment or hypothyroidism, myopathy or rhabdomyolysis
   A statin should not usually be started if the baseline creatine kinase concentration is more than 5 times the upper limit of normal, caution needs to be taken for those who are very physically active or who take part in rigorous exercise.

Hypothyroidism
Hypothyroidism should be managed adequately before starting treatment with a statin.

Hepatic impairment
In general, manufacturers advise caution (risk of increased exposure); avoid in active disease or unexplained persistent elevations in serum transaminases.

Renal impairment
Doses above 10 mg daily should be used with caution if estimated glomerular filtration rate is less than 30 ml/minute/1.73 m²

There are side effects which are common across all statins. These commonly include constipation, diarrhoea and flatulence alongside dizziness nausea and sleep disorders. Less commonly, alopecia and hepatic disorders are noted. Although uncommon, muscle myopathy and dyspnoea related to interstitial lung changes are serious and require further investigation immediately (BNFc, 2020).

Ezetimibe

Ezetimibe can be combined with statins or as an alternative, if statins are not tolerated. Ezetimibe inhibits the absorption of cholesterol in the intestine, and is only considered for use in children aged 10 years and up (Miller et al., 2015). Common side effects include gastrointestinal discomfort, whereas you may find chest pain, cough, hypertension and muscle complaints among the less common.

Evolocumab

Evolocumab can be used for children over the age of 12 years. Evolocumab binds to pro-protein which is involved in the protection of LDL receptors in liver cells, because these receptors are protected from damaging proteins the uptake of LDL cholesterol is increased, (JFC, 2021). This medication can be oral or subcutaneous and may be offered to children who are undergoing apheresis therapy due to familial hypercholesterolaemia and in conjunction with statin therapy. Side effects do include back pain and increased infection risk.

Anticoagulant Medications

Aspirin

This is an antiplatelet drug that is used to prevent thrombus formation after congenital cardiac surgery or in the case of inflammatory vascular disorders, such as Kawasaki disease to prevent coronary thrombosis. It is not recommended to give aspirin to children under 16 years due to the risk of Reye's syndrome (BNFc, 2020), which can cause dangerous cerebral and hepatic swelling. Therefore, it is very important to query the use of aspirin in children under 16 years, unless specifically recommended by a doctor.

Aspirin works inside platelets by blocking synthesis of thromboxane A2 from arachidonic acid, which reduces the aggregating properties of the platelet and lasts for 7–10 days with an irreversible effect (Hatchet and Thompson, 2002).

Common side effects of oral aspirin include dyspepsia and haemorrhage. Caution should also be given to those with asthma, allergies, previous peptic ulcers, thyrotoxicosis, anaemia, dehydration and uncontrolled hypertension (BNFc, 2020).

Clinical Consideration

It is best practice to investigate aspirin being prescribed to anyone under 16 years (BNFc, 2020).

Warfarin

Warfarin is a historical anticoagulant drug, responsible for reducing the chances of unwanted blood clot formation. Warfarin works as a competitive inhibitor, decreasing the effect of enzymes which activate vitamin K and ultimately reducing the synthesis of complex clotting factors.

Warfarin is most commonly taken orally, with initial onset duration of between 24–72 hours. Due to each patient experiencing individual effects of warfarin, a blood test must be regularly undertaken to quantify the therapeutic effect. This test is commonly termed a prothrombin time (PT) or international normalised ratio (INR).

When considering organs involved in clotting, the liver produces prothrombin (factor II), which becomes activated by vitamin K. Therefore, if liver dysfunction is present, there may be reduced coagulation prior to warfarin commencement. Table 7.4 shows warfarin/aspirin differences.

Table 7.4 Warfarin versus Aspirin ADME.

	WARFARIN	ASPIRIN
Absorption	Completely absorbed by GI tract	Generally rapid and complete via oral route, absorbed in stomach and proximal small intestine
Distribution	Within 6–12 hours, 99% bound to plasma proteins (mainly albumin)	50–90% plasma protein bound, particularly albumin bound
Metabolism	Metabolised by CYP2C9 enzyme	Generally within 24 hours via liver enzymes
Excretion	Almost entirely metabolised with 80% excretion via urine, 20% faeces	10–85% elimination via urine, however this is dependent upon urine pH. Acidic pH increases tubular reabsorption, alkali pH decreases tubular reabsorption

Angiotensin Converting Enzyme (ACE) Inhibitors

ACE inhibitors act by preventing or blocking the conversion of angiotensin I to angiotensin II. Angiotensin II is a potent vasoconstrictor which also stimulates aldosterone secretion, increasing vascular sodium retention, therefore increasing blood pressure and cardiac afterload (Klabunde, 2017). When taking ACE inhibitors, blood vessels should remain dilated, thus reducing the workload of the heart and lowering blood pressure (Peate, 2018).

Renal sodium reabsorption due to aldosterone increase can exacerbate symptoms of a failing heart, resulting in cardiac and vascular remodelling due to hypertension. Therefore, ACE inhibitors are useful for both hypertension and heart failure (Hatchett and Thompson, 2002). Contraindications and side effects of ACE inhibitors can be found in Table 7.5.

The three main ACE inhibitors used for children are:

1. Captopril
2. Enalapril
3. Lisinopril

Clinical Consideration

ACE inhibitors are common first line treatments for primary hypertension. A very common side effect is dry, non-productive cough, which is useful to know for medication history taking.

Table 7.5 Contraindication and side effects of ACE inhibitors.

Contraindications	Previous hypersensitivity Impaired renal function Bilateral renovascular disease Lower blood glucose with diabetes mellitus First dose hypotension associated with: high-dose diuretics, on a low-sodium diet, on dialysis, dehydrated, or with heart failure. Primary aldosteronism reduces effectiveness Caution with hypertrophic cardiomyopathy and severe or symptomatic aortic stenosis.
Side effects	10% of patients experience dry non-productive cough as the most common side effect, due to increased bradykinin. Hypotension is also common with heart failure patients (Klabunde, 2017). Hyperkalaemia is most common with impaired renal function. Therefore, baseline renal function, followed by regular monitoring, is essential. Arrythmia, angina pectoris, chest pain, sleep disorder, syncope, nausea and electrolyte imbalance are common

Angiotensin II Receptor Antagonists

Properties of Angiotensin II Receptor Antagonists (A2RA) are close to those of ACE inhibitors, however, they do not increase bradykinin, therefore are less likely to cause a dry cough. Therefore, they are a good alternative to ACE inhibitors. This said, serum potassium and creatinine should be checked to establish baseline levels, as per ACE inhibitor protocol (NHLBI, 2012).

Candesartan, Losartan Potassium and Valsartan are the most common A2RA. Losartan is available as a suspension, whereas others are primarily in tablet form (NHLBI, 2012).

Cautions for A2RA include patients with current left ventricular hypertrophy, hypertrophic cardiomyopathy, and patients with mitral, aortic or renal stenosis. The only contraindication noted is cholestasis. Common side effects include abdominal and back pain, diarrhoea, nausea, dizziness, hypotension and serum electrolyte changes (BNFc, 2020).

Peripheral Alpha Antagonist or Alpha-Adrenergic Blockers: 'Alpha Blockers'

Doxazosin and prazosin are the two most common alpha blockers (AB). They both have post-synaptic alpha blocking and vasodilator properties, therefore are effective for lowering blood pressure. Some of the most common side effects are an initial drop of blood pressure after the first dose so should be introduced with caution. They can be effectively combined with other antihypertensives, for an improved anti-hypertensive effect.

A contraindication for AB is a history of postural hypotension, while also noting aortic stenosis can contraindicate AB. Common side effects include arrythmia, chest pain, cough, dizziness and increased risk of infection, while side effects unique to prazosin only include nervousness, palpitations and blurred vision (BNFc, 2020).

Cardiovascular Drugs for Use in Acute Clinical Scenarios

Within the UK population, CVS disease is more associated with adults than children, however drug treatments are widely transferrable (Lawrenson et al., 2011). British Heart Foundation (BHF, 2020) suggest that 12 babies per day are diagnosed with congenital cardiovascular anomalies, with Mocumbi et al. (2011) suggesting a figure of 5–8 per 1000 births having some form of CVS anomaly within western countries. The UK National Congenital Heart Disease Audit (NCHDA, 2019) identifies a 1% prevalence of congenital cardiovascular anomaly among UK births – predominantly in the heart and great vessels. NCHDA (2019) confirming one third of these patients require intervention, often being surgical, requiring a period of intensive recuperation on an Intensive Care Unit (ICU).

Ritter et al. (2020) suggest there are a limited number of drugs which affect cardiovascular function directly. For more pragmatic classification, we can roughly clinically translate to the four following actions:

1. Antidysrhythmic drugs (which help control arrythmia)
2. Inotropic drugs (which affect contractility of each heart beat)
3. Chronotropic drugs (which affect heart rate)
4. Vasoactive drugs (which affect peripheral vascular system)

Table 7.6 will facilitate further understanding of the common terminology.

Electrophysiological System Recap

Within a healthy heart, an electrical action potential (AP) passes through a chronological pathway, leading to effective timing of cardiac contractility. Through stimulation of the sino-atrial node, the AP will pass through the internodal tracts, to Bachman's bundle in the left atrium and the atrioventricular node at the junction

Chapter 7 Medications Used in the Cardiovascular System

Table 7.6 Four main actions of cardiovascular system drugs.

Control arrythmia	*Vaughan-Williams classification* Drugs which act upon the electrophysiological apparatus of the heart	
Control cardiac contractility	*Negative inotrope* A drug which reduces the force of cardiac contraction	*Positive inotrope* A drug which increases the force of cardiac contraction
Control heart rate	*Negative chronotrope* A drug which actively reduces heart rate	*Positive chronotrope* A drug which actively increases heart rate
Control peripheral vascular system	*Vasodilator* A drug which increases the diameter of the peripheral arterioles – decreasing systemic vascular resistance	*Vasoconstrictor* A drug which decreases the diameter of the peripheral arterioles – increasing systemic vascular resistance

Source: Adapted from Lei et al., 2018.

between atria and ventricles. Upon passing through the atrioventricular node, the AP will pass along the bundle of His, into the left and right bundle branches into Purkinje fibres, finally stimulating contractility of both ventricles (Stanfield, 2017).

Clinical Consideration

Diagnosing arrythmia will require specialist analysis of an electrocardiogram. Common symptoms include:
- Disinterest in feeding, pale skin and irritability in younger children
- Lightheaded feeling and palpitations in older children

Antidysrhythmic Drugs

Ritter et al. (2020) supports the classification of four primary categories of antidysrhythmic drugs. These are largely based around the work of Miles Vaughan-Williams (1918–2016). Table 7.7 identifies the classifications.

Class 1 – 1a Quinidine, 1b Lidocaine, 1c Propafenone

Cardiac cells require an action potential to 'excite' the contractile cells, with sodium, potassium and calcium being the primary ions involved. Due to a large amount of these ions within the sarcoplasmic reticulum of the cardiac myocyte, the balance of action potentials within cardiac cells are rarely stable. This instability requires electrical depolarisation to activate, which triggers myocardial contraction.

Sodium channels consist of three main states: open, inactive and resting. During depolarisation (contraction), they are between resting and open states, sodium influx triggering contraction. Within class 1 antidysrhythmic drugs there are three sub-classifications: 1a, 1b and 1c. Moderate (1a), weak (1b) and marked (1c) sodium channel blocking is noted (Lei et al., 2018) (see Figure 7.2).

Table 7.7 Vaughan-Williams classification.

Class 1	drugs that block voltage sensitive sodium channels
Class 2	beta-adrenoreceptor antagonists (beta blockers)
Class 3	drugs that substantially prolong a cardiac action potential
Class 4	calcium antagonists

Source: Adapted from Lei et al., 2018.

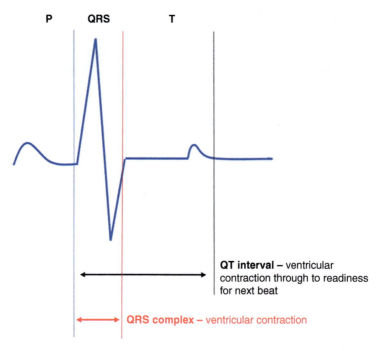

Figure 7.2 **QRS/QT type 1 affects.** *Source:* Adapted from Lei et al., 2018.

Class 2 – Atenolol, Metoprolol, Labetalol
Class 2 consists of beta-adrenergic inhibitors, which are popular anti-arrhythmic drugs. Interestingly, beta-adrenergic antagonists and beta-adrenergic inhibitors are used as semi-interchangeable terms within class 2 drugs. Due to this inhibitor process, these drugs are classically termed 'beta blockers' (BB).

Beta-adrenergic receptors are stimulated by hormones called catecholamines. Common catecholamines are adrenaline (epinephrine), noradrenaline (norepinephrine) and dopamine. Catecholamines are said to be endogenous (internal), producing a physiological response within the cardiovascular system. For example, adrenaline increases heart rate and cardiac contractility. This is done through activation of both beta-1 and beta-2 adrenergic receptors. If this action can be inhibited through class 2 BB, catecholamine effect is limited, reducing heart rate and contractility.

A smaller number of beta-1 and beta-2 adrenergic receptors within children with HF can make BB less effective compared to use in adult patients. This should be noted when caring for children with HF, as increasing dosage may not be effective (Miyamoto et al., 2014; Lipshultz and Wilkinson, 2014).

Importantly, contraindications of BB include asthma, hypotension and bradycardia. For those with a clinical history of asthma, bronchospasm or obstructive disease a cardio-selective BB can be chosen as a substitute. Notably, BB can reduce secretion of melatonin, so can have a negative effect upon sleep (Farzam and Jan, 2020). For ease of interpretation, a three-section classification has been adapted from the work of Farzam and Jan (2020) in Table 7.8. This demonstrates alternatives if a patient suffers side effects or if BB are contraindicated.

Class 3 – Amiodarone and Sotalol Hydrochloride
These drugs predominantly affect potassium channels, alongside lesser effects upon sodium and calcium channels. This leads to reduced excitability of myocardial membranes, meaning a negative chronotropic effect. In higher doses, some class 3 drugs block alpha and beta-adrenergic receptors, contributing to negative inotropic effect (Iyer, 2008).

Chapter 7 Medications Used in the Cardiovascular System

Table 7.8 Sub-classifications of beta blockers.

Type 1	Non-selective beta blockers (beta-1 and beta-2 receptors – acting 'globally')	propranolol, carvedilol, labetalol hydrochloride, sotalol hydrochloride
Type 2	Water-soluble beta blockers (less likely to cross the blood–brain barrier and cause sleep disturbance)	atenolol, sotalol hydrochloride
Type 3	Cardio-selective beta blockers (primarily acting upon beta-1 receptors in the heart)	atenolol, metoprolol

Source: Adapted from Farzam and Jan, 2020.

Amiodarone is most common, due be being a highly effective anti-arrhythmic drug, even in the presence of heart failure. Amiodarone is used primarily for supraventricular and ventricular tachycardias (BNFc, 2020). By blocking potassium currents, this slows the action potential, reducing cell excitability, reducing tachyarrhythmia risk (Florek and Girzadas, 2020). Amiodarone is contraindicated for rapid loading post-cardiac surgery, in patients with anatomical disturbances to the heart's conduction system (without pacemaker fitted) and sinus bradycardia.

A less common class 3 antidysrhythmic drug is sotolol hydrochloride. It is a non-selective BB in class 2, however, it also blocks the potassium channels so can be included in class 3. Sotalol has good oral absorption and effective transplacental passage, so can be used for the treatment of foetal arrythmia (Iyer, 2008).

Class 4 – Verapamil and Diltiazem

These drugs are calcium channel blockers (CCB), which act upon the sino-atrial and atrioventricular nodes. The effectiveness of these drugs in treatment of tachycardia can often be measured through the PR interval of an ECG (see Figure 7.2 – P wave to the R crest). Calcium channel receptors are also found in smooth muscle of blood vessels. This means calcium channel blockers can be multimodal in treatment, and can be used in the treatment of hypertension.

Verapamil has powerful effects in reducing heart rate but also strongly binds to alpha receptors, inhibiting catecholamine effects, mostly adrenaline and noradrenaline. Verapamil is used to treat supraventricular tachycardia, which is a sudden and transient increase in heart rate. Verapamil is useful for persistent left ventricular tachycardia and reducing blood pressure in hypertrophic cardiomyopathy.

Diltiazem is also a common CCB, acting more predominantly on the sino-atrial and atrioventricular nodes, although it has utility as treatment for hypertension. Diltiazem is also considered a useful drug for treatment of supraventricular tachycardia.

Drugs with an Inotropic Effect

Positive Inotropes

Within acute care, drugs which increase cardiac contractility and force of ejection are very useful (see Table 7.10 for more information). These drugs can be used in low cardiac output syndrome (LCOS), which can be a fairly common phenomena post-cardiac surgery, occurring in up to 25% of cases (Jones et al., 2005). Inotropic drugs can also be very useful in managing cardiovascular failure in critically unwell patients with conditions such as sepsis or cardiac arrest.

The heart has both sympathetic (rapid and involuntary) and parasympathetic (to balance sympathetic) innervation from the nervous system (Figure 7.3 shows receptor sites). Parasympathetic innervation remains mostly atrial, while sympathetic innervation is both atrial and ventricular.

Drugs with a positive inotropic effect are 'calcium mobilisers', loading cardiac myocytes with calcium ions. This increase in available calcium comes from the intracellular store within the sarcoplasmic reticulum and increased calcium influx (see Figure 7.4). Positive inotropic effect will increase cardiac contractility, but will also increase heart rate. This increase in heart rate will increase the oxygen consumption of the cardiac muscle, so patient arrythmia can be common (Nagy et al., 2014).

Milrinone

Milrinone is a drug with positive inotropic effects, used short-term for the improvement of cardiac function. Milrinone may be used longer term for patients awaiting heart transplantation and falls under a category of drug called Phosphodieterase (PDE) inhibitors. Milrinone has a vasoactive effect on both pulmonary and systemic arterial beds (Giaccone et al., 2017). This causes vasodilation, reducing peripheral vascular resistance (afterload) and reduces pressure of blood returning to the heart (preload).

Chapter 7 Medications Used in the Cardiovascular System

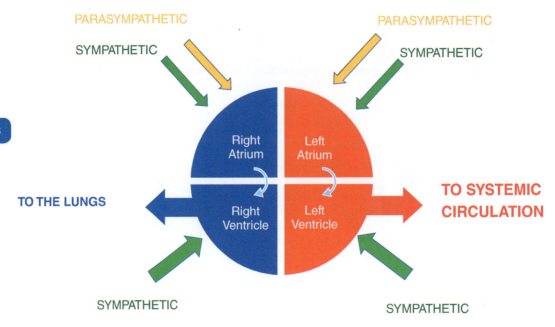

Figure 7.3 Areas of parasympathetic and sympathetic innervation.

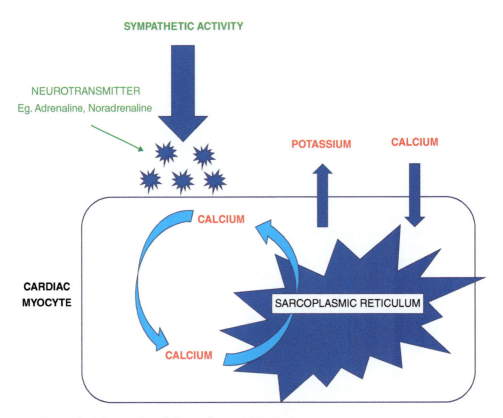

Figure 7.4 Sympathetic innervation of the cardiac myocyte.

The Prophylactic Intravenous Use of Milrinone post-operatively After Cardiac Operation in Paediatrics (PRIMACORP) study found milrinone to be useful in the prophylactic treatment of LCOS. Milrinone is an adjunct to cardiac surgery, which is a common treatment for congenital heart disease (Hoffman et al., 2002). Some common side effects of milrinone include arrythmia, headache and hypotension, while severe hypovolaemia is a contraindication.

Adrenaline (Epinephrine)

Adrenaline is produced in the adrenal glands, situated just above the kidney. Primarily, it will cause a positive inotropic effect, increasing the force of cardiac contraction, while stimulating transient increase in heart rate. In urgent cardiovascular events, synthetic adrenaline can be delivered intravenously to improve cardiac output, stimulating alpha-1 receptors to reverse vasodilation.

Stimulation of beta-1 and beta-2 receptors will increase cardiac contractility while receptors in vascular smooth muscle increase peripheral vascular resistance through vasoconstriction. Another benefit of Adrenaline is suppression of histamine release, particularly helpful in the treatment of anaphylaxis.

The administration of adrenaline works best through a central line, giving rapid access to cardiac tissue, although remains effective via a cannulated peripheral vein. Due to the powerful vasoconstrictive effects of adrenaline, it must not be delivered to extreme peripheries via adrenaline release device, due to increasing the chance of tissue malperfusion.

Skills in Practice

Adrenaline should be delivered via intramuscular injection. The suggested site for adrenaline is the anterolateral aspect of vastus lateralis (front outer third of the of thigh). If pre-prepared adrenaline release devices are not available, anything from a 16mm length 25G orange needle, to a 38mm length 21G green needle can be used.

An alternative site would be the deltoid muscle, roughly 2–3 centimetres below the acromion process (at the very top of the humerus, looking side on).

Source: Based on Resuscitation Council, 2008.

A secondary effect of adrenaline is bronchodilation, beta-2 binding causes respiratory smooth muscle dilation. Adrenaline is useful for treatment of anaphylaxis, through dilating airways and improving respiratory gas transfer, supporting Epipen use for respiratory distress with allergic reactions.

As discussed, hypotension, anaphylaxis and severe allergic reactions are indications for adrenaline use. Some contraindications include hyperthyroidism, diabetes mellitus and severe renal impairment. Interestingly, adrenaline is said to have no noted common side effects.

Dopamine Hydrochloride

Dopamine is a dose-dependent drug, changing its primary characteristics depending upon the dosage (see Table 7.9). Pharmacological dopamine is a synthetic catecholamine, meaning it has a reduced half-life in comparison to native biological catecholamines. At lower doses, it has a primary positive inotropic effect, alongside a secondary vasoconstrictive effect due to acting upon both the alpha and beta-adrenergic receptors (Wen and Xu, 2020). At low doses, there is a vasodilatory effect upon renal, mesenteric, coronary and intracerebral vascular beds.

At higher doses (>15 micrograms/kg/min) there is an increase in peripheral vascular resistance and renal vasoconstriction occurs. Furthermore, dopamine is contraindicated in pheochromocytoma and tachyarrhythmia, alongside having no common side effects.

Dobutamine Hydrochloride

Dobutamine is a selective beta-1 receptor stimulator, which increases cardiac contractility in both normally functioning hearts and hearts in failure. Dobutamine will also decrease peripheral vascular resistance (afterload) which in turn will reduce the ventricular filling pressure (preload).

Dobutamine does not have chronotropic effects and will not increase heart rate under typical circumstances. However, due to increased myocardial contractility, there will be an increase in stroke volume, meaning increased cardiac output (see Figure 7.5). This increase in cardiac output will increase the amount of urine being produced without vaso-actively affecting the renal blood flow.

Table 7.9 Dose-dependent dopamine hydrochloride actions.

DOSAGE	RECEPTOR SITES	PHYSIOLOGICAL ACTION
0.5–2 micrograms/kg/min	Dopaminergic – vasodilator	Renal, mesenteric, coronary and intracerebral arterial beds blood flow increase
5–10 micrograms/kg/min	Beta-1 – positive inotropic effect Dopaminergic – vasodilator	Positive inotropic effect increases cardiac contractility and cardiac output. Vasodilator effects same as above
10–15 micrograms/kg/min	Beta-1 – positive inotropic effect Alpha-1 – mild vasoconstrictive effect	Positive inotropic effect increases cardiac output, while stimulation of Alpha-1 receptors has mild vasoconstrictive effect
>15 micrograms/kg/min	Alpha-1 – powerful vasoconstrictive effect Beta-1 – minimal inotropic effect	Alpha-1 receptors are now the primary stimulus creating a powerful vasoconstrictive effect with minimal inotropic effect.

Source: Adapted from Wen and Xu, 2020

Table 7.10 Table of inotropic actions.

DRUG	RECEPTOR	MAIN PHYSIOLOGICAL EFFECT	PHASE OF CARDIAC CYCLE
Milrinone	Inhibits intracellular phosphodieterase (PDE)	Positive inotropy, vasodilation	Diastole
Adrenaline	Alpha-1, Beta-1, Beta-2	Positive inotropy, positive chronotropy, bronchodilation	Systole
Dopamine	Beta-1, Alpha-1	Positive inotropy, positive chronotropy	Systole
Dobutamine	Beta-1, Beta-2	Positive inotropy, positive chronotropy, vasodilation	Systole
Noradrenaline	Alpha-1, Beta-1	Mild positive inotropy, mainly vasoconstrictive	Systole

Source: Adapted from Giaccone et al., 2017; Wen and Xu, 2020.

Dobutamine is indicated in cardiomyopathy and LCOS, although is contraindicated in patients with pheochromocytoma. Side effects are numerous, with arrythmia, bronchospasm, fever and palpitations being common.

Noradrenaline (Norepinephrine)

The primary effect of noradrenaline is the stimulation of vasoconstriction in smaller arterial beds. Noradrenaline is an alpha receptor stimulator, having the physiological effect of increasing both systolic and diastolic blood pressures. Due to this powerful vasoconstriction, noradrenaline reduces peripheral blood flow. This is notable in both the renal and mesenteric circulation, while blood flow to skeletal muscle will also decrease.

A secondary effect of noradrenaline is stimulation of cardiac beta-1 receptors. This stimulation will induce a positive inotropic effect, therefore hypertensive patients are contraindicated. This is not often the primary desired therapeutic effect of noradrenaline. Noradrenaline will be discussed again in the vasoactive drug section.

Important risk factors in administering noradrenaline are line site necrosis when given through a central line, while extravasation necrosis and peripheral ischaemia are risk factors when given via peripheral cannula, which is the less preferred option.

Drugs with a Chronotropic Effect

Within the cardiovascular system, there are drugs which increase or decrease heart rate. The drugs which increase heart rate fall into the category of positive chronotropes while decreased heart rate categorise as negative chronotropes. To understand the importance of heart rate, it is useful to revisit the equation for cardiac output (see Figure 7.5).

Positive Chronotropes
Atropine Sulfate
Atropine is given to block the effect of acetylcholine as a neurotransmitter upon the sino-atrial (SA) and atrioventricular (AV) node. For this reason, it is a common treatment for low heart rate abnormal rhythms or bradyarrythmias.

Atropine increases conduction velocity through the cardiac action potential, alongside increasing the SA node discharge rate, which increases overall heart rate. This also reduces AV node refractory period, which allows the ventricle to keep up with the now higher atrial discharge rate more effectively.

Adrenaline (Epinephrine)
Adrenaline will couple with beta-adrenergic receptors (beta-1 and beta-2), which will increase heart rate. This is often a secondary affect, with adrenaline primarily chosen for its inotropic qualities. Due to its positive inotropic, positive chronotropic and vasoconstrictive affect, adrenaline is an extremely effective treatment during cardiac resuscitation.

Episode of Care

Karim is 8 years of age and is rushed to the emergency department requiring cardiac resuscitation and he is in asystole. Chest compressions have been started with patent peripheral cannula inserted by paramedics. The emergency department consultant requires adrenaline for the advanced life support algorithm in an attempt to stimulate cardiac contractility and heart rate.

This should be titrated depending upon Karim's weight to a dose of 10mcg kg^{-1} (alternatively 0.1ml kg^{-1} of 1 in 10,000 adrenaline solution). This will be delivered every 3–5 minutes intravenously depending upon cycle loops and presence of pulse. If intravenous access is unavailable central venous catheter (if available) or intra-osseous are alternative delivery methods.

Local policy should be adhered to – this is a generic example.

Based on Resuscitation Council, 2015.

CARDIAC OUTPUT =
HEART RATE X STROKE
VOLUME

• This equation lets us know that the amount of blood pumped by the left ventricle is dependent upon heart rate (in beats per minute) and stroke volume, or how much blood is ejected from the left ventricle with each ejection measured in millilitres (mL).

Figure 7.5 **Cardiac output.**

Dopamine Hydrochloride

Dopamine has both direct and indirect effects. Its direct affect is upon beta-1 receptors, which increase chronotropy, resulting in higher heart rate. Indirectly, Dopamine increases the release of the neurotransmitter Noradrenaline from sympathetic nerves creating positive inotropic and vasoconstrictive effects also.

Negative Chronotropes
Beta Blockers (BB)

BB inhibit adrenergic receptors and are classified into three modes of action: non-selective, cardio-selective and water-soluble. For the purposes of negative chronotropy, beta-1 receptors are the primary location of action. BB prescribed for chronotropic reasons inhibit the beta-1 receptors which are located within the heart, reducing the frequency of SA and AV node impulses.

Digoxin (Digitalis)

Digoxin reduces heart rate but also increase the force of cardiac contractility. Digoxin can be more commonly associated with antidysrhythmic action, for example in treating atrial fibrillation.

Digoxin is effective dysrhythmia treatment due to its stimulation of parasympathetic nerves (revisit Figure 7.3). This is most commonly done through the vagus nerve, which directly affects the SA node, therefore reducing AV node conduction. Digoxin also has utility in treating patients with HF, who show increase levels of the neurotransmitter noradrenaline, something which digoxin decreases.

Diltiazem Hydrochloride

Diltiazem is a potent vasodilator, but also effective for reducing heart rate. Although it has powerful therapeutic effects, diltiazem is said to have an intermediate specificity effect upon both cardiac and vascular smooth muscle. This means it acts upon a wider variety of receptor sites with reduced affinity to cardiac receptors.

Diltiazem inhibits the influx of calcium ions during the depolarisation phase of an action potential. This inhibition is in both cardiac and vascular smooth muscle. Within cardiac cells, it inhibits slow calcium channels, reducing calcium influx. This reduced influx prolongs the depolarisation or contraction phase, while also prolonging the AV node refraction period. Ultimately, this leads to negative chronotropy or decreased heart rate.

Vasoactive Drugs
Noradrenaline

Noradrenaline stimulates alpha receptors, causing a powerful vasoconstrictive effect. Due to this effect, it is a drug with great utility in the treatment of septic shock, reversing the systemic vasodilation associated with this reaction (Lampin et al., 2012). A primary risk of noradrenaline treatment is hypertension, which should be monitored closely, this reaction will reduce as the appropriate physiological dose is found.

Episode of Care

Julia is a 12-year old child and she was admitted as an inpatient with severe sepsis, Noradrenaline was given to Julia to increase blood pressure.

Preferred routes of administration (in order of preference):

1. Central venous catheter
2. Peripheral line
3. Intra-osseus

Initial nursing considerations: Noradrenaline causes vasoconstriction, so hypertension is a common side effect, alongside arrythmia (BNFc, 2020). This means continuous blood pressure monitoring and electrocardiogram (ECG) are required.

Further nursing considerations: Line site extravasation necrosis is a risk, (although mainly with peripheral lines). Line sites should therefore be monitored for any discoloration, this should be at least once daily via visual infusion phlebitis (VIP) score (Royal College of Nursing, 2016).

Monitoring of peripheral vascular state is also warranted due to vasoconstrictive effect. This can be effectively achieved through examination for peripheral cyanosis, effective capillary refill and temperature check of extremities.

Noradrenaline is contraindicated in patients who may be suffering peripheral vascular thrombosis or mesenteric thrombosis. This increases risk of further reduction in peripheral blood flow, increasing the risk of ischaemia. Notably, hypovolaemic hypotension cannot be treated with noradrenaline, so must be carefully considered.

Vasopressin (Pitressin)

Vasopressin is a posterior pituitary hormone, produced by hypothalamic cells but stored in the pituitary. It is also known as antidiuretic hormone (ADH) or pitressin when produced synthetically. Vasopressin has multiple physiological effects. For the purposes of this chapter, its primary action is vasoconstriction. Vasopressin also has an antidiuretic effect, which potentially increases circulating blood volume while narrowing peripheral vessels, resulting in blood pressure increase.

Due to its antidiuretic effect, vasopressin is often used as a pharmacological treatment for diabetes insipidus. This disorder is symptomatically classified as a large volume of dilute urine being passed (polyuria) and extreme thirst (polydipsia). Understanding this pathology and treatment is useful, as polyuria can lead to hypotension if not treated.

Additional Haemodynamic Effectors

Diuretics

There are three types of diuretics known as:
1. Potassium-sparing diuretics and aldosterone antagonists
2. Loop diuretics
3. Thiazide and related diuretics

Diuretics are primarily used in children for pulmonary oedema, congestive heart failure, and hypertension. Chapter 8 discusses diuretics and the renal system.

Clinical Consideration

When taking a medication history, it is useful to understand the classifications of diuretics which may be used to control hypertension or manage heart failure. These may be used in conjunction with CVS drugs mentioned previously in this chapter, in both chronic and acute cases.

Potassium-sparing diuretics – Weaker diuretics but are useful to maintain serum potassium levels (often lost in urine with diuretic use). Examples of these: spironolactone, amiloride and potassium canrenoate.

Loop diuretics – Quick acting and effective, often working best as an infusion to maintain haemodynamic stability (Miller et al., 2014). They also work well orally. Examples of these: furosemide, bumetadine and torsemide

Thiazide diuretics – Thiazide diuretics inhibit sodium reabsorption, increasing diuresis and are most commonly used as combination therapy (Akbari and Khorasani-Zadeh, 2020). Examples of these: bendroflumethiazide, chlorothiazide and chlortalidone

Conclusion

When revisiting the learning outcomes for this chapter, you should now feel more comfortable identifying physiological actions of CVS drugs, while distinguishing between CVS drugs for chronic versus acute care. Finally, you will also be able to identify less common or adjunct treatments which affect the CVS.

CVD is very common, and should not be considered as an adult only disease. CVS drugs are numerous and complex, meaning further learning during your nurse training is often worthwhile to fully understand their clinical utility. Hopefully this chapter has helped develop some further understanding.

Glossary

Asystole: absence of ventricular contraction
Arrythmia: an abnormal heart rhythm
Aorta: major blood vessel supplying blood from the left ventricle to the body.
Atria: upper two chambers of the heart.
Atrium: singular version of atria.
Bundle of His: alternative name for the atrioventricular bundle.
Congenital: something existing at birth.
Cyanosis: bluish discoloration of the skin caused by a lack of oxygen.
Diastole: represents the period of time when the ventricles are relaxed
Ductus arteriosus: a small vessel connecting the pulmonary artery to the aorta preventing blood flow to the lungs.
Endocardium: the lining of the inside of the heart.
Inferior vena cava: major blood vessel returning deoxygenated blood from the lower part of the body to the heart.
Myocardium: the contractile muscle of the heart.
Pacemaker: an artificial pacemaker is a battery-operated device that delivers electrical impulses to the heart muscle.
Pericardium: the outer layer of the heart.
Purkinje fibre: part of the conducting system of the heart.
Superior vena cava: major blood vessel returning deoxygenated blood from the upper body to the heart.
Systole: contraction of the atria or ventricles.
Ventricle: lower two chambers of the heart.

References

Akbari, P. and Khorasani-Zadeh, A. (2020). Thiazide Diuretics. www.ncbi.nlm.nih.gov/books/NBK532918/ (accessed 20 April 2021).

Ashworth, M.T. (2019). Aspects of paediatric cardiovascular pathology. *Diagnostic Histopathology* 25(8): 313–323.

Berenson, G.S., Srinivasan, S.R., Bao, W. et al. (1998). Association between multiple cardiovascular risk factors and atherosclerosis in children and young adults. The Bogalusa heart study. *New England Journal of Medicine* 38(23): 1650–1656.

Bloetzer, C., Bovet, P., Suris, J.C. et al. (2015) Screening for cardiovascular disease risk factors, beginning in childhood. *Public Health Reviews* 36: 9.

Braunwald, E. (2015) The path to an angiotensin receptor antagonist – neprilysin inhibitor in the treatment of heart failure. *Journal of the American College of Cardiology* 65(10): 1029–1041.

British Heart Foundation (2013). Children and young people statistics 2013. www.bhf.org.uk/informationsupport/publications/statistics/children-and-young-people-statistics-2013 (accessed 20 April 2021).

British Heart Foundation (2020). www.bhf.org.uk/what-we-do/our-research/heart-conditions-research/congenital-heart-disease-research (accessed 20 April 2021).

British National Formulary for Children BNFc (2020). https://bnfc.nice.org.uk/ (accessed 20 April 2021).

Drugbank (2020). www.drugbank.ca/drugs/DB01076 (accessed 20 April 2021).

Farzam, K. and Jan, A. (2020). Beta Blockers. www.ncbi.nlm.nih.gov/books/NBK532906/ (accessed 20 April 2021).

Florek, J.B. and Girzadas, D. (2020). *Amiodarone*. www.ncbi.nlm.nih.gov/books/NBK482154/ (accessed 20 April 2021).

Giaccone, A., Zuppa, A.F., Sood, B. et al. (2017). Milrinone Pharmacokinetics and Pharmacodynamics in Neonates with Persistent Pulmonary Hypertension of the Newborn. *American Journal of Perinatology* 34(8): 749–758.

Gormley-Fleming, E. and Peate, I. (2018). *Fundamentals of Children's Applied Pathophysiology: An Essential Guide for Nursing and Healthcare Students*. VitalSouce bookshelf version. Retrieved from vbk://9781119232674.

Hatchett, R. and Thompson, D.R. (2002). *Cardiac Nursing. A Comprehensive Guide*, 2e. Churchill Livingstone. Elsevier.

Hoffman, T.M., Wernovsky, G., Atz, A.M. et al. (2002). Prophylactic Use of Milrinone After Cardiac Operation in Paediatrics (PRIMACORP) study. *American Heart Journal*. 143: 15–21.

Iyer, V.R. (2008). Drug therapy considerations in arrythmias in children. *Indian Pacing Electrophysiology Journal* 8(3): 202–210.

Joint Formulary Committee (JFC) (2021) BNFc. https://bnfc.nice.org.uk/ (accessed 20 April 2021).

Jones, B., Hayden, M., Frazer, J.F., and Janes, E. (2005). Low cardiac output syndrome in children. *Current Anaesthesia and Critical Care* 16(6): 347–358.

Kavey, R.-E.W., Manlhiot, C., Runeckles, K. et al. (2020). Effectiveness and safety of statin therapy in children: A real-world clinical practice experience. *CJC Open*. doi: 10.1016/j.cjco.2020.06.002.

Klabunde, R.E. (2017). Angiotensin converting enzyme inhibitors. https://cvpharmacology.com/vasodilator/ACE (accessed 20 April 2021).

Lampin, M.E., Rousseaux, J., Botte, A. et al. (2012). Noradrenaline use for septic shock in children: doses, routes of administration and complications. *ACTA Paediatrica* 101(9): 426–430. doi: 10.1111/j.1651-2227.2012.02725.x.

Lawrenson, J., Pribut, H., and Zuhlke, L. (2011). Drugs for the paediatric heart, a scenario-based guide to practice. *Continuing Medical Education* 29(11): 471–474.

Lei, M., Wu, L., Terrar, D.A., and Huang, C.L.H. (2018). Modernized classification of cardiac antiarrhythmic drugs. *Circulation* 138: 1879–1896.

Li, Y., He, P.P., Zhang, D.W. et al. (2014). Lipoprotein lipase: from gene to atherosclerosis. *Atherosclerosis* 237(2): 597–608.

Lipshultz, S.E. and Wilkinson, J.D. (2014). Beta-adrenergic adaptation in idiopathic dilated cardiomyopathy: differences between children and adults. *European Heart Journal* 35(1): 10–11.

McGill, H.C., McMahon, C.A., and Gidding, S.S. (2008). Preventing heart disease in the 21st Century: implications of the pathobiological determinants of atherosclerosis in youth (PDAY) study. *Circulation* 117(9): 1216–1227.

McGill, H.C., McMahon, C.A., and Gidding, S.S. (2009). Are pediatricians responsible for prevention of adult cardiovascular disease?. *Nature Clinical Practice Cardiovascular Medicine* 6(1): 10–11.

Miller, J.L., Thomas, A.N., and Johnson, P.N. (2014). Use of continuous-infusion loop diuretics in critically ill children. *Pharmacotherapy* 34(8): 858–867.

Miyamoto, S.D., Stauffer, B.L., Nakano, S. et al. (2014). Beta-adrenergic adaptation in paediatric idiopathic dilated cardiomyopathy. *European Heart Journal* 35(1): 33–41.

Mocumbi, A.O., Lameira, E., Yaksh, A. et al. (2011) Challenges on the management of congenital heart disease in developing countries. *International Journal of Cardiology* 148: 285–258.

Nagy, L., Pollesello, P., and Papp, Z. (2014). Inotropes and inodilators for acute heart failure: Sarcomere active drugs in focus. *Journal of Cardiovascular Pharmacology* 64(3): 199–208. doi: 10.1097/FJC.0000000000000113.

National Congenital Heart Disease Audit (2019). 2019 Summary Report. www.nicor.org.uk/wp-content/uploads/2019/09/NCHDA-2019-Summary-Report-final.pdf (accessed 20 April 2021).

National Health Lung and Blood Institute (NHLBI) (2012). Integrated guidelines for cardiovascular health and risk reduction in children and adolescents. www.nhlbi.nih.gov/health-topics/integrated-guidelines-for-cardiovascular-health-and-risk-reduction-in-children-and-adolescents (accessed 20 April 2021).

National Institute for Health and Care Excellence (2020). *Dyslipidaemias*. https://bnf.nice.org.uk/treatment-summary/dyslipidaemias.html (accessed 20 April 2021).

Peate, I. (ed.) (2018). *Fundamentals of Applied Pathophysiology: An Essential Guide for Nursing and Healthcare Students*, 3e. Chichester: Wiley-Blackwell.

Resuscitation Council (2008). Emergency treatment of anaphylactic reactions. www.resus.org.uk/sites/default/files/2020-06/EmergencyTreatmentOfAnaphylacticReactions%20%281%29.pdf (accessed 20 April 2021).

Resuscitation Council UK (2015). Guidelines: Paediatric advanced life support. www.resus.org.uk/print/pdf/node/132 (accessed 2 April 2021).

Ritter, J., Flower, R., Henderson, G. et al. (2020). *Rang and Dale's Pharmacology*, 9e. Elsevier.

Royal College of Nursing (2016). Competence: an education and competence framework for peripheral venous cannulation in children and young people. file:///C:/Users/antho/Downloads/005699.pdf.

Stanfield, C. (2017). *Principles of Human Physiology*, 6e. Pearson Education Limited: Harlow.

Wen, L. and Xu, L. (2020). The efficacy of dopamine versus epinephrine for paediatric or neonatal septic shock: a meta-analysis of randomized controlled studies. *Italian Journal of Paediatrics* 46: 6.

World Health Organisation (2017). Cardiovascular Disease Fact Sheet. www.who.int/en/news-room/fact-sheets/detail/cardiovascular-diseases-(cvds) (accessed 20 April 2021).

Further Resources

Burnström Å, Mora MA, Öjmyr-Joelsson M et al. (2019) Ready for transfer to adult care? A triadic evaluation of transition readiness in adolescents with congenital heart disease and their parents. *Journal of Family Nursing*. 25, 3, 447–468. doi: 10.1177/1074840719864255

Children's Heart Federation www.chfed.org.uk/how-we-help/information-service/heart-conditions/

A charitable organisation that provides resources for patients, families and healthcare practitioners as well as an information phone line for support and advice.

Hambly, C. and Cockett, A. (2017) Understanding parents' experiences of caring for a child with congenital heart disease *Nursing People and Young People* https://rcni.com/nursing-children-and-young-people/careers/research-practice/understanding-parents-experiences-of-caring-a-child-congenital-heart-disease-124436#

Chapter 7 Medications Used in the Cardiovascular System

Multiple Choice Questions

1. Considering the anatomy of the heart, which of the following has the most powerful muscle?
   (a) Right atrium
   (b) Left atrium
   (c) Right ventricle
   (d) Left ventricle

2. The thickest layer of the heart is called?
   (a) Pericardium
   (b) Epicardium
   (c) Myocardium
   (d) Endocardium

3. Which of the following drugs reduces the contractile force of the heart most effectively?
   (a) Alpha blockers
   (b) ACE inhibitors
   (c) Angiotensin II receptor blockers
   (d) Thiazide diuretics

4. Cardiac and vascular smooth muscle is innervated mostly by which of the following ions?
   (a) Potassium
   (b) Magnesium
   (c) Sodium
   (d) Calcium

5. Which of the following cardiovascular drugs has dose-dependent effects
   (a) Dobutamine
   (b) Noradrenaline
   (c) Dopamine
   (d) Adrenaline

6. Which of the following is classed as a positive chronotrope?
   (a) Atropine
   (b) Atenolol
   (c) Spironolactone
   (d) Simvastatin

7. Antidiuretic hormone is also known as which of the following?
   (a) Epinephrine
   (b) Pitressin
   (c) Milrinone
   (d) Norepinephrine

8. Which of the following drugs will require regular blood testing and dose titration?
   (a) Aspirin
   (b) Furosemide
   (c) Warfarin
   (d) Verapamil

9. Which of the following mechanisms of actions best describes statins?
   (a) Decrease low-density lipoproteins
   (b) Increase high-density lipoproteins
   (c) Increase low-density lipoproteins
   (d) Decrease high-density lipoproteins

10. Which of the following medications should be carefully considered when prescribed to children under the age of 16?
    (a) Warfarin
    (b) Atorvastatin
    (c) Aspirin
    (d) Lisinopril

Chapter 7 Medications Used in the Cardiovascular System

11. If someone has just been prescribed ACE inhibitors for hypertension, which of the following is the most common potential side effect?
    (a) Itch of the lower legs
    (b) A dry non-productive cough
    (c) Tingling in the hands and feet
    (d) Difficulty with sleeping or sleep disturbance
12. The term 'positive inotropic effect' best describes which of the following statements?
    (a) A decrease in cardiac contractility
    (b) An increase in peripheral vascular resistance
    (c) A decrease in heart rate
    (d) An increase in cardiac contractility
13. Which of the following actions makes adrenaline a very effective treatment for cardiac arrest?
    (a) An increase in heart rate and cardiac contractility
    (b) A decrease in heart rate and increase in cardiac contractility
    (c) An increase in heart rate but a decrease in cardiac contractility
    (d) A decrease in heart rate and cardiac contractility
14. Which of the following is a risk of peripherally delivered noradrenaline?
    (a) Extreme vasodilation
    (b) Extravasation necrosis
    (c) Renal injury
    (d) Headaches
15. Beta blockers are part of which of the Vaughan-Williams classifications?
    (a) Class 1
    (b) Class 2
    (c) Class 3
    (d) Class 4

Find Out More

The following are a list of conditions that are associated with the cardiovascular system. Take some time and write notes about each of the conditions. Think about the medications that may be used in order to treat these conditions and be specific about the pharmacokinetics and pharmacodynamics. Remember to include aspects of patient care. If you are making notes about people you have offered care and support to, you must ensure that you have adhered to the rules of confidentiality.

THE CONDITION	YOUR NOTES
Infective endocarditis	
Patent ductus arteriosus	
Cardiac failure	
Aortic stenosis	
Wolff–Parkinson–White Syndrome	

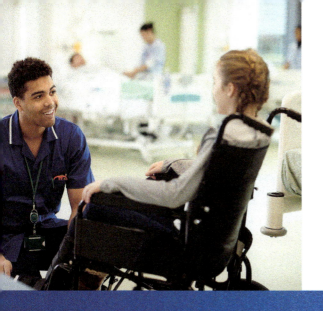

8
Medications Used in the Renal System

Katherine Drape, Sadie Diamond Fox and Alexandra Gatehouse

Aim

The aim of this chapter is to provide the reader with an introduction to some of the common renal conditions for children and young people that may be encountered within clinical practice and to explore medications used as part of their management and care.

Learning Outcomes

After reading this chapter the reader will:

- Have gained an understanding of renal physiology and some of the common renal conditions that effect children and young people
- Understand key classes of renal drugs and their pharmacology relating to renal conditions
- Understand the side effects of common renal medications
- Have gained knowledge and understanding in safe medicines management

Test Your Knowledge

1. Describe the main components of the renal system and its principal functions.
2. How is kidney function be measured?

Fundamentals of Pharmacology for Children's Nurses, First Edition. Edited by Ian Peate and Peter Dryden.
© 2022 John Wiley & Sons Ltd. Published 2022 by John Wiley & Sons Ltd.
Companion website: www.wiley.com/go/pharmacologyforCN

Chapter 8 Medications Used in the Renal System

3. **Name four common renal conditions.**
4. **Name some of the physiological functions that may be affected by renal disease.**
5. **List the common types of drugs used to treat renal disorders.**

Introduction

Renal or kidney disease can affect children and young people (CYP) in various ways. Acute kidney injury (AKI) can cause partial or complete loss of kidney function which may be temporary or longer-lasting. Chronic kidney disease (CKD) progressively gets worse over time and leads to kidney failure also described as end-stage renal disease (ESRD).

Around 3 million people in the UK have CKD, including around 1,000 CYP (Kidney Research UK, 2020), with people from black, Asian and minority ethnic communities five times more likely to experience kidney failure in their lifetime (Kidney Research UK, 2018). The impact upon healthcare services is significant; dialysis requirements in end-stage renal disease cost around £30,000 per patient per year. Of those patients in the UK that are fortunate enough to receive a kidney transplant, around £7,000 per year is required to fund the NHS services required per patient (Kidney Research UK, 2018).

For the purpose of this chapter, pharmacotherapy that is utilised in the management and treatment of electrolyte disorders will be explored as the renal system plays an essential role in maintenance of homeostasis, controlling fluid, electrolyte and acid-base balance. Consideration will be given to CYP with ESRD and some of the associated medications related to management of their disease.

Nephrotic syndrome will also be explored recognising a collection of symptoms that require pharmacological intervention and prevention of long-term renal damage. There will be episodes of care case studies and skills in practice features for the reader to consider theory in practice and recommended further reading to enhance knowledge in this area.

Anatomy and Physiology of the Renal System

The main function of the kidneys is maintenance of homeostasis (physiological stability) through excretory, regulatory and metabolic mechanisms. Waste products of metabolism, for example urea and creatinine, are eliminated via the production and excretion of urine. Fluid, electrolyte and acid-base balance is regulated through filtration, selective absorption and excretion of water, sodium, potassium, phosphate, calcium, hydrogen ions, bicarbonate ions and other substances. In addition, the kidneys have an endocrine function secreting hormones such as renin (blood pressure regulation) and erythropoietin, which stimulates the bone marrow to manufacture red blood cells. Vitamin D is metabolised, contributing to the regulation of calcium and phosphate, and prostaglandins are synthesised, resulting in renal protection from profound vasoconstriction.

The renal system comprises of the kidneys, which filter the blood to produce urine, the ureters, which convey urine to the urinary bladder, the urinary bladder, which stores the urine, and the urethra, which carries urine to the exterior. Each kidney receives its blood supply via the renal artery arising from the aorta, and once the blood is filtered, the renal vein takes the blood away. The renal vascular system and juxtaglomerular apparatus is supplied by the sympathetic nervous system. Urine formed by the kidney passes from the collecting duct to the renal pelvis via the papillary duct in the renal pyramid minor calyx, and major calyx. The kidney structure is depicted in Figure 8.1. Peristalsis facilitates the movement of urine along the ureter into the bladder.

The nephrons are the functional units of the kidney and they consist of several segments including: the Bowman's capsule, the glomerulus, the proximal convoluted tubule, the Loop of Henle, the distal convoluted tubule and the collecting ducts. Figure 8.2 demonstrates the structure of the nephron. The function of the nephron is filtration, selective reabsorption and excretion.

Development of the kidney begins within the first few weeks of embryonic life and although a newborn has their full complement of nephrons at birth, they are immature and less efficient than at later ages. Glomerular

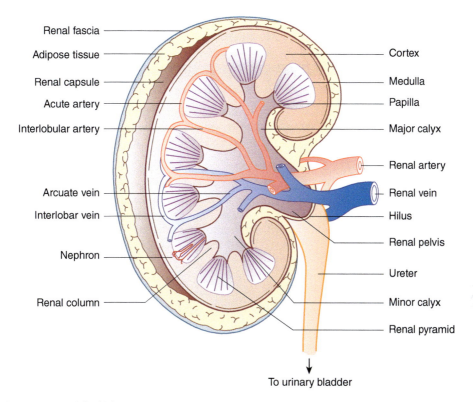

Figure 8.1 **Structure of the kidney.** *Source*: Ian Peate and Muralitharan Nair 2011/John Wiley & Sons.

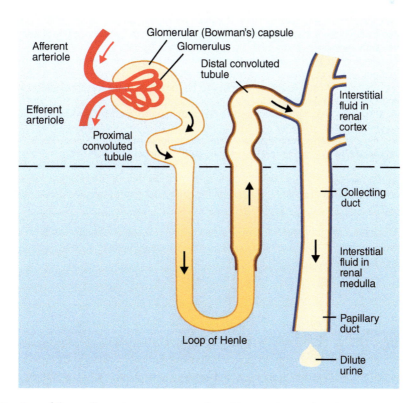

Figure 8.2 **Structure of the nephron.** *Source*: Ian Peate and Muralitharan Nair 2011/John Wiley & Sons.

Chapter 8 Medications Used in the Renal System

filtration and absorption are relatively low and do not reach adult values until the child is between 1 and 2 years old. As a result, newborns are unable to dispose of excess water and solute rapidly or efficiently.

Common Renal Conditions

Kidney disease can affect CYP in various ways from treatable conditions without long-term consequences to life-threatening. In addition, children and young people with CKD or kidney failure face other challenges such as delayed development with language skills and/or motor skills and may have delayed growth in comparison to their peers.

Considering the role and function of the kidney the common pathophysiological processes observed in renal disease include failure to maintain fluid and acid-base balance and electrolyte disturbances. From birth to around age 4, the most common causes of renal disease are birth defects and hereditary diseases. Between the ages of 5 to 14 years, hereditary diseases, nephrotic syndrome and systemic diseases are most common and as children progress into young adulthood, diseases which affect the glomeruli become the leading cause of renal failure (National Institute of Diabetes and Digestive and Kidney Diseases, 2020).

Skills in Practice

Urinalysis: Reagent Strip Procedure

Urinalysis using reagent strips is a rapid point-of-care test that is used as one of the primary diagnostic tests for multiple conditions. Urinalysis can aid in clinical decision making as to which advanced diagnostic tests are required to investigate for the presence of potential disease.

A clean catch urine sample is the recommended method for urine collection. If a clean catch urine sample is unobtainable, for example in infants and young children other non-invasive methods such as urine collection pads should be used. It is important to follow the manufacturer's instructions when using urine collection pads. Cotton wool balls, gauze and sanitary towels should not be used to collect urine in infants and children (National Institute for Health and Care Excellence (NICE) 2018).

How to Perform Urinalysis Using Reagent Strips

- If taking the specimen from a urinary catheter it should be collected using an aseptic technique
- For girls the labia should be separated and vulva wiped from front to back with clean water. Boys should clean the penis with soap and water
- Obtain a clean specimen of fresh urine from the patient which is to be analysed within 2 hours from collection. The patient should commence micturition and when a few millilitres of urine have been passed into the toilet a container or sterile receptacle should be introduced into the urine stream and then the remaining urine can pass into the toilet
- Check reagent strips have been stored in accordance with manufacturer's instructions. This is usually a dark dry place in an airtight container.
- Wearing gloves dip the reagent strip into the urine for no longer than 1 second. The strip should be completely immersed in the urine and then removed immediately. Run edge of strip along the container
- Hold the strip at an angle
- Wait the required time before reading the strip against the colour chart (usually 60 seconds)

Post Procedure

- Dispose of urine sample appropriately in either sluice or toilet. Dispose of urinalysis strip and gloves in correct wastage bin. Ensure cap to urine reagent strips is replace immediately and closed tightly.
- Document urinalysis readings and report any abnormal results

Source: Based on National Institute for Health and Care Excellence, 2018.

Nephrotic Syndrome

Nephrotic syndrome (NS) is an overarching term to describe a heterogeneous group of disorders. A triad of proteinuria, (greater than 40 mg/m^2 in children), hypoalbuminaemia and oedema are evident in the majority of cases and hyperlipdaemia can be an associated feature (Vivarelli et al., 2017; Ware, 2020). The cause may not always be obvious; however, the central issue appears to be glomerular dysfunction with increased permeability of the glomeruli. This may be due to a primary glomerular defect, circulating factors or an immunological abnormality. Complications of NS may include hypercoagulability, an increased risk of infection and end-stage renal failure

The annual incidence is estimated at 2–4 cases per 100,000 children in the UK. The majority of the patients are younger than 6 years of age (80%) and there is a male predisposition (Zolotas and Krishnan, 2016). Most cases are idiopathic, with only a small number of children developing NS secondary to infections or systemic diseases.

Long-term prognosis is often determined by steroid responsiveness with 80% of children having complete remission of symptoms within 4 weeks of treatment. These children are classed as steroid sensitive nephrotic syndrome (SSNS) with the vast majority having minimal change disease (MCD) however, this group of children will have at least one relapse and around half of them will have frequent relapses.

A relapse is defined as proteinuria, positive 3 on urinalysis of 3 consecutive days or positive 2 on urinalysis for 7 consecutive days. Treatment following a relapse is usually commenced at home; however, parents or carers are advised to contact their local hospital immediately if the child becomes unwell, particularly if complaining of abdominal pain, vomiting, diarrhoea or if they become oedematous.

Hypovolaemia is a common complication in children with NS and life-threatening as intravascular fluid shifts into the interstitial space; however, clinical assessment may be difficult, particularly in oedematous children and due to non-specific signs.

The remaining 20% of children who do not achieve remission after 4 weeks of steroid treatment are classed as steroid-resistant nephrotic syndrome (SRNS) suggesting on underlying cause other than MCD. Focal segmental glomerulosclerosis (FSGS) is the commonest cause of SRNS in young ages and mesangiocapillary glomerulonephritis (MCGN) tends to present in older children (Dolan and Gill, 2008). More than 15% of SRNS will progress to end-stage renal failure (ESRF), (Zolotas and Krishnan, 2016).

Clinical Consideration

A child or young person presenting with any of the following should be treated immediately considering hypovolaemia:

- Capillary refill time > 2 seconds, cool peripheries
- Reduced urine output
- Hypotension (<5th centile), and paradoxically hypertension (>95th centile) both can be features of hypovolaemia
- Persistent tachycardia
- Abdominal pain – abdominal pain can also be a symptom of peritonitis, renal vein thrombosis or steroid-induced gastritis

Remember: a child may still be hypovolaemic in the absence of all of these.

Episode of Care

Alexander, aged six years, lives at home in a sixth-floor flat with his single parent mother and his two siblings (Kofi who is 2 years and Wilson who is 8 years). Alexander has recently started to wake up in the morning with puffy eyes and extreme tiredness. His urine has become frothy and he has a reduced urine output. His mother had taken him to his GP today as he has a swollen abdomen and is complaining of abdominal pain. Alexander was referred to the local children's assessment unit at the district hospital and was found to have protein in his urine following urinalysis

Plan of care will include:

- A careful explanation to Alexander, his mum and if appropriate, his siblings regarding care and medical interventions
- Examination of Alexander and assess level of oedema. Note any swelling around the eyes, ankles, scrotal area and record the level of pitting
- Weigh on admission to gain a baseline and subsequent daily weights should be recorded to determine increase or decrease in weight as a result of fluid retention or successful diuresis
- Strict fluid balance monitoring
- Test all urine for protein losses daily (first morning urinalysis)
- Urinary sodium/osmolality concentration
- Observe for signs of hypovolaemia to include capillary refill time <2 seconds, cool peripheries, tachycardia and hypotension.
- No added salt diet whilst oedema present and proteinuria
- Oral prescribed prednisolone and penicillin and antacid such as omeprazole or ranitidine

Treatment of MCNS

Initial Presentation – Prednisolone

Prednisolone exerts predominantly glucocorticoid effects which include anti-inflammatory and immunosuppressant properties (Paediatric Joint Formulary Committee 2020a).

The effects of glucocorticoids are mediated by both genomic and non-genomic mechanisms. Genomic mechanisms implicate the activation or repression of specific genes encoding anti- and pro-inflammatory proteins, the genomic glucocorticoid action is characterised by a slow onset of the response. In contrast, non-genomic mechanisms do not influence gene expression and have a rapid onset and a short duration of the effect (Schijvens et al. 2019).

Standard therapy for the initial episode is to give 4–6 weeks of prednisolone daily followed by 4 weeks alternate days as per the International Study of Kidney Disease in Children (ISKDC) regimen. Many UK centres continue to use this regimen first described in the 1960s. Recent studies using randomised control trials have sought to determine if extending initial prednisolone treatment from eight to sixteen weeks improves the pattern of disease relapse, however they have found that although it does not significantly improve disease relapse, it has made a small improvement on the quality of life by reducing healthcare resources used (Webb et al., 2019).

Recommendations for Management of SRNS

Give prednisolone 60mg/m^2 orally daily for 4 weeks (maximum daily dose = 80mg) as a single morning dose. After this daily regimen, give prednisolone 40mg/m^2 orally on alternate days (maximum dose = orally/60mg/m^2 on alternate days) for a further 4 weeks

Clinical Consideration

To minimise side effects, give steroids in the morning as it mimics the timing of the body's own production of cortisone.

They are also best taken with or after food to reduce risk of gastric complications

Ranitidine/omeprazole can be given at initial presentation for 4–8 weeks in order to reduce gastric symptoms with reassessment as steroid dose is reduced

Contraindications

Live vaccines need to be avoided in those receiving immunosuppressive doses of prednisolone as the serum antibody response diminishes (Paediatric Formulary Committee, 2020a). Prolonged corticosteroid therapy may lead to side effects such as obesity and Cushingoid features developing, ocular complications and risk of osteoporosis also increases. The risk of adrenal atrophy may develop and persist even years after stopping with acute adrenal insufficiency, hypotension or death remaining a high risk after an abrupt withdrawal following prolonged use. It is advised that CYP on long-term corticosteroid treatment should carry a steroid treatment card which gives guidance on minimising risk and provides details of prescriber, drug, dosage and duration of treatment.

There is an increased susceptibility to infections as antibodies are lost and to severe infections following prolonged use of corticosteroids. Clinical presentation may be atypical, with serious infections reaching an advanced stage before being recognised, and for this reason infection is the leading cause of morbidity and mortality in children with NS. Peritonitis is the commonest serious infection, with an estimated incidence of 5% NS patients being affected (Zolotas and Krishnan, 2016; Noone et al., 2018). Prophylactic penicillin is often prescribed whilst CYP have proteinuria to guard against pneumococcal infection although there is scarcity of evidence to support its use. Children and young people receiving corticosteroids are at an increased risk of severe chickenpox and measles, with a risk of complications including pneumonia and hepatitis (Paediatric Formulary Committee, 2020a), with confirmed cases requiring immediate medical advice and treatment. Passive immunisation with varicella zoster immunoglobulin is needed for those non–immune patients exposed to chickenpox receiving systemic corticosteroids or for those who have used them within the previous 3 months. Prophylaxis with intramuscular normal immunoglobulin may be needed for children exposed to measles.

Behavioural changes have been reported in some cases of patients receiving high-dose corticosteroids including euphoria, insomnia, irritability, mood lability, suicidal thoughts and psychotic reactions. Although these changes often subside once the corticosteroid is reduced or stopped, patients and parents should be advised to seek medical advice if any symptoms occur as they may require specific management (Paediatric Formulary Committee, 2020a, Noone et al., 2018).

Furosemide

Furosemide is classified in a group of diuretics known as loop diuretics which inhibit reabsorption from the ascending limb of the loop of Henle in the renal tubule. Furosemide is actively secreted by the proximal tubules into the urine. Here it has a potent diuretic action via the inhibition of the sodium-potassium-chloride cotransporter, or the Na-K-Cl (NKCC2) cotransporter as it is otherwise known. The NKCC2 in normal physiology reabsorbs a high sodium and chloride load, therefore inhibition of this pump via a loop diuretic such as furosemide inhibits sodium and chloride reabsorption causing both diuresis and loss of sodium and chloride, mainly sodium (naturesis). In addition, potassium secretion is increased under the influence of aldosterone in the distal convoluted tubule, through the exchange of potassium for sodium. This eventually leads to increased potassium excretion and may result in lowered blood serum potassium levels (hypokalaemia).

Loop diuretics are highly protein bound to albumin, therefore during conditions such MCNS and extreme hypoalbuminaemia, the diuretic effect may be less effective due to the impaired delivery of the drug to the kidney. There are some renal conditions in which the co-administration of human albumin solution with a loop diuretic may prove useful, although there is a lack of strong evidence to support this (Noone et al., 2018).

As previously discussed, a proportion of children with NS may present as hypovolaemic, therefore the use of albumin alongside diuretics may be beneficial. Care should be taken, however, if the child is not exhibiting hypovolaemia, as an expansion in intravascular fluid could precipitate pulmonary oedema.

The pharmacokinetics of loop diuretics demonstrate a steep dose-response curve with little diuretic or naturetic effect below a certain threshold/plasma concentration. Once the plasma concentration reaches said threshold, a rapid increase in the response to the administered diuretic is observed. At high plasma concentrations of the drug, a plateau is reached and further dose increases no longer elicit a therapeutic effect (diuresis). Loop diuretics accumulate in the renal tubules via tubular secretion and it is this urinary concentration that determines the therapeutic threshold, not the serum/blood concentration (Anisman et al., 2019). The effects of both AKI and CKD on the pharmacokinetics and pharmacodynamics of loop diuretics can lead to a reduced diuretic response, including reduced tubular secretion and a blunted response of the NKCC2 cotransporter. Dose adjustment should therefore be taken into consideration particularly in CYP with reduced urine output (oliguria) and non-production of urine (anuria). Furosemide dosage for each age group is identified in Table 8.1.

Table 8.1 Furosemide dosage for CYP.

AGE	ORAL	SLOW INTRAVENOUS INJECTION	CONTINUOUS INTRAVENOUS INFUSION
Neonate	0.5–2 mg/kg every 12–24 hours, alternatively 0.5–2 mg/kg every 24 hours, if corrected gestational age under 31 weeks.	0.5–1 mg/kg every 12–24 hours, alternatively 0.5–1 mg/kg every 24 hours, if corrected gestational age under 31 weeks.	
1 month–11 years	0.5–2 mg/kg 2–3 times a day, alternatively 0.5–2 mg/kg every 24 hours, if corrected gestational age of under 31 weeks, higher doses may be required in resistant oedema; maximum 80 mg per day; maximum 12 mg/kg per day.	0.5–1 mg/kg every 8 hours (max. per dose 40 mg every 8 hours) as required; maximum 6 mg/kg per day.	
12–17 years	20–40 mg daily; increased to 80–120 mg daily, in resistant oedema.	20–40 mg every 8 hours as required, higher doses may be required in resistant cases.	0.1–2 mg/kg/hour.

Source: Paediatric Formulary Committee, 2020b/NICE/Public domain

Children who do not achieve remission after 4 weeks of steroid treatment are classed as steroid-resistant nephrotic syndrome (SRNS) or children who have frequently relapsing nephrotic syndrome (FRNS) may require a tailored approach to their treatment.

Steroid sparing agents such as levamisole or cyclophosphamide, are two of the more common steroid sparing agents used within this group of patients. Levamisole has a favourable side effect profile, with some evidence to suggest the reduced risk of relapse compared with placebo or no treatment. Unfortunately, the effect of levamisole is not sustained once it has been discontinued. Cyclophosphamide, an alkylating agent which works by interfering with DNA synthesis, has been shown to be effective in numerous Random Control Trials for the treatment of SDNS and FRNS and can achieve prolonged remission (Zolota and Krishan, 2016; Noone et al., 2018). Side effects of cyclophosphamide remain an important consideration including infertility, hepatic dysfunction, pulmonary fibrosis, myelosuppression, leucopenia and azoospermia with a cumulative dose, therefore its use in prepubertal patients should be avoided. Typically, lower doses of cyclophosphamide are prescribed intravenously rather than oral as there are less side effects. However, approximately 32% of NS patients developed leucopenia during treatment (Latta et al., 2001).

Calcineurin Inhibitors

This group of immunosuppressive drugs now discussed work mainly by blocking intracellular signalling pathways that are critical for the production of cytokines by lymphocytes. They inhibit phosphatase calcineurin production, a cellular enzyme responsible for activation of T cells.

Ciclosporin is now rarely used with CYP due to multiple side effects and evidence to suggest a high risk of dependency and higher risk of relapse following a period of interruption (El-Husseini et al., 2005). An increased risk of renal toxicity has also been identified, particularly in children after prolonged use of 2 years or more, therefore many specialist teams undertake renal biopsies to detect renal toxicity. Tacrolimus has a comparable mechanism of action to ciclosporin with both drugs being similar in effectiveness. It has been used with SSNS patients who have not responded to ciclosporin treatment however, renal toxicity remains a notable adverse side effect.

Mycophenolate Mofetil (MMF) works by selective inhibition of DNA replication in T and B lymphocytes. It is seen as less effective than cyclosporine but has a more favourable side effect profile with the absence of renal toxicity. There is, however, limited trial evidence for this group of patients (Noone et al., 2018).

Rituxamab is increasingly used with CYP, especially for those who frequently relapse following treatment with tacrolimus and MMF. Rituxamab is a monoclonal anti-CD20 antibody and is an effective steroid and calcineurin- sparing agent for children and young people with SDNS (NHS England, 2015). It is generally well tolerated in most children but can have potentially serious adverse side effects including hypo-gammaglobulinaemia and B cell deficiency (Noone et al., 2018).

Calcineurin inhibitors are discussed in Table 8.2. Please refer to British National Formulary for children for age/weight dosage.

As previously highlighted, from birth to around 4 years, the most common causes of renal disease are congenital abnormalities and hereditary diseases. Between the ages of 5 and 14, hereditary disease is most common. Congenital anomalies of the kidney and urinary tract as a disease group represent the most common reason for end-stage renal disease (ESRD) in children and adolescents (Isert et al., 2020). Congenital anomalies can include renal dysplasias, hypoplasias, agenesis, horseshoe kidneys, obstructions at the ureteropelvic junction or at the vesicoureteral junction, posterior urethral valves (PUV), and vesicoureteral reflux (VUR). Children with some of the conditions mentioned will be at a higher risk of developing kidney disease.

Hereditary or genetic diseases such as polycystic kidney disease characterised by clusters of fluid filled sacs can develop and destroy kidney tissue over time. Alport syndrome, characterised by glomerulonephritis, can develop in early childhood and lead to ESRD.

The renal system plays an essential role in maintenance of homeostasis, controlling fluid, electrolyte and acid-base balance. Renal disease may affect all of these processes, and the aim of the following section is to explore the impact of this and identify how pharmacotherapy may be utilised in management and treatment.

Fluid balance refers to the distribution of body fluid within the intracellular and extracellular (interstitial and intravascular) compartments. Total body volume, and therefore total body water, is regulated within a narrow range, through alteration of sodium and water content (O'Callaghan, 2017; Peate, 2017). Sodium excretion is controlled via the kidneys and regulated by neural and endocrine

Table 8.2 Calcineurin inhibitors monitoring and side effects.

DRUG	MONITORING	SIDE EFFECTS
Tacrolimus	Drug concentrations, creatinine, electrolytes, glucose, transaminases	Nephrotoxicity, hypertension, hyperglycaemia, seizures, diarrhoea, hypomagnesaemia
Ciclosporin	Drug concentrations, creatinine, electrolytes, glucose, transaminases	Nephrotoxicity, hypertension, hypertrichosis, gingival hyperplasia
Mycophenolate mofetil	Area under the curve measurements, full blood counts, creatinine, transaminases	Abdominal pain, diarrhoea, anorexia, leucopenia and raised transaminases are uncommon
Cyclophosphamide	Full blood count	Alopecia, marrow suppression, vomiting, haemorrhagic cystitis, risk of systemic infections. Long-term: cancer, infertility
Rituximab	Hepatitis B screen, CD19 cell count, full blood count. Monitoring of allergic reactions during infusion, immunosuppression	Risk of infections

Source: Paediatric Formulary Committee, 2020c, 2020d, 2020e, 2020f, 2020g

responses. The sodium-potassium pumps (Na^+-K^+) drive sodium from the tubular cells into the blood, and this creates a lower concentration gradient within the cell. Sodium and water then move, from the tubular infiltrate into the cell via various channels or co-transporters, according to the permeability of the cell membrane and the concentration gradient.

Renal tubulointerstitial disease although rare in children and Addison's disease (deficiency of the hormone aldosterone) both cause excessive sodium excretion, whilst primary hyperaldosteronism, renal failure or oedema syndromes such as nephrotic syndrome result in inadequate sodium excretion (O'Callaghan, 2017). The underlying cause should be identified and treated, however, pharmacotherapy manipulation of renal sodium through the use of diuretics may be useful.

Potassium is integral to the maintenance of an electrochemical gradient across the cell membrane, and the ability of nerves and muscle to create an action potential. Hypokalaemia and hyperkalaemia are life-threatening, causing cardiac dysrhythmias and potentially cardiac arrest, and the kidneys and adrenal glands are vital in the maintenance of potassium homeostasis. Within the nephron the majority of potassium is reabsorbed prior to the collecting duct, and excretion of potassium occurs in this segment through several mechanisms. The sodium-potassium pumps and the potassium channels in the cell membranes of the collecting duct are affected by the extracellular potassium concentration, the release of aldosterone, the pH, flow rates within the collecting duct, filtrate sodium concentration and intracellular magnesium. Renal tubular acidosis and primary or secondary hyperaldosteronism result in potassium loss and hypokalaemia, whilst renal failure and hyperaldosteronism cause hyperkalaemia. Life-threatening hyperkalaemia warrants emergency treatment as outlined in the UK Resuscitation Council Guidelines (Soar et al., 2015), and renal replacement therapy. Pharmacotherapy of longer-term potassium management may include potassium supplementation or potassium binding agents, both of which are discussed in subsequent sections.

Calcium and phosphate are inextricably linked and are essential to the maintenance of bone density. They are regulated by one of several mechanisms including gut reabsorption, bone reabsorption and renal handling. Calcium is regulated by the thyroid gland, and when levels fall parathyroid hormone (PTH) stimulates bone reabsorption (release of calcium and phosphate from bone), increases Vitamin D synthesis, increases renal phosphate excretion and increases renal calcium reabsorption. Vitamin D is synthesised within the kidney, increasing phosphate and calcium levels via reabsorption through the gut, bones and renal tubules. In renal failure bone disease can be caused by Vitamin D deficiency and renal phosphate retention. Due to lack of gut reabsorption and the formation of calcium phosphate deposits (due to hyperphosphataemia), the fall in calcium stimulates PTH, triggering further bone reabsorption and eventually hyperparathyroidism.

Pharmacotherapy aims to maintain normal calcium and phosphate levels, preventing hyperparathyroidism, bone pain, poorly mineralised bone and soft-tissue deposits as typically seen in chronic kidney disease.

Acid-base balance, and so pH, is controlled by the respiratory and renal systems. By regulating carbon dioxide (respiratory) and bicarbonate (renal) the pH may be normalised when acidosis or alkalosis occurs. In renal disease the kidneys are unable to effectively perform these processes and so metabolic acidosis occurs causing hyperkalaemia. Renal replacement therapy may be used to correct severe metabolic acidosis in both the acute and chronic setting of renal failure. Pharmacotherapy may be utilised to correct the acid-base balance and this is explored in subsequent sections of this chapter.

Drugs Used to Treat Electrolyte Disorders

Electrolyte disorders can occur as a result of altered homeostasis of the renal system, as a result of multiple other disease processes for example gastrointestinal dysfunction or iatrogenic causes such as a result of pharmacotherapy (i.e. potassium depletion due to loop diuretics). This can lead to multiple derangements in serum levels of measured ions and/or vitamins. The principal treatments of electrolyte disorders involve either replacement or the promotion of excretion of said ions or vitamins. Wherever possible the primary or underlying cause of the electrolyte and or/vitamin disturbance should be treated to avoid the potential for unnecessary long-term treatment strategies that only mask the underlying problem.

Phosphate Binders, Calcium Supplements and Vitamin D Supplements

Phosphate binders, calcium supplements and vitamin D supplements are commonly used in combination for children and young people with chronic renal disease due to the altered calcium and phosphate metabolism. This can lead to raised phosphate serum levels (hyperphosphataemia) and lowered serum levels of calcium (hypocalcaemia) and low vitamin D levels. Secondary hyperparathyroidism can also develop as a result of hyperphosphataemia leading to increased parathormone (parathyroid hormone; PTH) levels. Persistent overproduction of PTH leads to renal osteodystrophy, a defective or abnormal bone development leading to weakness, bone pain, and skeletal deformity. There are significant cardiovascular consequences as a result of increased PTH which increase morbidity and mortality rates among this population. Calcium and calcium phosphate deposits within the cardiovascular system, as a result of increased PTH, cause vascular calcification which mainly effects blood vessels, myocardial tissue and cardiac valves. This can lead to hypertension, myocardial infarction and heart failure (Jablonski and Chonchol, 2013).

Hypocalcaemia due to renal disease is due to two primary causes; phosphate retention and decreased renal production of 1,25-dihydroxyvitamin vitamin D. A spectrum of consequences can occur which may be life-threatening (coma, cardiac arrhythmias, seizures, laryngeal stridor) to more chronic, but debilitating (cataracts, extra-skeletal calcification and renal bone disease). Decreased production of 1,25-dihydroxyvitamin D leads to decreased absorption of calcium from the gut which in turn lowers serum calcium levels. PTH is then secreted from the parathyroid glands in response to lowered serum calcium levels which can eventually lead to hypertrophy of these glands and other disorders as explored above as the cycle continues until the underlying cause (decreased vitamin D) is treated.

Phosphate binders inhibit phosphate retention by binding to phosphate within the gut lumen and preventing its absorption, vitamin D supplements are converted rapidly in the liver to 1,25-dihydroxyvitamin D. The following tables 8.3 and 8.4 outline some of the commonly prescribed agents and their pharmacological properties within these drug classes.

Potassium Binders and Supplements

Potassium homeostasis is maintained via the kidneys and the adrenal glands. Potassium binders or supplements may be prescribed depending upon the underlying cause of the potassium imbalance. Potassium binders although rarely used in CYP can be used in chronic renal disease to manage hyperkalaemia associated with anuria, severe oliguria and children who are dialysis dependent. They are artificial resins containing either sodium or calcium, which is exchanged for potassium in the gastrointestinal tract, and then eliminated in the faeces.

Chapter 8 Medications Used in the Renal System

Table 8.3 **Phosphate binders and their related pharmacology.**

MEDICATION NAME	SEVELAMER	LANTHANUM
Mode of action	Reduction of phosphate absorption within gut lumen	
Route of administration	Oral	Oral
		Child
	Hyperphosphataemia in patients on haemodialysis or peritoneal dialysis	
	Hyperphosphataemia in chronic kidney disease	
Contraindications	Previous anaphylactic reaction to this agent	
	Bowel obstruction	
Cautions	Gastrointestinal disorders	Acute peptic ulcer
	Pregnancy and breast-feeding:	Bowel obstruction
	Manufacturer advises use only if	Crohn's disease
	potential benefit outweighs risk.	Ulcerative colitis
		Pregnancy and breast-feeding:
		Manufacturer advises avoid –
		toxicity in *animal* studies.
Side effects (common & very common *only*)	Constipation	
	Diarrhoea	
	Gastrointestinal discomfort	
	Gastrointestinal disorders	
	Nausea	
	Vomiting	
Interactions	Ciprofloxacin	Antacids
	Anti-arrhythmic medications	Chloroquine
	Anti-seizure medications	Hydroxychloroquine
	Levothyroxine	Ketoconazole
	Anti-rejection drugs	
	Warfarin	
	Proton pump inhibitors	
Absorption	Not absorbed from the gastrointestinal tract	Minimally absorbed following oral administration.
Distribution	No data	Extensively bound to plasma proteins (>99.7%)
Metabolism	No data	Not metabolised
Elimination	No data	Excreted mainly in the faeces

Source: Paediatric Formulary Committee, 2019h, 2019i; Electronic Medicines Compendium, 2019a, 2019b.

Potassium supplements may be required in conditions causing potassium depletion or hypokalaemia. The causes of which include drugs (diuretics, insulin, corticosteroids, laxatives), gastrointestinal losses (diarrhoea, vomiting), renal losses (diuretic phase of acute tubular necrosis), hyperaldosteronism and malnutrition. Treatment of hypokalaemia should aim to identify and manage the underlying disease or primary causative factor. Mild to moderate hypokalaemia may be treated with oral supplementation.

Tables 8.5 and 8.6 outline some of the commonly used potassium binders and potassium supplements.

Bicarbonate Supplements

The kidneys control bicarbonate levels, contributing to the maintenance of acid-base homeostasis. Metabolic acidosis occurs due to the loss of bicarbonate or the gain of hydrogen ions. Under normal circumstances sodium bicarbonate is reabsorbed, via the sodium gradient, and hydrogen ions are secreted in the proximal tubule. In the distal tubule, hydrogen ions either contribute to reabsorption of the remaining bicarbonate or are buffered by phosphate. Bicarbonate loss is caused by gut losses, increased sodium chloride administration and renal bicarbonate loss. Renal tubular acidosis results in the kidneys being either unable to excrete

Table 8.4 Vitamin D supplements and their related pharmacology.

MEDICATION NAME	ALFACALCIDOL	CALCITRIOL
Mode of action	1,25 (OH)2 vitamin D supplementation	
Route of administration	Oral	Oral
	Child	
	Persistent hypocalcaemia due to hypoparathyroidism or pseudohypoparathyroidism Prevention of vitamin D deficiency in renal or cholestatic liver disease	Vitamin D-dependent rickets Hypophosphataemic rickets Persistent hypocalcaemia due to hypoparathyroidism Pseudo-hypoparathyroidism (limited data)
Contraindications	Hypercalcaemia Metastatic calcification	
Cautions	Nephrolithiasis Take care to ensure correct dose in infants *Pregnancy and breast-feeding:* High doses teratogenic in *animals* but therapeutic doses unlikely to be harmful Caution with high doses; may cause hypercalcaemia in infant – monitor serum calcium concentration	
Side effects (common and very common *only*)	Abdominal discomfort Hyperphosphataemia Rash pustular	Abdominal pain Headache Hypercalcaemia Hypercalciuria Nausea Skin reactions
Interactions	Thiazide diuretics Other vitamin D containing preparations Anticonvulsants Magnesium-containing antacids Aluminium-contain preparations	
Absorption	Via intestines in a dose-related manner.	Rapidly absorbed from the intestine
Distribution	No data	Mostly bound to a specific vitamin D binding protein Bound to lipoproteins and albumin in a lesser degree
Metabolism	No data	Hydroxylated and oxidised in the kidney and in the liver by a specific cytochrome P450 enzyme
Elimination	No data	Excreted in the bile

Source: Paediatric Formulary Committee, 2019j, 2019k; Electronic Medicines Compendium, 2019c, 2019d.

hydrogen ions and reabsorb bicarbonate ions due to disorders of the proximal tubule (rare), or secrete hydrogen ions or absorb sodium ions due to secretory, permeability and voltage defects as well as hypoaldosteronism in the distal tubule (O'Callaghan, 2017). The gain of hydrogen ions occurs in lactic acidosis, ketoacidosis, poisoning and renal failure. Metabolic acidosis becomes more common with advancing CKD. Damage to both the glomerulus and renal tubules significantly reduces the number of functioning nephrons and as CKD progresses ammonia excretion is impaired (less hydrogen ions are excreted), bicarbonate absorption is reduced and there is insufficient production of renal bicarbonate (Adamczak et al., 2018).

Table 8.5 Potassium binders and their related pharmacology.

MEDICATION NAME	SODIUM POLYSTYRENE SULFONATE	CALCIUM POLYSTYRENE SULFONATE
Mode of action	Gastrointestinal potassium binding resin	
Route of administration	Oral or rectal	
	Child	
	Hyperkalaemia associated with anuria or severe oliguria, and in dialysis patients	
Contraindications	Obstructive bowel disease Reduced gut motility in neonates Hypersensitivity to polystyrene sulfonate resins	Hyperparathyroidism Metastatic carcinoma Multiple myeloma Obstructive bowel disease Sarcoidosis Reduced gut motility in neonates Hypersensitivity to polystyrene sulfonate resins
Cautions	Congestive heart failure Hypertension Oedema Children – hypertension, impact of resin with excessive dosage or inadequate dilution, should only be given to neonates rectally *Pregnancy and breast-feeding:* Manufacturers advise only if potential benefit outweighs risk	Children – Impact of resin with excessive dosage or inadequate dilution *Pregnancy and breast-feeding:* Manufacturers advise only if potential benefit outweighs risk
Side effects (common and very common *only*)	Severe hypokalaemia, administration should cease once serum potassium level falls to 5mmol/L Electrolyte deficiency – calcium or magnesium Constipation	Severe hypokalaemia, administration should cease once serum potassium level falls to 5mmol/L Electrolyte deficiency – calcium or magnesium Constipation
Interactions	Manufacturers advise to take other drugs 3 hours before or after, with a 6-hour separation considered in gastroparesis Gastointestinal stenosis, intestinal ischaemia and complications if administered with sorbitol Binding effect reduced with cation-donating agents Aluminium hydroxide – intestinal obstruction Toxic effects of digitalis if hypokalaemia occurs Possible decreased absorption of lithium or levothyroxine	
Absorption	Not absorbed	
Distribution	As above	
Metabolism	As above	
Elimination	Excreted in the faeces	

Source: Paediatric Formulary Committee, 2019l, 2019m; Electronic Medicines Compendium, 2019e, 2019f.

Table 8.7 outlines the commonly used sodium bicarbonate supplement.

One of the most common sequelae for children and young people with chronic kidney disease is hypertension (Hadstein and Scaefer, 2007, Gallibois et al., 2017). Hypertension is associated with a more rapid decline in kidney function and often, due to a lack of acute symptoms, goes undetected for a period of time. Active screening is recommended for children and young people within this population, as some evidence suggests early recognition and treatment of hypertension can slow renal progression and in some cases reverse cardiovascular changes.

Chapter 8 Medications Used in the Renal System

Table 8.6 **Potassium supplements and their related pharmacology.**

MEDICATION NAME	POTASSIUM CHLORIDE
Mode of action	Potassium supplementation
Route of administration	Oral
	Child
	Prevention of hypokalaemia (patients with normal diet)
	Potassium depletion
Contraindications	Plasma potassium above 5mmol/L
	Severe renal impairment
	Inadequately treated Addison's disease
Cautions	Cardiac disease
	With modified-release preparations – hiatus hernia, history of peptic ulcer, intestinal stricture
	Pregnancy and breast-feeding:
	No clinical problems encountered but benefit and risks must be considered in pregnancy
Side effects (common and very common *only*)	Hyperkalaemia
	Abdominal cramps
	Diarrhoea
	Gastrointestinal disorders
	Nausea and vomiting
Interactions	Risk of hyperkalaemia increased with potassium-sparing diuretics and ACEi
Absorption	Readily absorbed from the gastrointestinal tract
Distribution	Not applicable
Metabolism	Not applicable
Elimination	Excretion of potassium via the distal tubules of the kidney, by the faeces and a smaller amount in the perspiration

Source: Paediatric Formulary Committee, 2019n; Electronic Medicines Compendium, 2019g.

Table 8.7 **Bicarbonate supplementation and the related pharmacology.**

MEDICATION NAME	SODIUM BICARBONATE
Mode of action	Bicarbonate supplementation
Route of administration	Oral
	Child
	Chronic acidotic states such as uraemic acidosis or renal tubular acidosis
Contraindications	Salt-restricted diet
	Metabolic or respiratory alkalosis
	Hypocalcaemia
	Hypochlorydia
Cautions	May affect stability or absorption of other drugs if administered at the same time, allow 1-2 hours before other oral drug administration
	Avoid prolonged use in urinary conditions
	Cardiac disease
	Patients on sodium-restricted diet
	Respiratory acidosis
	Pregnancy and breast-feeding:
	Not recommended in pregnancy or women of child bearing potential not using contraception
	Risk to a child who is breast-feeding cannot be excluded

Table 8.7 (Continued)

MEDICATION NAME	SODIUM BICARBONATE
Side effects (common and very common *only*)	Abdominal cramps Burping Flatulence Hypokalaemia Metabolic alkalosis
Interactions	Corticosteroids Increases excretion of lithium, aspirin and methotrexate Decreases excretion of quinidine and ephedrine May reduce the absorption of antibacterials, antifungals, dipyridamole, phenothiazines, chloroquine, phenytoin and penicillamine Readily absorbed from the gastrointestinal tract
Distribution	Present in all body fluids
Metabolism	Not significantly metabolised
Elimination	Bicarbonate is absorbed if not involved in gastric acid neutralisation, in the absence of a deficit it is excreted in the urine

Source: Paediatric Formulary Committee, 2019o; Electronic Medicines Compendium, 2019h.

As the kidneys are the primary regulator of blood volume, their function is critical in the maintenance of blood pressure. Fluid overload and activation of the angiotensin system are two of the main pathophysiological pathways associated with hypertension. However, sympathetic hyperactivation, endothelial dysfunction and chronic hyperparathyroidism have also been identified as important contributing factors.

The renin angiotensin aldosterone system (RAAS) is a complex hormone system that regulates blood pressure and fluid balance. The juxtaglomerular cells (baroreceptors) located in the afferent arterioles of the kidney identify low blood volume and will secrete renin directly into the circulation. Renin then converts angiotensinogen released by the liver to angiotensin I. Angiotensin I is then converted to angiotensin II in the lungs by an enzyme called angiotensin converting enzyme or ACE. Angiotensin II is a strong vasoactive peptide which causes blood vessels to constrict, leading to increased blood pressure. Angiotensin II also stimulates the secretion of the hormone aldosterone from the zona glomerulosa in the adrenal cortex. Aldosterone then acts on the distal convoluted tubules and the cortical collecting ducts of the kidneys, increasing the reabsorption of sodium and water into the blood. This increases the volume of fluid in the body, which also increases blood pressure.

Clinical Consideration

In addition to medication, low salt diet can be considered for children with hypertension and chronic kidney disease. Research has demonstrated that each 1000mg/day sodium intake has been associated with a 1.0mmHg increase in systolic BP

Source: Based on Yang et al., 2012.

ACE inhibitors and angiotensin II receptor antagonists are more commonly used to treat hypertension, although there is limited information on the use of receptor antagonists in children (NICE, 2020). ACE inhibitors work by inhibiting the conversion of angiotensin I to angiotensin II. By doing so they help widen blood vessels to allow blood to flow more easily, which lowers blood pressure. Recommendations advise that therapy should be initiated with a single drug at the lowest recommended dose, particularly in children who are volume depleted, as ACE inhibitors can cause a very rapid fall in blood pressure. The dose can be increased until the target blood pressure is achieved (NICE, 2020).

Some of the most common ACE inhibitors are listed in Table 8.8. Please refer to British National Formulary for children for age/weight dosage.

Table 8.8 Common ACE inhibitors used for CYP, monitoring and side effects.

DRUG	MONITORING	SIDE EFFECTS
Captopril	Renal function Electrolytes Blood pressure	**For all** Hyperkalaemia, alopecia, angioedema, arrhythmias, asthenia, chest pain, constipation, cough, diarrhoea, dizziness, drowsiness, dry mouth, dyspnoea, electrolyte imbalance, gastrointestinal discomfort, headache, hypotension, myalgia, nausea, palpitations, paraesthesia, renal impairment, rhinitis, skin reactions, sleep disorder, syncope, taste altered, tinnitus, vertigo, vomiting **For Captopril** Common or very common; Insomnia; peptic ulcer Uncommon; Appetite decreased; flushing; malaise; pallor; Raynaud's phenomenon Rare or very rare; Anaemia; aplastic anaemia; autoimmune disorder; cardiac arrest; cardiogenic shock; cerebrovascular insufficiency; depression; gynaecomastia; hepatic disorders; hypoglycaemia; lymphadenopathy; nephrotic syndrome; oral disorders; proteinuria; urinary disorders; vision blurred
Enalapril	Renal function Electrolytes Blood pressure	**For Enalapril** Common or very common Depression; hypersensitivity; vision blurred Uncommon Anaemia; appetite decreased; asthma; bone marrow disorders; flushing; gastrointestinal disorders; hoarseness; hypoglycaemia; malaise; muscle cramps; nervousness; proteinuria; rhinorrhoea; sleep disorders; throat pain Rare or very rare Autoimmune disorder; gynaecomastia; hepatic disorders; lymphadenopathy; oral disorders; Raynaud's phenomenon; toxic epidermal necrolysis
Lisinopril	Renal function Electrolytes Blood pressure	**For Lisinopril** Common or very common Postural disorders Uncommon Hallucination; mood altered; Raynaud's phenomenon Rare or very rare Anaemia; autoimmune disorder; azotaemia; bone marrow depression; gynaecomastia; hepatic disorders; hypersensitivity; hypoglycaemia; lymphadenopathy; olfactory nerve disorder; syndrome of inappropriate antidiuretic hormone secretion (SIADH); sinusitis; toxic epidermal necrolysis

Source: Paediatric Formulary Committee 2020p, 2020q and 2020r.

Skills in Practice

Measuring Blood Pressure with Doppler
- Incorrect cuff size is a major source of error. An under-sized cuff can significantly overestimate BP.
- Incorrect cuff placement can also be a major source of error. The cuff should be placed on the arm with the centre of the bladder over the brachial artery.

Blood Pressure Monitoring
- Wash hands.
- Ensure the child is comfortable and introduce self.
- Apply the cuff, ensure the internal bladder encircles 90–100% of the upper arm circumference.
- The arrow on the cuff should be placed over the brachial artery.
- The first BP reading should be estimated by placing a doppler over the pulse and pumping up the cuff. When the pulse sound disappears this is your estimated BP. Now deflate the cuff quickly.
- Keep the doppler over the pulse; pump the cuff up to a pressure 30 mmHg higher than the estimated BP.
- Reduce the pressure slowly.
- The first repetitive sound is recorded as the systolic BP.
- If you need to repeat the BP you should wait 1 minute to give the vessels a chance to refill.
- Record the systolic BP measurement immediately.
- To obtain a diastolic reading use a stethoscope rather than Doppler.
- Ensure CYP is comfortable.
- Wash hands.
- Record BP and report changes or recordings outside of normal parameters for age of child.

Conclusion

This chapter has provided an overview of the anatomy and physiology of the kidney and considered its main functions. The importance that the kidney plays in maintaining homeostasis has been explored and common renal conditions highlighted that can affect the function of the kidneys. Nephrotic syndrome has been explored in depth and subsequent management of the disease with associated medications. Medications commonly used in children have then been discussed in the management and treatment of children with ESRD and CRD.

It is important to highlight that only some of the conditions and associated medications have been explored within this chapter, therefore the importance of further reading and reflection of practice is vital to continuing professional development.

Glossary

Diuresis: Increased or excessive production of urine.
Glomerulosclerosis: Scarring or hardening of the glomeruli.
Homeostasis: Ability to maintain a relatively stable internal state that continues even if there are changes in the world outside.
Hypercoagulability: State or condition marked by an increased tendency to form blood clots within a blood vessel.
Metabolism: The bodily processes needed to maintain life.
Nephrotoxicity: The harmful effect of substances on renal function.
Oedema: Swelling caused by a build-up of fluid in the spaces between the cells.
Peristalsis: The involuntary constriction and relaxation of the muscles in a tubular structure (i.e. the ureters), creating wave-like movements pushing the contents of the structure forward.
Prophylaxis: Treatment that is given or action taken to prevent disease.
Syndrome: A group of symptoms which consistently occur together.

References

Adamczak, M., Masajtis-Zagajewska, A., Mazanowska, O. et al. (2018). Diagnosis and treatment of Metabolic acidosis in Patients with Chronic Kidney Disease – Position statement of the Working Group of the Polish Society of Nephrology. www.karger.com/Article/Pdf/490475 (accessed September 2019).

Anisman, S., Erickson, S., and Morden, N. (2019). *How to prescribe loop diuretics in oedema*. www.bmj.com/content/364/bmj.l359?hwoasp=authn%3A1569172103%3A4058629%3A1467218820%3A0%3A0%3ABxWwOYLM8njIrRWgakDdKQ%3D%3D (accessed September 2019).

Dolan, N.M. and Gill, D. (2008). 'Causes of nephrotic syndrome in childhood' *Paediatrics and Child Health* 8(18): 369–374.

Electronic Medicines Compendium (2019a) *Sevelamer hydrochloride* www.medicines.org.uk/emc/product/207/smpc (accessed September 2019).

Electronic Medicines Compendium (2019b) *Lanthanum* www.medicines.org.uk/emc/product/7494/smpc (accessed September 2019).

Electronic Medicines Compendium (2019c) *Alfacalcidol* www.medicines.org.uk/emc/product/5516/smpc (accessed September 2019).

Electronic Medicines Compendium (2019d) *Calcitriol* www.medicines.org.uk/emc/search?q=%22calcitriol%22 (accessed September 2019).

Electronic Medicines Compendium (2019e) *Sodium Polystyrene Sulfonate* www.medicines.org.uk/emc/product/1461 (accessed September 2019).

Electronic Medicines Compendium (2019f) *Calcium Resonium* www.medicines.org.uk/emc/product/1439 (accessed September 2019).

Electronic Medicines) Compendium (2019g) *Sando K* www.medicines.org.uk/emc/product/959 (accessed September 2019).

Electronic Medicines) Compendium (2019h) *Sodium bicarbonate* www.medicines.org.uk/emc/product/10531/smpc (accessed September 2019).

El-Husseini, A., El-Basuony, F., Mahmoud, I. et al. (2005). Long-term effects of cyclosporine in children with idiopathic nephrotic syndrome: a single-centre experience. *Nephrology Dialysis Transplantation* 20(11): 2433–2438.

Gallibois, C.M., Jawa, N.A., and Noone, D.G. (2017). Hypertension in pediatric patients with chronic kidney disease: management challenges. *International Journal of Nephrology and Renovascular Disease* 10: 205.

Hadstein, C. and Schaefer, F. (2008). 'Hypertension in children with chronic kidney disease: pathophysiology and management'. *Pediatric Nephrology* 23(3): 363–371.

Isert, S., Müller, D., and Thumfart, J. (2020). 'Factors associated with the development of chronic kidney disease in children with congenital anomalies of the kidney and urinary tract' *Frontiers in Pediatrics* 8: 298.

Jablonski, K.L and Chonchol, M. (2013). *Vascular Calcification in End-Stage Renal Disease*. www.ncbi.nlm.nih.gov/pmc/articles/PMC3813300/#!po=30.0000 (accessed September 2019).

Kidney Research UK (2018). *Annual Report and Financial Statements*. https://kidneyresearchuk.org/about-us/annual-reports/ (accessed September 2019).

Kidney Research UK (2020). https://kidneyresearchuk.org/ (accessed July 2020).

Latta, K., von Schnakenburg, C., and Ehrich, J.H. (2001). 'A meta-analysis of cytotoxic treatment for frequently relapsing nephrotic syndrome in children'. *Pediatric Nephrology* 16(3): 271–282.

National Institute of Diabetes and Digestive and Kidney Diseases (2020). www.niddk.nih.gov/health-information/kidney-disease (accessed July 2020).

National Institute for Health and Care Excellence (2018). *Urinary Tract Infection in Under 16s: Diagnosis and Management*. www.nice.org.uk/guidance/cg54 (accessed July 2020).

NHS England (2015). *Clinical Commissioning Policy: Rituximab for the Treatment of Relapsing Steroid Sensitive Nephrotic Syndrome*.www.england.nhs.uk/commissioning/wp-content/uploads/sites/12/2015/10/e03pb-rituxmb-nephrtc-syndrm-chld-oct15.pdf (accessed July 2020).

Noone, D.G., Iijima, K., and Parekh, R. (2018). Idiopathic nephrotic syndrome in children. *The Lancet* 392(10141): 61–74.

O'Callaghan, C. (2017). *The Renal System at a Glance*, 4e. Chichester: John Wiley & Sons.

Paediatric Formulary Committee (2020a) *BNF for Children* (online) *Prednisolone*. London: BMJ Group, Pharmaceutical Press, and RCPCH Publications. https://bnfc.nice.org.uk/drug/prednisolone.html (accessed September 2020).

Paediatric Formulary Committee (2020b) *BNF for Children* (online) *Furosemide*. London: BMJ Group, Pharmaceutical Press, and RCPCH Publications. https://bnfc.nice.org.uk/drug/furosemide.html (accessed September 2020).

Paediatric Formulary Committee (2020c) *BNF for Children* (online) *Tacrolimus*. London: BMJ Group, Pharmaceutical Press, and RCPCH Publications. https://bnfc.nice.org.uk/drug/tacrolimus.html (accessed September 2020).

Paediatric Formulary Committee (2020d) *BNF for Children* (online) *Ciclosporin*. London: BMJ Group, Pharmaceutical Press, and RCPCH Publications. https://bnfc.nice.org.uk/drug/ciclosporin.html (accessed September 2020).

Paediatric Formulary Committee (2020e) *BNF for Children* (online) *Mycophenolate mofetil*. London: BMJ Group, Pharmaceutical Press, and RCPCH Publications. https://bnfc.nice.org.uk/drug/Mycophenolate-mofetil.html (accessed September 2020).

Paediatric Formulary Committee (2020f) *BNF for Children* (online) *Cyclophosphamide*. London: BMJ Group, Pharmaceutical Press, and RCPCH Publications. https://bnfc.nice.org.uk/drug/cyclophosphamide.html (accessed September 2020).

Paediatric Formulary Committee (2020g) *BNF for Children* (online) *Rituximab*. London: BMJ Group, Pharmaceutical Press, and RCPCH Publications. https://bnfc.nice.org.uk/drug/rituximab.html (accessed September 2020).

Paediatric Formulary Committee (2019h) *BNF for Children* (online) *Sevelamer*. London: BMJ Group, Pharmaceutical Press, and RCPCH Publications. https://bnfc.nice.org.uk/drug/sevelamer.html (accessed September 2019).

Paediatric Formulary Committee (2019i) *BNF for Children* (online) *Lanthanum*. London: BMJ Group, Pharmaceutical Press, and RCPCH Publications. https://bnfc.nice.org.uk/drug/lanthanum.html (accessed September 2019).

Paediatric Formulary Committee (2019j) *BNF for Children* (online) *Alfacalcidol*. London: BMJ Group, Pharmaceutical Press, and RCPCH Publications. https://bnfc.nice.org.uk/drug/alfacalcidol.html (accessed September 2019).

Paediatric Formulary Committee (2019k) *BNF for Children* (online) *Calcitriol*. London: BMJ Group, Pharmaceutical Press, and RCPCH Publications. https://bnfc.nice.org.uk/drug/calcitriol.html (accessed September 2019).

Paediatric Formulary Committee (2019l) *BNF for Children* (online) *Sodium Polystyrene sulfonate*. London: BMJ Group, Pharmaceutical Press, and RCPCH Publications. https://bnfc.nice.org.uk/drug/sodium-polystyrene-sulfonate.html (accessed September 2019).

Paediatric Formulary Committee (2019m) *BNF for Children* (online) *Calcium Polystyrene sulfonate*. London: BMJ Group, Pharmaceutical Press, and RCPCH Publications. https://bnfc.nice.org.uk/drug/calcium-polystyrene-sulfonate.html (accessed September 2019).

Paediatric Formulary Committee (2019n) *BNF for Children* (online) *Potassium Chloride*. London: BMJ Group, Pharmaceutical Press, and RCPCH Publications. https://bnfc.nice.org.uk/drug/potassium-chloride.html (accessed September 2019).

Paediatric Formulary Committee (2019o) *BNF for Children* (online). *Sodium Bicarbonate*. London: BMJ Group, Pharmaceutical Press, and RCPCH Publications. https://bnfc.nice.org.uk/drug/sodium-bicarbonate.html (accessed September 2019).

Paediatric Formulary Committee (2019p) *BNF for Children* (online). *Captopril*. London: BMJ Group, Pharmaceutical Press, and RCPCH Publications. https://bnfc.nice.org.uk/drug/captopril.html (accessed September 2019).

Paediatric Formulary Committee (2019q) *BNF for Children* (online). *Enalapril Maleate*. London: BMJ Group, Pharmaceutical Press, and RCPCH Publications. https://bnfc.nice.org.uk/drug/enalapril-maleate.html (accessed September 2019).

Paediatric Formulary Committee (2019r) *BNF for Children* (online). *Lisinopril*. London: BMJ Group, Pharmaceutical Press, and RCPCH Publications. https://bnfc.nice.org.uk/drug/lisinopril.html (accessed September 2019).

Peate, I. (2017). Fluid and electrolyte balance and associated disorders. In: *Fundamentals of Applied Pathophysiology: An Essential Guide for Nursing and Healthcare Students* (ed. Peate, I.), 506–533. Hoboken, NJ: John Wiley & Sons.

Peate, I. and Nair, M. (2011). *Fundamentals of Anatomy and Physiology for Student Nurses*. John Wiley & Sons.

Schijvens, A.M., ter Heine, R., De Wildt, S.N., and Schreuder, M.F. (2019). 'Pharmacology and pharmacogenetics of prednisone and prednisolone in patients with nephrotic syndrome'. *Pediatric Nephrology* 34(3): 389–403.

Soar, J. Deakin, C. Lockey, A. et al. (2015). *Resuscitation Guidelines 2015 Adult Life Support* London: Resuscitation Council UK.

Vivarelli, M., Massella, L., Ruggiero, B., and Emma, F. (2017). Minimal change disease. *Clinical Journal of the American Society of Nephrology* 12(2): 332–345.

Ware, T. (2020). Nephrotic syndrome. *InnovAiT* 13(3): 159–163.

Webb, N.J., Woolley, R.L., Lambe, T. et al. (2019). Long term tapering versus standard prednisolone treatment for first episode of childhood nephrotic syndrome: phase III randomised controlled trial and economic evaluation. *BMJ*, 365.

Yang, Q., Zhang, Z., and Kuklina, E.V. (2012). Sodium intake and blood pressure among US children and adolescents. *Pediatrics* 130(4): 611–619.

Zolotas, E. and Krishnan, R. (2016). Nephrotic syndrome. *Paediatrics and Child Health* 26(8): 349–352.

Further Resources

KDIGO Guidelines (https://kdigo.org/guidelines/): KDIGO is *the* global nonprofit organisation developing and implementing evidence-based clinical practice guidelines in kidney disease. KDIGO guidelines are created, reviewed, published and implemented following a rigorous scientific process.

National Institute of Health and Care Excellence (NICE) Guidelines (www.nice.org.uk/): NICE provides national guidance and advice to improve health and social care. They provide a number of guidelines concerning all aspects of healthcare delivery. Their aim is to improve health and social care through evidence-based guidance.

Chapter 8 Medications Used in the Renal System

Multiple Choice Questions

1. Which of the following is NOT a function of the kidney?
   (a) Removal of the waste product of metabolism, including urea and creatinine
   (b) Fluid balance via selective absorption of sodium and water
   (c) Regulation of potassium via the secretion of aldosterone
   (d) Glucose homeostasis via gluconeogenesis and reabsorption of glucose
2. What are the three main features of nephrotic syndrome?
   (a) Tachycardia, proteinuria and excessive thirst
   (b) Proteinuria, hypoalbuminaemia and oedema
   (c) Oedema, hypertension and hyperkalaemia
   (d) Proteinuria, hyponatraemia and oedema
3. What is the initial treatment for minimal change nephrotic syndrome?
   (a) Prednisolone
   (b) Rituximab
   (c) Albumin
   (d) Alfacalcidol
4. The genomic glucocorticoid action is characterised by
   (a) A rapid onset of the effect
   (b) Short duration of the effect
   (c) A slow onset of the effect
   (d) Long duration of the effect
5. What is a calcineurin inhibitors and how does it work?
   (a) A group of immunosuppressive drugs which inhibit phosphatase calcineurin
   (b) An alkylating agent which works by interfering with DNA synthesis
   (c) Is a loop diuretic which inhibits reabsorption
   (d) Is a glucocorticoid, mediated by both genomic and non-genomic mechanisms.
6. Hypokalaemia is:
   (a) High potassium
   (b) High calcium
   (c) Low phosphate
   (d) Low potassium
7. ACE inhibitors:
   (a) Work by inhibiting the conversion of angiotensin I to angiotensin II
   (b) Stop the production of vitamin D
   (c) Are prescribed at maximum dose
   (d) Work by blocking the effect of angiotensin II
8. Loop diuretics exert their effect upon which part of the nephron?
   (a) Proximal convoluted tubule
   (b) Collecting
   (c) Loop of Henle
   (d) Glomerulus
9. Furosemide has a potent diuretic effect via the inhibition of which of the following?
   (a) Sodium-potassium-chloride cotransporter, or the Na-K-Cl (NKCC2)
   (b) Phosphodiesterase type 5
   (c) Sodium-potassium ATPase pump
   (d) Aldosterone antagonism
10. Which segment of the nephron is critical in the excretion of potassium ions?
    (a) Proximal convoluted tubule
    (b) Collecting duct
    (c) Thick ascending Loop of Henle
    (d) Thin descending Loop of Henle
11. Secondary hyperparathyroidism can lead to which of the following?
    (a) Hypercalcaemia
    (b) Hyperphosphataemia

(c) High vitamin D levels

(d) Diabetes

12. An under-sized BP cuff can:

(a) Underestimate a BP

(b) Significantly overestimate a BP

(c) Make no difference

(d) Cause harm to the child

13. Angiotensin II receptor antagonists:

(a) Block the effect of angiotensin II

(b) Constrict blood vessels

(c) Increase blood pressure

(d) Work by inhibiting the conversion of angiotensin I to angiotensin II

14. The juxtaglomerular cells (baroreceptors) located in the afferent arterioles of the kidney identify low blood volume and will secrete:

(a) Potassium

(b) Renin

(c) Parathyroid hormone

(d) Aldosterone

15. A common side effect of captopril is:

(a) Weight gain

(b) Increased risk of infection

(c) Electrolyte imbalance

(d) Polyuria

Find Out More

The following is a list of conditions that are associated with the renal system. Take some time and write notes about each of the conditions. Think about the medications that may be used in order to treat these conditions and be specific about the pharmacokinetics and pharmacodynamics. Remember to include aspects of patient care. If you are making notes about people you have offered care and support to, you must ensure that you have adhered to the rules of confidentiality.

THE CONDITION	YOUR NOTES
Haemolytic uremic syndrome	
Systemic lupus erythematous (juvenile)	
Henoch-Schönlein purpura	
Alport syndrome	
Addison's disease	

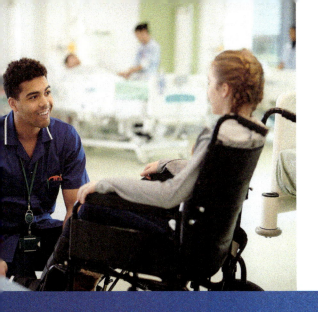

9

Medications Used in the Endocrine System

Jackie O'Sullivan

Aim

The aim of this chapter is to provide an introduction to the medications used in endocrine disorders in childhood

Learning Outcomes

After reading this chapter the reader will be able to:
- Name endocrine glands and the hormones produced and their systemic actions
- Describe a feedback loop in relation to production of a specific hormone
- Discuss the pharmacology related to the endocrine system and the problems that some endocrine drugs treat in children and young people (CYP)
- Describe medications commonly used for endocrine conditions in CYP

Test Your Knowledge

1. List the endocrine glands, identify where they are in the body and list the hormones they produce
2. Make a list of all the hormone medications you already know. What format do they come in?

Fundamentals of Pharmacology for Children's Nurses, First Edition. Edited by Ian Peate and Peter Dryden.
© 2022 John Wiley & Sons Ltd. Published 2022 by John Wiley & Sons Ltd.
Companion website: www.wiley.com/go/pharmacologyforCN

Chapter 9 Medications Used in the Endocrine System

3. What is the relevance of screening programmes in neonatal period and early childhood for endocrine conditions?
4. What is the long-term benefit for patients and society of early recognition and treatment of hypothyroidism in childhood?
5. At what ages are specific types of endocrine dysfunction likely to present?

Introduction

The endocrine system maintains internal homeostasis through the use of hormones. A hormone is generally described as a chemical messenger that is released into the bloodstream where it causes an effect on target cells that are located some distance from the hormonal release site.

Hormones can be seen as medicines that the patient's body makes. The use of medicines that regulate and control endocrine function is an important aspect of pharmacology and as such has important implications for nursing and healthcare provision. Patients take drugs as replacement therapy when there is a hormonal deficiency, such as the administration of insulin in diabetes mellitus. Steroids (glucocorticoids) to replace adrenal production in congenital adrenal hyperplasia. Antithyroid drugs, on the other hand, can be used to treat endocrine hyperactivity in treatment of hyperthyroidism (Birrell and Cheetham, 2004).

The chapter provides a fundamental overview of the basic aspects of how the endocrine system functions, as well as hormones and their effects. How medicines can be used to alter endocrine function is discussed. It is not possible in a chapter of this of this size to discuss all aspects of pharmacology and the endocrine system. A general discussion of the pharmacology related to the endocrine system and the problems that some endocrine drugs that are used to treat children and young people (CYP) is provided. The reader is advised to delve deeper into the pharmacology associated with endocrine system and specific conditions.

The Endocrine System

The endocrine system maintains internal homeostasis throughout the body through the release of hormones into the blood supply. The target cells that a hormone acts on are usually located at a distance from the site of release. Endocrine glands produce and release specific hormones that regulate reproduction, growth, energy metabolism, fluid balance and response to injury or stress. Feedback loop systems are a common feature of the regulation of hormone requirements. Some hormones such as the luteinising hormone (LH) and follicle-stimulating hormone (FSH) or cortisol are produced in a cyclical pattern over short or longer periods of time; this cyclical pattern is also linked in with a feedback loop system.

Health conditions related to hormone production can occur due to an excess or under-production of the hormone with short- and long-term effects. Drugs used in endocrinology may be direct replacements for hormones that are not being produced in sufficient quantity such as levothyroxine or androgens, or medications that block the action of a hormone or its production such as carbimazole when used in hyperthyroidism. Doses required are managed by ensuring sufficient is administered to replace the usual level of a hormone which may vary over the lifespan of the CYP. In infancy much higher levels of circulating thyroid hormone are seen than occur in adults. Thyroid hormone is an essential element during the critical brain growth that occurs in the first two years of life. Low levels of thyroid hormone in infancy results in long-term neurodisability. Globally, untreated congenital hypothyroidism, mainly due to iodine deficiency, is the commonest cause of preventable learning disability (WHO, 2007).

The homeostatic regulation of body systems generally follows an order of signal and response.

- A signal is received in a gland
- A response is made and hormones are produced
- A reaction occurs in a target tissue

Almost all systems use a negative feedback loop where the production of hormone up to a set level will suppress the signal for it being produced. Once levels fall below the desired level the signal hormone level rises again.

Chapter 9 Medications Used in the Endocrine System

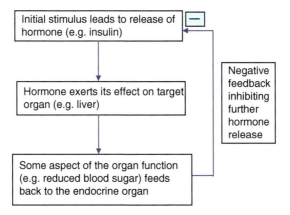

Figure 9.1 **The negative feedback system.** *Source: Ian Peate and Suzanne Evans 2020/John Wiley & Sons.*

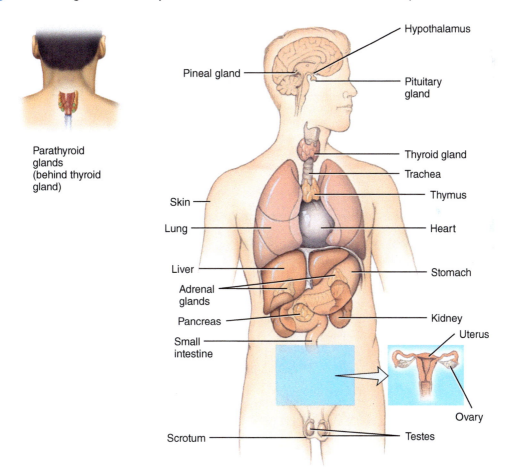

Figure 9.2 **The location of the endocrine glands.** *Source: Ian Peate and Suzanne Evans 2020 / John Wiley & Sons.*

There is one positive feedback loop in the endocrine system. In this case the stimulus for production of prolactin is suckling at the breast, rising levels of prolactin lead to lactation, further suckling leads to increased lactation. The process of feeding an infant therefore stimulates the production of the required amount of food. As weaning commences and suckling decreases, prolactin declines reducing milk produced. Figure 9.1 demonstrates the negative feedback loop.

Chapter 9 Medications Used in the Endocrine System

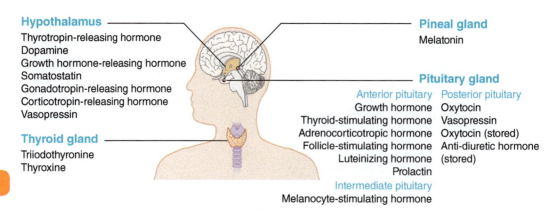

Figure 9.3 **Endocrines glands and hormones that are locates in the head and neck.** Source: Peate and Gormley-Fleming, 2015/John Wiley & Sons.

Figure 9.2 shows the location of the endocrine organs and Figure 9.3 the endocrine glands and hormones of the head and neck.

Other tissues also produce hormones in an endocrine and paracrine fashion. The hypothalamus largely produces paracrine hormones that stimulate the pituitary gland. Most tissues respond to GH to produce insulin-like growth factor 1 (IGF-1) which acts locally as a paracrine hormone to induce growth and metabolic effects. The digestive system produces some endocrine hormones involved in appetite regulation such as leptin, ghrelin and peptide YY. The function of these hormones is the subject of current research into their role in obesity but as yet has not led to realistic therapeutic options. Common terminology used in relation to the endocrine system can be found in Table 9.1.

Medications Used in Endocrine Disorders Affecting Growth

Somatropin: (Growth Hormone) (GH)

Natural GH is synthesised and secreted by somatotroph cells in the anterior pituitary gland. It is a protein consisting of 190 amino acids and it has major effects on bone growth as well as a number of metabolic effects in the regulation of blood glucose levels, utilisation of fat and muscle function.

Prior to the early 1980s GH was extracted from homogenised human cadaveric pituitary glands and used only for the most severely growth restricted CYP. Supply was erratic and of variable quality with dosing regimens of three times a week being common due to the supply problems. In the early 1980s it was recognised that some adults previously treated with human GH were developing and dying from Creutzfeldt–Jacob disease (CJD). All GH treatments were suspended until drug companies were able to provide a regulated, pure product.

Since 1985 production of GH using recombinant DNA techniques has allowed a ready supply of good quality product. The number of growth conditions in which the treatment has proved useful has increased, there are six licensed indications for use of GH in the UK. National Institute for Health and Care Excellence (NICE) also allows individual trials of GH for those outside of the stated conditions as long as parameters for 'success' are decided at the outset of treatment by clinicians so that treatment is not continued for prolonged periods without evidence of a good result.

Uses: as Licensed by NICE (2010)
1. GH deficiency in children and adults
2. Turner syndrome in girls before epiphyseal fusion
3. Prader–Willi syndrome in children
4. Chronic renal failure in children with glomerular filtration rate below 50ml/min/L.
5. Children born small for gestational age with failure to catch up by 4 years of age
6. Children with short stature homeobox-containing gene (SHOX) deficiency

Table 9.1 Some common terminology used in relation to the endocrine system.

TERM	DISCUSSION
Hyper-	An overproduction of a hormone, most commonly seen as thyrotoxicosis from excess production of thyroid hormone. Treatment involves blocking the activity of the overproduced hormone, preventing production of the hormone by interfering with receptors on the target tissues, medically destroying the function of the gland using radioactive iodine or removing the gland.
Hypo-	Under-production of a hormone, commonly seen in thyroid conditions. Can be congenital or acquired and may be genetic or autoimmune. In congenital conditions the national neonatal screening programme aims to identify all babies with insufficient thyroid hormone production and ensure they commence appropriate hormone replacement within 7 days of a positive screening test. Replacement of the under-produced hormone is the simplest means of treatment in these conditions.
Dyshormonogenesis	A group of inherited disorders of thyroid hormone synthesis leading to low levels of thyroid hormone and high levels of thyroid-stimulating hormone
Primary conditions	A hormone production problem where the tissue producing the hormone is unable to do so, resulting in high level of the stimulating hormone for that tissue and low or absent levels of the hormone that should be being produced. In primary disorders the only treatment option is to replace the hormones that should be present. In Addison's disease this involves administering a glucocorticoid such as hydrocortisone and a mineralocorticoid replacement such as fludrocortisone.
Secondary conditions	Secondary hormone failure is due to lack of a signalling hormone. Commonly, this relates to a series of disorders affecting the pituitary gland, these may be congenital disorders of the development of the pituitary gland itself and may affect a single hormone or multiple hormones. It is also the case in surgery or radiotherapy treatments which are used for management of a variety of brain tumours. Treatment in secondary conditions is usually to replace the final hormone in the feedback chain such as thyroxine or cortisol.
Tertiary conditions	While the pituitary gland itself is seen as the master control gland regulating hormone production, an area above the pituitary, the hypothalamus, is involved in stimulating the pituitary gland itself. In this case it is the pituitary gland that is a secondary failure due to lack of stimulation from the hypothalamus. Tertiary disorders also develop over time after radiotherapy for some brain tumours and these need to be considered when using some provocation tests stimulating the end organ where a response to the hormone stimulus will appear normal.
Paracrine	Describes a hormone that only has an action close to the area of its secretion. Growth hormone stimulates the production of IGF1 in bone cells. This hormone (IGF-1) when produced by bone cells acts on the growth plate of the bone to stimulate growth. Other hormones with a paracrine effect are testosterone produced by the Leydig cells in the testes and oestrogen produced in ovaries, which is important in the development of ovarian follicles before ovulation
Normal ranges	Most endocrine treatments are titrated according to normal ranges of hormone levels for age and stage of development. Ranges vary between services according to the type of testing kits used in analysis, local reference ranges should be consulted when interpreting blood results for medication monitoring purposes

Growth hormone is given by subcutaneous daily injection using a pen injector device, similar to insulin pens. There is one electronic device which is useful for concordance monitoring.

Each device can only be used with the GH produced by that specific drug company. The selection of which GH to use is therefore linked to lifestyle factors within a family which will influence the choice of device. Some products are stable at room temperature while others are not. Monitoring of concordance is a requirement. Where needle phobia is a problem, then the needle free device is often the preferred option.

Poor concordance with a daily injection is a common feature of treatment with GH. Patient involvement in the choice of injection device has been shown to improve concordance (Gau and Takasawa 2017).

As most GH is produced during sleep it is advised that doses should be injected in the evening although some families find it easier to establish a routine with the injection being administered earlier in the day. The best response rate is seen in those who administer 6 or 7 doses per week with a sharp decline in growth velocity seen in those administering 5 or fewer doses per week (Arecini et al., 2013).

Growth hormone binds to cell surfaces on a GH receptor. This stimulates the secretion of IGF-1. Most IGF-1 is produced in the liver but many other tissues will also generate smaller amounts. IGF-1 from the liver acts as an endocrine hormone and the smaller amounts produced in other tissues acts locally on those tissues in a paracrine fashion.

An important function of GH besides the control of growth is to provide a mechanism to cope with periods of food deprivation. In this way, GH stimulates lipolysis and provides free fatty acids and glycerol as substrates for energy metabolism. Growth hormone promotes the 'browning' of adipose tissue and inhibits the deposition of white adipose tissue. Children and young people with GH deficiency have a characteristic appearance that includes centrally deposited adipose tissue making them heavy for their height. Once treated with GH they use this adipose tissue in a far more metabolically efficient way and lose their truncal obesity.

In muscle tissues GH promotes an increase in mitochondrial capacity for oxidation. It prevents muscle atrophy and reduces the change from slow twitch to fast twitch muscle fibres which tire more easily. This function of GH appears to be most effective in children with Prader–Willi syndrome who have low muscle tone before commencing treatment. Exercise is known to increase the secretion of GH and the use of a treadmill to induce additional GH secretion has sometimes been used in place of other stimulation tests (Farhad et al., 2018).

Clinical Consideration

Growth-promoting agents such as GH and mecasermin are associated with two significant side effects.

1. Benign intracranial hypertension (BIH): An increase in fluid in the dural space which results in a pseudo-tumour syndrome of severe persistent headache, and visual disturbance from raised intracranial pressure, occurring soon after initiation of treatment. Growth hormone supplements should be discontinued until intracranial pressure returns to normal. The drug is reintroduced in a more gradual series of dose increments.
2. Slipped upper capital femoral epiphysis (SUFE): The rapid skeletal growth that occurs during puberty can cause the growth plate at the upper end of the femur to shear, often occurring in adolescents, especially those who are overweight. Other risk factors for SUFE are hypothyroidism and treatment for more than 2 years with gonadotrophin-releasing hormone analogues for early puberty. Onset of hip or knee pain and limping where there is no associated physical injury should be reported and radiological investigations to rule out SUFE are required.

Source: Based on NICE, 2010.

Mecasermin (Increlex®)

Recombinant IGF-1 is a protein 70 amino acids in length produced mainly in the liver under the action of GH. IGF-1 has growth-promoting effects on nearly all cells, especially skeletal muscle and bone.

This medication is used to treat those with GH resistance or disorders of primary IGF-1 deficiency. Laron syndrome is a recessively inherited form of dwarfism due to a lack of GH receptors. They have characteristically high GH levels with low or absent levels of IGF-1 and severe growth retardation. Growth hormone insensitivity can also occur as a secondary problem in some chronic nutritional disorders and as a result of the development of antibodies to GH (Fintini et al., 2009).

Mecasermin is administered as a subcutaneous injection twice daily as the action of the drug lasts for approximately 5 hours. The drug is provided as a multidose vial and medication is withdrawn using 1ml syringes and 25g needles. Initiation of treatment is managed in hospital for the first week due to the significant risk of hypoglycaemia from the injections. Treatment starts at a very low dose and is increased in small increments over the first month as tolerated. If hypoglycaemia occurs, the dose is reduced back to the previously tolerated level. During this inpatient stay parents and CYP can be taught how to assemble and use the correct needles and syringes, how to draw up the correct dose and how to give a subcutaneous injection.

Skills in Practice

Injection Devices for Subcutaneous injections

- **Insulin syringe:** Holds a maximum of 1 ml of medicine, has markings from 10 to 100 units. The marking at 100 is the same as 1 ml. The marking at 50 is the same as ½ ml. They should only be used for insulin, coming with an integral 30g needle usually 12mm in length.
- **Tuberculin syringe:** Holds up to 1 ml of medicine. It has a needle slightly longer than an insulin syringe. The syringe is marked every 0.1 ml.
- **Reusable pen devices:** Designed to hold cartridges of insulin or growth hormone. Each drug company has a dedicated device for their own drug product. Cartridges have a threaded end to which single-use fine needles can be attached. Cartridges are multidose and must be discarded when empty or when the maximum number of days' use is reached. This varies dependent on storage conditions and excipients in the cartridge.
- **Disposable pen devices:** Used for growth hormone, insulin, FSH and HCG. Designed to function with single-use fine-bore needles attached to a screw thread at the tip. The entire pen is discarded after multiple injections.

   When giving injections, rotation of sites is important to avoid damage over time to the subcutaneous fat which disrupts absorption of injected medication due to reduced numbers of capillaries. It can also result in noticeable dips or lumps in the affected area.

Parents and the patient need to be able to recognise and respond to signs of hypoglycaemia. Injections should always be given with a meal; if the patient is unable to eat, then doses should be omitted.

In target tissues, the Type 1 IGF-1 receptor is activated by IGF-1, leading to intracellular signalling which stimulates multiple processes, resulting in growth. The metabolic actions of IGF-1 stimulate the uptake of glucose, fatty acids, and amino acids so that metabolism supports growing tissues.

Skeletal growth occurs at the cartilage growth plates of the epiphyses of bones where stem cells divide to produce new cartilage cells or chondrocytes. The growth of chondrocytes is under the control of IGF-1 and GH. The chondrocytes become calcified so that new bone is formed, allowing the length of the bones to increase. This results in skeletal growth until the cartilage growth plates fuse at the end of puberty.

IGF-1 receptors are present on most types of cells and tissues. IGF-1 has mitogenic activities that lead to an increased number of cells in the body.

IGF-1 suppresses hepatic glucose production and stimulates peripheral glucose utilisation and therefore has a hypoglycaemic potential. IGF-1 has inhibitory effects on insulin secretion.

In Table 9.2. medications that are used in endocrine disorders affecting growth are outlined, this table also provides a discussion on the absorption, distribution, metabolism and excretion of somatropin and mecasermin (Increlex ®).

Endocrine Disorders of Puberty

Puberty is a period of growth and development where maturation and development of sexual organs occurs. In boys changes start to happen between 9 and 14 years and in girls development usually starts between 8 and 13 years. There is a tempo and order of development which takes between 2 and 5 years to complete.

Chapter 9 Medications Used in the Endocrine System

Table 9.2 Medications used in endocrine disorders affecting growth.

MEDICATION	DRUG FORM AND DOSES	ABSORPTION AND DISTRIBUTION	METABOLISM AND EXCRETION
Somatropin (growth hormone)	Available as dry powder and liquid forms for subcutaneous injection using pen devices autoinjectors. Dosing in growth hormone deficiency: prepubertal children $0.7mg/m^2$ daily Pubertal children $1mg/m^2$ daily. Use in supraphysiological doses for other conditions: $1-1.4mg/m^2$ daily Aiming to maintain serum IGF-1 levels within upper half of normal range for age. Doses in post pubertal young adults with confirmed growth hormone deficiency is titrated to an IGF-1 level within the normal range.	Somatropin is rapidly absorbed from subcutaneous tissue into the blood stream at a rate of 600ng/hr/ml. Peak levels occur about 3 hours after injection. Bioavailability is approximately 80%.	Somatropin is a potent metabolic hormone of importance for the metabolism of lipids, carbohydrates and proteins. In children with inadequate endogenous growth hormone it stimulates linear growth and increases growth rate. In adults, as well as in children, it maintains a normal body composition. Visceral adipose tissue is particularly responsive to somatropin. There is also a decrease in uptake of triglycerides into body fat stores. Serum concentrations of IGF-I, and IGFBP3 (Insulin-like Growth Factor Binding Protein 3) are increased by somatropin. Subcutaneous injection shows a half-life of 2–3 hours. The drug is excreted in urine with approximately 0.1% of it being unchanged.
Mecasermin (Increlex®)	Available in vials of 10mg Mecasermin for multiple doses. Administered as a subcutaneous injection using insulin syringes. Treatment initiation is managed in a hospital setting due to the high risk of hypoglycaemia.	In healthy subjects the bioavailability is reported as 100%. The absolute availability in primary IGF deficiency has not been determined. Administered as a subcutaneous injection.	Mecasermin has widespread metabolic effects. Skeletal growth occurs at epiphyseal plates in direct response to IGF-1. Glucose production from the liver is suppressed by mecasermin. This means there is a risk of hypoglycaemia in response to its use. As primary IGF-1 deficiency is very rare there is limited evidence on the excretion of mecasermin. Small studies show a half-life of 5.8 hours. To maintain adequate growth from circulating IGF-1 a twice daily dosing regimen is required.

Source: Based on Joint Formulary Committee, 2020

Evaluation of the current stage of puberty refers to Tanner stages of development (Emmanuel and Bokor, 2020). Endocrine dysfunction can cause early pubertal development or lack of pubertal development. Some conditions such as Klinefelter syndrome can mean initial development of pubertal progress and then an arrest in development as the gonadal tissue is unable to maintain sufficient hormone production (Growth Foundation, ND).

Endocrine medications related to puberty are largely aimed at replacing sex hormones or suppression of production of gonadotrophins. Replacement of gonadotrophins to stimulate testicular and penile growth in boys during the mini puberty of infancy is a new development aimed at improving fertility of gonadotrophin-deficient young men in adulthood by simulating a natural physiological process that has an importance in testicular development (Papadimitriou et al. 2019).

Direct Hormone Replacements

Administration of end organ hormones in cases of deficiency is usually easier to manage than attempting to stimulate their production. In delayed puberty small doses of sex steroids can initiate the negative feedback processes involved in the development of secondary sexual characteristics.

Oestrogen and Progesterone

Used in girls for the initiation of puberty in small incremental doses over 2 years as either tablets or transdermal patches. Maintenance doses are usually given in the form of a combined contraceptive pill (OCP) or a hormone replacement therapy (HRT) format with a cyclical introduction of progesterone as well as the oestrogen to give rise to menstrual bleeding. British Society for Paediatric Endocrinology and Diabetes (BSPED) have detailed guidance on induction of puberty and maintenance therapies for those requiring long-term hormone replacement (Matthews et al., 2016)

Testosterone

Used in boys to increase genital size and to induce puberty when delayed. Medication is available in various formats; tablets, intramuscular injections and transdermal gels. The commonest use is the injectable format given monthly in incremental doses. For those requiring continued medication as an adult there are depot injections (Nebido – testosterone preparation) which provide a longer action of testosterone within the usual adult range. The convenience of infrequent doses is attractive to adolescents who at times struggle to remember multiple oral doses or application of gels daily (El-Khairi et al., 2016).

Dihydrotestosterone (DHT)

This is a powerful androgen which has significant effect on virilisation of male genitalia at puberty. The presence of the enzyme 5 Alpha reductase is essential for the production of DHT from testosterone. A rare inborn deficiency in 5 Alpha reductase leads to severe under-virilisation of males at birth such that many infants are assigned female gender until testes further descend into what are thought to be labia but are actually scrotal folds a few weeks after birth. In this condition topical DHT gel as a 2.5% preparation is administered to the thighs daily for several months. This promotes the growth of the micropenis to a size permitting surgical correction of hypospadias. Families are advised that pubic hair will also develop in response to the presence of DHT, once treatment is discontinued the pubic hair becomes finer but does not completely regress.

Human Chorionic Gonadotrophin (HCG)

This drug is used as an analogue for luteinising hormone, it shares a transmembrane receptor on ovarian theca cells and in Leydig cells in the testes. It is primarily prescribed in adulthood to women undergoing assisted reproduction therapy. In CYP it is used in boys to stimulate testicular production of testosterone. The drug is given by subcutaneous injection twice weekly at a dose of 1500 to 2000 international units for 3 weeks as part of an HCG test. It has been available as a prefilled pen device, parents can be taught to administer the medications at home reducing the need for multiple hospital visits. In boys with undescended testes HCG stimulation is used to determine the presence of testicular tissue, there will be a rise in serum testosterone levels from a pre-treatment to post treatment level if testes are present. Some boys with gonadotrophin deficiency will achieve descent of testes and an increase in their size as a response to the stimulation of endogenous testosterone production. This process makes surgical fixation of testes into the scrotum easier and less likely to cause damage with a long-term effect on their function in adulthood (Kucharski and Neildziski, 2013). Many countries are starting to offer a course of gonadotrophin treatment to males with gonadotrpophin deficiency due to pituitary hormone deficiency or Kallman's syndrome to simulate a mini puberty as there is increasing evidence that this improves their fertility as adults (Papadimitriou et al., 2019).

Menotrophin or Follicle-Stimulating Hormone (FSH)

This drug is derived from human menopausal gonadotrophin and almost all preparations are a combination drug with HCG. It is most commonly used in adult females undergoing assisted reproductive therapy; however, this is also of use in stimulating testicular development leading to spermatogenesis in adolescent boys with secondary hypogonadism. Injections are given subcutaneously three times a week of increasing doses until there are measurable levels of FSH in the normal range for age. In stimulating mini puberty in boys with hypogonadotrophic hypogonadism it is used in combination with HCG for up to 3 months. Spermatogenesis requires a high level of intratesticular testosterone and while FSH alone will stimulate some Sertoli cell proliferation the complete process of spermatogenesis requires locally produced testosterone by Leydig cells. The medication is available in a range of strengths in single-use vials which require reconstitution and injection with 25g size needles. It is also available in a multi-dose pen device which is used with smaller pen needles similar to insulin pens.

Drugs Used to Block Puberty or the Action of Sex Steroids

Gonadotrophin-Releasing Hormone Analogues (GnRha)

This group of drugs includes a range of injectable medications intended to suppress the release of LH and FSH from the pituitary gland. There is an initial surge of hormone release after the first injection but subsequent injections given at the correct interval will maintain the suppression of hormone production. These medications are primarily used in CYP who enter puberty early. Their licensed use in the UK is to treat central precocious puberty occurring before the age of 8 years in girls or 10 years in boys. There is increasing use outside of its licence for blocking natural hormone production in adolescents with gender dysphoria. The most commonly used preparation for CYP in the UK is triptorelin acetate. This is available in 3.75mg, 11.25mg and 22.5mg doses administered either monthly, every 12 weeks or every 24 weeks. Lower dose preparations can be administered intramuscularly or subcutaneously, the largest dose is given intramuscularly.

Treatment is commenced after investigations to ensure the pubertal progress is due to the production of pituitary gonadotrophins. GnRh analogues will not suppress puberty where the testosterone or oestrogen is being produced independent of pituitary feedback. The medication must be carefully prepared following the guidance provided with it and administered using 20g needles which are provided with the medication. The medication has a tendency to form a gel which can block the needles so must be administered very soon after it is reconstituted. Preparation of the child for the process and good parental/carer involvement in helping to maintain a suitable position for the injection to take place is essential. The use of local pain relief such as topical anaesthetic creams or ethyl chloride cold spray at the injection site can help with co-operation of the child. The surge of oestrogen in girls after the first injection is followed by a drop to negligible levels which can induce a menstrual bleed, parents/carers and the girl need to be advised that this may happen so that they can prepare for it.

Treatment in precocious puberty continues until the average age of the stage of puberty the child is in at commencement of treatment. This would be an average of 11 years in girls and 12 years in boys. Once treatment is discontinued, production of pubertal hormones starts again, leading to a continuation and completion of the transition through puberty. In girls menses usually occur 12 months after treatment is stopped.

Unwanted effects in CYP are rare the most common being obesity. This is thought to be due to continued hypothalamic drive to increase calorie intake required for pubertal growth which is not directly linked to the production of testosterone or oestrogen. Families are advised that the only element of puberty being suppressed is the production of sex steroids and that careful attention to food intake and exercise levels is needed to prevent weight gain while being treated. Those treated long term have an increased risk of SUFE, particularly if treated for longer than 2 years and if they are overweight. This is thought to be due to a weakening of the epiphyseal plate due to low levels of oestrogen. While this is a rare side effect, recognition and rapid treatment are required to reduce the risk of long-term problems with hip joints. Long-term use will reduce bone mineral density, this is of importance for those being treated for gender dysphoria as they may be treated for many years before cross-gender sex hormone replacement is introduced which will promote the production of bone.

Drugs Used to Reduce the Action of Sex Steroids

In some conditions such as congenital adrenal hyperplasia (CAH) where there is excess production of sex steroids, medications that block or inhibit their action on target tissues are used if usual treatments to suppress their production are insufficient. Production of testosterone from the adrenal glands can lead to rapid growth and skeletal maturation in early childhood which can have a major impact on final adult height. Use of aromatase inhibitors or anti-androgenic drugs preserve skeletal growth in these CYP (see Table 9.3).

Table 9.3 **Aromatase inhibitors or anti-androgenic drugs.**

MEDICATION	DRUG FORMS AND DOSES	ABSORPTION AND DISTRIBUTION	METABOLISM AND EXCRETION
Flutamide An anti-androgen which is a highly specific antagonist to testosterone.	Available as 250mg tablets. Dosages in children are usually 125mg twice daily. Carers should be advised to minimise handling of the medication especially women who may be pregnant due to potential harmful effects to the foetus. Monitoring of liver function regularly throughout treatment is recommended.	Acts directly on receptors of tissues that respond to testosterone thereby blocking local action of testosterone either by inhibiting androgen uptake or by blocking cytoplasmic and nuclear binding of androgen. Flutamide is rapidly and extensively absorbed and almost completely metabolised following oral administration.	Approximately 45% of the administered dose is excreted in the urine and 2% in faeces during the first two days. The excretion and metabolism is essentially complete within two days. The elimination half-life in plasma is 5 to 6 hours in adults, there are no studies in paediatric populations.
Letrozole An aromatase inhibitor used to reduce the conversion of testosterone to oestrogen and oestradiol. Used in children with CAH where excess adrenal testosterone production is having an effect on skeletal maturation which may lead to reduced final adult height.	Available as 2.5mg film-coated tablets. The pharmacological action is to reduce oestrogen production by aromatase inhibition.	A non-steroidal aromatase inhibitor. Inhibits the aromatase enzyme by competitively binding to the aromatase cytochrome P450. Letrozole is rapidly and completely absorbed from the gastrointestinal tract. Letrozole is rapidly and extensively distributed to tissues.	Letrozole is eliminated after conversion to carbinol metabolites which have an active role in the liver in reducing the action of oestrogen. The drug half-life is 2–4 days and a steady state level is achieved and maintained after 2–4 weeks of treatment

Source: Joint Formulary Committee, 2020 and The Royal Pharmaceutical Society, 2020.

Chapter 9 Medications Used in the Endocrine System

Episode of Care

Hypothyroidism

Layla was referred by her GP to a paediatrician with concerns about short stature when she was 9 years old. Parent-held health records showed that at the age of 2 years her height had been recorded as 50th centile. Her current height was now below the 0.4th centile. The paediatrician noted that Layla had dry skin and dry, brittle hair. Her parents reported that she was always complaining about being cold. The GP felt that clinically Layla had hypothyroidism, blood for thyroid function tests were taken before prescribing levo-thyroxine 50 micrograms daily. Her thyroid-stimulating hormone level on those initial tests was reported as greater than 1000mU/L, confirming diagnosis. Three-month review of treatment showed TSH level had not normalised as would have been expected, thyroxine was increased to 75 micrograms daily, referral made to a specialist endocrine service.

On referral thyroxine was again increased to 100 micrograms daily as TSH level was still high at 9.5mU/L. The family were provided with written information about hypothyroidism as well as a discussion in clinic about the role of thyroxine in growth and development and the importance of remembering to take medication daily. At her next review Layla had a normal TSH level with a high T4 level of 23.5pmol/L (range 12.6–21pmol/L) This shows much improved concordance with medication. Height increased from below the 0.4th centile to the 3rd centile and she remained prepubertal at 10 years and 4 months, which had good implications for her final adult height being within the expected range. Over the next year and a half TSH level gradually increased and by the age of 11 years and 8 months she had a TSH of 73mU/L with a T4 of 17pmol/L. Her dose had been increased twice and was now at 175micrograms daily. At clinic she admitted to missing two doses per week. Mum had been trying to let Layla take more responsibility for managing her medications but Layla did not fully understand the implications of missing doses.

An education session was arranged with Layla and her mum to find out what she already knew about her hypothyroidism and her medication. An explanation of how her monitoring blood tests could show how effectively she had been taking her medication was also explained. Strategies for managing daily doses using a weekly tablet box and mum ensuring the box was refilled on a specific day each week were agreed upon.

Levothyroxine

Levothyroxine is used in the control of hypothyroidism, congenital hypothyroidism in infants, acquired hypothyroidism in children and juvenile myxoedema. The chief action of levothyroxine is to increase the rate of cell metabolism.

It is highly active within the blood stream with a long half-life of 72 hours. It is a medication that is safe to double up doses when one day is forgotten and to even take a whole week of medication all at once. When faced with chronic poor concordance that is denied by the patient arranging for a weekly dose to be administered under supervision in a healthcare setting can rapidly normalise and stabilise thyroid function tests. Offering options of how to manage taking this medication several times per week rather than daily by doubling up on doses if forgotten or taking all the remaining tablets on a set day per week when a dosing box is refilled can very rapidly lead to a normalisation of TSH and T4 levels and a greater feeling of well-being. Over time this pattern of permitting missed doses as long as they are taken later allows a CYP to learn to trust health professionals and to engage in discussions about how they are managing their condition now and what can be done to improve this. Encouraging a CYP with a long-term health condition to develop their own strategies for managing their condition improves concordance with medication and engagement with healthcare services.

Medications Used in Disorders of the Adrenal Glands

Hydrocortisone, prednisolone and dexamethasone (corticosteroids) are the most commonly used corticosteroids for replacement of adrenal cortisol in states of deficiency. This can be due to congenital adrenal disorders, autoimmune disorders or suppression of adrenal function related to treatment of other systemic conditions with steroids.

Children and young people who are using regular corticosteroid medications should be provided with an emergency plan of when and by how much to increase their corticosteroid dose during episodes of physiological stress from illness or injury. Carers and older children should be taught how to administer an injection of hydrocortisone when they are severely unwell. All patients are advised to wear or carry some kind of medical alert stating adrenal insufficiency, steroid-dependent (Miller et al., 2019).

Mineralocorticoids are used as partial replacement therapy for primary adrenocortical insufficiency in Addison's disease and for the treatment of salt-losing congenital Adrenal Hyperplasia (CAH). Sodium chloride corrects mild to moderate hyponatraemia in infants in the first year. Some older children may get insufficient sodium chloride in their diet and may need to add sachets of salt to food in order to avoid hyponatraemia.

Table 9.4 outlines medications used in disorders of the adrenal glands, drug formulae and doses along with absorption, distribution, metabolism and excretion.

Medications Used in the Management of Diabetes

There are over 50 drugs available to be used in the treatment of diabetes in the UK. The commonest ones used in paediatric populations are insulin, metformin, glucagon and sulfonylureas. There are rapid advances in medications for management of type 2 diabetes using a range of manufactured peptide hormones including GLP-1 analogues which may find a place in paediatric populations in coming years.

Insulins are used in the management of type 1 diabetes and occasionally in those with type 2 diabetes. There are multiple pen devices and strengths of insulin available which have varying degrees of onset and length of action. Insulin infusion pumps are medical devices able to deliver programmed doses of insulin continuously and with booster doses as needed according to serum blood sugar levels or carbohydrate content of food being eaten is an increasing part of managing type 1 diabetes in CYP. Comprehensive management guidelines are available at national levels (NICE, 2016).

Human glucagon is indicated for treatment of severe hypoglycaemic reactions, which may occur in the management of insulin treated children and adults with diabetes mellitus.

Metformin is a biguanide which prevents the liver from producing glucose, helping to improve the body's sensitivity towards insulin. Metformin is commonly used as a first line treatment for type 2 diabetes and may occasionally be prescribed, in combination with insulin. In Table 9.6 a number of medications used in the treatment of diabetes are discussed.

Conclusion

The management of endocrine conditions requires knowledge of normal hormone production and control processes and an understanding of normal patterns of growth and development. Endocrine dysfunction can occur at any time in life and may be congenital or develop as a result of autoimmune processes, tumour growth within a gland or as a result of injury to a gland directly or from treatments used to manage cancers.

Treatments offered are intended to stimulate, supplement or replace the usual hormonal and biochemical control of growth and development. Doses and types of medication that are most appropriate will change over the lifespan of a child and young adult.

Where a gland is removed, absent or unable to produce essential hormones replacement of the end product is the easiest method of managing a condition. Since many hormones are produced in cycles using feedback loops and requirements can vary over hours, days or weeks, replacement in a physiological manner is not always possible. However, experience over time and the availability of newer medications are making this more feasible.

Where the pituitary or hypothalamic control of hormone release is the problem again the easiest option is to replace the end product hormone, however the availability of pituitary hormones can stimulate organs such as the ovaries and testes and is used for short periods only to achieve production of sperm or ova in fertility treatments.

Treatments may be given to block the action of hormones that are being produced in excess or at the wrong time in a child's life. This blockade is usually a temporary process.

Table 9.4 Medications used in disorders of the adrenal glands.

MEDICATION	DRUG FORMS AND DOSES	ABSORPTION AND DISTRIBUTION	METABOLISM AND EXCRETION
Corticosteroids: hydrocortisone, prednisolone and dexamethasone.	The most commonly used replacement corticosteroid in childhood is hydrocortisone, available as 10mg or 20mg tablets, as suspensions containing 1mg or 2mg/ml and as capsules containing measured doses of granules as 0.5mg, 1mg, 2mg and 5mg strengths. And as vials of 100mg/ml for injection in times of life-threatening adrenal crisis. Hydrocortisone has the least effect on bone growth and is the preferred option for long-term replacement in children who are still growing. Replacement doses are aimed at providing 7–10mg/M^2/day aiming for the lowest dose possible. Doses are given 3 or 4 times daily, aiming to reproduce the usual diurnal variation in cortisol production from the adrenal cortex. At standard replacement doses there should be no undesirable effects which may be seen in the supraphysiological doses seen in treatment of inflammatory conditions. Prednisolone and dexamethasone are longer-acting corticosteroids used in young people with congenital adrenal hyperplasia who are at or approaching their final adult height. They have a greater effect at suppressing the morning surge of ACTH which leads to testosterone secretion from the adrenal glands which are unable to generate cortisol. Prednisolone as a replacement hormone is commonly used as 1mg, 2mg or 5mg tablets with a larger dose in the morning and a smaller early afternoon dose. Dexamethasone as a replacement steroid is usually administered daily as a 0.25mg to 0.75mg dose. See Table 9.5 for a comparison of potency of steroid medications.	Glucocorticoids are adrenocortical steroids, both naturally occurring and synthetic, which are readily absorbed from the gastrointestinal tract. Naturally occurring glucocorticosteroids (hydrocortisone and cortisone), which also have salt-retaining properties, are used as replacement therapy in adrenocortical deficiency states. Glucocorticoids cause profound and varied metabolic effects. In addition, they modify the body's immune responses to diverse stimuli. *Hydrocortisone* is readily absorbed from the gastrointestinal tract. *Prednisolone* is readily and almost completely absorbed from the GI tract after oral administration. *Dexamethasone* After oral administration, dexamethasone is rapidly and almost completely absorbed in the stomach and small intestine.	*Hydrocortisone* is metabolised in the liver and most body tissues and then excreted in the urine, together with a very small proportion of unchanged hydrocortisone. Hydrocortisone has a plasma half-life of about 100 minutes. *Prednisolone* is mainly metabolised in the liver and has a usual plasma half-life of 2–3 hours. Its initial absorption, but not its overall bioavailability, is affected by food, hepatic or renal impairment and certain drugs. It is excreted in the urine. *Dexamethasone:* The average (serum) elimination half-life of dexamethasone in adults is 250 minutes (+ 80 minutes). Due to its long biological half-life of more than 36 hours, daily continuous administration of dexamethasone can lead to accumulation and overdosing. The elimination is largely renal. Dexamethasone crosses the placenta and its use as a means of supressing genital virilisation in female foetuses with CAH is associated with babies being born small for gestational age and may have effects on their brain development.

Mineralocorticoids	Available as 0.1mg tablets which should be stored in a refrigerator. Administered as a once daily dose usually in the morning. Doses range from 50 to 400 micrograms, with higher doses being needed in babies and infants under 1 year of age due to less responsive renal function and a greater renal sodium loss. As fludrocortisone acetate is a potent mineralocorticoid both the dosage and salt intake should be carefully monitored to avoid the development of hypertension, oedema or weight gain. Periodic checking of serum electrolyte levels is advisable during prolonged therapy. Because corticosteroids and mineralocorticoids can suppress growth, the growth and development of infants, children and adolescents on prolonged corticosteroid therapy should be carefully monitored. The comparative degree of potency is shown in Table 9.5.	Fludrocortisone is rapidly and completely absorbed after oral administration. Fludrocortisone is widely distributed throughout the body.	Fludrocortisone is hydrolysed to produce the non-esterified alcohol; after administration of the acetate, only the non-esterified alcohol is detectable in blood. The blood level reaches a peak between 4 and 8 hours. Elimination half-life after intravenous administration was 30 minutes. Excretion through urine was about 80%, and it was concluded that about 20% were excreted by a different route. It is likely that, as for the metabolism of other steroids, excretion into the bile is balanced by reabsorption in the intestine and some part is excreted with the faeces.
Sodium chloride	Available as sodium chloride 1 mmol/ml oral solution. 3 to 5 mmol (3 to 5 ml of sodium chloride 1mmol/ml (oral solution) per kg daily in divided doses. Dosages are adjusted according to patient requirements. Example dilutions are 2 mmol (2 ml) diluted in 100ml formula feed, or 3 to 4 mmol (3 to 4 ml) diluted in 100 ml breast milk. The product is added and thoroughly mixed into the drink, breast milk or formula feed immediately before administration. Babies and infants with salt wasting CAH readily drink this solution, once weaned they start to find it less palatable as they gain additional sodium chloride in their diet. Older children may be prescribed individual sachets to add to food several times daily to maintain normal serum sodium levels.	Oral or enteral sodium chloride is actively transported across gastrointestinal membranes. Widely distributed in extracellular and intracellular fluids.	In infancy, sodium chloride is mainly eliminated in the urine.

Source: Based on Joint Formulary Committee, 2020

Chapter 9 Medications Used in the Endocrine System

Table 9.5 Comparison of the potency of various corticosteroid medications where hydrocortisone is the baseline of comparison.

DRUG	GLUCOCORTICOID POTENCY	MINERALOCORTICOID POTENCY	HOURS OF ACTION
Hydrocortisone/cortisol	1	1	8–12
Cortisone	0.8	0.8	8–12
Methylprednisolone	5	0.5	12–36
Fludrocortisone	15	150	24–36
Prednisolone or Prednisone	4	0.8	12–36
Dexamethasone or betamethasone	30	0	36–54

Source: Based on Samuel et al., 2017

Table 9.6 Medications used in the treatment of diabetes are discussed.

MEDICATION	DRUG FORMS AND DOSES	ABSORPTION AND DISTRIBUTION	METABOLISM AND EXCRETION
Insulins	All insulin is presented as a solution of 100 international units per ml for subcutaneous injection. Dosages are highly individualised and range between 0.3 and 1 international units per kg in divided doses throughout the day. Treatment regimens are individualised to the lifestyle of the patient and may vary throughout their life as factors influencing their ability to manage their diabetes change. Poor glycaemic control leads to multiple systemic problems including renal impairment and blindness. Common insulin products in the UK: *Humalog:* An extremely rapid-acting, usually begins working within 15 minutes. *Lantus:* A long-acting analogue insulin. *Levemir:* A long-acting analogue insulin. Tends to have a slightly shorter duration than Lantus, is often taken twice daily. *Novorapid:* The active ingredient is insulin aspart. When injected, it is extremely fast-acting, works rapidly to normalise blood glucose levels. Begins working after 10–20 minutes, lasts for between 3 and 5 hours. *Humulin:* Short-acting insulins, intermediate-acting and premixed humulin insulins are available. *Insuman:* Comes in several different forms. Insuman basal is an intermediate-acting insulin with the active ingredient isophane insulin. *Insulatard:* Comes in preloaded pens, penfill cartridges and vials based around the active ingredient human isophane insulin.	Absorption rates of insulin vary dependent on the form. See Table 9.7 for a comparison of absorption rates and length of action. The primary action of all insulins is regulation of glucose metabolism in all cells. Insulin regulates how the body uses and stores glucose and fat, it also has anabolic and anti-catabolic actions on a variety of different tissues. Within muscle tissue this includes increasing glycogen, fatty acid, glycerol and protein synthesis and amino acid uptake, while decreasing glycogenolysis, gluconeogenesis, ketogenesis, lipolysis, protein catabolism and amino acid output.	The kidney plays an important role in insulin metabolism and clearance. Insulin is filtered by the glomeruli and reabsorbed in the proximal tubule.

(*Continued*)

Table 9.6 (Continued)

MEDICATION	DRUG FORMS AND DOSES	ABSORPTION AND DISTRIBUTION	METABOLISM AND EXCRETION
Glucagon	GlucaGen HypoKit 1 mg powder and solvent for solution for injection. Dosage for paediatric patients: Administer 0.5 mg (children below 25kg or younger than 6–8 years) or 1 mg (children above 25kg or older than 6–8 years). Administer by subcutaneous or intramuscular injection. When the patient has responded to the treatment, give oral carbohydrate to restore the liver glycogen and prevent relapse of hypoglycaemia. If the patient does not respond within 10 minutes, intravenous glucose should be administered.	*Mechanism of action* Glucagon is a hyperglycaemic agent, mobilising hepatic glycogen, which is released into the blood as glucose. Glucagon inhibits the tone and motility of the smooth muscle in the gastrointestinal tract. When used in treatment of severe hypoglycaemia, an effect on blood glucose is usually seen within 10 minutes. Onset of inhibitory effect on gastrointestinal motility occurs within 1 minute after an intravenous injection and can cause vomiting. Duration of action is 5–20 minutes depending on dose.	Glucagon is degraded enzymatically in the blood plasma and in the organs to which it is distributed. The liver and kidney are major sites of glucagon clearance. Glucagon has a short half-life in the blood of about 3–6 minutes.
Metformin	Available in a range of tablets for immediate release and sustained release formulations. Usual starting dose is 500 mg or 850 mg metformin hydrochloride 2 or 3 times daily during or after meals. After 10 to 15 days dose should be adjusted on the basis of blood glucose measurements. The maximum recommended dose of metformin hydrochloride is 3g daily, taken as three divided doses. Metformin and insulin may be used in combination to achieve better blood glucose control. Metformin hydrochloride is given at the usual starting dose of 500 mg or 850 mg 2 or 3 times daily, while insulin dosage is adjusted on the basis of blood glucose measurements.	Metformin has antihyperglycaemic effects. It does not stimulate insulin secretion and therefore does not produce hypoglycaemia. Metformin may act via three mechanisms: • reduction of hepatic glucose production by inhibiting gluconeogenesis and glycogenolysis. • in muscle, by increasing insulin sensitivity, improving peripheral glucose uptake and utilisation. • delaying absorption of glucose from the intestine. Metformin stimulates intracellular glycogen synthesis by acting on glycogen synthase. Metformin increases the transport capacity of all types of membrane glucose transporters (GLUTs) known to date. Maximum effect is achieved after approximately 2.5 hours. At the recommended metformin doses and dosing schedules, steady state plasma concentrations are reached within 24 to 48 hours and are generally less than 1 microgram/ml. Food decreases the extent and slightly delays the absorption of metformin.	Metformin is excreted unchanged in the urine. Renal clearance of metformin is > 400 ml/min, indicating that metformin is eliminated by glomerular filtration and tubular secretion. Following an oral dose, apparent terminal elimination half-life is approximately 6.5 hours. When renal function is impaired, renal clearance is decreased in proportion to that of creatinine and half-life is prolonged, leading to increased levels of metformin in plasma.

Source: Based on Joint Formulary Committee, 2020

Table 9.7 Comparison of absorption rates and length of action of insulin types.

TYPE OF INSULIN	ONSET OF ACTION	PEAK OF ACTIVITY	DURATION OF ACTION
Rapid analogues	Within 15 minutes	15 minutes to 1 hours	3–4 hours
Short-acting	Within 30 minutes	1–3 hours	6–8 hours
Intermediate	Within 2 hours	2–12 hours	18–24 hours
Long-acting analogue	Within 1 hour	No peak	18–24 hours
Ultra-long-acting analogue	Within 1 hour	No peak	More than 42 hours

Source: Adapted from British Diabetes.co.uk, 2019.

Glossary

Benign: A condition, tumour, or growth that is not cancerous.
Concordance: An agreement reached after negotiation between a patient and a healthcare professional, respecting the beliefs and wishes of the patient in determining whether, when and how medicines are to be taken.
Congenital: A disease or physical abnormality present at birth.
Endocrine: Relating to glands that secrete hormones or other products directly into the blood.
Exocrine: Relating to glands that secrete their products through ducts opening on to an epithelium as opposed to directly into the blood.
Hormone: Chemical substance produced in the body that controls and regulates the activity of certain cells or organs.
Hyperplasia: Enlargement of an organ or tissue caused by an increase in the reproduction rate cells, often an initial stage in the development of cancer.
Precocious puberty: When a child's body begins changing into that of an adult (puberty) too soon.
Spermatogenesis: The biological process of producing mature sperm cells.

References

Arecini, C., Assunta, A., Casey, A. et al (2013). Children and adolescents initiating growth hormone therapy for children and adolescents. *British Journal of Nursing* 21(18):

Birrell G. and Cheetham T. (2004). Juvenile thyrotoxicosis; can we do better? *Archives of Disease in Childhood* 89: 745–750.

British Diabetes.co.uk (2019). Insulin actions and duration. www.diabetes.co.uk/insulin/insulin-actions-and-durations.html (accessed November 2020).

El-Khairi, R., Shaw, N., and Cowne, E. (2016). Testosterone replacement therapy. BSPED Clinical Committee Clinical Guideline. www.bsped.org.uk/media/1375/testosteronereplacementguideline.pdf (accessed November 2020).

Farhad, D., Lee, C.M.M., Johan, M., and Brooks, A.J. (2018) The growth hormone receptor: Mechanism of receptor activation, cell signaling, and physiological aspects. *Frontiers in Endocrinology* 9. doi:10.3389/fendo.2018.00035.

Fintini, D., Brufani, C., and Cappa, M. (2009) Profile of mecasermin for the long-term treatment of growth failure in children and adolescents with severe primary IGF-1 deficiency. *Therapeutic Clinical Risk Management* 5(3): 553–559.

Gau, M. and Talasawa (2017). Initial patient choice of a growth hormone device improves child and adolescent adherence to and therapeutic effects of growth hormone replacement therapy. *Journal of Pediatric Endocrinology and Metabolism* 30(9). doi: 10.1515/jpem-2017-0146.

Gormley-Fleming, E. and Peate, I. (2015). *Fundamentals of Children's Anatomy and Physiology*. Chichester: John Wiley & Sons.

Growth Foundation (ND). Puberty and the Tanner Stages developed by Professor James M Tanner. https://childgrowthfoundation.org/wp-content/uploads/2018/05/Puberty-and-the-Tanner-Stages.pdf (accessed 20 April 2021).

Joint Formulary Committee (2020). *British National Formulary*, 80e. London: BMJ Group and Pharmaceutical Press.

Kucharski, P. and Niedzielski, J. (2013) Neoadjuvant human Chorionic Gonadotropin (hCG) therapy may improve the position of undescended testis: a preliminary report. *Central European Journal of Urology* 66(2):224–228. doi:10.5173/ceju.2013.02.art29.

Chapter 9 Medications Used in the Endocrine System

Matthews, D., Bath, L., Holger, W. et al (2016). Guidance Statement: hormone supplementation for pubertal induction in girls. BSPED Clinical Committee Clinical Guideline. www.bsped.org.uk/media/1378/hormonesupplementationforpubertalinductioningirls.pdf (accessed November 2020).

Miller, B.S., Spencer, S.P., Geffner, M.E. et al. (2019). Emergency management of adrenal insufficiency in children: advocating for treatment options in outpatient and field settings. *Journal of Investigative Medicine* 68(1): 16–25. doi: 10.1136/jim-2019-000999.

NICE (2010). Human growth hormone (somatropin) for the treatment of growth failure in children. Technology appraisal guidance [TA188]. www.nice.org.uk/guidance/ta188/resources/human-growth-hormone-somatropin-for-the-treatment-of-growth-failure-in-children-pdf-82598502860485 (accessed November 2020).

NICE (2016). Diabetes (type 1 and type 2) in children and young people: diagnosis and management.

NICE guideline [NG18]Published date: 01 August 2015 Last updated: 08 November 2016.

Papadimitriou, D.Y., Diontsios, C., Nyktari, G. et al. (2019). Replacement of male mini puberty. *Journal of the Endocrine Society* 3(7): 1275–1282. doi: 10.1210/js.2019-00083.

Peate, I. and Evans, S. (2020). *Fundamentals of Anatomy and Physiology For Nursing and Healthcare Students.* John Wiley & Sons.

Samuel, S., Nguyen, N., Choi, H.A. (2017) Pharmacologic characteristics of corticosteroids. *J Neurocrit Care.* 10(2): 53–59.

WHO (2007). *Assessment of Iodine Deficiency Disorders and Monitoring their Elimination: A Guide for Programme Managers*, 3e. https://apps.who.int/iris/bitstream/handle/10665/43781/9789241595827_eng.pdf (accessed November 2020).

Further Resources

NHS Lothian Endocrinology Teaching Resources: https://services.nhslothian.scot/Endocrinology/Pages/EndocrinologyTeachingResources.aspx

Hormone Health Network: www.hormone.org/support-and-resources

You and Your Hormones: www.yourhormones.info/

Multiple Choice Questions

1. Which of the following is not a NICE-licensed indication for the use of growth hormone?
   (a) Turner's Syndrome
   (b) Renal disease
   (c) Birth weight under 2kg

2. What time of day is it advised to administer growth hormone?
   (a) Morning
   (b) Lunch time
   (c) Evening

3. What is the half-life of levothyroxine in someone with a thyroid profile within reference range?
   (a) Less than 24 hrs
   (b) 2–3 days
   (c) 6–7 days

4. What is a common side effect indicating a patient is receiving too much levothyroxine?
   (a) Diarrhoea
   (b) Skin rash
   (c) Feeling cold

5. Which of the following drugs is not a glucocorticoid?
   (a) Hydrocortisone
   (b) Fludrocortisone
   (c) Prednisolone

Chapter 9 Medications Used in the Endocrine System

6. Which of the following drugs is not a steroid used in the treatment of adrenal insufficiency?
   (a) Hydrocortisone
   (b) Prednisolone
   (c) Oxandrolone
7. Intramuscular oily medications such as Nebido should be administered slowly to avoid
   (a) Pain on administration
   (b) Oil embolism
   (c) Sudden painful erection
8. atients taking carbimazole for the treatment of hyperthyroidism should contact their specialist nurse or doctor for an urgent blood test should they
   (a) Develop a sore throat
   (b) Gain an unexpected amount of weight
   (c) Develop a rash
9. Desmopressin is used in the treatment of diabetes insipidus; over treatment can cause
   (a) Hyponatraemia
   (b) Polyuria
   (c) Polydipsia
10. What medication is used in the treatment of hypoparathyroidism?
    (a) Parathyroid hormone
    (b) Vitamin D
    (c) Sodium chloride
11. Which fast-acting insulin would be given before a meal?
    (a) Novorapid
    (b) Glargine
    (c) Degludec
12. How do you store unopened vials of insulin?
    (a) At room temperature
    (b) In the fridge
    (c) In a cool dark place away from direct sunlight
13. Which of these drugs can cause hypoglycaemia?
    (a) Sulfonamide
    (b) Growth hormone
    (c) GNRH analogue
14. What should be discussed with female patients commencing GNRH analogue injections?
    (a) withdrawal bleed
    (b) Weight gain
    (c) Slipped upper femoral epiphysis
15. How can oestrogen be given for pubertal induction?
    (a) Oral
    (b) Injection
    (c) Transdermal

Chapter 9 Medications Used in the Endocrine System

Find Out More

The following is a list of conditions that are associated with the endocrine system. Take some time and write notes about each of the conditions. Think about the medications that may be used in order to treat these conditions and be specific about the pharmacokinetics and pharmacodynamics. Remember to include aspects of patient care. If you are making notes about people you have offered care and support to, you must ensure that you have adhered to the rules of confidentiality.

THE CONDITION	YOUR NOTES
Hypercalcaemia	
Diabetes insipidus	
Hyperthyroidism	
Congenital hypothyroidism	
Gender dysphoria	

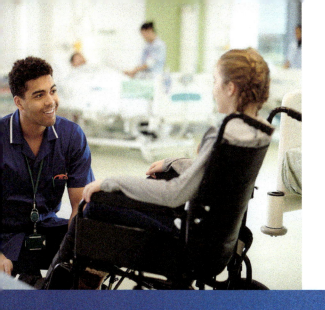

10

Medications Used in the Respiratory System

Claire Fagan, Janis Bloomer, Alison Sewell, Carol Sharpe and Harriet Minto

Aim

The aim of this chapter is to introduce the reader to medications commonly used in the treatment of respiratory conditions in children and young people, in order to develop knowledge and skill in their administration and mode of action.

Learning Outcomes

On completion of this chapter, the reader will be able to
- Describe basic mechanism of illness in the commonly encountered respiratory conditions: asthma, croup, bronchiolitis, pneumonia and cystic fibrosis
- Explain mode of action of medicines used to treat these conditions
- Understand potential side effects of common respiratory medicines
- Discuss correct inhaler technique

Fundamentals of Pharmacology for Children's Nurses, First Edition. Edited by Ian Peate and Peter Dryden.
© 2022 John Wiley & Sons Ltd. Published 2022 by John Wiley & Sons Ltd.
Companion website: www.wiley.com/go/pharmacologyforCN

Chapter 10 Medications Used in the Respiratory System

Test Your Knowledge

1. Name four respiratory conditions commonly seen in children
2. List some commonly used drugs used to treat respiratory conditions
3. Describe how to administer an inhaler
4. Name the common triggers of asthma
5. Name three ways to administer prescribed oxygen

Introduction

Respiratory illnesses are very common in children due to developmental differences in the respiratory system of children and infants compared with adults. Children, especially those under 5 years of age, have the highest burden of respiratory symptoms of all age groups in the general population (European Respiratory Society, 2020).

The primary function of the respiratory system is gas exchange between environmental air and the blood to ensure the cells of the body are supplied with oxygen and carbon dioxide is efficiently removed. Gas exchange occurs in the alveoli in the lungs. Young children have significantly fewer alveoli and therefore have less surface area for gas exchange.

They are also at increased risk of respiratory illness due to:

- An immature immune system, making them vulnerable to infection
- Increased oxygen requirement due to a higher metabolic rate
- Anatomical differences associated with airway resistance such as: large tongue, small oral cavity, nasal breathing, small airways and a compliant chest wall (this requires the infant to perform more work than an adult chest to move a similar amount of air; see Figure 10.1 to compare the adult and child airway)
- Children having less efficient respiratory muscles, which can rapidly become fatigued

Oedema of the airways from infection or inflammation can have a large impact on overall airway resistance. Poiseuille's law states that airway resistance is inversely proportional to the diameter of the airway, for example halving the radius of an airway would cause a 16-fold increase in resistance (Glasper and Richardson, 2006). Therefore a relatively small amount of mucus or oedema in the airway can cause significant obstruction, resulting in increased work of breathing.

For the registered nurse, administration of medicines is a core responsibility. Individuals administering medications should have an awareness of the various routes of administration, indications and contraindications of a drug and its side effects.

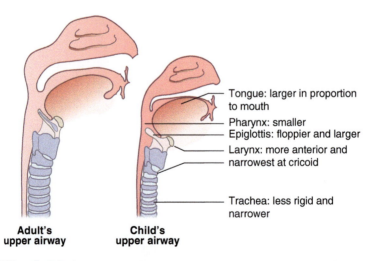

Figure 10.1 **The child and adult airway.** *Source:* Elizabeth Gormley-Fleming and Ian Peate 2014/John Wiley & Sons.

Medicines targeting the respiratory system can be delivered by inhalation, oral or parenteral routes. Inhalation is often the preferred route as the drug is delivered directly into the airways, limiting systemic side effects (Joint Formulary Committee, 2020).

Respiratory drugs have varying mechanisms of action such as relaxing bronchial smooth muscle or moderating inflammatory responses. This chapter will outline some common respiratory conditions seen in paediatrics. Medications used in the treatment of these conditions and their mode of action will then be explored in more depth.

Asthma

Asthma is the most common lung condition in children and affects around 1 in 11 children in the UK (Asthma UK, 2020). It affects people of all ages and often starts in childhood, but can develop at any age and is the most common reason for urgent admissions to hospital in children and young people in England (NHS England, 2020).

Asthma is caused by inflammation in the airways of the lungs. The airways become hypersensitive, leading to bronchospasm and an increase in production of sticky mucous (phlegm). This causes narrowing of the bronchial walls, which is reversible with prompt treatment. The main symptoms of asthma include wheeze, breathlessness, chest tightness and coughing. Symptoms may occur randomly or after exposure to a trigger. Common asthma triggers include allergies (e.g. house dust mite, animal fur or pollen), environment (e.g. smoke, pollution and cold air), exercise and respiratory infections.

There is currently no cure for asthma, but along with identifying and avoiding triggers, there are treatments which can help to keep the symptoms under control. The current concept of asthma treatment is based on a stepwise approach, depending on disease severity. The aim is to reduce the symptoms that result from airway obstruction and inflammation, to prevent exacerbations and to maintain normal lung function. In general, asthma medication can be divided into two groups (Table 10.1)

The administration of prescribed bronchodilators and steroids via inhalers is the most effective means of controlling asthma symptoms. The oral corticosteroid prednisolone may also be used in short courses.

As part of the nursing management, all people with asthma (and/or their parents or carers) should be offered self-management education, which should include a written personalised asthma management plan. This should include advice on how to manage symptoms at home, which medicines to take each day and when to contact a health professional for further advice.

Inhalers should only be prescribed after patients have received training in the use of the device and have demonstrated satisfactory technique (British Thoracic Society (BTS), 2019). All children should be trained in the use of their specific inhaler device at least annually. All metred dose inhalers (MDIs) should be administered via a spacer device. Different types of spacer are available but the principles of use are the same. Guidance is given below for a large volume spacer. Refer to Asthma UK/Beat Asthma websites for further detailed instructions/videos and advice for children/families.

Most children's nurses will encounter childhood asthma during an acute exacerbation. This can be a potentially stressful situation depending on the severity of the episode. Table 10.2 outlines proposed management of an acute asthma exacerbation in children over 5. Inhaled beta$_2$ agonists are the first line treatment in acute asthma, Oral steroids should also be given early in an exacerbation. Particular care should be taken when preparing intravenous (IV) bronchodilators due to very small doses and volumes. Care should be taken to follow local guidance on medication preparation, checking and administration. Use of IV bronchodilators is relatively rare as nebulised forms of the drug are usually very effective.

Table 10.1 Classes of asthma medication.

PREVENTERS	RELIEVERS
Inhaled corticosteroids taken daily on a long-term basis to get and keep persistent asthma under control. They help stop asthma symptoms developing by protecting the airways but can take up to 4 weeks to become effective in the airway. When taken regularly they can prevent asthma symptoms. They can also reduce the risk of a potential life-threatening asthma attack (Beat Asthma, 2020).	Inhaled bronchodilators e.g. beta$_2$-adrenoceptor agonists (salbutamol) that act quickly to relieve bronchoconstriction and its accompanying acute symptoms such as cough, chest tightness and wheezing. People with asthma should be advised to ALWAYS carry a reliever inhaler and spacer to ensure that it is available in an emergency.

Table 10.2 The management of acute asthma in children 5 years and over.

	MID-MODERATE	SEVERE	LIFE-THREATENING
1. Assess clinical signs	Assess ABC Oxygen saturations >92% Peak flow rate >50% predicted No clinical features of severe asthma	Assess ABC Oxygen saturations <92% Too breathless to talk/eat Heart rate > 140/min Respiratory rate >40/min Use of accessory muscles	Assess ABC Oxygen saturations <92% Silent chest Poor respiratory effort Agitation Altered consciousness Cyanosis
2. Treatment	Salbutamol 10 puffs via spacer Reassess after 20 mins	Oxygen to achieve normal saturations Salbutamol nebuliser 5mg Consider prednisolone 30–40mg or intravenous hydrocortisone 4mg/kg **Poor response?** Add ipratropium bromide 250mcg, nebulised	Oxygen to achieve normal saturations Salbutamol nebuliser 5mg AND ipratropium bromide 250mcg Consider intravenous hydrocortisone 4mg/kg or 100mg

3. Assess response
Record respiratory rate, heart rate, oxygen saturation and peak flow rate 1–4 hourly

4. Action if responding:	4. Action if not responding:
Continue to administer inhaled salbutamol 1–4 hourly Consider oral prednisolone Discharge on 4 hourly treatment when stable	Repeat salbutamol every 20–30 mins **And** ipratropium bromide every 20–30 mins for 2 hours then repeat 6 hourly Urgent discussion with consultant paediatrician **Consider:** Chest x-ray and blood gases Cardiac monitor Intravenous infusion of magnesium over 20 mins 40mg/kg (max2g) Intravenous salbutamol 15mcg/kg as bolus over 10 mins (max 250mcg) followed by continuous infusion 1–2mcg/kg/min (max 60 mcg/min) Child may require admission to PICU Following discussion between consultants – intravenous aminophylline 5mg/kg (max500mg) loading dose over 20 mins (omit this if taking oral theophylline), followed by continuous infusion 1mg/kg/hr

5. Discharge Plan (when stable on 4 hourly inhaled treatment):
Check inhaler technique
Consider prednisolone daily for 3 days
Provide and discuss written asthma management plan
Review regular treatment
Arrange hospital follow-up or at GP within 1 week-inform child's consultant of admission

Skills in Practice

How to Use a Large Volume Spacer

1. If using for the first time, wash the spacer in warm soapy water. Do not rinse, leave to air dry. This removes the static from the device and once dry is ready to use. This should be repeated monthly.
2. Shake the inhaler well and put it in the hole at the end of the spacer
3. Help the child to put the mouthpiece into their mouth, encouraging them to make a seal with their teeth and lips.
4. Push the top of the inhaler to release a dose of medication – a puff.
5. Encourage them to breathe in and out at a normal rate 4 to 5 times or for a count of 10, making the valve click.
6. Wait 30 seconds and repeat the above until the correct number of 'puffs' have been given.
7. Encourage child to have a drink or clean teeth if using the spacer for inhaled steroids, to help prevent the risk of side effects.

Clinical Consideration

Poor inhaler technique is a common cause of asthma symptoms. It is important to distinguish this from a true exacerbation.

Children over 4 years of age should use a spacer with a mouthpiece and not a facemask to ensure optimal deposition of the inhaled medication.

Croup

Croup (laryngotracheobronchitis) is a common acute respiratory illness of childhood. It affects approximately 3% of children per year usually between the ages of 6 months and 3 years (NICE, 2019). It causes inflammation and narrowing of the subglottic region of the larynx resulting in upper airway obstruction. It is characterised by a barking 'seal-like' cough, inspiratory stridor and respiratory distress which may include raised respiratory rate, intercostal and sub-costal recession, nasal flaring. A pyrexia is also commonly present. Croup is primarily caused by a virus typically parainfluenza.

The treatment of croup depends on the severity of the symptoms. See Table 10.3.

Table 10.3 Treatment of croup.

SEVERITY	SYMPTOMS	TREATMENT
Mild	The child is clinically well but cough and stridor are present when the child is upset or active.	Administer oral dexamethasone 0.15mg/kg in a single dose (British Medical Journal (BMJ), 2020) Patient information about croup should be given to the family.
Moderate	Cough, stridor and signs of increased work of breathing when the child is at rest.	Administer oral dexamethasone 0.15kg/kg in a single dose OR 2 mg nebulised budesonide (BMJ, 2020) and observe in the Emergency Department for 2–3 hours, if symptoms desist, discharge home with croup information sheet.
Severe	Child presents in severe respiratory distress with possible cyanosis and signs of exhaustion and dehydration.	Administer nebulised adrenaline 5 ml 1:1000 (repeat dose if necessary). Give oral/I/V dexamethasone. Administer oxygen via a face mask

Chapter 10 Medications Used in the Respiratory System

Clinical Consideration

A hands-off approach for assessment of the child with suspected croup is recognised to reduce fear. Children should be examined/treated on a parent's knee if possible. It is very common for symptoms to increase with agitation and this is seen in all levels of severity of croup.

Source: Based on BMJ, 2020.

Episode of Care

Daljit is an 18-month-old child who is brought to the emergency department (ED) by his parents with a three-day history of runny nose and increased barking cough, which parents describe as seal-like. His parents say he has had intermittent high temperatures and a stridor is heard. Parents have become increasingly concerned as his cough has worsened and he is not feeding. He is normally a well child. He has recently started nursery and this is his second respiratory illness in the last three months.

Daljit was assessed by the ED nurse. His vital signs were:

- Pulse: 120 beat per minute
- Respiratory rate: 40 per minute
- Oxygen saturations: 98% in air
- Temperature: 37.5°C

Reflect on this case and consider:

1. What could be the most likely diagnosis?
2. What if any medication may be offered and what dose?
3. What information do parents require?

Bronchiolitis

Bronchiolitis is the most common lower respiratory tract infection in the first two years of life, with 1 in 3 infants developing it in their first year (NICE, 2015). It is usually caused by the respiratory syncytial virus (RSV) although not exclusively. It presents with cough and increased work of breathing and may affect a child's ability to feed. The majority of infants diagnosed with bronchiolitis can be cared for by their parents at home and require no medical intervention apart from support and advice about feeding as well as information about 'red flags' e.g. apnoea, central cyanosis and severe respiratory distress.

Approximately 3% of children with bronchiolitis will require hospital admission (NICE, 2015). Treatment is largely supportive to ensure adequate hydration and oxygen therapy in those with persistent saturation levels below 92%. NICE (2015) suggest that it is inappropriate to treat with antibiotics or nebulised bronchodilators, steroids or adrenaline.

Pneumonia

Community-acquired pneumonia (CAP) is the inflammation of the alveoli in one or both lungs due to infection from bacteria, virus or rarely fungus. This leads to the alveoli becoming filled with fluid and pus, so hindering gaseous exchange. Children may present with pyrexia, tachypnoea, breathlessness, cough, and wheeze or chest pain. Abdominal pain, vomiting and headache may also feature.

It is often difficult to establish a causative organism and it is suggested that in children who have a persistent or repeated temperature above 38.5°C with recession and tachypnoea, bacterial pneumonia should be considered (Harris et al., 2011) and as such should receive treatment with antibiotics.

The choice of which antibiotic, length of course and route of administration of antibiotics will depend on the severity of symptoms the child presents with. Most children can be cared for at home and be treated with oral antibiotics. Harris et al. (2011) recommend amoxicillin is used as first line treatment as it is effective against the majority of organisms that cause CAP and is well tolerated and relatively cheap. Other antibiotics that may be appropriate are co-amoxiclav (recommended if associated with influenza), erythromycin, azithromycin and clarithromycin. Macrolides may be added if there is limited response to first line treatment (Harris et al., 2011, Paediatric Formulary Committee, 2019).

The administration of oral antibiotics should be considered as first line treatment as they are safe, convenient and effective, even in severe CAP. However, intravenous (IV) administration may be necessary if a child is unable to tolerate oral fluids e.g. due to vomiting and so will not absorb oral antibiotics. Intravenous antibiotics will be necessary in children who develop signs of septicaemia or complicated pneumonia. The use of IV antibiotics should be reviewed after 48 hours and changed to the oral route if tolerated and there are signs of improvement (Paediatric Formulary Committee, 2019).

Cystic Fibrosis

Cystic fibrosis (CF) is an autosomal recessive genetic disorder which affects more than 10,500 people in the UK (CF Trust, 2020). It affects the movement of salt and water across cell membranes in the body resulting in the production of thick viscous secretions which have an impact on multiple organ systems including the lungs, pancreas, liver, gastrointestinal tract, and the reproductive organs.

Respiratory disease accounts for most of the morbidity and mortality in patients with CF (Chalmers, 2020), with repeated lung infections and large amounts of viscous secretions leading to irreversible lung damage. The respiratory treatment of cystic fibrosis is based on the prevention of lung infections, loosening and removal of secretions and the maintenance of lung function.

Non-Pharmaceutical Management

Airway clearance is essential to the respiratory management of CF. All patients with CF should be reviewed by a specialist physiotherapist and taught appropriate airway clearance techniques. Physical activity and exercise are good for general health and to clear mucus.

Pharmaceutical Management

Medicines commonly used in the routine treatment of CF respiratory disease largely fall into two classes;

- *Mucolytics:* These are medicines which make the mucus in the lung less thick and sticky and easier to cough up. They are administered via nebuliser. It is important that these drugs are administered prior to airway clearance as they loosen mucus to make it easier to move. Commonly used mucolytics include dornase alfa and hypertonic saline. These will be addressed in detail later in the chapter.
- *Antibiotics:* These are medicines which are either used prophylactically to prevent lung infections, or to actively treat bacterial lung infections. These may be delivered orally, intravenously or via nebuliser or dry powder inhaler.
- *Flucloxacillin:* Most children with CF will take prophylactic flucloxacillin to prevent colonisation of staphylococcus aureus. This is taken orally every day. Practices vary between centres so be sure to follow local guidelines.
- *Intravenous antibiotics* are usually given to treat acute respiratory symptoms or in response to specific bacterial isolation. Those commonly used in CF include ceftazidime, tobramycin, cefuroxime and meropenem.
- *Inhaled antibiotics* are most commonly used in the eradication or suppression of Pseudomonas aeruginosa. The antibiotics of choice are usually colomycin or tobramycin. They are commonly administered using a compressor nebuliser with a filter system. Alternatively, both colomycin and tobramycin are available as dry powder inhaler devices; these are often preferred by older children. They should be given after airway clearance.

Clinical Consideration

When administering nebulised antibiotics the most common side effects are cough and bronchospasm. A supervised test dose should be given in hospital before patients are discharged home on these medications. Some patients require a bronchodilator via a spacer before taking inhaled antibiotics due to bronchospasm.

Chapter 10 Medications Used in the Respiratory System

Other drugs commonly used in the treatment of CF include steroids and antifungal medications.

Skills in Practice

How to Administer a Nebuliser

A nebuliser device is a machine that turns liquid medicine (usually antibiotics, bronchodilators or mucolytics) into a mist which can be inhaled. The machine or compressor pressurises air which is pulled through it, this compressed air passes through the liquid medication turning it into a mist which can be inhaled via a facemask or a mouthpiece. It is important that the nebuliser used is able to produce a small enough particle size so there is a good deposition of the medication into the lungs (Boe et al. 2001). Larger droplets are more likely to deposit in the upper airways. Devices producing large droplets are ineffective at delivering antibiotics/mucolytics into the lungs.

If clinically indicated and the patient has an oxygen requirement, bronchodilators can be nebulised via piped oxygen in a medical environment. Antibiotics and mucolytic drugs should not be administered this way.

There are many different devices available and those supplied vary from location to location. The basics of how to use a compressor remain the same:

1. Explain procedure to the patient and parent.
2. Wash hands.
3. Prepare equipment as per local guidelines; i.e. compressor, device appropriate accessories and tubing, mouthpiece/facemask, filter set (if nebulising antibiotics) and medication.
4. Prepare and check medication as per local medicine administration guidelines, being sure to check correct patient, date, time, drug name, dose and route of administration.
5. Assemble nebuliser and plug compressor into the mains.
6. Connect the tubing between the nebuliser and the compressor.
7. Add the medication to the nebuliser chamber and replace the lid
8. Ensure the patient is as upright as possible and apply an appropriate facemask or mouth piece.
9. Turn on the compressor and the solution should begin to mist.
10. The patient should be encouraged to breathe through their mouth and not talk. Once the nebuliser has finished (misting stops), switch off the compressor and remove the facemask or mouth piece.
11. Encourage the patient to have a drink once the nebuliser has finished.
12. Wash the nebuliser components as per local guidelines dependent on the compressor used. Usually this involves washing all components in warm soapy water after use and leaving to air dry. Most nebuliser components should also be sterilised at least weekly, but local and manufacturer guidelines should be followed.
13. Evaluate the effectiveness of the treatment (particularly if a bronchodilator has been administered) by monitoring the patient's vital signs and work of breathing. In the case of antibiotics or mucolytics you may be monitoring for adverse effects such as wheeze or increased cough.
14. Document according to local policies including any observations about the effectiveness of the medication.

Clinical Considerations

Always use separate nebuliser sets (mouthpiece/mask and pots) for nebulised antibiotics and other nebulised medications

Always be aware of the need to add filter when nebulising antibiotics. Follow local guidance.

Respiratory Medicines

All qualified nurses in the UK should have knowledge of the pharmacology, potential side effects, indications for and interactions of any medication they administer (Nursing and Midwifery Council (NMC), 2018). They should also be able to recognise prescribing errors and have knowledge of appropriate routes of administration. The following section will provide a more in depth discussion of the common respiratory drugs briefly identified in relation to the various respiratory conditions above.

Oxygen Therapy

Oxygen is a drug and must be treated as such. Oxygen is probably the most common drug used in medical emergencies. It should be prescribed initially to achieve normal or near-normal oxygen saturation (Joint Formulary Committee, 2020).

Oxygen therapy is indicated when there are abnormally low concentrations of oxygen in arterial blood, which may be due to trauma, acute illness or long-term chronic respiratory conditions such as CF. Oxygen is required by tissues to metabolise carbohydrates and for the production of adenosine triphosphates (ADP) (Walsh and Smallwood, 2017). Inadequate oxygenation will ultimately result in tissue hypoxia, organ dysfunction and, in severe circumstances, death.

Oxygen enters the body via the lungs during respiration, where it diffuses across the alveolar membrane in the process of gaseous exchange. Oxygen and carbon dioxide move across the membranes from areas of higher partial pressure to lower partial pressure. Oxygen is then absorbed into the blood stream by combining with haemoglobin. The oxygen saturation (SaO_2) indicates the average saturation of haemoglobin and is demonstrated in the oxygen-haemoglobin dissociative curve (Akers, 2015). Figure 10.2 shows the oxygen dissociation curve.

The curve displays the relationship between the partial pressure of arterial oxygen (PaO_2) and oxygen saturation of haemoglobin (SaO_2). The relationship is not linear, it has a sigmoidal shape, and it does not remains constant. It is determined by how readily haemoglobin acquires and releases oxygen from its surrounding tissue. Haemoglobin's affinity for oxygen increases as more molecules of oxygen bind to the protein. The partial pressure continues to increase as more molecules bind until the maximum amount that can be bound is reached.

Above pressures of 60mmHg the curve is almost flat and at this point the oxygen content of the blood does not change significantly. As the partial pressure falls below 60mmHg (the steep portion of the curve) haemoglobin's affinity for oxygen decreases as oxygen is unloaded into the surrounding tissues.

Clinical conditions which alter haemoglobin's affinity for oxygen can impact the oxygen-haemoglobin dissociation curve and cause what is described as a shift of the normal-shaped curve of healthy individuals. A shift to the right reduces haemoglobin's affinity for oxygen at a given PaO2 value. Therefore, the SaO2 value will drop below normal because the demand for oxygen is higher than normal and haemoglobin releases oxygen more readily to the tissues in an attempt to keep tissue well oxygenated. A shift to the right can be caused by an increase in body temperature or reduced blood pH (acidosis).

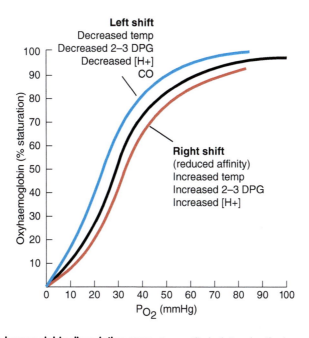

Figure 10.2 **The oxygen-haemoglobin dissociation curve.** *Source:* Elizabeth Gormley-Fleming and Ian Peate 2014/John Wiley & Sons.

A shift to the left increases the haemoglobin's affinity for oxygen. This can be as a result of decreased body temperature, a rise in blood pH, reduced PaCO2 levels or reduced 2,3-DPG levels (2,3-DPG is a phosphate which forms when red blood cells break down glucose into ATP).

The role of haemoglobin and the oxygen-haemoglobin dissociation curve are important when trying to understand the relationship of oxygen saturations and arterial oxygen and its partial pressure in a clinical situation. It is important to understand the factors which can influence the curve and the elements which may impact and help explain clinical problems.

There are very few contraindications to oxygen therapy although in some children with congenital heart disease caution is necessary as oxygen therapy may cause over-circulation within the pulmonary system (Walsh and Smallwood, 2017). Care should also be taken when using oxygen therapy in neonates as oxygen toxicity may result in retinopathy of prematurity or bronchopulmonary dysplasia.

The administration of oxygen to children requires an appropriate delivery route which takes into account the child's age, size, clinical condition and goal of treatment. The lowest flow rate of oxygen to achieve desirable saturation level should be given.

Table 10.4 shows commonly used oxygen delivery systems in children.

Ideally a prescription should include a range of deliverable litres/minute as well as the desired oxygen saturation level. Oxygen therapy should be monitored to ensure adequate response to therapy is achieved. This is usually done by using non-invasive pulse oximetry to measure oxygen saturation percentage. The usual acceptable oxygen saturations in children are above 94% (Hiley et al. 2019).

Bronchodilators

Bronchodilators are medicines usually administered via inhalation to treat bronchoconstriction primarily seen in asthma in children. They fall into four categories: short-acting beta$_2$ agonists (SABA), long-acting beta$_2$ agonists (LABA), antimuscarinic bronchodilators and xanthines.

Adrenoceptor Agonists

Selective beta$_2$ agonists cause bronchodilation and can be divided into either short-acting beta$_2$ agonists (SABA) or long-acting beta$_2$ agonists (LABA). Examples of SABAs include salbutamol or terbutaline and examples of LABAs include formoterol, vilanterol or salmeterol. SABAs are the first line treatment for acute asthma ideally given via a metered dose inhaler and a spacer.

The mode of action is to bind to the beta$_2$-adrenoceptor of the bronchial muscle: this results in relaxation of the smooth muscle (bronchodilation), reduction in oedema and increased mucociliary clearance (Barker et al., 2019).

Table10.5 summarises some commonly used beta$_2$ agonists.

Doses often vary depending on the inhaler used and age of the patient. These can be found in the British National Formulary for Children. For all beta agonists common side effects include fine tremor (especially in the hands), muscle cramp, tachycardia and headache. High doses are associated with hypokalaemia.

Different forms of inhalers are available for use depending on the patient's age, capabilities and personal preference. As previously mentioned it is important that patients use good inhaler technique to obtain the most benefit from their inhaled medicines and the technique should be assessed at least annually by a healthcare professional.

Antimuscarinic Bronchodilators

Ipratropium is a competitive antagonist of muscarinic acetylcholine receptors which result in smooth muscle relaxation and bronchodilation. It exerts greatest potency on the bronchial receptors when inhaled or nebulised. The onset of action is fast and occurs within a few minutes of inhalation (eMC, 2020).

Ipratropium is summarised in Table 10.6.

Each actuation from the ipratropium inhaler delivers a 20 microgram dose. Common side effects include arrhythmias, cough, dizziness, dry mouth, headache and nausea (Paediatric Formulary Committee, 2020).

Tiotropium is a long-acting antimuscarinic licensed for those over 6 years of age with asthma, but is rarely used in practice.

Leukotrienes

Leukotrienes are produced as part of the inflammatory process; they are involved in increasing mucus production, bronchoconstriction, oedema and an increase in eosinophil levels (Berger, 1999).

Table 10.4 Oxygen delivery methods in children.

DEVICE		DESCRIPTION	INDICATIONS	NURSING CONSIDERATIONS
Low flow nasal cannula		Lightweight tubing with two small prongs that fit in the child's nostrils. Different sizes of cannula are available. Usually fastened with appropriate tape.	Children who require relatively low oxygen concentration	Most commonly used delivery system. Maximum flow rate 4 l/min. At higher flow rates may require humidifying. Allows child to eat and drink normally. Careful assessment of skin integrity under the fixing tape is essential.
High flow nasal cannula		Humidified high flow nasal cannula. Oxygen titrated from flow rate of 4L/min to 40L/min.	Used when higher flow rates are required and when some end expiratory pressure is required.	Flow rate may be adjusted according to the child's respiratory effort. Cannula sizes vary according to size of child. Devices provide humidity.
Simple face mask		Semi-rigid mask that fits over the nose and mouth and has an elastic strap.	Low flow device for children. Delivers 35–60% oxygen concentration.	Minimum of 4l/min flow to ensure adequate oxygen delivery. Mask needs to be removed for eating. Select mask size suitable for the child's face.
High concentration mask (non-rebreathe mask)		A non-rebreathing face mask has an oxygen reservoir bag and one-way valve system which prevents exhaled gases mixing with fresh gas flow.	Used for emergency situations. It allows the delivery of the highest concentration of oxygen via a mask.	To ensure the highest concentration of oxygen is delivered to the patient the reservoir bag needs to be inflated prior to placing on the patients face. The bag should remain inflated during the whole respiratory cycle (i.e. inspiration and expiration). Non-rebreathing face masks are not designed to allow added humidification.
Tracheostomy		Tracheostomy masks and Swedish nose can be used to deliver oxygen via tracheostomies depending on requirement.	Children with a tracheostomy who develop an oxygen requirement.	Patients may also need suction to remove mucus from the airway. Patient may need humidity as oxygen can dry secretions.

Table 10.5 Beta$_2$ agonists.

DRUG	ONSET OF ACTION	DURATION OF ACTION	DOSE	ABSORPTION/DISTRIBUTION/METABOLISM/EXCRETION (ADME)
Salbutamol	5 mins	4–6 hours	1–2 puffs of 100 microgram per spray inhaler up to 4 times daily when required for breathlessness, although some patients may need to use up to 10 puffs when having an asthma exacerbation (Paediatric Formulary Committee, 2020). The nebulised dose is 2.5 mg to 5 mg salbutamol up to four times a day	Salbutamol has a fast onset of action and is fully absorbed about 1–4 hours after administration. It is not metabolised in the lung. Most of the inhaled dose is swallowed and undergoes first pass metabolism where it is degraded by the liver. About 10–25% of the dose is distributed to the lungs. Protein binding of the drug is 10%. Salbutamol and its metabolites are rapidly excreted in the urine and faeces. The half-life is 2.7–5.5 hours after administration.
Terbutaline (dry powder inhaler)	5 mins	3–5 hours	500mcg (1 dose) up to 4 times a day for breathlessness for those over 5 years old (Paediatric Formulary Committee, 2020).	Bioavailability of terbutaline is about 16% of the delivered dose. Approximately 60% of the drug is metabolised by conjugation in the liver. Terbutaline has a half-life of 12 hours. About 90% of the drug is excreted in the urine as either unchanged drug or as conjugates.
Formoterol (available as a dry powder combination inhaler with budesonide or fluticasone)	3 mins	12 hours	6–12 micrograms twice a day (depending on the age of the child). Not licensed in those less than 6 years of age.	About 80% of the administered dose is swallowed and then absorbed by the GI tract. The dose that reaches the respiratory tract is readily absorbed within 0.5–1 hour. Plasma protein binding of formoterol is 61–64%. Formoterol is mainly eliminated by metabolism catalysed by multiply CYP450 enzymes. Half-life of the drug at twice a day dosing is 2–3 hours and is excreted in the urine and faeces.
Salmeterol (nebuliser, MDI, DPI alone or with fluticasone)	20 mins	12 hours	50mcg twice a day (for over 5 years of age). These should not be used on an as required basis, but should be used regularly alongside an inhaled corticosteroid.	Salmeterol is oxidised by CYP3A4 and hydrolysed which is subsequently eliminated mainly in the faeces. The full pharmacokinetics of salmeterol are still not fully known.

Chapter 10 Medications Used in the Respiratory System

Table 10.6 Ipratropium bromide.

AGE	IPRATROPIUM DOSE	ONSET OF ACTION	DURATION OF ACTION	ADME
1month – 5 years	Inhaler: 20micrograms three times a day Nebuliser: 125–250 micrograms as required (max 1mg per day).	15 minutes	4 hours	Depending on the formulation, device and inhalation technique, about 10–30% of the dose is deposited in the lungs. The drug reaches systemic circulation within minutes. The drug is minimally bound to protein (20%). About 2.8% of the drug is metabolised through the kidneys and 48% through the faeces. The half-life is 2–3.8 hours.
6–11 years	Inhaler: 20–40 micrograms three times a day. Nebuliser: 250micrograms as required (max 1mg per day).			
12–17 years	Inhaler: 20–40 micrograms three to four times a day Nebuliser: 500micrograms as required (max 2mg per day).			

Table 10.7 Montelukast.

MONTELUKAST INDICATION	DOSE	AVAILABLE FORM	ADME
Asthma	Age 6 months to 5 years: 4mg once a day in the evening Age 6–14 years: 5mg once a day in the evening Age 15 years: 10mg once a day in the evening	Tablet: 10mg Chewable tablet: 4mg and 5mg Granules: 4mg sachets	It is rapidly absorbed after administration and reaches peak concentration after 3 hours. Bioavailability is 64% and is about 99% to plasma proteins. The main CYP450 enzyme involved in metabolism is 2C8, but 3A4 and 2C9 are also involved.
Allergic rhinitis	Age over 15 years: 10 mg once a day in the evening.		

Montelukast is a leukotriene receptor agonist. It works by binding to the leukotriene receptors in the airway which blocks the effects of cysteinyl leukotrienes therefore inhibiting that inflammatory process. Common side effects include gastrointestinal discomfort, headache and sleep disturbance (Paediatric Formulary Committee, 2020). Montelukast is useful in patients with exercise-induced asthma and those with concomitant rhinitis, but less useful in patients with severe asthma who are also on high doses of other drugs. Table 10.7 summarises montelukast.

Xanthines

Xanthines are phosphodiesterase 3 and 4 inhibitors and have similar effects to beta $_2$ agonists. Theophylline and aminophylline belong to the xanthine class of drugs and are bronchodilators used as add on therapy for hard to control asthma. In addition to this, they affect a number of cells which are involved in the inflammatory processes linked with asthma. They suppress T-lymphocyte activity, reduce eosinophil count and also neutrophil function. These all have a beneficial anti-inflammatory effect in patients with asthma.

Xanthines have a narrow therapeutic index and adverse effects can occur within therapeutic concentrations. For most patients, the plasma theophylline concentration should be between 10 and 20 mg/litre. When patients are given intravenous aminophylline, a blood test should be taken 4–6 hours after starting treatment to monitor the plasma concentration of the drug. With oral aminophylline or theophylline, this test should be taken 5 days after starting treatment and 3 days after a dose change.

Overdoses of aminophylline or theophylline can cause vomiting, restlessness, dilated pupils, seizures, hypokalaemia, hyperglycaemia and tachycardia. Caution is therefore needed in patients with epilepsy and in those using high doses of beta agonist therapy, for example during acute exacerbation, due to the potentiation of hypokalaemia (eMC, 2020). IV aminophylline should only be considered in children with severe or life-threatening asthma which is unresponsive to maximum doses of bronchodilators and steroids.

Chapter 10 Medications Used in the Respiratory System

Table 10.8 Aminophylline and theophyline.

DRUG	DOSE	AVAILABLE FORM	ADME
Aminophylline	IV: 5mg/kg (maximum 500mg) given over 20 minutes followed by an IV infusion based on the age of the patient. Oral (for those over 40kg): Initially 225 mg twice daily for 1 week then increased if necessary to 450 mg twice daily. Doses are adjusted according to plasma-theophylline concentration.	M/R tablet: 225mg or 350mg Solution for injection: 250mg/10ml	After oral administration of aminophylline (theophylline), it is delivered to systemic circulation in a controlled and steady state; peak concentrations are seen after about 5 hours. It is bound 60% to plasma proteins and is metabolised by the liver and excreted in the urine. Therapeutic drug monitoring Is essential if doing intravenous loading and can be helpful for those established on oral treatment. A blood plasma level of 10–20 mg/litre is desired, but adverse effects can still occur during this range, so a lower target of 5–15 mg/litre may be used.
Theophylline	Age 2–11 years: 9mg/kg (max. 200mg per dose)(can be increased to 10–16mg/kg max. 400mg per dose) Age 12–17 years: 200mg every 12 hours adjusted to response (can go up to 400mg twice a day.	M/R Tablet (Uniphyllin): 200mg, 300mg or 400mg	

Aminophylline and theophylline are summarised in Table 10.8.

Theophylline is available orally as a modified-release preparation and dosing varies based on the age of the child and on the brand of theophylline prescribed. All preparations are modified-release and should be given twice a day.

Smoking can reduce drug levels by increasing the clearance of the drug in the body so doses may need to be changed if the patient starts to smoke or stops smoking during treatment. For those patients who are obese, ideal body weight should be used for dosing to avoid excessive dosing. Alcohol consumption can also increase the clearance of the drug (Paediatric Formulary Committee, 2020).

Corticosteroids

Corticosteroids can be sub-categorised into either mineral corticosteroids or glucocorticoids. In respiratory medicine glucocorticoids are predominantly used. Prednisolone and dexamethasone are used systemically and others such as beclomethasone, budesonide and fluticasone via the inhaled route.

Glucocorticoids bind to glucocorticoid receptors; this causes up regulation of anti-inflammatory genes and down regulation of pro-inflammatory genes.

Prednisolone is usually used as short courses for flare-ups of asthma for 3 days if aged from 1 month to 11 years old; for those over 12 years of age a course of at least 5 days is used (Paediatric Formulary Committee, 2020). Longer courses may be required for those who have severe asthma. Tablets are normally prescribed; if patients are unable to swallow tablets, the tablets are soluble so they can be crushed and dispersed in sterile water prior to administration.

Dexamethasone is first line treatment for croup and is available as a tablet or oral solution for those unable to swallow tablets.

Oral steroids are summarised in Table 10.9.

Hydrocortisone should be used via the IV route in severe cases of acute asthma when patients are unable to take medicine orally.

Chapter 10 Medications Used in the Respiratory System

Table 10.9 **Oral steroids.**

DRUG	DOSE	PHARMACOKINETICS
Prednisolone	Age 1 month – 11 years: 1–2 mg/kg once a day (maximum of 40 mg per dose) Age over 12 years: 40–50mg once a day	Prednisolone is readily absorbed into the GI tract and has a bioavailability of about 82%. Half-life is normally 2–4 hours. The duration of action is about 12–36 hours. Metabolism is mainly via the liver.
Dexamethasone	150 micrograms/kg as a single dose (this can be repeated on admission to hospital if required).	Dexamethasone is rapidly and almost completely absorbed in the stomach and small intestine; bioavailability is 80–90%. It has a long half-life of 36 hours which means that continuous daily dosing can lead to accumulation and toxicity. Elimination occurs mainly by the kidneys.

Fluticasone, budesonide and beclomethasone all come as inhalers on their own or as combination preparations with long-acting beta agonists. These are commonly referred to as preventer medications. There is little difference in efficacy between the inhaled corticosteroids, although some are more potent than others. These are designed to be used regularly to prevent an asthma flare-up so should be taken even when the patient feels well. More detailed dosing information depending on the different inhalers is available in the BNFc.

Side effects of glucocorticoids can include growth retardation, mood or behaviour changes, increased hunger, immunosuppression, adrenal suppression, oral candidiasis and fluid retention among others.

Steroid cards should be issued to patients when appropriate, especially those on long-term maintenance therapy. They can be used to alert others to consider corticosteroid replacement during episodes of stress such as illness or operation.

Clinical Considerations

Steroids may sometimes need to be reduced gradually, especially with repeat courses, prolonged courses or high doses to reduce withdrawal symptoms due to reduced cortisol levels or renewed symptoms of the disease.

Steroids can sometimes increase blood glucose levels in patients. If a high blood glucose level is detected in a patient without confirmed diabetes, advice should be sought from the endocrine team. Patients with existing diabetes may need their insulin regime adjusted.

Children should be encouraged to brush their teeth or have a drink after inhaled steroids or antibiotics to minimise the risk of oral candida infection.

Antibiotics

One of the most common antibiotics used in respiratory infections is amoxicillin and the second line is usually co-amoxiclav; these are both available orally and as an IV preparation. Dosing is based on the age and weight of the child as well as severity of the infection; more information can be found in the BNFc. Co-trimoxazole and azithromycin are sometimes used as prophylactic antibiotics for certain patients at higher risk of respiratory tract infections. As well as being an antibiotic, azithromycin also has anti-inflammatory effects which are useful in respiratory patients. Antibiotics and their modes of action are discussed in detail in Chapter 18.

Young people with respiratory conditions (particularly those with CF or bronchiectasis) can repeatedly isolate Pseudomonas aeruginosa on respiratory specimens (sputum samples or cough swabs). These patients can become chronically infected with this organism and require long-term treatment with inhaled antibiotics, usually colomycin or tobramycin.

Preparations available include colomycin powder, which can be reconstituted with sodium chloride or water for injection based on local practice, or Colobreathe which is a dry powder preparation; some patients find this harder to tolerate (Teva, 2016).

When nebulised colomycin and tobramycin are initiated, the first dose should be given in hospital and their lung function should be measured before and after the dose to observe for possible reactive bronchoconstriction or allergic reaction.

Mucolytics

Hypertonic saline (sodium chloride 7%) inhalation via a nebuliser increases the ion concentration in the airway surface liquid and this draws water into the airway lumen by osmosis. This reduces the viscosity of the fluid layer of the airway surface liquid and increases mucus clearance. This treatment is particularly useful in cystic fibrosis patients where increased viscosity of the airway mucus increases the risk of infection (Elkins and Bye, 2006, Robinson et al., 1997).

The dose is normally 4ml either once a day or twice a day. Some patients may require a bronchodilator such as salbutamol prior to using hypertonic saline. Side effects are rare; however, some patients cannot tolerate the salty taste.

In certain conditions such as CF or chronic lung disease, viscous purulent secretions in the airways can lead to reduced lung function and increased risk of infection.

Dornase alfa is a nebulised enzyme which hydrolyses the extracellular DNA in purulent secretions; this reduces the viscosity of the sputum making it easier to expectorate.

Dornase is licensed for over-5s at 2.5 mg once a day. Side effects are not common, but include chest pain, conjunctivitis and dyspepsia.

Other mucolytics including mannitol and acetylcysteine are also used in paediatric practice but are less common.

The exact mechanism of action of mannitol is not completely understood, but it is thought to work as a hyperosmotic agent. It increases the hydration of the mucus layer and this makes it easier to clear through mucociliary activity (eMC, 2020).

The licensed use of mannitol inhaler is 400 mg (10 capsules) twice a day.

Acetylcysteine is not used commonly as a mucolytic, but can be used when other mucolytics fail. It acts by breaking down the mucoprotein complexes and nucleic acids as well as having a direct antioxidant action. This reduces the viscosity of the sputum and other secretion as well as offering a protective element from the treatment (eMC, 2020). It is available as either granules for oral administration or IV solution which can be nebulised. Dosing regimens vary according to age and should be checked locally. Often oral acetylcysteine is not tolerated by patients due to the foul smell when opening the sachet packet.

Other Respiratory Drugs

Monoclonal Antibodies

Omalizumab is licensed for patients aged over 6 years for prophylaxis of persistent allergic asthma. This monoclonal antibody selectively binds to human immunoglobulin E (IgE); this prevents the IgE from binding to the IgE receptor on basophils and mast cells thus reducing the amount of free IgE to trigger the allergic cascade (eMC, 2020). Doses can vary based on the patient's IgE levels and weight and are usually given once every four weeks by subcutaneous injection. After administration, omalizumab is absorbed slowly, reaching a peak after about 6–8 days; bioavailability is about 62%.

Palivizumab is a monoclonal antibody used throughout the winter months to prevent lower respiratory tract disease caused by respiratory syncytial virus (RSV) in children considered to be high risk due to underlying respiratory conditions. This includes infants who were born at under 35 weeks gestation and are less than 6 months old, those less than 2 years who have had bronchopulmonary dysplasia in the last 6 months and those who are less than 2 years with significant congenital heart disease are eligible.

Pavilizumab works by binding to the RSV surface which prevents cell to cell and virus to cell fusion thus neutralising the effects of the virus. The dose is 15mg per kg of body weight and is administered intramuscularly (usually into the thigh) for a total of five doses at one month intervals. If the volume of the dose works out as more than 1ml then it should be given as a divided dose (eMC, 2020).

CFTR Modulators

There are three drugs that have recently become available to cystic fibrosis patients called Kalydeco, Orkambi and Symkevi. The age and genotype of the patient determines whether they are eligible for treatment with one of these modulators.

In cystic fibrosis, patients have a mutation in the gene which codes for the CFTR channel; this channel allows salt and water to move in and out of the cells. The mutation means that the CFTR channel does not work correctly and creates thick sticky mucus which blocks many cells in the body. Each of the three drugs targets the defective CFTR protein in a different way. They each target a different mutation, which is why each drug is only suitable for individuals with certain mutations (Rowe et al., 2005). As these drugs are quite new, long-term data is being collected, but the main things to monitor are liver function tests and ophthalmic tests.

Doses should be taken with fat containing foods and patients should be advised not to have Seville oranges or grapefruit as they effect metabolism and so can increase exposure to the drug (Vertex, 2019).

There is a fourth CFTR modulator called Kaftrio which has just received a licence and will be available to CF patients in the UK soon.

Episode of Care

Joey is a 9-year-old boy who presents with his Mum in the accident and emergency department with a wheeze, shortness of breath and a feeling of tightness in his chest. His Mum states that his symptoms started after he played football with his friends that afternoon. He is normally fit and well and his asthma is generally well controlled. He weighs 29kg and his height is 130cm.

His current medicines are:

- Salbutamol 100micrograms per dose 2–4 puffs four times a day as required
- Seretide Evohaler 50micrograms 1 puff twice a day

His SpO2 is 94% in air, Peak expiratory flow (PEF) is 64%, heart rate is 120 beats per minute and respiratory rate is 28 per minute.

After being assessed, he is diagnosed with an acute exacerbation of asthma and started on a short course of prednisolone and an appointment is made to be followed up in the nurse-led asthma clinic.

1. What symptoms of asthma is Joey showing on admission?
2. What dose can his salbutamol be increased to during the exacerbation?
3. You decide to assess his inhaler technique, how would you counsel Joey on how to use his salbutamol and seretide inhalers?
4. What are the criteria for diagnosing a mild-moderate asthma exacerbation?
5. What would you expect a normal oxygen saturation to be (SaO2)?
6. What dose of prednisolone should Joey be started on and how long should he have it for?
7. Are there any ways we could optimise this patient's normal medications?
8. If this patient deteriorated further and required PICU admission and IV aminophylline, what initial dose would you expect to be prescribed and how would you give it?

Conclusion

This chapter has examined the most common respiratory illnesses in children and the medicines routinely used in their treatment. Prompt recognition of respiratory symptoms and initiation of appropriate management is paramount in the nursing care of children. As a health professional it is essential that before administering any medications you must have an overall understanding of the medicine being administered, its potential effects and modes of administration (Royal Pharmaceutical Society, 2019). There are a variety of resources available for further study to enable greater understanding of respiratory illness in children. These are listed at the end of this chapter.

Chapter 10 Medications Used in the Respiratory System

Glossary

Half-life: The time required for a drug concentration to decrease to half of the starting dose in the body

First pass metabolism: A process where the concentration of a drug (when administered orally) is greatly reduced before reaching systemic circulation due to metabolism by the gut and or liver.

Protein binding: This refers to the degree in which medications attach to proteins within the blood; this affects the efficiency of the drug. If the binding is low, then this increases efficiency of the drug.

Bioavailability: The fraction of the administered drug which reaches systemic circulation. When a medicine is administered intravenously it has 100% bioavailability.

References

Akers, E. (2015). The respiratory system. In: *Fundamentals of Children's Anatomy and Physiology* (ed. Peate, I. and Gormley-Fleming, E), 216–232. Wiley, Oxford.

Asthma UK (2020). www.asthma.org.uk/advice/understanding-asthma/what-is-asthma/ (accessed June 2020).

Barker, C. Turner, M., Sharland, M. (2019). *Prescribing Medicines in Children*. Pharmaceutical Press: London.

Beat Asthma (2020). www.beatasthma.co.uk/resources/young-people-with-asthma/ (accessed May 2020).

Berger, A. (1999). What are leukotrienes and how do they work in asthma? *BMJ* 319: 90.

BMJ (2020). BMJ Best Practice: Croup. https://bestpractice.bmj.com/topics/en-us/681/treatment-algorithm (accessed June 2020).

British Thoracic Society/SIGN (2019). British guideline on management of asthma. SIGN 158 first published 2003. www.sign.ac.uk/sign-158-british-guideline-on-the-management-of-asthma (accessed June 2020)

Boe, J., Dennis, J.H., O'Driscoll, B.R. et al. (2001). European Respiratory Society Guidelines on the use of nebulizers. European respiratory Journal. 18: 228–242.

Chalmers, J.D. (2020). Cystic fibrosis lung disease and bronchiectasis. *The Lancet Respiratory Medicine* 8(1): 12–14.

Cystic Fibrosis Trust (CF Trust) (2020). www.cysticfibrosis.org.uk/what-is-cystic-fibrosis (accessed 20 February 2020).

Electronic Medicines Compendium (eMC) (2020). www.medicines.org.uk/ (accessed June 2020).

Elkins, M.R. and Bye, P.T. (2006). Inhaled hypertonic saline as a therapy for Cystic Fibrosis. *Current Opinion in Pulmonary Medicine* 12: 445–452.

European Respiratory Society (2020). European lung white book. www.erswhitebook.org/chapters/paediatric-respiratory-medicine/ (accessed 4 March 2020).

Glasper, A. and Richardson, J. (2006). *A Textbook of Children's and Young People's Nursing*. Churchill Livingstone, Elsevier.

Harris, M., Clark, J., Coote, N. et al. (2011) British Thoracic Society guidelines for the management of community-acquired pneumonia in children: update 2011. *Thorax* 66(ii): 1–23.

Hiley, E., Rickards, E., Kelly, C.A. (2019). Ensuring the safe use of emergency oxygen in acutely ill patients. *Nursing Times* 115: 18–21.

Joint Formulary Committee (2020). British National Formulary (online) London: BMJ Group and Pharmaceutical Press. https://bnf.nice.org.uk/treatment-summary/respiratory-system-drug-delivery.html (accessed September 2020).

National Institute for Health and Care Excellence (NICE) (2015). Bronchiolitis in children: diagnosis and management. NICE Guidelines [NG9]. www.nice.org.uk/guidance/ng9/resources/bronchiolitis-in-children-diagnosis-and-management-pdf-51048523717 (accessed 12 May 20).

National Institute for Health and Care Excellence (NICE) (2019). Clinical Knowledge Summary: Croup. https://cks.nice.org.uk/croup (accessed June 2020).

NHS England (2020). www.england.nhs.uk/childhood-asthma/ (accessed May 2020).

Nursing and Midwifery Council (2018). Future nurse: Standards of proficiency for registered nurses. www.nmc.org.uk/globalassets/sitedocuments/standards-of-proficiency/nurses/future-nurse-proficiencies.pdf (accessed September 2020).

Paediatric Formulary Committee (2019). *British National Formulary. For Children*, 2019–2020 ed. London: BMJ Group and Pharmaceutical Press.

Paediatric Formulary Committee (2020). *BNF for Children (online)*. London: BMJ Group, Pharmaceutical Press, and RCPCH Publication. https://bnfc.nice.org.uk/ (accessed May 2020).

Robinson, M., Hemming, A.L., Regnis, J.A. et al. (1997). Effect of increasing doses of hypertonic saline on mucociliary clearance in patients with cystic fibrosis. *Thorax* 52: 900–903.

Rowe, S.M., Miller, S., Sorcher, E.J. (2005). Cystic Fibrosis. *New England Journal of Medicine* 352: 1992–2001.

Royal Pharmaceutical Society (2019). *Professional Guidance on the Administration of Medicines in Healthcare Settings*. www.rpharms.com/Portals/0/RPS%20document%20library/Open%20access/Professional%20standards/SSHM%20and%20Admin/Admin%20of%20Meds%20prof%20guidance.pdf?ver=2019-01-23-145026-567 (accessed July 2020).

Teva UK. (2016). Colobreathe 1,662,500 IU inhalation powder, Hard Capsules. www.medicines.org.uk/emc/product/3063#EXCIPIENTS (accessed 25 June 2020).

Vertex (2019). How to take your Symkevi and Kalydeco Combination Treatment. Vertex Pharmaceuticals.

Walsh, B.K., Smallwood, C.D. (2017). Paediatric oxygen therapy: a review and update. *Respiratory Care* 26(6): 645–659.

Further Resources

CF Trust: www.cysticfibrosis.org.uk/

NICE guideline CF: www.nice.org.uk/guidance/ng78

National Consensus standards for the nursing management of CF (2001)

BEAT Asthma: www.beatasthma.co.uk/

Standards of Care and Good Clinical Practice for the Physiotherapy Management of Cystic Fibrosis, 3e (2017). London: Cystic Fibrosis Trust.

Asthma UK: www.asthma.org.uk/

Respiratory assessment of children. NICE guidelines: www.evidence.nhs.uk/search?q=respiratory+assessment+of+children

Asthma BTS Guidelines: www.guidelines.co.uk/respiratory/sign-and-bts-management-of-asthma-in-children-guideline/454880.article

Multiple Choice Questions

1. Select three common symptoms of asthma:
   - (a) Cough
   - (b) Pyrexia
   - (c) Wheeze
   - (d) Breathlessness
   - (e) Stridor

2. Inhaled corticosteroid treatment for asthma should only be given during an exacerbation. True or false?
   - (a) True
   - (b) False

3. Croup mainly affects which section of the airway?
   - (a) Pharynx
   - (b) Alveoli
   - (c) Trachea
   - (d) Larynx
   - (e) Bronchus

4. All children presenting with symptoms of croup should be given nebulised adrenaline. True or false?
   - (a) True
   - (b) False

5. What approximate percentage of infants with bronchiolitis requires hospital admission?
   - (a) 42%
   - (b) 90%
   - (c) 60%
   - (d) 3%
   - (e) 10%

6. Which virus most commonly causes bronchiolitis?
   - (a) Adenovirus
   - (b) Respiratory syncytial virus
   - (c) Metapneumo virus

7. Community-acquired pneumonia is only caused by bacterial organisms. True or false?
   - (a) True
   - (b) False

Chapter 10 Medications Used in the Respiratory System

8. Which one of these is NOT a common symptom of pneumonia?
   (a) High fever
   (b) Tachypnoea
   (c) Breathlessness
   (d) Cough
   (e) Stridor

9. Flucloxacillin is an antibiotic commonly used in CF to prevent which common childhood infection?
   (a) Haemophilus influenza
   (b) Pseudomonas aeruginosa
   (c) Staphylococcus aureus
   (d) Aspergillus
   (e) Influenza

10. What is an acceptable oxygen saturation level for a healthy child?
    (a) 90% or above
    (b) 94% or above
    (c) 85% or above
    (d) Below 90%
    (e) Above 80%

11. Which 3 of the following are included in a personalised asthma management plan?
    (a) Guidelines for medical management when admitted to hospital
    (b) Advice on how to manage symptoms at home depending on severity
    (c) When to contact a health professional for advice
    (d) Which medicines to take each day
    (e) Specific guidelines for school as to use of oral steroids

12. Salbutamol is the most common beta$_2$ agonist used and has a quick onset of action of about 5 minutes. How long does this bronchodilator effect last?
    (a) 2 hours
    (b) 30 mins – 1 hour
    (c) between 4–6 hours
    (d) 12 hours

13. Children should be encouraged to have a drink and brush their teeth after inhaled steroids and antibiotics. This is to:
    (a) Take away the taste of the medication
    (b) Encourage good dental care
    (c) Prevent oral candida infection

14. Dexamethasone is first line treatment for croup. What dosage is given?
    (a) 150 micrograms/kg for a single dose
    (b) 150 micrograms/kg three times a day
    (c) 125 micrograms/kg 4 hourly

15. Dornase alfa, (d'nase) is an inhaled mucolytic. It acts by;
    (a) Breaking down infection in the phlegm
    (b) Making the patient cough and expectorate sputum
    (c) Reducing the viscosity of the sputum, making it easier to expectorate.

Find Out More

The following is a list of respiratory conditions that you may encounter when working with children. Take some time and write notes about each of the conditions. Think about the medications that may be used in order to treat these conditions and be specific about the pharmacokinetics and pharmacodynamics. Remember to include aspects of patient care. If you are making notes about people you have offered care and support to, you must ensure that you have adhered to the rules of confidentiality.

THE CONDITION	YOUR NOTES
Asthma	
Cystic fibrosis	
Bronchiolitis	
Croup	
Pneumonia	

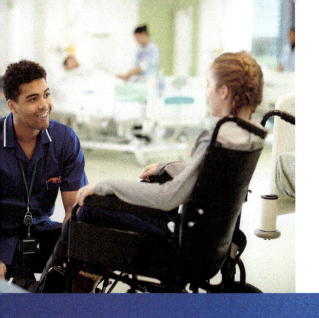

11

Medications Used in the Gastrointestinal System

Liz Gormley-Fleming

Aim
The aim of this chapter is to provide the reader with knowledge to develop an understanding of the fundamental principles of relevant pharmacology when caring for a child or young person (CYP) with gastrointestinal dysfunction. This will enable the CYP's nurse to provide evidenced-based, patient-centred care.

Learning Outcomes
On completion of this chapter the reader will be able to
- Apply knowledge and understanding of the fundamental principles of relevant pharmacological agents when caring for children and young people with gastrointestinal dysfunction
- Have a broad understanding of the action, interactions, side effects of a select range of medication used in the treatment of common gastrointestinal conditions
- Identify safe practice when administering medication to children and young people with gastrointestinal dysfunction
- Develop and apply knowledge of normal and altered anatomy and physiology of the gastrointestinal system when planning nursing care for children and young people who require pharmacological treatments within a family-centred care context
- Critically reflect on and evaluate learning and experiences to inform future practice

Fundamentals of Pharmacology for Children's Nurses, First Edition. Edited by Ian Peate and Peter Dryden.
© 2022 John Wiley & Sons Ltd. Published 2022 by John Wiley & Sons Ltd.
Companion website: www.wiley.com/go/pharmacologyforCN

Chapter 11 Medications Used in the Gastrointestinal System

Test Your Knowledge
1. Describe and explain the principle function of the gastrointestinal system
2. Identify the effects of Crohn's disease or ulcerative colitis on growth and development of the CYP
3. Identify the common causes of constipation in childhood
4. Explain the pharmacokinetics of proton pump inhibitors
5. List and explain the risk associated with mediation administration via an enteral tube
6. Identify and explain the action of stimulant laxatives

Introduction

This chapter will present an overview of the anatomy and physiology of the gastrointestinal tract. Following on from this a range of gastrointestinal disorders will be presented as episodes of care. Some of the associated nursing skills will be included. Pharmacology will be considered from the perspective of the knowledge required by those administering medication to CYP with gastrointestinal disorders.

Overview of the Anatomy and Physiology of the Gastrointestinal System

This section will provide an overview of the anatomy and physiology of the gastrointestinal system.

The gastrointestinal system (GI) comprises of the gastrointestinal tract and the accessory organs which are the liver, pancreas and gallbladder. The GI tract is referred to as the alimentary tract or digestive system. The GI tract commences at the oral cavity (mouth) and it extends through to the anus (Figure 11.1). This is

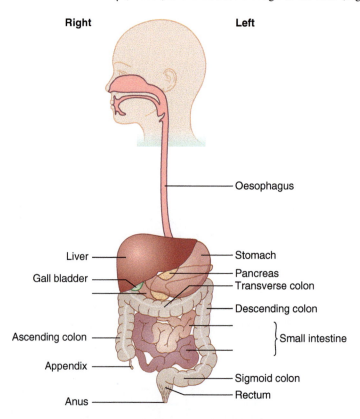

Figure 11.1 Gross anatomy of the GI tract. *Source:* Peate and Gormley-Fleming, 2015/John Wiley & Sons.

a complex system and it has a range of functions. The main function is to retrieve nutrients from food and convert them into a format that is then soluble in the blood or lymph. These are then transport to the part of the body where they are required and then eliminated as waste products. The common nutrient groups that are gained from ingestion of food and drink are carbohydrate, fats and proteins. These are broken down by the processes of mechanical and chemical digestion.

Mechanical digestion is movement of food, it is broken into smaller particles and mix digestive enzymes. This is achieved through chewing.

Chemical digestion is the use of the chemicals, both acids and enzymes, in digestive juices to break down food matter into its constituent components. This is then absorbed into the blood and lymph.

The mouth (buccal cavity) is responsible for both mechanical and chemical digestion. Mechanical digestion begins with chewing and the teeth. Chewing is controlled by cranial nerve V (trigeminal nerve).

Mechanical digestion is aided by the teeth. Food is physically broken into smaller particles, and the movement of the tongue enables a small ball or 'bolus' to be formed. This is passed to the back of the throat (pharynx) for swallowing. The chewing of food allows it to be mixed with the digestive enzymes in the mouth, starting the process of chemical digestion.

Food is transported via the oesophagus to the stomach via the mechanical process of peristalsis. The oesophagus is lined with epithelial cells, interspersed with mucus-secreting goblet cells that lubricate the food during its passage.

The Stomach

The stomach receives food and fluids from the oesophagus which joins the stomach at the cardiac or lower oesophageal sphincter (LOS). This is a circular muscle which prevents food from travelling back up the oesophagus (reverse peristalsis). The stomach is a j-shaped, muscular sac which is located on the left side of the abdomen. It performs both mechanical and chemical digestion, and passes its partially digested contents into pylorus before it moves through to the duodenum via the pyloric sphincter (Peate and Gormley-Fleming, 2015, 2021).

There are three layers of smooth muscles, a longitudinal muscular outer layer, a middle circular layer and an inner oblique layer. This musculature structure enables the churning of food and the expansion of the stomach.

The inner mucous membrane is stratified columnar epithelium which permits expansion of the stomach. There are goblet cells interspersed with the columnar epithelium, and these secrete mucus to assist in the breaking down and lubrication of solid food particles into semi-solid matter called *chyme*. The presence of chyme stimulates the entero-endocrine cells to release secretin and cholecystokinin which play a role in completing the digestion of food before it enters the jejunum and then the ileum.

The gastric mucosal barrier consists of surface mucosal cells which are located in the pyloric region. These secrete a thick, alkaline rich mucous that protects the epithelium of both the stomach and duodenum from the acid conditions of the lumen. These cells are stimulated by mechanical and chemical irritation and parasympathetic nerve input. This protective mucous barrier may be damaged by infection: bacterial and viral, and, medications e.g. aspirin. The pH is 7 at the surface of the mucosal barrier.

The parietal cells produce hydrochloric acid. Water and carbon dioxide combine with the cytoplasm of the parietal cell and carbonic acid is produced. Carbonic acid then dissociates into a hydrogen ion (H+) and a bicarbonate ion (HCO^3-) (Marieb and Hoehn, 2019) The hydrogen ion is transported into the stomach lumen via H^+, -K^+, ATPase. The ATP energy is exchanged into potassium ions in the stomach with the hydrogen ions in the parietal cells. The bicarbonate ion is transported out of the cell into the blood via a anion exchanger in exchange for a chloride ion. Chloride ions are then transported into the stomach lumen through the chloride cuniculus. Now both hydrogen and chloride ions are present in the stomach lumen. The associate with each other and from hydrochloric acid (HCl). Hydrochloric acid assists in the breakdown of the cell walls of the plant and animal matter ingested, allowing the nutrition from the cell contents to be released (Figure 11.2)

Chapter 11 Medications Used in the Gastrointestinal System

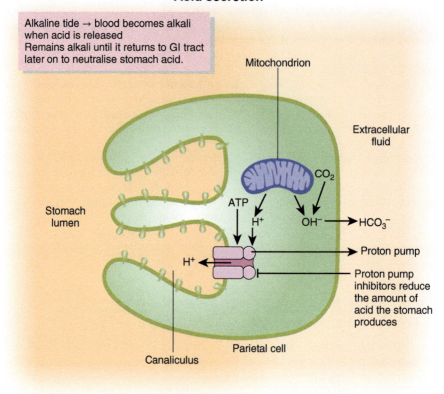

Figure 11.2 **The mechanism that produces hydrochloric acid.**

Small Intestines

The small intestine is divided into three sections: the duodenum, the jejunum and the ileum. The bile duct (from the gallbladder), and the exocrine pancreatic duct empty into the duodenum.

Duodenum
This is the proximal part of the small intestine, joining the stomach to the jejunum. It is approximately 5 cm long. From an anatomical perspective it is divided into four segments and each has a role to play in the digestion and absorption of food and nutrients. The common bile duct from the gallbladder empties into the duodenum. The pancreatic duct empties directly into the duodenum. The function of the duodenum is to receive partially digested food from the stomach-chyme and commence the absorption of nutrients. Some medication is designed to pass through the stomach before it is absorbed in the duodenum e.g. proton pump inhibitors

Jejunum
The jejunum is the portion of the small intestine between the duodenum and the ileum. It is approximately 8cm long. It is here that the pH of the digestive contents has changed from pH 3–5 in the stomach, to pH 8–9 in the jejunum. This allows for different enzymes become active and break down food into various groups.

Ileum
The ileum is the longest part of the small intestine and is approximately 8 metres long in adults. It is here that the majority of nutrients are absorbed from the partially digested chyme passing from the jejunum. Carbohydrates, proteins, and some vitamins and minerals pass into the blood stream here as the gut is highly vascularised. Lipids and vitamins ADEK pass into the lymph. Its surface area is increased by the presence of villi.

Chapter 11 Medications Used in the Gastrointestinal System

The ileum is responsible for the absorption nutrients, and some absorption of water. It leads to the large intestine, the junction of which is called the ileocaecal valve.

The Liver

The liver is responsible for the following functions:
1. Metabolism and excretion of proteins
2. Breakdown and excretion of red blood cells
3. Synthesis of clotting factors
4. Synthesis of bile
5. Storage of blood

The liver has 2 lobes; a large superior anterior lobe, and a smaller posterior inferior lobe.

The Gallbladder

The liver continuously produces bile, which is stored in the gallbladder and released when food is ingested. The gallbladder contracts and empties the bile into the duodenum. The role of bile is to emulsify fats and it breaks it down into smaller globules. These globules are of a size where they can be surrounded by the digestive juices from the pancreas and broken down into lipids which can be absorbed into the lymph. If bile is not released, then pancreatic enzymes can only work on the outer part of the large fat molecules. This leads to inadequate amounts of lipids being absorbed. The child then has difficulty gaining weight and also difficulty absorbing the fat-soluble vitamins ADEK, and the excess fat is excreted in the stools (steatorrhea).

The Pancreas

The pancreas has two functions: endocrine and exocrine. The endocrine function is the release of insulin in response to a rise in blood glucose levels, and the release of glucagon in response to a drop-in blood glucose levels.

The exocrine function is the release of alkaline digestive enzymes.

The Large Intestine

The large intestine begins at the ileocaecal junction and ends at the anus. It is responsible for the final absorption of nutrients and water, and for compaction and defecation of waste products.

The caecum is the blind ending of the large intestine. Located on the inferior surface of the caecum is the vestigial appendix. This contains limited lymphoid tissue and it has a role in immunity (Azzouz and Sharma, 2020). Infectious material may get trapped in the lumen which will lead to appendicitis. Surgical treatment may be required and there are no adverse effects as humans can live perfectly well without an appendix.

The digestive process takes to 16 hours to complete in the large intestine. Gut flora assist with this process and digest the remaining food matter and assist with the synthesis vitamins such as Vitamin K, B12, thiamine and riboflavin. Water is absorbed from the chyme as it passes through the large bowel. Fermentation via the gut flora occurs and any of the substances that remain after digestive process in the small intestines will be broken down by this method. What is not absorbed as nutrients is then prepared for excretion as faeces. As the lumen of the colon is larger than the ileum, it requires the bolus of faeces to be a reasonable size and consistency in order to be passed by peristalsis. If the stools are too watery, they will pass through too quickly, with inadequate time for water to be absorbed, and diarrhoea will result. If the stools are too hard, then it takes longer for them to pass, resulting in more water absorption and more compaction of additional faecal material, resulting in a large, hard stool that is difficult to pass which is constipation (Figure 11.3).

Once the stool has passed through the ascending, transverse, descending, and sigmoid colons, it is stored in the rectal ampulla which acts as a temporary reservoir.

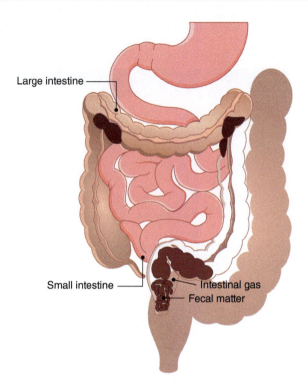

Figure 11.3 Large bowel and the passage of faeces.

When the rectum is full, the stretch receptors in the wall of the rectum send a signal to constrict the muscles of the rectum. The internal anal sphincter relaxes, and faeces enters the anus. A signal is sent to the brain identifying the urge to defecate and then the forcing the stored faeces through the anal sphincter. Once the voluntary signal to defecate is returned from the brain, the external anal sphincter relaxes, and defecation occurs. This is an involuntary response in the younger child and as they develop, they learn that they can control the constriction of the rectal muscles through the process of toilet training.

The physical aspect of defecation is often complicated by social and emotional aspects e.g. need for privacy, familiar environment to defecate in. Retention of faeces in the rectum may result in constipation.

This section has provided an overview of the anatomy and physiology of the GI system that is most relevant to the topic of discussion in this textbook. The nurse, nursing associate (NA) and healthcare worker needs a good understanding of the anatomy of the GI system in order to begin to understand associate dysfunction and the medication used in their management.

Gastro-Oesophageal Reflux Disease (GORD)

Gastro-oesophageal reflux (GOR) is a normal physiological process that occurs spontaneously after eating. The reflux of the gastric contents is managed by two mechanisms-peristalsis of the oesophagus which returns the contents to the stomach and neutralisation of the acidic fluid by the weakly alkaline saliva which has been swallowed. The third protective mechanism is the presence of epithelial cells in the lining of the oesophagus.

Alternatively, GORD occurs when the effects of GOR exacerbate or when the gastro-oesophageal sphincter becomes chronically lax and the gastric contents reflux into the oesophagus (Rudolf et al., 2011, NICE 2015). The presentation may be from mild posseting to that of a life-threatening event. 50% of infants will be symptomatic. The most common cause is functional immaturity of the gastro-oesophageal sphincter. The persistent refluxing of gastric acid into the oesophagus will cause irritation, leading to oesophagitis. If left untreated bleeding, ulceration and chronic scarring may occur.

GORD is a common disorder of infancy and childhood. It is often difficult to differentiate between GOR and GORD and the terms may be used interchangeably. GORD is more common in premature infants and CYP with severe and complex neuro-disabilities. The clinical manifestations are presented in Table 11.1.

Chapter 11 Medications Used in the Gastrointestinal System

Table 11.1 **GOR and GORD clinical manifestations.**

GOR	GORD
• Very common	• Severe pain and discomfort (retrosternal and epigastric pain)
• Affects 40% of infants	• Excessive crying
• 6 or more regurgitations per day	• Occult reflux
• Frequency diminishes as child increases in age with 90% resolved by the age of one year	• Overt regurgitation
• Irritability	• Eructation (belching)
• Infant has normal weight gain	• Sandifer's syndrome – dystonic posturing caused by reflux
	• Dysphagia
	• Haematemesis
	• Occult blood in stools
	• Pneumonia secondary to aspiration
	• Apnoea and bradycardia
	• Apparent life-threatening episodes (ALTEs)
	• Sleep disturbance
	• Refusal to feed/eat
	• Weight loss
	• Recurrent episodes of wheezing, coughing, stridor

There are several contributing factors that lead to GORD:

- Infants and children with chronic lung disease have been noted to have a greater incidence of GORD (Nettina, 2010)
- Obesity is thought to contribute to GORD
- Infants who present with gastro-oesophageal abnormalities (pyloric stenosis, oesophageal atresia) are pre-disposed to GORD even after surgical repair
- Extreme changes in position – from lying flat to then sitting with a greater than 30% incline – change the intra-abdominal pressure and this is thought to lead to reflux
- Anatomical and physiological conditions pre-dispose some infants and children to GORD. These include:
  - Short and narrow oesophagus
  - Delayed gastric emptying
  - Shorter and lower oesophageal sphincter-sits slightly above the diaphragm rather than below it.
  - Liquid, high calorie diet which increases the strain on gastric capacity
  - Larger ratio of gastric volume to oesophageal volume (Dogra et al., 2011)

It is essential that infants, children and young people who present with vomiting or regurgitation have a thorough assessment to exclude other disorders other than GORD (NICE, 2015).

Diagnosis is based systematic assessment, detailed history (feeding, sleep patterns, growth assessment) and possibly some simple investigations: urinalysis to exclude UTI and blood test for urea and electrolytes and coeliac screen (if weaned).

For suspected cases of GORD, abdominal X-ray, upper GI contrast studies, pH impedance study, oesophageal manometry, upper GI endoscopy and allergy testing will be performed.

Episode of Care

Glenn is a four-year-old boy who was born prematurely at 30 weeks. He had a grade 4 intraventricular bleed during the neonatal period which has resulted in spastic quadriplegia cerebral palsy. Glenn attends a pre-school for children with special needs. He has very restricted mobility, difficulty in controlling his movements and has frequent upper and lower respiratory tract infections. He is being treated for GORD and epilepsy. He has been feed orally. He has now lost weight and it has been agreed that he will have a percutaneous endoscopic gastrostomy (PEG) inserted. His parents have declined this in the past but after his last admission to ITU, following aspiration, they now feel that it will be safer to have a PEG inserted. He will be feed via his PEG and has been prescribed omeprazole, phenytoin and multivitamins.

You are his nurse/NA. How will you administer his medication? What do you need to consider?

Management of GOR and GORD

The management of GOR and GORD should follow best practice guidance (NICE, 2015). The CYP nurse, NA and healthcare support worker will all play a significant role in supporting the parents and CYP.

Mild uncomplicated cases without any associated symptoms may be managed with minimal intervention: thicken feeds, careful winding post feeding and nursing the infant in an upright position post feeding.

Specific care will include:

- Feeding regimes (feeding pattern, a trial of smaller volume feeds and a trail of, thickened feeds and alginate therapy (Gaviscon™) if thickened feeds do not work).
- Breast-feeding should be continued, and alginate therapy considered for 1–2 weeks (NICE, 2015). To administer alginate, the powered dose should be mixed with cooled boiled water and given by oral syringe or spoon to the infant.
- Positioning during and after feeding-feeding in a upright position, elevate head of cot/bed (bed blocks to tilt-pillows must never be used). Sleep management for infants should for follow NHS advise, they should be placed on their backs with their feet at the foot of their cots.
- Enteral tube feeding may be required to promote weight gain. A specific individualised feeding plan will be required and there should be a strategy in place to return to oral feeding as soon as possible. Oral stimulation should be provided during the period of enteral feeding.
- Growth monitoring – this includes management of obesity for the CYP who are obese.
- The mainstay of nursing care is support for the CYP and their parents/carers, through these lifestyle changes
- Medication administration: local policy must always be adhered to when administering medication.

Pharmacological Treatment for GORD

There are two primary medications that are used to treat overt regurgitation in children and young people. These are Proton Pump Inhibitors (PPIs) and H^2 receptor antagonist (H^2RA). These are not recommended for overt reflux or isolated symptoms (NICE, 2015). In this chapter PPIs will be discussed as they are more commonly used.

PPIs are recommended for use for moderate, non-erosive oesophagitis. In the presence of persistent heartburn, epigastric or retrosternal pain a four-week trial of either PPIs or H^2RAs should be implemented. Likewise, for infants and CYP who are pre/nonverbal and who have overt regurgitation in the presence of one of the following:

- Unexplained feeding difficulties
- Distressed behaviour or faltering growth

a four-week trial of PPIs or H^2RAs should be prescribed (NICE, 2015).

If the CYP has had endoscopically confirmed erosive, ulcerative or structuring disease then treatment with PPIs is recommended (British National Formula for Children (BNFc), 2020). The treatment should be maintained at the minimum effective dose.

Proton Pump Inhibitors

Proton Pump Inhibitors are one of the most frequently prescribed medications worldwide. When clinically indicated they are effective in managing GORD, oesophagitis and peptic ulceration with limited risk of harm. CYP who may be on long-term non-steroidal anti-inflammatory medication may be prescribed PPIs concurrently as prophylaxis against upper gastrointestinal injury. In the long term, the prolonged use of PPIs can lead to adverse effects (Marks, 2016). These are outlined in Table 11.2.

The parietal cells secret gastric acid and PPIs have been developed to target these cells directly and to inhibit the secretion of gastric acid. PPIs have dramatically influenced the management of acid related disorders in CYP.

Pharmacokinetic Properties of PPIs

PPIs act by inhibiting gastric acid secretion. They are acid labile and as an oral preparation, they are designed to avoid contact with the stomach. PPIs are a prodrug and have an acid resistant coating which protects them from premature degradation by gastric acid and they pass through the stomach intact. This coating is dissolved in the duodenum as the pH is 6. The PPI cross the cell membranes. The prodrug is absorbed in the alkaline duodenum and then transported to the parietal cells (Figure 11.4). The parietal cells are the only

Table 11.2 Side effects of PPIs.

Gastrointestinal disturbances – nausea, vomiting, abdominal pain, flatulence, diarrhoea, constipation

Headaches

Dry mouth

Dizziness, tiredness, sleep disturbances

Paranaesthesia, arthralgia, myalgia

C-difficile associate diarrhoea

Fracture risk

Interstitial nephritis

Chronic kidney disease

Increase risk of drug interaction for patients with comorbidity was and polypharmacy

Source: Modified from BNFc, 2020/BNF Publications.

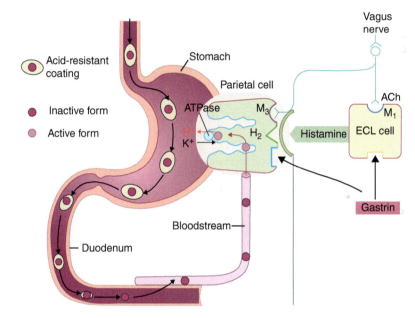

Figure 11.4 The transportation of PPIs.

membrane-enclosed space in the body with a pH of less than 4. The PPIs accumulate in the secretory canaliculus of the parietal cell.

The PPI blocks the gastric hydrogen (H$^+$), potassium (K$^+$) and ATPase enzyme. This is known as the gastric proton pump and is in the parietal cells of the stomach wall. By binding to the H$^+$, K$^+$ -ATPase enzyme system (proton pump) of the parietal cells, the secretion of hydrogen ions into the gastric lumen is suppressed, resulting in inhibition of the secretion of gastric acid (Litalien et al., 2005). In the parietal cells the PPIs are converted into an active form. It forms a stable covalent bond with H$^+$, K$^+$ -ATPase. The diagram (Figure 11.5) demonstrates the action of the PPI (omeprazole in this example). The resynthesis of H$^+$, K$^+$ -ATPase is approximately 18 hours.

PPIs are relatively slow in achieving a steady state of inhibition of gastric acid secretion and may typically take three days.

Pharmacodynamics of PPIs

PPIs have a relatively short half-life. They are rapidly absorbed in the GI tract following oral administration. Half-life is usually one hour but for a maximum plasma concentration it has been noted that this may be from one hour and up to a maximum of five hours. This is in part due to the drug formulation and also the effect

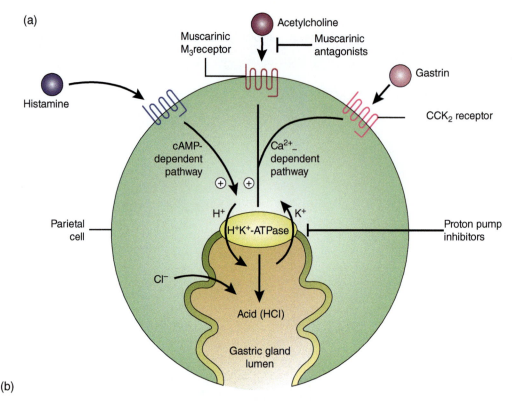

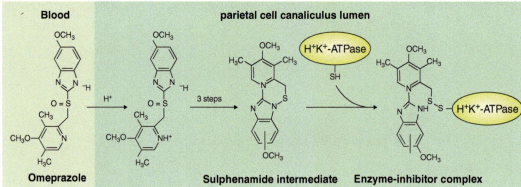

Figure 11.5 The action of PPIs in the parietal cell. *Source:* Redrawn from Gormley-Fleming and Martin, 2018.

of food in the stomach. Hepatic first pass rate is relatively low and oral bioavailability is between 77–90% depending on the formulation (Litalien et al., 2005).

PPIs inhibit >90% of the total daily gastric production (Moo Shin and Kim, 2013). There is little difference in gastric acid suppression between some contemporary formulations e.g. omeprazole and lansoprazole.

Metabolism of PPIs occurs in the liver and they are eliminated via the urine and faeces. Twice a day dosage has been shown to demonstrate greater acid suppression than once a day (Sachs et al., 2006) but most PPIs are prescribed once a day for CYP.

Enteral Feeding Tubes and Medication Administration

Feeding and medication administration should ideally be through the oral route. There are medically indicated needs to provide nutrition via other routes, namely the enteral route. There are a few routes where enteral tubes may be inserted, and these are outlined in the diagram below (Figure 11.6)

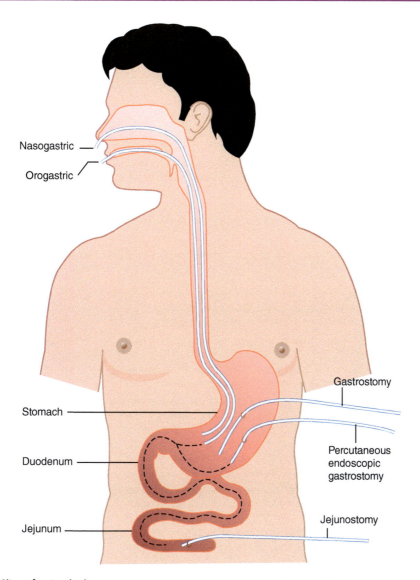

Figure 11.6 **Sites of enteral tubes.** *Source:* Redrawn from Gormley-Fleming and Martin, 2018.

Primarily, orogastric, nasogastric (NG) and percutaneous endoscopic gastrostomy (PEG) tubes are designed to administer fluids and liquid food administration and not medication. Nasojejunal tubes (NJ) require special consideration when administering medication. This is due to the tip of the tube bypassing the stomach so absorption may be impaired. If the CYP has an NJ tube and this is the only route for the administration of medication, the absorption characteristics must be verified before it may be used for this purpose.

Prescribing medication for CYP is complex and the issue of the use of unlicensed further adds to its complexity. The legal implications of administering medication for oral route via NG tube or PEG must be considered. The registered nurse and NA must be able to undertake all aspects of evidenced-based medicines administration competently (Nursing and Midwifery Council (NMC), 2018a, 2018b, 2018c, 2018d). The four themes of the Code of Conduct (NMC, 2018a) – prioritise people, practise effectively, preserve safety and promote professionalism and trust – are all equally applicable to this aspect of medication management.

Administration of medication via enteral tubes is complex and error prone. Most medication is not licensed or designed to be administered via enteral feeding tubes. Currently there is no medication licensed in the UK for administration via a nasojejunal tube. The clinical response to any medication administered via an enteral tube must be monitored.

Chapter 11 Medications Used in the Gastrointestinal System

Healthcare professionals may have limited alternatives other than to use off-label and unlicensed medication (Terry and Sinclair, 2012). Increasingly, licensed formulations are becoming available. This means that the medication will have been tested specifically for use with NG and PEG tubes. The manufactures instructions must be followed, this includes reconstitution volume and fluid, flush volume and occasionally the type of tube (Wright et al., 2019). In addition, the hospital- or community-based pharmacist's instructions must be adhered to.

When a medication is only available in a tablet or capsule format they must be reformulated before administration via an enteral tube is possible. Altering the medication may have undesirable consequences. The nurse/NA must be aware of this as they are accountable for this aspect of practice. Local guidelines on the administration of medication via enteral tubes must be followed and patient care records reflective of the care given. Competency-based training must be completed before the healthcare professional administers medication via an enteral feeding tube (NHS Improvement, 2016) and it is recommended that regular competency assessment is undertaken (National Patient Safety Agency (NSPA), 2011; Care Quality Commission, 2020). Some of the potential consequences are presented in Table 11.3 below.

Table 11.3 Risks associated with medication administration via an enteral tube.

RISK	CONSEQUENCE TO THE CHILD AND YOUNG PERSON	CONTROL
Incompatible route	Crushing tablets may be clinically unsafe. Pharmacokinetics or pharmacodynamic properties may be changed Toxic dose may be released from crushed tablets.	Refer to Pharmacist
	Possible risk of toxicity to the person crushing the tablet if inhaled. Sensitisation or anaphylaxis in the susceptible individual (administrator) if crushing tablets is a potential risk.	Appropriate Personal and Protective Equipment must be worn
Altered absorption	Bioavailability is not guaranteed. Reduced effectiveness of the medication e.g. ciprofloxacin forms insoluble chelates with the divalent iron in enteral feeds. This will reduce the absorption of ciprofloxacin significantly. Increased gastric surface area available for drug interaction and absorption rate is altered.	Medication review. Refer to Pharmacist.
Preparation errors	Modified-release or enteric-coated medication must never be crushed and administered via enteral tube (White and Bradnam, 2015; Wright, 2019). Liquid-filled capsules – it is very difficult to be certain that all the liquid has been removed, so a dose error may occur (Grissinger, 2013). Unanticipated interaction with feeding products. Particle adhesion to interior surface of enteral tube reducing the amount of medication the child will receive.	Medication review. Refer to Pharmacist.
	Enteral tube blockage. For example, sucralfate forms bezoars which will block the tube. Inadequate flushing of enteral tube so drug remains in tube, resulting in medication administration error (Kelly et al., 2011).	Competency-based training for all staff who administer medication via enteral feeding tubes.
	Increased number of 'feed breaks' required if multiple medications required at different times.	Medication review. Refer to Pharmacist. Dietician review.
	Medication that must be administered before or after food in order to optimise the bioavailability should be administered immediately after the feed and not during the feed break. Difference in excipients between formulations e.g. alcohol in liquid formula which may be an issue for some patients, sorbitol may lead to gastrointestinal disturbances. Dispersible/dissolvable mediation required large volumes of water and also contain large amounts of sodium. This may impact on serum sodium levels.	Medication review. Refer to Pharmacist.

Chapter 11 Medications Used in the Gastrointestinal System

Table 11.4 Impact of a blocked enteral tube on the CYP and their family.

- Child is unable to receive liquids, food and medicine so impact on physical well-being
- Risk of morbidity due to lack of access to medicines
- Trauma of having to have new NG tube inserted-psychological upset.
- May have to attend hospital to have new tube inserted. Costs associated with this.
- Potential radiation exposure if x-ray required to confirm the position of tube

Table 11.5 Legal aspects of medication administration via enteral tubes.

- Once prescribed, liability is transferred from the manufacturer to the prescriber and to the administrator-nurse/NA.
- The administrator is accountable if the prescriber has not authorised the process, e.g. crushing or dissolving the medication.
- The administrator is answerable to their profession regulator, employer and the law.
- Any manipulation of the drug (crushing) will render it unlicensed under the Human Medicines Regulation (2012) (Aronson and Ferner, 2017)
- Consent of the child and parents should be sought before administration.
- Child and family should be aware that medication is being administered via NG/NJ/PEG tube to avoid any suggestion that medication administration is covert. Care plan should be updated to reflect this.

Source: Human Medicines Regulation, 2012 and Aronson and Ferner, 2017.

A review of the child or young person's medication should occur if enteral administration is required. This should include frequency of administration, volume of medication, number of medicines and the risks and benefits of each medication should be considered. This discussion should involve the prescriber, pharmacist and nursing staff.

There are a number of drug formulations that must never be via an enteral feeding tube, so it is important that the CYP nurse/NA refers to the British National Formulary for Children at all times.

The risk of blocking the enteral feeding tube increases with the number of medications administered and the duration of the administration (Heineck et al., 2009). The impact of blocked NG tube on the child and family are outlines in Table 11.4

The nurse and NA must be aware of their responsibility from a professional, regulatory and legal perspective when administering medication via enteral tubes. It is not possible to discuss the full extent of the legal aspects of medication administration in this chapter, but the pertinent points are included in Table 11.5.

Skills for Practice

Administration of Medication Via an Enteral Tube
- Medication should only be administered via an enteral tube if it is not feasible for the CYP to take them orally.
- Medicines must be administered individually. If enteral nutrition is administered continuously, it must be stopped for the prescribed time frame pre and post drug administration as advised by the dietician/pharmacist.
- Medication should be prepared as instructed by the pharmacist and should not be prepared in advance for administration later.
- Once prepared it must not be left unattended.
- The volume of flush used should be recorded.
- Oral syringes must be used where possible.
- Local policies should be followed-medication administration and enteral tube management and record-keeping.
- Assemble all equipment.
- Wash hands and apply apron and gloves.
- Before administering any medication, the position of the tube must be confirmed. This will include noting the length of the NG tube at the nostril each time also.
- Connect the 20ml syringe to the port of the NG tube and aspirate 0.5–1 ml of gastric contents.
- Drop onto the pH paper, wait for 10 seconds and match the colour to the comparison chart. Read within 60 seconds of placing the aspirate on the pH paper. The pH should be below 5.5 for infants (term), children and young person. Do not proceed if it is greater than pH is 5.5.

Chapter 11 Medications Used in the Gastrointestinal System

- If the CYP is receiving any medication that may alter the pH of the gastric contents this should be noted, and an agreed course of action recorded in their plan of care.
- Flush the tube with the prescribed volume of water.
- Administer each drug one at a time and flush with the prescribed volume in between until all the medication has been administered and again flush after the last drug has been given.
- Have a feed break if required.
- Resume the feed as soon as appropriate.

Record-Keeping
- The CYPs care plan should be updated to reflect that their medication is administered via their enteral tube.
- The volume of fluid used to flush should be recorded on their feed or fluid balanced chart.
- Their medication administration record must be completed in full.
- Any adverse drug reactions/interactions should be reported via the 'Yellow Card' system to the Medicines and Healthcare Products Regulatory Agency (MHRA). A low tolerance should be maintained when administering medication via enteral tube for any reactions.
- The expected outcome from supportive care and medication is that the infant, CYP with GORD will be able to feed, thrive and engage in their normal activities. If this cannot be achieved the further intervention e.g. surgery may be required.

Source: Based on Gormley-Fleming and Martin, 2018.

Constipation

The frequency of bowel action in CYP varies and there is no set pattern. Some will have their bowels open twice a day whereas for others it may be once every two days or longer. The normal frequency of defecation is age-specific. A newborn baby may pass on average four stools a day in the first few weeks of life and by the age of four the child will pass on average three per week. The diagnosis of constipation is based hardness of the stool and pain associated with defecation (Rudolf et al., 2011). A common diagnosis, constipation is usually functional (idiopathic) in nature, meaning it cannot be explained by any anatomical abnormalities. These are outlined in Figure 11.7. However, it is essential to rule out serious disease before functional constipation is diagnosed.

The factors that may contribute to constipation are:

- Abdominal pain
- Fever
- Inadequate fluid intake
- Inadequate dietary fibre
- Toilet training issues
- Psychosocial issues
- Effects of medication
- Family history

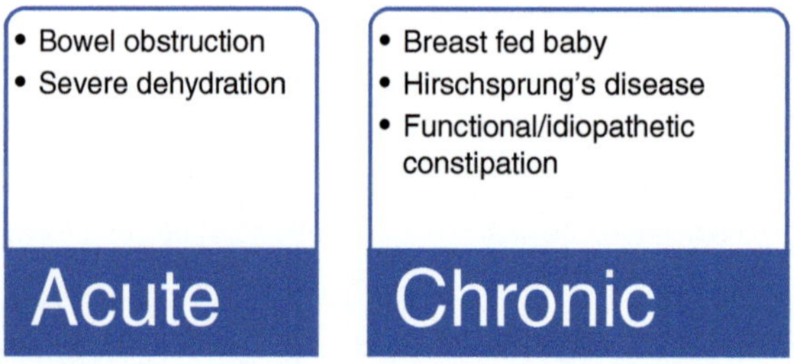

• Bowel obstruction • Severe dehydration	• Breast fed baby • Hirschsprung's disease • Functional/idiopathic constipation
Acute	**Chronic**

Figure 11.7 Causes of constipation.

Management of constipation will be dependent on the cause and the degree of constipation. Underlying conditions should be considered (e.g. coeliac disease, hypothyroidism) if ongoing constipation has not been resolved by laxative treatment.

Suppositories

A suppository is a solid dose of medication that is administered into the rectum or as a laxative to enable the CYP to defecate. The administration of a suppository may be unpleasant for the CYP.

Glycerine suppositories may be used to treat temporary constipation only. They are used to remove faeces by stimulating the bowel and this will usually provide rapid relief to the child. Before being administered these must be prescribed and the medication administration process followed as per local policy.

Clinical Skill

Suppository Administration

A suppository is a solid dose of medication that is administered into the rectum. Privacy and dignity must be maintained when administration medication per rectum.

The child should be asked to void urine first and then once returned to their bed, asked to lie on their left side with their legs flexed. If possible, ask the child to breathe deeply as this will help to relax them. Hold the buttock to one side and identify the anus. Lubricate the suppository with some aqueous gel, insert the blunt end of the suppository first. Use one finger to gently push the suppository into anus (approximately 1–1.5 cms) (Figure 11.8). Hold the buttock gently together as this will help the child retain the medication.

Wipe the anus and gently lower the child's legs to a comfortable position and ask them to remain on their side for 15 minutes. This will help them to retain the suppository as they will often feel like pushing it out. If it is expelled immediately it is likely that it was not inserted high enough. A toilet or commode should be near by for the child to access if required. Dispose of all waste, wash hands and document administration of this medication. Record the effectiveness of the suppository in the CYP's care record.

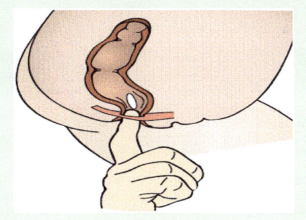

Figure 11.8 **Insert the suppository into the anus using one finger.** *Source:* Gormley-Fleming and Martin, 2018. John Wiley & Sons.

Once functional constipation has been diagnosed the management will include medication, behavioural interventions and support. Laxatives are usually the first line of treatment and these will need to be taken over several months. If the child has faecal impaction, a disimpaction regimen will need to commence. This involve the administration of a macrogol e.g. Movicol ®Paediatric Plain or Movicol ® using an escalating regimen. A stimulant laxative may be added to this regimen if the macrogol is not tolerated and not successful after two weeks (Figure 11.9). The CYP should be reviewed weekly until disimpaction is achieved. Maintenance laxatives drug treatment will commence once impaction has been treated (NICE, 2019a).

Chapter 11 Medications Used in the Gastrointestinal System

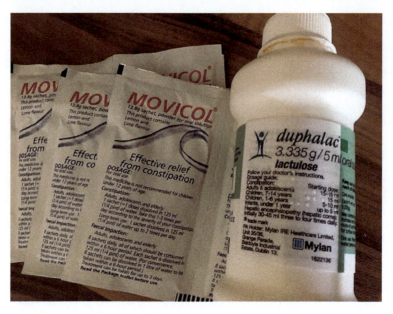

Figure 11.9 A macrogol and stimulant laxative for use in faecal disimpaction.

The choice of laxatives will depend on the age of the child, their preference and the preferred formulation. Laxatives are a group of drugs that either accelerate the movement of faecal matter from the body or decrease the consistency of faecal matter. There are four main groups of laxatives:

- Bulk-forming
- Lubricant
- Osmotic
- Stimulant

When treating functional constipation in CYP, the choice is either osmotic laxatives or stimulant laxatives (National Institute for Clinical Excellence, 2018). While these are the front-line choice of medication it is important that lifestyle changes are initiated simultaneously: dietary review, increase in fluid intake and exercise should be considered as part of the holistic treatment plan for the child or young person. Psychological intervention is not recommended for idiopathic constipation unless there is likely to be a perceived benefit (NICE, 2018). If not the CYP will become constipated once medication is stopped.

Osmotic Laxatives

Osmotic laxatives increase the amount of fluid in the large bowel by drawing fluid into the lumen of the bowel (Figure 11.10). These are administered via the oral route and most will reach the bowel unchanged. They contain substances that are poorly absorbable but gently attracts water into the bowel through the process of osmosis The increased fluid has a threefold action: softens the faeces by drawing water into it, it distends the large intestine, triggering the defecation reflex which in turn promotes peristalsis and thus easing the passage of the faeces into the rectum and then the anus.

Stimulant Laxatives

Stimulant laxatives include formulations such as sodium picosulfate and formulations from the anthraquinone group such as senna. They work by causing peristalsis which stimulates the colonic and rectal nerves (Figure 11.10). The myenteric plexus and Auerbach plexus in the intestinal mucosa are stimulated. This increases intestinal secretions and motility (Tack and Müller-Lissner, 2009) and decreases absorption of water from the lumen of the bowel. Stimulant laxatives generally take six to twelve hours to be effective and may cause abdominal pain

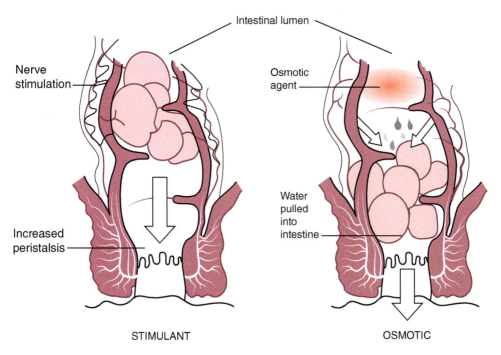

Figure 11.10 **Action of stimulant and osmotic laxatives.**

Pharmacokinetics

Laxatives are either administered orally or rectally. When taken orally, most will reach the target site, the intestines, unchanged. Stimulant laxatives are excreted in the faeces. There may be minimal absorption of stimulant laxatives during first pass. They are metabolised in the liver and excreted via the kidneys in the urine. Long-term use of stimulant laxatives can lead to muscle weakness and prolonged diarrhoea which may cause hyponatraemia, hypokalaemia and dehydration (CKS, 2019).

Osmotic laxatives are metabolised by the bacteria in the intestines. This forms lactic and acetic acid which forms a softer stool and alters the pH of the stool also. If saline compounds are used sodium and magnesium ions are excreted in the urine. Osmotic compounds that contain magnesium can cause electrolyte disturbances particularly in the presence of renal disease so should be used with caution (Liu, 2011). As osmotic compounds result in volume load, caution is required when using with CYP with renal or cardiac dysfunction (Bashir et al., 2020)

Chronic constipation is constipation lasting greater than eight weeks duration. Diet, particularly recommended fluid intake and lifestyle advice should be provided early on in the management of the child or young person. Laxative treatment should not be stopped abruptly, and laxatives may be administered long term. If treatment is unsuccessful then surgical procedures may be required (manual evacuation, whole gut lavage, antegrade colonic enema administration) along with psychological and behavioural interventions. The CYP may be referred to Child and Adolescent Mental Health Services if it is felt to be of value.

Crohn's Disease

Crohn's disease (CD) is a chronic inflammatory disease that may affect any part of the intestinal tract and also extra-intestinal tissue. It is one of the conditions that sits within the umbrella term Inflammatory Bowel Disorders (IBD). This is a debilitating disease that often has life changing consequences for the child and their family. The incidence of CD in children and young people is increasing with approximately 4.5–5.7 cases per 100,000 population and the cause of this increase is not known (Crohn's & Colitis UK, 2020). It is slightly more common in females than males and in those who smoke.

Crohn's disease is categorised according to which part of the gut is most affected. The main types are:

- Terminal ileal and ileocaecal (most common type)
- Small bowel, ileitis or jejunoileitis (common in CYP)
- Colonic: large intestine affected.
- Gastroduodenal
- Perianal: may occur on its own or at the same time with inflammation elsewhere in the body
- Oral Crohn's – although rare it is more likely to affect CYP; it is referred to as orofacial granulomatosis (OFG). The lips become swollen and mouth fissures occur. People with CD frequently develop mouth ulcers during flare-ups.

CYP who present with CD may have the following symptoms:

- Diarrhoea
- Abdominal pain
- Reduced growth
- Rectal bleeding

Extra-intestinal involvement may include:

- Skin – most common problem is erythema nodosum (raised red or purple swelling 1.5 cm in diameter and generally found on the legs).
- Eyes – episcleritis, the episcleral is a layer of tissue between the conjunctiva and the sclera. This becomes red and inflamed. Scleritis (inflammation of the sclera) and uveitis (inflammation of the middle layer of the eye made of the iris, ciliary body, and choroid) may also occur and the latter may lead to blindness.
- Musculoskeletal system – arthritis is a common complication of CD. Osteoporosis is also found in people with CD.
- Hepatobiliary system – gallstones are common in people who have CD. Some of the medication used to treat CD may impact negatively on the liver e.g. methotrexate. Primary Sclerosing Cholangitis is rare but can lead to liver damage (Crohn's and Colitis UK, 2020)

The onset is often insidious and by the time diagnosis is confirmed, the CYP may well have advanced CD. The entire intestinal tract may be affected and transmural inflammation may result in stricture formation. Fistulisation between the bowel and other abdominal organs including the skin may occur (Kammermeier et al., 2016). Specialist referral is required once the disease is suspected. Table 11.6 outlines the expected investigations.

Treatment of Crohn's Disease

The treatment aim of CD is to induce remission, optimise nutrition, optimise growth, define bone status, progress puberty and overall, to minimise the adverse effects of pharmacological agents. The desired outcome is long-term intestinal mucosal healing without relapse. The treatment strategy is the early introduction of immunomodulatory and biological therapy.

Pharmacological Treatment for Crohn's Disease

Initially, the child will be exclusively enterally fed (EEF). Polymeric feeds (whole protein) are the feed of choice as they are better tolerated (Garrick et al., 2011). There is some evidence to suggest that maintenance enteral feeding is advantageous for some children (Duncan et al., 2014). The aim of enteral feeding is to promote healing of the lumen of the bowel and it will provide nutrition to the child or young person.

Corticosteroids will be used to induce a remission if enteral feeding has not been successful. This will be administered by the oral or intravenous route. The location of the disease will determine the type of steroid

Table 11.6 Investigations required to confirm Crohn's disease.

- Upper gastrointestinal endoscopy
- Ileocolonoscopic with histology
- Small bowel imaging (MRE or VCE)
- Bloods: FBC, ESR, CRP, albumin, liver function tests, immune assay
- Stools for faecal calprotectin

used. Active luminal disease will be treated with oral prednisolone – 1mg/kg up to a maximum of 40 mg per day. This must be tapered over an 8- to 10-week period. For ileocaecal disease, budesonide may be used and a maximum dose of 12 mg per day tapered over 2–4 weeks is recommended (BNFc, 2020). In very severe cases, intravenous methylprednisolone or hydrocortisone may be prescribed.

Aminosalicylates (5-ASAs)-these include mesalazine, sulphasalazine and valsalazide. Aminosalicylates are used for mild to moderate relapse and only if the CYP does not respond to glucocorticosteroids (NICE, 2020). Each 5-ASA act in different parts of the bowel so the choice of drug is dependent on the location of the disease.

Immunosuppressant medication supresses the immune system and thus reduces the level of inflammation. Thiopurines (6-mecaptopurine or azathioprine) are commenced to maintain remission. Methotrexate may be introduced if the CYP has not responded effectively to thiopurines (NICE, 2020). The CYP will require careful monitoring and lifestyle advice appropriate for patients receive long-term immunosuppressants.

Biological drugs are the latest group to be added to treat CD. These are Anti TFN α antibody group.

Anti TFN-α antibody treatment is recommended to either induce a remission or maintaining a remission in CYP with steroid refractory disease or luminal disease which has not responded to maximum immunosuppressant therapy (Kammermeier et al., 2016). The disease will usually be severe, active and fistulating (NICE, 2019b) with the CYP in a general state of very poor health. The effect of using this treatment has been shown to be very beneficial with up to 71% of CYP responding to biologicals (Gasior and Maltz, 2020). Infliximab is currently the only drug in this group that is within its licensed indication recommended for use in CYP between the ages of 6–17 years of age (NICE, 2019b; BNFc, 2020).

Infliximab is a chimeric mouse monoclonal antibody (Ig) G1. It inhibits the pro-inflammatory cytokine tumour necrosis factor alpha (TNF-α). The mechanism of action is not entirely understood and it is thought that TNF-α blocking agents is mediated via apoptosis (death of cells which occur as a normal part of an organism's growth or development) of TFN-α expressing inflammatory cells (Figure 11.11).

The mucosal cells of patients with CD are thought to be highly resistant to apoptosis. There is overexpression of one of the inhibitory proteins called FLICE and impairment of caspase (protease enzymes) mediated pathway of apoptosis (Levin and Shibolet, 2008). Infliximab can induce apoptosis on the inflammatory cells including T cells and monocytes.

The distribution of infliximab is low and corresponds to the available intravascular space. The elimination half-life is 7–12 days, hence why the systemic clearance is low 11–15 ml/hr (Ternant et al., 2008).

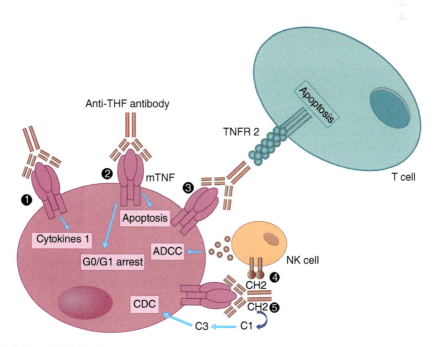

Figure 11.11 Action of infliximab.

The mechanisms of how infliximab is cleared from the intravascular space is not well understood but it is thought to be like that of all circulating proteins. IgGs are encocyted (devoured) by the vascular endothelial cells and then directed to lysosomes where they are degraded. They are then transported into the circulation (Ternant and Paintaud, 2005). The concentration of infliximab is variable in individual patients and this influences this clinical response. It is thought that this is in part due to the development of antibodies in some patients that are directed towards infliximab. The antibodies have been found in patients where the medication is not administered regularly. Hence the prescribed regime must be adhered to if it is to be effective. The effect of these antibodies is threefold: infusion reaction are more likely, lower infliximab trough levels and reduced duration of effect (Cameron et al., 2015). The use of concomitant immunosuppressant therapy is advised as this is thought to counteract the development of antibodies (Kammermeier et al., 2016).

Infliximab is administered intravenously, and hypersensitive reactions have been reported (BNFc, 2020). All children and young people must be observed very closely for the first one-two hour of the infusion and local policy must be adhered to.

This treatment should be continued for a year and then reviewed. If the CYP develops antibodies to it or has a severe hypersensitive reaction, it may need to be discontinued prior to the twelve-month review period.

Episode of Care

Jamal, aged 16 years, has presented with an exacerbation of his Crohn's disease. He is having frequent bouts of bloody diarrhoea – up to 25 episodes per day. He is very pale and lethargic on admission. He is now having severe abdominal pain. He has lost 5 kilos in weight since his last outpatients appointment, which was seven weeks ago. His GP has referred him for urgent review by the Paediatric Gastroenterology team. He is admitted to your ward. During admission he tells you he has been unable to attend school of late as he needs to be in close proximity to the toilet at all times. He is very anxious about this as he is due to do take his GCSEs soon. He is very tearful. He has had numerous admissions to the ward so is well known to the staff. He has had enteral feeding previously and corticosteroids to which he responded to well initially and which did put his Crohn's disease into remission.

He was diagnosed with Crohn's disease 18 months ago. He has had a sub-total colectomy six months ago and he really does not want to have more surgery at this stage as he will be studying for his A levels. He wants to go to university and be 'like all the other young people there'. He knows he is going to need enteral feeding again due to his weight loss. The Gastroenterology team have decided to commence infliximab (dose 5mg/kg, then 5mg/kg two weeks and six weeks after initial dose 5mg/kg every eight weeks (BNF, 2020)). He was having oral mesalazine 2 grams daily prior to this flare-up (maintenance dose for remission).

Conclusion

This chapter has presented an overview of the anatomy and physiology of the GI system. It is important that the nurse, NA and other healthcare workers understand the associated anatomy and physiology if they are to understand the interaction of the medication that the child or young person is prescribed. Some common gastrointestinal disorders of childhood have been presented. The current medication regimes for these conditions, the route of administration and the associated clinical skills have been addressed. Reference to legal, professional and regulatory bodies have been included. The nurse, NA and healthcare professional must always practice in accordance with employer policy and the guidance and frameworks provided by the NMC. Competence in medication management and optimisation of treatment are essential for safe and effective patient-centred care.

Glossary

Atresia: Absence or closure of a natural passage or tube
Apoptosis: death of cells which occur as a normal part of an organism's growth or development.
Bezoars: a mass/bolus that is found in a feeding tube composed of food/medication.
Crohn's disease: a long-term chronic condition characterised by inflammation in the GI tract.

Constipation: infrequent bowel motions and difficulty in passing stools

Diarrhoea: loose, watery bowel stools

Enteral: passing through the intestine either naturally or through artificial means via the mouth or oesophagus.

Fistula: an abnormal connection between two epithelised surfaces.

Fundoplication: Wrapping (plication) of the fundus of the stomach around the lower end of the oesophagus.

Half-life: the time taken for a specific substance in the body to decrease by half.

Monoclonal antibody: a laboratory produce molecule to act as substitute antibodies that can restore, mimic or enhance the immune systems attack on target cells.

Osmotic: the spontaneous movement of molecules through a selective permeable membrane.

Reflux: the flow of fluids through a vessel in the opposite direction to normal.

Peristalsis: involuntary constriction and relaxation of the muscles creating a wave like action.

Pyloric stenosis: thickening of the pylorus causing obstruction of the flow of gastric contents.

Suppository: a solid dose of medication that is administered into the rectum

References

Aronson, J.K., and Ferner, R.E. (2017). Unlicensed and off-label use of medicines: definitions and clarification of terminology. *British Journal of Pharmacology* 83(12): 2615–2625.

Azzouz, L.L. and Sharma, S. (2020). *Physiology: Large Intestines*. Treasure Island, FL: StatPearls Publishing.

Bashir, A., Shadrav, A., and Siza, S. (2020). *Laxatives*. Treasure Island, FL: StatPearls Publishing.

British National Formulary for Children (2020). *British National Formulary for Children*. Basingstoke: RP Publishing.

Cameron, F.L., Wilson, M.L., Basheer, N., et al. (2015). Anti TFN therapy for paediatric IBD. Scottish National Experience. *Archive of Disease of Childhood* 100: 399–405.

Care Quality Commission (2020). *Enteral Feeding and Medicines Administration*. CQC. www.cqc.org.uk (accessed 20 April 2021).

Crohn's & Colitis UK (2020). www.crohnsandcolitis.org.uk (accessed August 2020).

Dogra, H., Lad, B. Sirisena, D. (2011). Paediatric gastro-oesophageal reflux disease. *British Journal of Medical Practitioners* 4(2): 234–241.

Duncan, H., Buchanan, E., Cardigan, T. et al. (2014). A retrospective study showing maintenance treatment options for paediatric CD in the first year following diagnosis after induction of remission with EEN: supplemental enteral nutrition is better than nothing! *BMC Gastroenterol* 14: 50.

Garrick, V., Buchanan, E. Bishop, J. et al. (2011). Specialist nurse and dietician care pathway for exclusive enteral nutrition in paediatric Crohn's Disease – a tertiary experience. *Journal of Pediatric Gastroenterology* 52. (Supplement 2) E2.

Gasior, A.C. and Maltz, R. (2020). Ulcerative colitis and indeterminate colitis in children. In: *Pediatric Colorectal and Pelvic Reconsruction Surgery* (ed. Vilanova-Sánchez, A. and Levitt, M.A.), 193–196. CRC Press. Taylor Francis Group.

Gormley-Fleming, E., Martin, D. (2018). *Children's and Young People's Nursing Skills at a Glance*. Wiley-Blackwell.

Grissinger, M. (2013). Preventing errors when drugs are given via enteral feeding tubes. *P T* 38(10): 575–576.

Heineck, I., Bueno, D., Heydrich, J. (2009). Study on the use of drugs in patients with enteral feeding tubes. *Pharam. World Sci* 31(2): 145–148.

Human Medicines Regulation (2012). *The National Archives*. Legislation.gov.

Kammermeier, J., Morris, M.A., Garrick, V. et al. (2016). Management of Crohn's disease. *Arch Dis Child* 101: 475–480.

Kelly, J. Wright, D. Wood, J. (2011). Medicine administration errors in patients with dysphagia in secondary care – a multi-centre observational study. *Journal of Advanced Nursing* 2615–2627.

Levin, A. and Shibolet, O. (2008). Inflixmab in ulcerative colitis. *Biologicals: Targets and Therapy* 2(3): 379–388.

Litalien, C., Théorêt, Y., and Faure, C. (2005). Pharmacokinetics of proton pump inhibitors in children. *Clinical Pharmacokinetics* 44(5): 441–466.

Liu, L.W. (2011). Chronic constipation: current treatment options. *Can. J. Gasterenterol*. Oct 25. Supplement B. 22–28.

Marks, D.B. (2016). Time to halt the over prescription of proton pump inhibitors. *Clinical Pharmacist* August 2016.

Marieb, E.N. and Hoehn, K. (2019). *Human Anatomy and Physiology*, 11e. San Francisco, CA: Pearson International.

Moo Shin, J. and Kim, N. (2013). Pharmacokinetics and Pharmacodynamics of the Proton Pump Inhibitors. *Journal of Neurogastroenterology and Motility* 19(1) 25–35.

National Institute for Health and Care Excellence (2015). *Gastro-oesophageal Reflux Disease in Children and Young People: Diagnosis and Management*. NICE.

National Institute for Health and Care Excellence (2018). *Constipation in Children and Young People: Diagnosis and Management. Clinical Guideline (CG99)*. NICE.

Chapter 11 Medications Used in the Gastrointestinal System

National Institute for Health and Care Excellence (2019a). Clinical Knowledge Summary: Constipation in Children. https://cks.nice.org.uk/topics/constipation/ (accessed August 2020).

National Institute for Health and Care Excellence (2019b). *Crohn's Disease Management. Clinical Guideline NG129*. NICE.

National Patient Safety Agency (NPSA) (2011). Patient Safety Alert NPSA/2011/PSA002 Reducing the harm caused by misplaced nasogastric feeding tubes in adults, children and infants. London: NPSA.

Nettina, S.M (2010). *Lippincott Manual of Nursing Practice*, 9e. Philadelphia, PA: Wolter Kluwer.

NHS Improvement (2016). Nasogastric tube misplacement: continued risk of death and severe harm. Patient Safety. http://improvement.nhs.uk/resources/patient-safety-alerts (accessed 20 April 2021).

Nursing and Midwifery Council (2018a). *The Code: Professional Standards of Practice and Behaviour for Nurses, Midwives and Nursing Associates*. London: NMC.

Nursing and Midwifery Council (2018b). *Standards of Proficiency for Nursing Associates*. London: NMC.

Nursing and Midwifery Council (2018c). *Future Nurse: Standards of Proficiency for Registered Nurses*. London: NMC.

Nursing and Midwifery Council (2018d). *Realising Professionalism: Standards for Education and Training*. London: NMC.

NHS Improvement (2016). *Resource Set. Initial Placement Checks for Nasogastric and Orogastric Tubes*. Leeds: NHS Improvement.

Peate, I. and Gormley-Fleming, E. (2015). *Fundamentals of Children's Anatomy and Physiology: A Textbook for Nursing and Healthcare Students*. Wiley-Blackwell.

Peate, I. and Gormley-Fleming. E. (2021). *Fundamentals of Children's Anatomy and Physiology: A Textbook for Nursing and Healthcare Students*, 2nd edition. Oxford: Wiley-Blackwell.

Rudolf, M., Lee, T., Levene, M. (2011). *Paediatrics and Child Health*, 3e. Oxford: Wiley Blackwell Publishing.

Sachs, G., Shin, J.M., and Howden, C.W (2006). Review article: the clinical pharmacology of proton pump inhibitors. *Alimentary Pharmacology and Therapeutics* 23(Supp 2): 2–8.

Tack, J. and Müller-Lissner, S. (2009). Treatment of chronic constipation: current pharmacological approaches and future directions. *Clin. Gastroenterol. Hepatol.* 7(5) 502–508.

Ternant, D., and Paintaud, G. (2005). Pharmokinetics and concentration effects relationships of therapeutic monoclonal antibodies and fusion proteins. *Expert Opinion Biological therapies* 5(Supplement 1): S37–47.

Ternant, D., Aubourg, A., Beuzelin, C.M. et al. (2008). Infliximab Pharmokinetics in Inflammatory Bowel Disease Patients. *Therapeutic Drug Monitoring* 30(4): 523–529.

Terry, D. and Sinclair, A. (2012). Prescribing for children at the interfaces of care. Arch Dis *Child Educ Pract Ed.* 97(4): 152–156.

White, R. and Bradnam, V. (2015). *Handbook of Drug Administration via Enteral Feeding Tubes*, 3e. London: Pharmaceutical Press.

Wright, D., Griffith, R., Merriman, H. et al. (2019). Medication management of patients with nasogastric (NG), percutaneous gastrostomy (PEG), or other enteral feeding tube. Guideline.

Further Resources

Peate, I. and Gormley-Fleming, E. (2015). *Fundamentals of Children's Anatomy and Physiology: A Textbook for Nursing and Healthcare Students*. Oxford: Wiley Blackwell.

Gormley-Fleming, E. and Peate, I. (2019). *The Fundamentals of Applied Pathophysiology: Child. An Essential Guide for Nursing and Healthcare Students*. Wiley.

British National Formulary for Children (2020).

NICE clinical guidelines:

National Institute for Health and Care Excellence (2015). *Gastro-oesophageal Reflux Disease in Children and Young People: Diagnosis and Management*. NICE.

National Institute for Health and Care Excellence. (2018). *Constipation in Children and Young People: Diagnosis and Management. Clinical Guideline (CG99)*. NICE.

National Institute for Health and Care Excellence (2019). *Crohn's Disease Management. Clinical Guideline NG129*. NICE.

Multiple Choice Questions

1. Pharmacokinetics is the branch of pharmacology that:
- **(a)** Details how the drug is manufactured
- **(b)** Determines the dose and frequency of administration
- **(c)** Identifies the movement of the drug into and out of the body
- **(d)** Identifies the side effects and interactions with other medication.

Chapter 11 Medications Used in the Gastrointestinal System

2. Increased sympathetic nervous stimulation in the gastrointestinal tract may cause:
(a) Constipation
(b) Diarrhoea
(c) Pain
(d) Flatulence

3. A long-term side effect of Proton Pump Inhibitors is:
(a) Weight gain
(b) Uric acid retention
(c) Osteoporosis
(d) Gastric ulceration

4. Patients who have oesophagitis should be prescribed Proton Pump Inhibitors for:
(a) Life long
(b) 4–8 weeks
(c) As instructed by the manufacturers
(d) Discontinues as soon as the symptoms disappear.

5. Is there a drug interaction between PPIs and NSAIDs?
(a) Yes
(b) No
(c) Only when taken on an empty stomach
(d) Occasionally if medication is crushed

6. PPIs are absorbed in the:
(a) Duodenum
(b) Ileum
(c) Jejunum
(d) Stomach

7. Medication that needs to be crushed to administer via a nasogastric tube is
(a) Off-label
(b) Licensed
(c) Unlicensed
(d) Legal

8. When administering medication via an enteral feeding tube the
(a) Drugs can be administered all at once
(b) Can be added to the enteral feed
(c) Be administered immediately after the feed has been stopped
(d) Must be administered individually, must never be added to feeds and must wait sufficient time after the feed has stopped before administering.

9. Infliximab belongs to which drug group?
(a) Corticosteroid
(b) Immunosupresant
(c) Aminosalicylate
(d) Biological

10. Receptors are:
(a) Located on the outer membrane of the cell
(b) Are deactivated by drugs
(c) Permits the drug entry via diffusion
(d) Not drug specific

11. The best time of day to administer omeprazole is:
(a) Morning
(b) Morning or evening
(c) Evening
(d) Does not matter-anytime of day

12. Idiopathic constipation is most likely caused by:
(a) Congenital defects
(b) Immobility
(c) No known cause
(d) Inadequate nutrition.

Chapter 11 Medications Used in the Gastrointestinal System

13. Children and young people who are treated with glucocorticoids should:
   (a) Have a short course only
   (b) Taper the dose before cessation
   (c) Take them with food
   (d) Stop them when they start to feel better
14. Osmotic laxatives:
   (a) Are metabolised by the bacteria in the intestines
   (b) Are metabolised by the liver
   (c) Absorbed by the microvilli
   (d) Absorbed in the lumen of the large bowel.
15. Glycerine suppositories should be inserted into the anus
   (a) Blunt end first
   (b) Pointed tip first
   (c) Does not matter
   (d) They are not recommended for children

Find Out More

The following is a list of conditions that are associated with the gastrointestinal tract. Take some time and write notes about each of the conditions. Think about the medications that may be used in order to treat these conditions and be specific about the pharmacokinetics and pharmacodynamics. Remember to include aspects of patient care. If you are making notes about people you have offered care and support to, you must ensure that you have adhered to the rules of confidentiality.

Coeliac disease

Gastro-oesophageal reflux

Crohn's disease

Ulcerative colitis

Hirschsprung's disease

Appendicitis

Gastroenteritis

Trachea-oesophageal fistula

Constipation

Pyloric stenosis

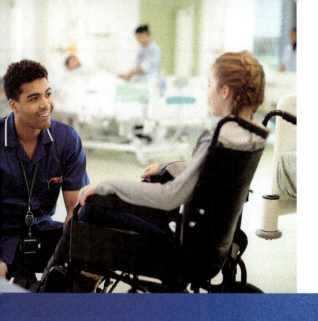

12

Medications Used in the Nervous System

Sophie Gilmour-Ivens

Aim
The aim of this chapter is to provide the reader with an introduction to some of the common neurological conditions affecting Children and Young People (CYP) and to explore the pharmacological therapies utilised in their management.

Learning Outcomes
After reading this chapter the reader will:
- Have gained an understanding of the causes of common neurological disorders
- Explain the use, side effects and contraindications, of medications used in the management of common neurological conditions
- Understand the current evidence base underpinning key recommendations of pharmacological management of common neurological conditions
- Appreciate the importance of family/carer involvement in managing neurological conditions effectively

Fundamentals of Pharmacology for Children's Nurses, First Edition. Edited by Ian Peate and Peter Dryden.
© 2022 John Wiley & Sons Ltd. Published 2022 by John Wiley & Sons Ltd.
Companion website: www.wiley.com/go/pharmacologyforCN

Chapter 12 Medications Used in the Nervous System

Test Your Knowledge

1. Why should sodium valproate be avoided in females of childbearing potential?
2. What antiepileptic drugs are recommended in the acute management of a seizure?
3. What are the two main treatments used in the management of Guillain–Barré Syndrome?
4. Why are drugs that avoid the gastrointestinal system of benefit in the acute treatment of migraine?
5. When would a preventative migraine treatment be considered for a young person?

Introduction

The nervous system is the major controlling, regulatory and communicating system in the body. The central nervous system is made up of the brain and spinal cord and the peripheral nervous system is made up of nerves that branch off from the spinal cord and extend to all parts of the body (Figure 12.1)

A neurological disorder is one that affects the nervous system and results in physical and/or psychological symptoms. There are over 470 neurological conditions (Brain & Spine Foundation, 2020) and the cause can be congenital (present at birth) or acquired later in childhood.

The focus of this chapter will be on the pharmacological management of just three neurological conditions that affect CYP: epilepsy, migraine and Guillain–Barré Syndrome. Each section will include an overview of

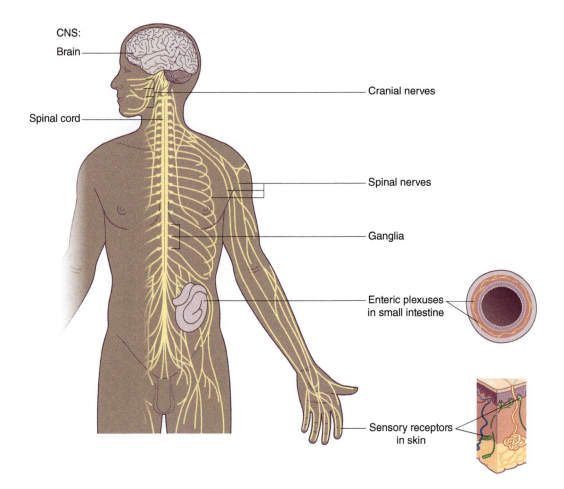

Figure 12.1 The main parts of the nervous system. *Source*: Ian Peate et al. 2014/John Wiley & Sons.

the neurological disorder, how medications work to treat the disorder and consideration of other issues important to managing the disorder effectively.

Epilepsy

Epilepsy is a condition defined by a person having at least two unprovoked seizures occurring >24 hours apart; the probability of further seizures occurring over the next 10 years and or diagnosis of an epilepsy syndrome (Fisher et al., 2014). In United Kingdom (UK), approximately one in every 220 CYP has a diagnosis of epilepsy (Epilepsy Action, 2018).

Normal human brain function involves communication between millions of neurons (nerve cells). Each neuron consists of a cell body and branches called axons and dendrites which join other neurons at junctions called synapses (Figure 12.2). Electrical signals, resulting from ion (sodium, potassium or calcium) currents in the cell membrane are sent from the cell body via the axon to the synapse. Chemical signals (neurotransmitters) jump across the synaptic gap between neurons and connect to the receptor site of the adjoining neuron. Neurotransmitters are either excitatory (excite the joining neuron to send another electrical signal) or inhibitory (inhibit electrical signals passing down that neuron) and it is by these electrical and chemical pathways that neurons within the brain communicate and normal function is maintained.

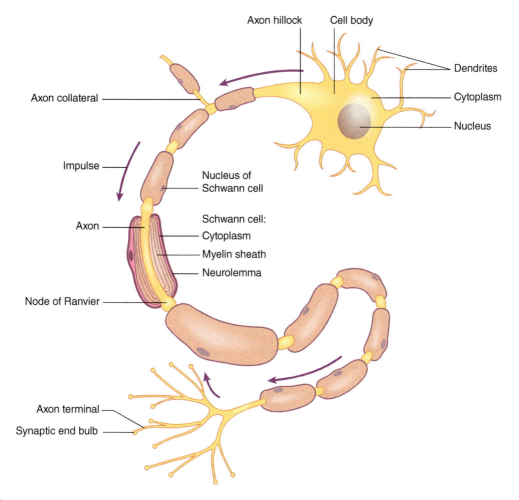

Figure 12.2 A neuron. *Source:* Ian Peate et al. 2014/John Wiley & Sons.

Focal Onset		Generalised Onset	Unknown Onset
Aware	**Impaired Awareness**	**Motor** Atonic Clonic Epileptic spasms Myoclonic Myoclonic-atonic Myoclonic-tonic-clonic Tonic Tonic-clonic	**Motor** Epileptic Spasms Tonic-clonic
Motor Onset Automatisms Atonic Clonic Epileptic Spasms Hyperkinetic Myoclonic Tonic			**Nonmotor** Behaviour arrest
Nonmotor Onet Aytonomic Behaviour arrest Cognitive Emotional Sensory		**Nonmotor (absence)** Atypical Eyelid myoclonia Myoclonic Typical	**Unclassified**

Figure 12.3 **Classification of seizure types.** *Source*: Adapted from Fisher et al. 2017.

If an imbalance occurs between the excitatory and inhibitory circuits in the brain, neurons will cease to communicate in an ordered fashion and 'fire-off' in an abnormal way; causing a transient occurrence of signs and/or symptoms known as an epileptic seizure.

Epileptic seizures are categorised by where in the brain they start and can be described as 'focal' or 'generalised' (Figure 12.3). Focal seizures can start in a small area of one lobe or a wider area in one hemisphere and they are described as either 'focal aware' seizures if the person remains conscious or 'focal impaired awareness' seizures if the person's consciousness is affected. They are further classified by whether they have 'motor onset' (seizures with physical movement) or 'non-motor onset' (seizures without physical movement but involving behaviour arrest, autonomic, cognitive, sensory or emotional symptoms). Generalised seizures affect both cerebral hemispheres and consciousness is always lost, albeit briefly for some seizures. Again, these are classified as being either 'motor' or 'non-motor' seizures.

When a focal seizure spreads to involve wider brain networks, this is known as a 'focal to bilateral tonic-clonic seizure' and the resulting seizure will have tonic (stiff) and clonic (rhythmical jerking) features. There is an 'unknown' category to describe seizures where the exact location of onset within the brain is not known.

Antiepileptic Drugs (AEDs)

Although there are non-pharmacological treatments for epilepsy (Vagal Nerve Stimulation (VNS), ketogenic diet and surgery), the mainstay of treatment is medication. AEDs work either by decreasing excitation or enhancing inhibition within the brain. This can be achieved by modifying electrical activity in neurons by affecting ion (sodium, potassium, calcium, chloride) channels in the cell membrane or by affecting neurotransmitters (glutamate and gamma-aminobutyric acid (GABA)) in order to alter chemical transmission between neurons. The mechanism of action of some AEDs is not yet fully understood.

AEDs have been used since 1857 when potassium bromide was used to treat 15 women with 'hysterical' epilepsy (an outdated term for epilepsy related to menstruation) (Brodie, 2010) and there are currently 28 AEDs used regularly in UK in the treatment of childhood epilepsy. AEDs are taken once or twice daily, usually orally or via an enteral feeding tube unless a CYP is nil by mouth, when some AEDs can be given intravenously.

The aim of epilepsy treatment is for a CYP to take the fewest number of AEDs, at the lowest dose possible in order to achieve seizure control with the fewest side effects. Approximately 70% of people with epilepsy will become seizure-free with the right medication.

Chapter 12 Medications Used in the Nervous System

AED choice should be individualised according to the seizure type, epilepsy syndrome, co-medication and comorbidity, the CYP's lifestyle and preferences of the CYP and their family and/or carers (NICE, 2020) as this will achieve concordance and improve adherence, thereby maximising seizure control.

Clinical Consideration

How to Prescribe AEDs for CYP

AEDs are prescribed by weight in CYP and each drug will have a range of doses (mg per kg per day) that are considered to be effective.

Starting drugs at the lower end of the range and increasing slowly enables seizure control to be achieved at the lowest dose possible and minimise side effects. Rapid escalation is more likely to be associated with dose-related side effects and families can lose faith in a medication before its efficacy has been fully established.

Clinical Consideration

Branded and Generic Drugs

Some AEDs should always be prescribed by brand name rather than generic substitutions, which could affect the bio-equivalency of the drug and reduce the therapeutic effect, resulting in seizures or increase side effects.

More information can be found here: www.gov.uk/drug-safety-update/antiepileptic-drugs-updated-advice-on-switching-between-different-manufacturers-products.

Sodium Valproate

Sodium valproate (VPA) is an AED with a mixed mechanism of action and is currently licensed for the treatment of all types of epileptic seizures from birth onwards. The wide range of formulations (oral solution and oral syrup (200mg/5ml), tablets, gastro-resistant tablets, prolonged-release tablets, capsules, granules, chronospheres (modified-release granules), and solution for injection or infusion) means that VPA is suitable for all ages and can be administered via a nasogastric tube or gastrostomy device and intravenously for CYP who are nil by mouth. The prolonged-release tablets, granules and chronospheres can be taken once daily which may improve adherence and the granules and chronospheres come as single sachets which are more portable than a bottle of liquid or box of tablets, for overnight stays outside the home.

The maintenance dose of VPA for CYP 1 month to 11 years is 25–30mg/kg daily in 2 divided doses and doses up to 60mg/kg daily may be used in infantile spasms (BNFc, 2019). For CYP 12–17 years, the maintenance dose is 1–2g daily in 2 divided doses; maximum 2.5g per day (BNFc, 2019).

After oral administration VPA is absorbed in the gastrointestinal tract, 15–60 minutes after oral solution or syrup; 1–4 hours after tablets and 3–7.5 hours after enteric tablets (prolonged or modified release) (Beatriz and Fagundes, 2008). It is metabolised by glucuronidation, β oxidation in the mitochondria and cytochrome P450 (CYP)-mediated oxidation (Ghodke-Puranika et al., 2013) and 30–50% is excreted in urine. The half-life is 8–15 hours, or 5–12 hours in patients taking concomitant enzyme-inducing drugs (drugs that induce liver enzymes and increase the metabolism of other drugs).

There is a link between maternal VPA use and foetal abnormalities. Approximately 10% of babies born to females taking VPA during pregnancy will have a congenital malformation and approximately 30–40% of CYP will have neurodevelopmental problems. There is also a link between maternal sodium valproate use and autism spectrum disorders and attention deficit hyperactivity disorder (ADHD) (Medicines and Healthcare products Regulatory Agency, 2019).

The Medicines and Healthcare products Regulatory Agency (MHRA)'s current position is that VPA should only be used in females of childbearing age (a pre-menopausal female who is capable of becoming pregnant) if other treatments are ineffective or not tolerated and when VPA is prescribed, females must be enrolled in the pregnancy prevention programme called 'Prevent'.

Lamotrigine

Lamotrigine (LTG) is a sodium channel blocker and may also inhibit the excitatory neurotransmitter glutamate. It is used to treat focal seizures, generalised tonic-clonic seizures and seizures associated with an

Chapter 12 Medications Used in the Nervous System

epileptic encephalopathy called Lennox–Gastaut syndrome, where the epilepsy adversely affects development. LTG is available as tablets and dispersible tablets for CYP unable to swallow tablets. The dispersible tablets can also be chewed and used with a nasogastric tube/gastrostomy device as they do not interact with enteral feeds.

After oral administration LTG is rapidly and completely absorbed from the gut with no significant first-pass metabolism. Peak plasma concentrations occur after approximately 2.5 hours and metabolism is predominantly in the liver by glucuronidation, with less than 10% excreted unchanged in the urine. The half-life of lamotrigine is 15–35 hours (Patsalos, 2013). However, this is reduced by other glucuronidation-inducing medications and increased to approximately 70 hours when co-administered with VPA (Medicines. org, 2020).

Up to 10% of patients taking LTG develop a rash, usually within the first eight weeks of treatment. The risk is 10 times higher in CYP than adults and rash is the most commonly reported adverse event (Egunsola et al., 2015). 1% of CYP with LTG rash require hospitalisation and life-threatening severe cutaneous adverse reactions such as Stevens–Johnson syndrome have been reported in relation to LTG. LTG must be stopped if a rash occurs.

Research suggests that lamotrigine can lower progestogen but not oestrogen blood levels in females taking the combined oral contraceptive pill. However, there is currently no conclusive evidence that lamotrigine reduces the effectiveness of the Pill. The combined contraceptive pill can reduce LTG blood levels and this could lead to reduced seizure control therefore any young woman taking LTG and considering contraceptive choices should be seen by a specialist.

Levetiracetam

Levetiracetam (LEV) is indicated for monotherapy of focal seizures with or without secondary generalisation (where a focal seizure evolves into a bilateral tonic-clonic seizure) in 16- to 17-year-olds; for adjunctive treatment of focal seizures with or without secondary generalisation in CYP aged 1 month to 17 years; and for adjunctive treatment of myoclonic seizures and tonic-clonic seizures in young people aged 12–17 years (BNFc, 2019). The maintenance dose of LEV is 60mg/kg/day (BNFc, 2019). However, in practice some clinicians use higher doses with good efficacy and in cases of accidental overdose, doses of 300mg/kg/day have not resulted in toxicity (Yayici Köken et al., 2019).

LEV has a unique mechanism of action as it binds to SV2A, a synaptic vesicle glycoprotein, inhibits pre-synaptic calcium channels and reduces neurotransmitter release. This is believed to inhibit impulse conduction across synapses however the exact mechanism by which LEV exerts its anticonvulsant effect is still under investigation.

LEV is rapidly and almost completely absorbed following oral administration, resulting in a bioavailability of more than 95% and time to peak plasma concentration is approximately 1 hour in babies and CYP below 12 years and 1.3 hours in adolescents (Medicines.org.uk, 2019a). The elimination half-life is 5–7 hours and steady state in blood is reached 24–48 hours after initiation of treatment (Patsalos, 2004).

LEV is available as tablets, granules, oral solution and concentrate for solution for infusion. This range of formulations makes it suitable for all ages as well as being able to be administered via an enteral feeding tube and intravenously for CYP who are nil by mouth. Desitrend® granules can be sprinkled on to a spoonful of cold food such as yoghurt for CYP who cannot swallow tablets or tolerate the taste of the oral solution.

The most common adverse events with LEV are somnolence, asthenia (abnormal physical weakness or lack of energy), dizziness and headache. However, in CYP and adolescents, behavioural adverse events (BAEs) including irritability, aggression, depression and suicidal ideation are also a significant issue.

When LEV-related BAEs are intolerable one option is to switch the child to brivaracetam (BRV) which is an analogue of LEV, with a similar mechanism of action. BRV has similar common adverse effects to LEV (somnolence, dizziness, fatigue, nausea and irritability). However, 93.1% patients switched to BRV had clinically meaningful reductions in BAEs (Yates et al., 2015).

The maintenance dose of BRV in CYP 4–17 years below 50kg is 1 mg/kg twice daily (max. per dose 2 mg/kg twice daily) (BNFc, 2019) therefore a child who is taking 40mg/kg/day of LEV could be swapped immediately to BRV 4mg/kg/day due to the close relationship between the two drugs.

Another option is to introduce pyridoxine (vitamin B6) alongside LEV. It is unclear how pyridoxine improves BAEs. However, 83.3% of CYP aged 2 to 10 years supplemented with an average dose of 7mg/kg/day (maximum dose 350 mg/day) had their behavioural symptoms controlled (Miller, 2002); and with smaller doses of 100mg pyridoxine daily, 93.3% patients remained on LEV as they had significant improvement in their BAEs (Sajja et al., 2017).

Cannabidiol

One of the newest AEDs is medical-grade cannabidiol (CBD), marketed in the UK as Epidyolex. It is derived from the Cannabis sativa plant and does not contain any tetrahydrocannabinol, the psychoactive chemical compound in marijuana. Epidyolex was commissioned by NHS England in January 2020 for the treatment of seizures in adults and CYP ≥ 2 years of age with Dravet Syndrome and Lennox–Gastaut Syndrome, in combination with clobazam (CLB).

Dravet syndrome (DS) and Lennox–Gastaut Syndrome (LGS) are both epileptic encephalopathies, where the presence of frequent epileptiform activity adversely impacts development, typically causing regression or slowing of developmental skills, and usually associated with frequent seizures.

Myoclonic, focal and generalised tonic-clonic seizures (GTCS) are most commonly seen in DS and in trials of Epidyolex more than 40% of patients with DS had convulsive seizure-frequency reductions of ≥50% (Devinsky et al., 2018). Tonic, atonic and atypical absence seizures are seen most regularly in LGS and patients taking Epidyolex had a reduction from baseline in 'drop' (tonic and atonic) seizure frequency of 48% to 60%. (Thiele et al., 2019). In both groups >80% of patients/caregivers reported an improvement in the patients' overall condition.

CBD has been shown to act on multiple molecular targets which play a key role in neuronal excitability however the exact mechanism of anticonvulsant action is not yet fully understood (Sekar and Pack, 2019). Co-administration of CBD and CLB leads to increased plasma levels of active metabolites of both drugs which may result in enhanced anticonvulsant effects, but the CLB dose may need to be reduced if increased plasma levels lead to the emergence of adverse effects.

Epidyolex is available as a strawberry-flavoured oral solution 100mg/ml. After administration it reaches maximum plasma concentration within 2.5 to 5 hours; is metabolised in the liver and the gut (primarily in the liver) by CYP2C19 and CYP3A4 enzymes; the half-life in plasma is 56 to 61 hours and it is excreted in faeces (Epidiolex.com 2020).

The most common adverse events are diarrhoea, pyrexia, decreased appetite and somnolence (Devinsky et al., 2018). However, status epilepticus and suicidal behaviours/ideation are also associated with CBD use. Epidyolex can cause dose-related elevations of liver enzymes, particularly in patients also taking VPA, therefore serum transaminases and total bilirubin levels should be monitored for the first 6 months after initiation of treatment (Medicines.org.uk 2019b), if a patient becomes symptomatic or if drugs are added that are known to be hepatotoxic.

There has been a lot of interest in Epidyolex from families of CYP with other epilepsy syndromes or unclassified, intractable epilepsy. However, currently it is not available to any child except those with DS and LGS.

Episode of Care

Sally is 5 years old. She had an intracranial haemorrhage in utero and has focal seizures, hydrocephalus and a left hemiplegia. She has a learning difficulty and attends main stream school with one-to-one support.

Sally weighs 22kg.

Sally had tried four AEDs but continued to have seizures therefore she was started on lacosamide.

The maintenance dose of lacosamide is 6–12mg/kg/day and Sally was advised to increase the dose using the following plan:

- 20mg twice daily for 2 weeks
- 40mg twice daily for 2 weeks
- 60mg twice daily for 2 weeks
- 80mg twice daily to continue

When Sally increased the dose from 20mg twice daily to 40mg twice daily, she started experiencing nausea, vomiting and dizziness (all of which are common side effects of lacosamide) and because of her pre-existing hemiplegia the dizziness meant she was falling several times a day and had sustained minor injuries. She was unable to attend school as she was vomiting and there were concerns that she could injure herself during a fall so Sally's mum, Alison, had to take time off work.

Alison spoke to the epilepsy specialist nurse and they negotiated slowing down the lacosamide dose increases to 10mg every 2 weeks instead of 20mg.

This reduced Sally's nausea and she no longer felt dizzy or fell over. She was able to return to school a week later and Alison returned to work.

Emergency Medications

Convulsive status epilepticus (CSE) is the most common life-threatening neurological emergency in CYP, with an incidence of 20 per 100,000 CYP per year. CSE occurs when a seizure does not stop spontaneously and the current International League Against Epilepsy (ILAE, 2014) definition of CSE gives two time points:

- (t1) is the time period after which the seizure should be considered 'continuous seizure activity'
- (t2) is the time after which there is a risk from ongoing seizure activity of long-term consequences such as neuronal death or injury, and functional deficits

For generalised convulsive seizures t1 is 5 minutes and t2 is 30 minutes therefore convulsive seizures are usually treated at 5 minutes.

Medicines used to treat CSE are referred to as 'rescue' or 'emergency' medications. Benzodiazepines (diazepam, lorazepam, midazolam), which enhance the inhibitory action of the neurotransmitter gamma-aminobutyric acid (GABA), are traditionally regarded as first line medications and the choice of medication and route of administration will be determined by a child's location, presence or absence of venous access, response to previous use, or existing sensitivity or allergy.

Any child who has 'rescue' medication should have an Individualised epilepsy care plan which moves between settings (home/school/hospital) with them and contains details of the child's epilepsy syndrome (if known), description of their seizures and when to administer rescue medication. The plan should be reviewed at least annually (NICE, 2020).

Drugs that are suitable for use out of hospital without venous access are buccal midazolam, buccal lorazepam, rectal diazepam and rectal paraldehyde. The ambulance service uses rectal diazepam. However, this is less effective than buccal midazolam at achieving and maintaining seizure cessation (Sánchez Fernández et al., 2017; Moretti et al., 2019) and also less socially acceptable, therefore most CYP will be given buccal midazolam for use in the community.

Buccal midazolam is given via a syringe into the space between the cheek and the gums and onto the buccal mucosa (the inner lining of the cheeks and the back of the lips) where it is absorbed through the network of capillaries and enters the systemic circulation (Figure 12.4).

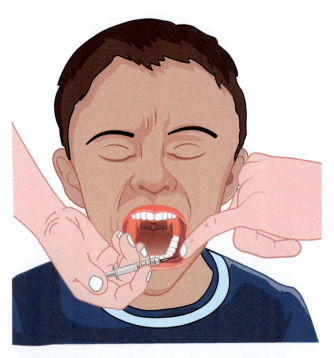

Figure 12.4 CYP buccal administration. *Source:* Redrawn from Medicines for Children, 2017.

Chapter 12 Medications Used in the Nervous System

Buccal lorazepam is given in the same way, via a syringe, as buccal midazolam. Lorazepam is associated with a much lower risk of seizure recurrence than midazolam, with duration of anticonvulsant effect of 24–48 h (Anderson, 2011) and therefore it may be preferable for CYP who have multiple seizures every day and want a longer break between seizures in order to improve quality of life.

The most common and clinically relevant side effect of benzodiazepine use is respiratory depression, therefore families/carers would be advised to ring 999 if they were using 'rescue' medication for the first time and not to repeat the dose of 'rescue' medication if the seizure did not terminate. The exception to this is if the young person has an epilepsy care plan which prescribes an additional dose or an alternative drug in addition to a benzodiazepine.

Another drug that is effective and safe in treating CSE out of hospital is rectal paraldehyde. The precise mechanism of action of paraldehyde is unknown. However, it is a central nervous system depressant and is effective in terminating over 60% of convulsive seizures within 10 minutes of its administration (Rowland et al., 2009). It does not cause respiratory depression at therapeutic doses and is therefore useful for treating CYP who have had previous respiratory depression following a benzodiazepine, who have a benzodiazepine allergy or for whom benzodiazepines are ineffective at curtailing seizures.

It comes as a premixed solution of paraldehyde in olive oil in equal volumes and is given at a dose of 0.8ml/kg (maximum 20ml). Approximately 70 to 90% of a dose of paraldehyde is hepatically metabolised. Unmetabolised paraldehyde (11 to 28%) is excreted via exhalation and trace amounts are excreted in the urine.

Paraldehyde is contraindicated in CYP with colitis as it is a rectal irritant and in CYP with severe hepatic insufficiency as altered metabolism may result in higher blood levels and increased side effects.

Once a child is in hospital and venous access has been established, the most commonly used drugs are intravenous (IV) lorazepam, phenytoin and phenobarbital (see NICE guideline Table 12.1).

Recently there have been trials comparing IV levetiracetam (LEV) to the more commonly used drugs. No significant difference in efficacy was found between IV LEV and IV lorazepam however patients given IV LEV had significantly lower need for ventilatory assistance (Chu et al., 2020). Adverse reactions were less frequent in CYP treated with LEV than phenytoin and because LEV is administered more rapidly (5–10 min) than phenytoin (a minimum of 20 min), earlier termination of CSE may be achieved (Lyttle et al., 2019).

Table 12.1 Treating convulsive status epilepticus.

Time		
0 mins (1st step)	Seizure starts. Check ABC, high flow O_2 if available. Check blood glucose.	Confirm clinically that it is an epileptic seizure.
5 mins (2nd step)	Midazolam 0.5 mg/kg buccally or Lorazepam 0.1 mg/kg if intravenous access established	Midazolam may be given by parents, carers or ambulance crew in non-hospital setting.
15 mins (3rd step)	Lorazepam 0.1 mg/kg intravenously	This step should be in hospital. Call for senior help. Start to prepare phenytoin for 4th step. Re-confirm it is an epileptic seizure.
25 mins (4th step)	Phenytoin 20 mg/kg by intravenous infusion over 20 mins or (if on regular phenytoin) Phenobarbital 20 mg/kg intravenously over 5 mins	Paraldehyde 0.8 ml/kg of mixture may be given after start of phenytoin infusion as directed by senior staff. Inform intensive care unit and/or senior anaesthetist.
45 mins (5th step)	Rapid sequence induction of anaesthesia using thiopental sodium 4 mg/kg intravenously	Transfer to paediatric intensive care unit.

When the protocol is initiated it is important to consider what prehospital treatment has been received and to modify the protocol accordingly.

Source: NICE 2020/Public domain

Chapter 12 Medications Used in the Nervous System

If treatment with IV phenytoin, phenobarbital or levetiracetam does not terminate the seizure, the child would require rapid sequence induction with anaesthetic agent thiopental sodium and transfer to a paediatric intensive care unit (PICU) for ongoing management.

Guillain–Barré Syndrome

Guillain–Barré Syndrome (GBS) is a rapidly progressive flaccid tetraparesis (weakness or paralysis of all four limbs with reduced muscle tone) with reduced reflexes and an increased protein level (> 45mg/dL) without an increased white blood cell count (< 10 cells/mm³) in the cerebrospinal fluid (CSF). It is an autoimmune condition that results from T and B cell activated immune response to a preceding infection; it usually occurs 2–4 weeks after a gastroenteritis or respiratory illness and is the most common cause of acute flaccid paralysis in healthy CYP. GBS has an incidence of 1–2/100,000 CYP each year. The most common type of GBS is acute inflammatory demyelinating polyradiculoneuropathy (AIDP). In AIDP myelin, the covering that protects axons and promotes the efficient transmission of nerve impulses is damaged by the immune response.

Infections linked to GBS are campylobacter jejuni, cytomegalovirus (CMV), human immunodeficiency virus (HIV), variola virus (smallpox), mycoplasma pneumoniae, herpes simplex virus (HSV), varicella zoster virus (chickenpox), Zika virus and Epstein–Barr virus (glandular fever). GBS can also be associated with vaccination with rabies vaccine, flu vaccine, polysaccharide meningococcal vaccine, measles vaccine, tetanus toxoid, measles-rubella vaccine, hepatitis B vaccine and oral polio vaccine; and can also be related to bone-marrow transplantation. GBS linked to Campylobacter jejuni infection is associated with a more severe course (Forsyth and Newton, 2018).

GBS starts with bilateral weakness and reduced reflexes in the lower limbs. Weakness typically progresses over hours to a few days and follows an ascending pattern involving trunk, upper limbs and finally bulbar muscles (muscles supplied by the medulla (tongue, pharynx, larynx, sternomastoid and upper trapezius)) and can evolve into muscle paralysis.

GBS involves mainly motor but also sensory and autonomic nerves. Sensory nerve involvement can lead to tingling, numbness and pain, and autonomic nervous system dysfunction can result in abnormal sweating, tachycardia, cardiac arrhythmias and blood pressure instability.

The mortality rate in GBS in CYP is approximately 3–5% (van Doorn, 2008) and deaths are usually related to dysautonomic complications such as respiratory failure, pneumonia and cardiac arrhythmias (Van der Linden et al., 2010; Goodfellow and Willison, 2016).

Respiratory failure occurs in approximately 15% of CYP with GBS and is more likely in CYP whose disease progression has been rapid, are unable to stand and cannot lift their head, have bilateral facial weakness and/or bulbar dysfunction. This would be managed with mechanical ventilation on a Paediatric Intensive Care Unit (PICU).

There are two treatment options for GBS: intravenous immunoglobulin (IVIG) and plasmapheresis/therapeutic plasma exchange (TPE). IVIG is thought to work by blocking antibody production and TPE is believed to work by removing circulating antibodies.

IVIG

Human immunoglobulin is a sterile preparation of concentrated antibodies (immune globulins) recovered from pooled human plasma or serum. Human normal immunoglobulin (HNIG) is prepared from pools of at least 1000 donations of human plasma; it contains immunoglobulin G (IgG) and antibodies to hepatitis A, measles, mumps, rubella, varicella, and other viruses that are currently prevalent in the general population (BNFc, 2019).

IVIG is given as an infusion through a peripheral venous cannula and can be given on a paediatric ward. Common dosing regimens are 0.4gram/kg/day for 5 days; 1gram/kg/day for 2 days; or a single 2gram/kg dose. There is more than one brand of IVIG and the brands are *not* interchangeable therefore once a child has started treatment with one brand, this must be maintained for the duration of their treatment. One brand of IVIG is Octagam® 10%, which contains 100mg human normal immunoglobulin in 1ml and is available as 2g in 20ml; 5g in 50ml; 6g in 60ml; 10g in 100ml; 20g in 200ml and 30g in 300ml (Medicines.org.uk, 2019c). It is stored in a refrigerator (2°C – 8°C) but should be brought to room temperature before being infused.

Octagam® 10% is given via an infusion pump at an initial infusion rate of 0.6ml/kg/hour for 30 minutes and if this is tolerated, the rate of infusion is gradually increased to a maximum of 7.2ml/kg/hour for the remainder of the infusion.

Clinical Consideration

Care of a Child During an IVIG Infusion

Prior to an IVIG infusion a child should have temperature, blood pressure, pulse and respiratory rate monitored and this should be repeated throughout the infusion and for one hour after the first infusion or 20 minutes after subsequent infusions.

As Octagam® has a pH of 4.5–5.0 (very strongly acidic) it may cause tissue damage in the event of extravasation therefore the peripheral cannula site must be monitored closely during the infusion and re-sited at the first signs of inflammation.

Common adverse reactions to IVIG are diarrhoea, dizziness, drowsiness, fatigue, gastrointestinal discomfort, headaches, hypotension, local reaction, myalgia, nausea, pain, skin reactions and the most frequent adverse reaction observed in the paediatric population is headache (Medicines.org.uk, 2019c).

Therapeutic Plasma Exchange

During TPE, a CYP's vascular system is connected to an apheresis device which removes and replaces blood plasma (which contains antibodies causing GBS) with a colloid solution (typically albumin/plasma) or a combination of crystalloid/colloid solution (saline in addition to albumin).

Common adverse reactions to TPE are hypertension, hypotension, pruritis (itching) breathlessness, shivering, dizziness, nausea, cold hands/feet and feeling tired afterwards. Bleeding, infection and allergic reaction to the replacement plasma are more serious but less common complications of TPE.

Medication is also required to manage the symptoms of GBS. CYP can develop bladder and bowel dysfunction and lactulose, a laxative that works by softening the stool, can be used if constipation is an issue.

Pain in GBS is commonly experienced in the limbs, back, head, extremities and abdomen (Yao et al., 2018) and can be radicular pain (pain that radiates from an inflamed or compressed nerve root), muscle pain, dysaesthesia (an abnormal unpleasant sensation felt when touched, caused by damage to peripheral nerves) or pain caused by stiff joints. Analgesics paracetamol and ibuprofen are usually prescribed for mild to moderate pain and oral morphine is prescribed for pain not adequately managed by paracetamol and ibuprofen.

Gabapentin, an anticonvulsant, is used to treat dysaesthesia. The mechanism of action is at the voltage-activated calcium channels in the central nervous system (CNS), but the mode of action in neuropathic pain is still not fully understood. The starting dose is 10mg/kg/24 h (max 300mg) once daily on day 1, twice daily on day 2 then three times daily thereafter, with a maintenance dose of 30–40mg/kg/24 hours. Up to 60mg/kg/24h have been used with benefit (Forsyth and Newton, 2018).

Gabapentin is available as tablets, capsules and oral solution (50mg/ml) and all three formulations are schedule 3 controlled drugs which means they are subject to special prescription requirements. The capsules can be opened and given in water if the oral solution is not available and the bitter taste can be disguised with blackcurrant (Forsyth and Newton, 2018)

Following oral administration, peak plasma gabapentin concentrations are observed within 2 to 3 hours. Gabapentin bioavailability decreases with increasing dose and the bioavailability of a 300mg capsule is approximately 60%. There is no evidence of gabapentin metabolism in humans and it is eliminated unchanged solely by renal excretion. The elimination half-life of gabapentin is independent of dose and averages 5 to 7 hours (Medicines.org.uk, 2019d).

Gabapentin has been associated with a rare risk of severe respiratory depression even without concomitant opioid medicines. Young people with underlying respiratory or neurological disease, renal impairment, and concomitant use of drugs causing central nervous system (CNS) depression may be at higher risk of experiencing severe respiratory depression and these patients may require dose adjustments (BNFc, 2019).

Episode of Care

Sam is 8 years old. He weighs 30kg.

Two weeks previously Sam had a 'cold': cough, sore throat and pyrexia (up to 38.2°C) and he was admitted via the ED after complaining of tingling in his feet and difficulty walking for 2 days. On admission he was unable to stand unaided.

Lumbar puncture confirmed a diagnosis of Guillain–Barré Syndrome and Sam received IVIG 30g daily for two consecutive days on the paediatric ward.

Sam was very distressed with pain during the admission and was prescribed regular paracetamol 370mg 6-hourly and gabapentin 300mg three times daily. He was also prescribed PRN ibuprofen 200mg 3 times daily and oral morphine 6mg 4 times daily.

He was nursed on a pulse oximeter and although he continued to take oral diet and fluids the head of the bed was elevated to 30–45° to minimise the risk of aspiration.

In addition to monitoring Sam's temperature, pulse, respiratory rate and blood pressure, he had -4-hourly peak flow measurements to assess any deterioration in expiratory muscle strength.

Sam did not require admission to the PICU.

Once he moved into the rehabilitation phase of the condition Sam was given daily physiotherapy which included hydrotherapy three times weekly and when he was discharged 4 weeks after admission, he could walk 25 metres unaided and climb stairs with assistance.

Migraine

Migraine is a form of primary headache: a headache that is not the result of an underlying medical condition. The exact cause of migraine is unknown but they are thought to be the result of temporary changes in blood vessels, nerves and chemicals in the brain (NHS, 2019). Migraine affects 12–15% of the world's population and is the second most disabling condition worldwide (Chua et al., 2019). Prior to puberty, migraine is more common in boys than girls, but this changes with the onset of hormonal changes (Straube and Andreou, 2019). Of CYP with primary headache, 50–80% have an affected parent and certain migraine genes have been identified. Psychological triggers can include stress, anxiety, and depression; physiological triggers may include illness and pyrexia, sleep deprivation, fatigue and missing a meal and environmental triggers include lighting, overexertion and participation in sport (Youssef and Mack, 2019).

In CYP and adolescents a diagnosis of migraine is made using the criteria in the International Classification of Headache Disorders 3rd edition (ICDH-3) (2019), which includes: at least five headaches over the last year that last 2–72 hours when untreated, with two out of four additional features (pulsatile quality, unilateral, worsening with activity or limiting activity, moderate to severe in intensity), and association with at least nausea, vomiting, photophobia or phonophobia (increased sensitivity to light or sound) (Oskoui et al., 2019).

Rescue Treatment

Rescue treatment aims to reduce the symptoms of migraine and drugs such as paracetamol and ibuprofen, taken early enough after the onset of headache and before nausea/vomiting become a significant problem, can be effective at treating pain. Ibuprofen at doses up to 10mg/kg/dose has been shown to have superior efficacy than paracetamol therefore paracetamol should be reserved for CYP in whom ibuprofen is contraindicated. Paracetamol is available as effervescent tablets and ibuprofen is available as effervescent granules, both of which are absorbed quickly and have a more rapid effect than non–dispersible tablets. Paracetamol is also available as suppositories for those CYP whose nausea/vomiting prevents oral administration of drugs.

If pain cannot be adequately controlled by over the counter analgesia or a child is unable to tolerate these drugs, a triptan may be prescribed. Triptans are Selective Serotonin 5-HT1-Receptor Agonists which work by stimulating serotonin, a neurotransmitter found in the brain, to reduce inflammation and constrict blood vessels, thereby stopping the migraine. All triptans have a similar molecular structure however their efficacy and tolerability differ due to pharmacokinetic differences between drugs, therefore an alternative should be tried if the first triptan is ineffective or causes side effects. Triptans work best when taken early into a migraine when pain is mild and non-steroidal anti-inflammatory drugs (NSAIDs) have been found to reinforce triptans' effectiveness (Barbanti et al., 2019).

Rizatriptan, sumatriptan and zolmitriptan are triptans indicated for use in CYP. In addition to tablets rizatriptan and zolmitriptan are available as orodispersible tablets which avoid the need for fluids in nauseated CYP and may improve bioavailability as hepatic first-pass metabolism is avoided. Sumatriptan and zolmitriptan are available as a nasal spray which is useful in CYP with nausea/vomiting as it avoids the gastrointestinal system; and sumatriptan is available as solution for injection prefilled pens for subcutaneous use which also avoid the gastrointestinal system.

Due to the triptans' vasoconstrictor action, which can extend beyond the central nervous system, they are contraindicated in CYP with cardiovascular diseases, and because triptans undergo hepatic metabolism they should be avoided in CYP with pre-existing liver conditions. Triptans should also be avoided in anyone being treated for depression with a selective serotonin reuptake inhibitor (SSRI) or monoamine oxidase inhibitor (MAOI) as this combination can lead to serotonin syndrome: a medical emergency characterised by neuromuscular hyperactivity (tremor, hyperreflexia, clonus, myoclonus, rigidity), autonomic dysfunction and altered mental state (agitation, confusion, mania) (BNF, 2019)

An antiemetic (anti-sickness drug) may also be added as part of a rescue treatment plan and because slowed digestion during a migraine can affect drug absorption, prochlorperazine which is available as a buccal tablet and ondansetron, which is available as a suppository, are effective choices. Both are only available on prescription and ondansetron should be prescribed with caution alongside a triptan as both can cause serotonin syndrome.

Preventative Treatments

Preventative treatments for migraine are medications that are taken daily and should be considered when CYP suffers at least two attacks a month; suffers an increasing frequency of headaches; suffers significant disability despite suitable treatment for migraine attacks; or cannot take suitable treatment for migraine attacks (BNFc, 2019).

Beta Blockers

Beta blockers bind to beta-adrenoceptors on cells and thereby block the binding of norepinephrine and epinephrine; resulting in decreased heart rate and blood pressure. Propranolol is widely used in the treatment of paediatric migraine. It can take up to 12 weeks of treatment with propranolol to be effective and after 3 months of treatment with 1mg/kg/day, 62% of patients had ≥ 50% reduction in monthly headache frequency (Fallah et al., 2013).

Propranolol is available as tablets, modified-release capsules and oral solution and after administration is almost completely absorbed from the gastrointestinal tract. It is metabolised in the liver therefore the dose should be reduced in hepatic impairment and the metabolites are excreted in the urine. Peak plasma levels are achieved 1–3 hours after ingestion. Side effects are nausea, dizziness, hypotension, bradycardia, drowsiness or sleep disorders and it should be avoided in CYP with asthma, bronchospasm, hypotension and certain cardiac conditions (heart block/bradycardia).

Clinical Consideration

Propranolol Oral Solution

Propranolol oral solution comes in a range of strengths (5mg/5ml; 10mg/5ml; 40mg/5ml and 50mg/5ml) therefore families should be counselled to check that their previous prescription was for the same strength otherwise this could result in under or overdose.

Overdose can result in life-threatening hypotension and bradycardia.

Calcium Channel Blockers

Calcium channel blockers inhibit the movement of calcium ions across cell membranes and this prevents mechanical contraction of the muscle wall of the artery.

Flunarizine is a calcium channel blocker which is widely prescribed in Europe and is used at specialist CYP's headache clinics. It is not licensed in UK for this indication. There are very few trials of flunarizine use in CYP with migraine but Peer et al. (2012) reported that doses of 5mg to 10mg given once daily resulted in ≥50% reduction in attack frequency in 57% of patients (41/72).

Flunarizine is well absorbed from the gastrointestinal tract, reaching peak plasma concentrations after two to four hours and steady state within 5–6 weeks. It is metabolised in the liver and primarily excreted through faeces via bile. <1% is excreted unchanged in the urine.

Chapter 12 Medications Used in the Nervous System

The most frequent side effects of flunarizine are sedation and weight increase. Depression, mood swings, abdominal pain and nausea are also possible.

Serotonin Modulators

Pizotifen is a serotonin modulator which blocks serotonin (5H-T) receptors in the brain and addresses the pain of migraine attacks by preventing blood vessels in the brain from dilating and contracting.

Pizotifen is also marketed as an appetite stimulant for adults and CYP over 2 with low body weight therefore one of the main side effects experienced by people taking pizotifen for migraine is an increase in appetite and weight; irrespective of dose or the pre-treatment BMI of the child (Briars et al., 2008). The weight gain associated with pizotifen use may make it a less desirable option for a child who is already overweight or any young person keen to avoid weight gain, and a suitable alternative should be chosen.

Pizotifen is available as tablets and special-order manufacturers can supply oral solution. The total daily dose is usually given in divided doses although up to 1mg has been given as a single dose at night. Following oral ingestion pizotifen is absorbed in the gastrointestinal tract and maximum blood levels are reached after 4–5 hours. Metabolism is in the liver mostly through glucuronidation and approximately one third of the dose is excreted in the faeces with the remainder being eliminated as metabolites in the urine.

Antiepileptic Drugs

Topiramate and sodium valproate are indicated in the treatment of paediatric migraine. Both drugs enhance GABAergic inhibition and block excitatory ion channels in the brain however the exact mechanisms by which they are effective in migraine have not been established.

Sodium valproate has been shown to reduce frequency, intensity and duration of migraine episodes by ≥50% in CYP (Ashrafi et al., 2005; Hesami et al., 2018; Amanat et al., 2019) and although there is a lack of evidence for topiramate's efficacy in many trials (Winner et al., 2005; Lakshmi et al., 2007; Lewis et al., 2009; Powers et al., 2017;) Oskoui et al. (2019) found that topiramate was superior to placebo in treating paediatric migraine.

Topiramate is available as tablets, oral suspension and sprinkle capsules; making it possible to administer to CYP of all ages. After oral administration bioavailability is greater than 80%. Maximum plasma levels are reached after 1.3–1.7 hours, the half-life is 19–23 hours and 50%–80% of the drug is excreted unchanged in the urine. Weight loss is a common side effect, as are impaired concentration and cognition, nausea, diarrhoea and paraesthesia.

Topiramate and sodium valproate must be used with caution in girls of childbearing potential as 4% of pregnancies exposed to topiramate and 10.3% of pregnancies exposed to sodium valproate resulted in major congenital malformations (Vossler, 2019) (as previously discussed in the section on Antiepileptic drugs).

Melatonin

Melatonin is a hormone secreted by the pineal gland and its main role is regulating sleep cycles. The level of melatonin may be decreased in migraine headaches and treatment with a synthetic form is thought to be effective due to its anti-inflammatory, hypnotic, analgesic and antioxidative effects (Fallah et al. 2018). Although not widely used. Melatonin 0.3mg/kg once daily at bedtime was found to be safe and effective at reducing headache frequency by ≥50% in 62.5% of CYP aged 5–15 years with migraine (Fallah et al., 2018).

Antidepressant Drugs

Amitriptyline hydrochloride is a tricyclic antidepressant. It works to treat migraine by increasing the level of serotonin neurotransmission by inhibiting its reuptake.

After oral administration amitriptyline is rapidly absorbed from the gastrointestinal tract and maximum plasma levels are reached after approximately 4 hours with steady state reached within a week. It is metabolised in the liver by cytochrome P450 isozymes CYP2D6 and CYP2C19 to the active metabolite nortriptyline and excreted mainly in urine.

Amitriptyline is usually given once daily which usually improves adherence (Srivastava et al., 2013). It is available as tablets which should be swallowed whole and taste bitter if crushed so should be given with jam or fruit juice if the off licence use of crushing them is required. It is also available as an oral liquid which is orange/fruit cup flavoured. Absorption may be decreased by high fibre enteral feeds.

Common side effects are drowsiness, hypotension and antimuscarinic effects (dry mouth, tachycardia, constipation, bladder issues, blurred vision and dilated pupils). Amitriptyline also causes QT interval prolongation therefore must be avoided in CYP with heart block and arrhythmias.

When cognitive behavioural therapy (CBT) was offered alongside amitriptyline treatment to CYP aged 10–17 years, more CYP had a reduction in their headache days per month than those offered headache education plus amitriptyline (Kroner et al., 2016). This highlights the value of non-pharmacological interventions for migraine and as we all CBT, measures such as avoiding dehydration, eating regularly, regular exercise, limiting caffeine and good sleep hygiene can be used alongside medication to manage migraine.

Neurotoxins

OnabotulinumtoxinA (botulinum toxin) is a neurotoxin which relaxes involuntarily muscle spasm by blocking the release of the neurotransmitter acetylcholine at the neuromuscular junction. It is widely used in the treatment of migraine and temporarily inhibits pain by blocking neurotransmitters that carry pain signals from the brain. It is recommended that patients should have failed at least two other preventative drugs before onabotulinumtoxinA is used and is particularly helpful when drug side effects have led to discontinuation or comorbidities have prevented drug use.

The head/neck region is divided into seven specific regions and OnabotulinumtoxinA is injected into several sites within each of the regions (Figure 12.5).

In addition to these sites, a 'follow the pain' strategy of additional injections in areas in which patients particularly have pain can be used. The effect is usually seen within 3–7 days.

Trials that used 100–150 units of OnabotulinumtoxinA in the treatment of paediatric migraineurs reported decreased pain scores (Chan et al., 2009); decreased frequency, duration and severity/intensity of headache (Ahmed et al., 2010; Kabbouche et al., 2012; Schroeder et al., 2012; Choi and Bae, 2016; Pezzuto et al., 2016; Calderon et al., 2017; Shah, 2018) and improved QOL (Chan et al., 2009).

There have also been statistically significant improvements in depression symptoms, anxiety symptoms and cognitive measures of speed and accuracy in patients administered OnabotulinumtoxinA for migraine (Ho et al., 2020).

Clinical Consideration

OnabotulinumtoxinA injection may spread beyond the area of injection and relax muscles in other areas of the body. This would be dangerous if the muscles involved in breathing or swallowing were affected and patients should be advised to seek medical advice if they experience any muscle weakness; double or blurred vision; drooping eyelids or brow; difficulty swallowing or breathing; hoarseness or change or loss of voice; difficulty speaking or saying words clearly; or inability to control urination.

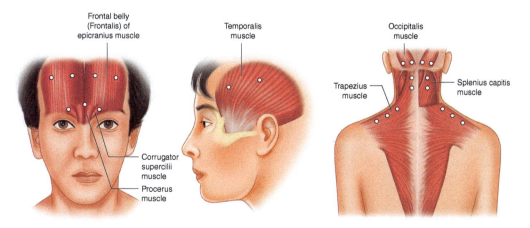

Figure 12.5 **The seven specific regions of the head and neck.** *Source*: Redrawn from Robertson and Garza, 2012.

Status Migrainosus

Status Migrainosus (SM) is 'a debilitating migraine attack lasting for more than 72 hours' (International classification of Headache Disorders, 3rd edition (ICHD-3), 2019) and often results in admission to the emergency department (ED) where drugs to treat pain and nausea can be administered intravenously (IV). This is of benefit as IV drug administration results in 100% bioavailability, speed of onset is increased and it avoids the gastrointestinal system in CYP who have nausea/vomiting as a symptom of their migraine. IV fluids are also given in the ED to CYP with SM. They prevent dehydration from repeated vomiting but do not lead to improvement in pain (Richer et al., 2014).

Conclusion

This chapter has provided an overview of medication used in the treatment of three common neurological conditions experienced by CYP, to help student nurses understand the importance of pharmacology in their treatment. A brief overview of each neurological condition has been given followed by the evidence to support the use of specific drugs, their actions, side effects and contraindications; all of which will contribute to the delivery of safe and effective care.

Glossary

Cognition: The mental action or process of acquiring knowledge and understanding through thought, experience and the senses.
Hydrotherapy: The internal and external use of water in the treatment of disease.
Hyperkinetic: Describes motion beyond the usual.
Migraine: A recurrent throbbing headache, typically affecting one side of the head and is often accompanied by nausea and disturbed vision.
Neurodevelopment: A term that refers to the brain's development of neurological pathways that influence performance or functioning, such as, intellectual functioning, reading ability, social skills, memory, attention or focus skills.
Psychoactive: Affecting the mind. Chemical substances (medications) that change a person's mental state by affecting the way the brain and nervous system work.
Seizure: A sudden attack or convulsion due to involuntary electrical activity in the brain.
Somnolence: Sleepiness, drowsiness.
Stevens-Johnson syndrome: A rare but serious disorder that affects the skin, mucous membrane, genitals and eyes.

References

Ahmed, K., Oas, K.H., Mack, K.J., and Garza, I. (2010). Experience with botulinum toxin type A in medically intractable pediatric chronic daily headache. *Pediatric Neurology.* 43: 316–319.

Amanat, M., Togha, M., Agah, E. et al. (2019) Cinnarizine and sodium valproate as the preventive agents of pediatric migraine: A randomized double-blind placebo-controlled trial. *Cephalalgia.* doi: 10.1177/0333102419888485.

Anderson, M. (2011). Benzodiazepines for prolonged seizures. *Archives of Disease in Childhood – Education and Practice* 95(6): 183–189.

Ashrafi, M.R., Shabanian, R., Zamani, G.R., and Mahfelati, F. (2005). Sodium valproate versus propranolol in paediatric migraine prophylaxis. *European Journal of Paediatric Neurology* 9(5): 333–338.

Barbanti, P., Grazzi, L., and Egeo, G. (2019). Pharmacotherapy for acute migraines in children and adolescents. *Expert Opinion on Pharmacotherapy* 20(4): 455–463. doi: 10.1080/14656566.2018.1552941.

Beatriz. S and Fagundes, R. (2008). Valproic acid review. *Reviews in the Neurosciences* 16(2): 130–6.

Brain & Spine Foundation (2020). What is a neurological problem? www.brainandspine.org.uk/information-and-support/what-is-a-neurological-problem/# (accessed 6 May 2020).

Briars, G.L., Travis, S.E., Anand, B., and Kelly, A.M. (2008). Weight gain with pizotifen therapy. *Archives of Disease in Childhood* 93(7): 590–593.

Brodie, M.J. (2010). Antiepileptic drug therapy the story so far. *Seizure* 19(10): 650–5. doi: 10.1016/j.seizure.2010.

Calderon, M.D., Wu, W., Ma, M. et al. (2017). A longitudinal evaluation on the effectiveness of Botox® in pediatric patients experiencing migraines: A five-year retrospective study. Poster presented at: The Anesthesiology Annual Meeting; 23 October 2017; Boston, MA.

Care Quality Commission (2019). High risk medicines: valproate. www.cqc.org.uk/guidance-providers/adult-social-care/high-risk-medicines-valproate (accessed 6 January 2020).

Chan, V.W., McCabe, E.J., and MacGregor, D.L. (2009). Botox treatment for migraine and chronic daily headache. *Journal of Neuroscience Nursing* 41: 235–243.

Choi, Y. and Bae, C. (2016). OnabotulinumtoxinA as one of the preventative treatments for chronic migraine in Korean adolescents. In: *5th European Headache and Migraine Trust International Congress*. Glasgow.

Chu, S-S., Wang, H-J., Zhu, L.N. et al. (2020). Therapeutic effect of intravenous levetiracetam in status epilepticus: A meta-analysis and systematic review. *Seizure* 74: 49–55.

Chua, A.L., Grosberg, B.M., and Evans, R.W. (2019). Status migrainosus in children and adults. *Headache: The Journal of Head and Face Pain* 59(9): 1611–1623.

Devinsky, O., Nabbout, R., Miller, I. et al. (2018). Long-term cannabidiol treatment in patients with Dravet syndrome: An open-label extension trial. *Epilepsia* 60: 294–302. doi: 10.1111/epi.14628.

Egunsola, O., Choonara, I., and Sammons, H.M. (2015). Safety of lamotrigine in paediatrics: a systematic review. *BMJ open* 5(6). doi: 10.1136/bmjopen-2015-007711.

Epidiolex.com (2019). Full prescribing information. www.epidiolex.com/sites/default/files/EPIDIOLEX_Full_Prescribing_Information.pdf (accessed 21 February 2020).

Epilepsy Society (2017). How anti-epileptic drugs work. www.epilepsysociety.org.uk/how-anti-epileptic-drugs-work#.Xd0qXXd2s74 (accessed 26 November 2019).

Fallah, R., Akhavan Karbasi, S., Shajari, A., and Fromandi, M. (2013). The efficacy and safety of topiramate for prophylaxis of migraine in children. *Iranian Journal of Child Neurology* 7: 7–11.

Fallah, R., Fazelishoroski, L., and Sekhavat, L. (2018). A randomized clinical trial comparing the efficacy of melatonin and amitriptyline in migraine prophylaxis of children. *Iranian Journal of Child Neurology* 12(1): 47–54.

Fisher, R.S., Acevedo, C., Arzimanoglou, A. et al. (2014). A practical clinical definition of epilepsy. *Epilepsia* 55(4): 475–482. doi: 10.1111/epi.12550.

ILAE (2014). Official Report. www.ilae.org/guidelines/definition-and-classification/the-2014-definition-of-epilepsy-a-perspective-for-patients-and-caregivers (accessed 20 April 2021).

Fisher, R.S., Cross, H., D'Souza, C. et al. (2017). Instruction manual for the ILAE 2017 operational classification of seizure types. *Epilepsia* 58(4): 531–542. doi: 10.1111/epi.13671.

Forsyth, R. and Newton, R. (2018). *Paediatric Neurology*, 3e. Oxford: Oxford University Press.

Goodfellow, J. and Willison, H. (2016). Guillain-Barré syndrome: a century of progress. *Nature Reviews Neurology*. 12(12): 723–731.

Gov. UK (2019). (b) Valproate use by women and girls. www.gov.uk/guidance/valproate-use-by-women-and-girls (accessed 6 January 2020).

Hesami, O., Shams, M.R., Ladan Ayazkhoo, L. et al. (2018). Comparison of pregabalin and sodium valproate in migraine prophylaxis: a randomized double-blinded study. *Iranian Journal of Pharmaceutical Research* 17(2): 783–89.

Ho, S., Darby, D., and Bear, N. (2020). Cognitive effects of onabotulinumtoxinA in chronic migraine. *BMJ Neurology Open* 2:e000014. https://neurologyopen.bmj.com/content/2/1/e000014 (accessed 16 April 2020).

Joint Formulary Committee (2019). *British National Formulary for Children 2019–2020*. London: BMJ Publishing and the Royal Pharmaceutical Society.

Kabbouche, M.A., O'Brien, H., and Hershey, A.D. (2012). OnabotulinumtoxinA in pediatric chronic daily headache. *Current Neurology and Neuroscience Reports* 12: 114–117.

Kroner, J.W., Hershey, A.D., Kashikar-Zuc, S.M. et al. (2016). Cognitive behavioral therapy plus amitriptyline for children and adolescents with chronic migraine reduces headache days to ≤ 4 per month. *Headache: The Journal of Head and Face Pain* 56(4): 711–716.

Lakshmi, C.V.S., Singhi, P., Malhi, P., and Ray, M. (2007). Topiramate in the prophylaxis of pediatric migraine: a double-blind placebo-controlled trial. *Journal of Child Neurology* 22(7): 829–835.

Lewis D., Winner P., Saper J. et al. (2009). Randomized, double-blind, placebo-controlled study to evaluate the efficacy and safety of topiramate for migraine prevention in pediatric subjects 12 to 17 years of age. *Pediatrics* 123(3): 924–934.

Lyttle, M.D., Rainford, N.E.A., Gamble, C. et al. (2019). Levetiracetam versus phenytoin for second-line treatment of paediatric convulsive status epilepticus (EcLiPSE): a multicentre, open-label, randomised trial. *Lancet* 393: 2125–2134.

Medicines and Healthcare products Regulatory Agency (2019). Valproate use by women and girls. www.gov.uk/guidance/valproate-use-by-women-and-girls (accessed 6 January 2020).

Medicines for Children.org.uk (2017). Midazolam for stopping seizures. www.medicinesforchildren.org.uk/midazolam-stopping-seizures (accessed 25 May 2020).

Medicines.org.uk (2019a). Keppra 100 mg/ml oral solution – Summary of Product Characteristics (SPC) – (eMC). www.medicines.org.uk/emc/product/2295/smpc (accessed 11 February 2020).

Medicines.org.uk (2019b). Epidyolex 100 mg/ml oral solution – Summary of Product Characteristics (SPC) – (eMC). www.medicines.org.uk/emc/product/10781/smpc (accessed 20 February 2020).

Medicines.org.uk (2019c). Octagam 10%, solution for infusion. www.medicines.org.uk/emc/product/4701/smpc (accessed 27 February 2020).

Medicines.org.uk (2019d). Gabapentin Rosemont 50mg/ml Oral Solution. www.medicines.org.uk/emc/product/2868/smpc (accessed 4 March 2020).

Miller, G.S. (2002). Pyridoxine ameliorates adverse behavioural effects of levetiracetam in children. *Epilepsia* 43 (supplement 7): 1.

Moretti, R., Julliand. S., Rinaldi, V.E., and Titomanlio, L. (2019). Buccal midazolam compared with rectal diazepam reduces seizure duration in children in the outpatient setting. *Pediatric Emergency Care* 35(11): 760–764.

National Institute for Health and Care Excellence (2020). *Epilepsies: Diagnosis and Management Clinical Guideline [CG137].* www.nice.org.uk/guidance/cg137 (accessed 22 March 2020).

NHS (2019). Migraine. www.nhs.uk/conditions/migraine/ (accessed 20 June 2020).

Oskoui, M., Pringsheim, T., Holler-Managan, Y. et al. (2019). Practice guideline update summary: Acute treatment of migraine in children and adolescents. *Neurology* 93: 487–499.

Patsalos, P.N. (2004). Clinical pharmacokinetics of levetiracetam. *Clinical Pharmacokinetics* 43(11): 707–724.

Patsalos, P.N. (2013). *The Epilepsy Prescriber's Guide to Antiepileptic Drugs.* Cambridge University Press.

Peer, M.B., Goadsby, P.J., and Prabhakar, P. (2012). Safety and efficacy of flunarizine in childhood migraine: 11 years' experience, with emphasis on its effect in hemiplegic migraine. *Developmental Medicine and Child Neurology* 54: 274–7.

Pezzuto, T., Beyderman, L., Chugani, D., and Xie, L. (2016). Is less more? Pediatric intractable migraine and botox treatment. *Annals of Neurology* 80: S299–S300.

Powers, S.W., Coffey, C.S., Chamberlin, L.A., et al. (2017). Trial of amitriptyline, topiramate, and placebo for pediatric migraine. *New England Journal of Medicine* 376(2): 115–124.

Richer, L., Craig, W., and Rowe, B. (2014). Randomized controlled trial of treatment expectation and intravenous fluid in pediatric migraine. *Headache* 54: 1496–1505.

Robertson, C.E and Garza, I. (2012). Critical analysis of the use of onabotulinumtoxinA (Botulinum Toxin Type A) in migraine. *Neuropsychiatric Disease and Treatment* 8: 35–48.

Rowland, A.G., Gill, A.M., Stewart, A.B. et al. (2009). Review of the efficacy of rectal paraldehyde in the management of acute and prolonged tonic-clonic convulsions. *Archives of Disease in Childhood* 94: 720–723.

Sajja K., Sankaraneni R., Galla K., and Singh, S.P. (2017). *Role of Pyridoxine (Vitamin B6) in the Treatment of Levetiracetam Induced Behavioral Effects in Epilepsy Patients.* Presented at AES annual meeting in Washington, DC. Abstract 1.308.

Sánchez Fernández, I., Gaínza-Lein, M., and Loddenkemper, T. (2017). Nonintravenous rescue medications for pediatric status epilepticus: a cost-effectiveness analysis. *Epilepsia* 58: 1349–1359.

Schroeder, A.S., Huss, K., Blaschek, A. et al. (2012). Ten-year follow-up in a case series of integrative botulinum toxin intervention in adolescents with chronic daily headache and associated muscle pain. *Neuropediatrics* 43(6): 339–45.

Sekar, K. and Pack, A. (2019). Epidiolex as adjunct therapy for treatment of refractory epilepsy: a comprehensive review with a focus on adverse effects. *F1000 Research.* 8(F1000 Faculty Rev) 234. doi: 10.12688/f1000research.16515.1.

Shah, S. (2018). Effectiveness of onabotulinumtoxinA (Botox®) in pediatric patients experiencing migraines: A randomized double blinded placebo crossover study in the pediatric pain population. In: *ASRA Chronic Pain Grant Update.* Pittsburgh. PA: American Society of Regional Anesthesia and Pain Medicine.

Srivastava, K., Arora, A., Katharine, A. et al. (2013). Impact of reducing dosing frequency on adherence to oral therapies: a literature review and meta-analysis. *Patient Preference and Adherence* 3(7): 419–434.

Straube, A. and Andreou, A. (2019). Primary headaches during lifespan. *The Journal of Headache and Pain* 20: 35. https://thejournalofheadacheandpain.biomedcentral.com/track/pdf/10.1186/s10194-019-0985-0 (accessed 21 March 2020).

The International Classification of Headache Disorders, 3e (2019). https://ichd-3.org/ (accessed 20 March 2020).

Thiele, E., Marsh, E., Mazurkiewicz-Beldzinska, M. et al. (2019). Cannabidiol in patients with Lennox–Gastaut syndrome: Interim analysis of an open-label extension study. *Epilepsia* 60(3): 419–428.

Van der Linden, V., Albino da Paz, J., Casella, E.B., and Marques-Dias, M.J. (2010). Guillain-Barré syndrome in children: clinic, laboratorial and epidemiologic study of 61 patients. *Arquivos de Neuro-Psiquiatria* 68(1): 12–17.

Van Doorn, P.A., Ruts, L., and Jacobs, B.C. (2008).Clinical features, pathogenesis, and treatment of Guillain-Barré syndrome. *Lancet Neurology* 7(10): 939–950.

Vossler, D.G. (2019). Comparative risk of major congenital malformations with 8 different antiepileptic drugs: a prospective cohort study of the EURAP Registry. *Epilepsy Currents* 19(2): 83–85.

Winner, P.K., Kabbouche, M., Yonker, M. et al. (2020). A randomized trial to evaluate OnabotulinumtoxinA for prevention of headaches in adolescents with chronic migraine. *Headache: The Journal of Head and Face Pain* 60(3): 564–575.

Yao, S., Chen, H., Zhang, Q. et al. (2018). Pain during the acute phase of Guillain–Barré syndrome. *Medicine (Baltimore)* 97(34): 1–5. www.ncbi.nlm.nih.gov/pmc/articles/PMC6113041/ (accessed 4 March 2020).

Yates, S.L., Fakhoury, T., Liang, W. et al. (2015). An open-label, prospective, exploratory study of patients with epilepsy switching from levetiracetam to brivaracetam. *Epilepsy & Behavior* 52: 165–168.

Yayici Köken, Ö., Öztoprak. U., Danis, A. et al. (2019). Three pediatric cases of accidental levetiracetam overdose administration for long term. *Turkiye Klinikleri Journal of Pediatrics* 28(1): 51–54.

Youssef, P.E. and Mack, K.J. (2019). Episodic and chronic migraine in children. *Developmental Medicine and Child Neurology* 62(1): 34–41.

Further Resources

Pregnancy Prevention Programme: 1988 https://assets.publishing.service.gov.uk/government/uploads/system/uploads/attachment_data/file/708850/123683_Valproate_HCP_Booklet_DR15.pdf

Multiple Choice Questions

1. What percentage of patients with epilepsy will become seizure-free with the right medication?
  (a) 30%
  (b) 50%
  (c) 70%
  (d) 90%

2. What two types of infections are the most common causes of Guillain–Barré Syndrome?
  (a) Respiratory and urinary tract infections
  (b) Respiratory and gastrointestinal infections
  (c) Respiratory and skin infections
  (d) Urinary tract and gastrointestinal infections

3. What percentage of babies born to females taking VPA during pregnancy will have a congenital malformation?
  (a) Approximately 5%
  (b) Approximately 10%
  (c) Approximately 15%
  (d) Approximately 20%

4. Which AED would be the first choice to swap a young person to if they were experiencing behavioural adverse effects from levetiracetam?
  (a) Sodium valproate
  (b) Cannabidiol
  (c) Lamotrigine
  (d) Brivaracetam

5. How much tetrahydrocannabinol does cannabidiol (CBD) contain?
  (a) None
  (b) 2%
  (c) 4%
  (d) 6%

6. What are the most common seizures seen in Lennox–Gastaut Syndrome (LGS)?
  (a) Myoclonic, focal and generalised tonic-clonic seizures
  (b) Focal, absence and atonic seizures
  (c) Tonic, atonic and atypical absence seizures
  (d) Myoclonic, absence and generalised tonic-clonic seizures

7. Which family of drugs is traditionally regarded as first line medications for convulsive status epilepticus?
  (a) Benzodiazepines
  (b) Antibiotics

Chapter 12 Medications Used in the Nervous System

    (c) Steroids
    (d) Beta blockers

8. What is the dose of phenytoin given in the treatment of convulsive status epilepticus?
    (a) 10mg/kg over 10 minutes
    (b) 10mg/kg over 20 minutes
    (c) 20mg/kg over 10 minutes
    (d) 20mg/kg over 20 minutes

9. How long can propranolol take to be effective in the treatment of childhood migraine?
    (a) Up to 4 weeks
    (b) Up to 8 weeks
    (c) Up to 12 weeks
    (d) Up to 16 weeks

10. How many preventative drugs should be trialled and failed before onabotulinumtoxinA is used in the treatment of paediatric migraine?
    (a) 1
    (b) 2
    (c) 3
    (d) 4

11. Why does treatment with IV lidocaine hydrochloride for status migrainosus require an admission to a paediatric intensive care unit?
    (a) Side effects include arrhythmias, atrioventricular block and cardiac arrest
    (b) IV lidocaine may cause seizures
    (c) IV lidocaine must be given through an arterial line
    (d) Side effects include respiratory depression

12. How often is amitriptyline usually given in the treatment of paediatric migraine?
    (a) Once daily
    (b) Twice daily
    (c) Three times daily
    (d) Four times daily

13. What is the maintenance dose of gabapentin used to treat dysaesthesia in GBS?
    (a) 5–10mg/kg/24 hours
    (b) 20–30mg/kg/24 hours
    (c) 30–40mg/kg/24 hours
    (d) 40–50mg/kg/24 hours

14. How common is respiratory failure in CYP with GBS?
    (a) Approximately 5%
    (b) Approximately15%
    (c) Approximately 25%
    (d) Approximately 35%

15. How many milligrams of human normal immunoglobulin does Octagam® 10% contain in 1ml?
    (a) 1mg
    (b) 10mg
    (c) 100mg
    (d) 1000mg

Chapter 12 Medications Used in the Nervous System

Appendix 1: AEDs Used in Treatment of Childhood Epilepsy

DRUG	INDICATION (SEIZURE TYPE/ SYNDROME)	MECHANISM OF ACTION/TARGET	FORMULATIONS
Acetazolamide	Generalised tonic-clonic seizures Catamenial epilepsy	Carbonic anhydrase inhibitor	Tablets Capsules Solution for injection
Brivaracetam	Focal seizures with or without secondary generalisation	SV2A (a synaptic vesicle glycoprotein)	Tablets Oral solution Solution for injection
Cannabidiol	Lennox–Gastaut syndrome Dravet syndrome	Multiple mechanisms of action	Oral solution
Carbamazepine	Focal and generalised tonic-clonic seizures	Sodium channel blocker	Tablets Prolonged-release tablets Oral suspension Liquid
Clobazam	All forms of epilepsy Catamenial (menstruation) seizures	Enhance GABA transmission	Tablets Oral suspension
Clonazepam	All forms of epilepsy	Enhance GABA transmission	Oral solution
Eslicarbazepine	Adjunctive therapy of focal seizures with or without secondary generalisation	Sodium channel blocker	Tablets Oral suspension
Ethosuximide	Absence seizures, Atypical absence seizures Myoclonic seizures	Calcium channel blocker	Capsules Oral solution
Everolimus	Tuberous sclerosis complex	mTor inhibition	Tablets Dispersible tablets
Gabapentin	Focal seizures with or without secondary generalisation	Enhance GABA transmission	Tablets Capsules Oral solution
Lacosamide	Focal seizures with or without secondary generalisation	Sodium channel blocker	Tablets Syrup Solution for infusion
Lamotrigine	Focal seizures Primary and secondary generalised tonic-clonic seizures Seizures associated with Lennox–Gastaut syndrome	Sodium channel blocker Inhibits glutamate	Tablets Dispersible tablets
Levetiracetam	Focal seizures with or without secondary generalisation Myoclonic seizures Tonic-clonic seizures	SV2A (a synaptic vesicle glycoprotein)	Tablets Granules Oral solution Concentrate for solution for infusion
Oxcarbazepine	Focal seizures with or without secondary generalised tonic-clonic seizures	Sodium channel blocker	Tablets Oral suspension

(Continued)

Chapter 12 Medications Used in the Nervous System

DRUG	INDICATION (SEIZURE TYPE/ SYNDROME)	MECHANISM OF ACTION/TARGET	FORMULATIONS
Perampanel	Focal seizures with or without secondary generalised seizures Primary generalised tonic-clonic seizures	AMPA antagonist	Tablets Oral suspension
Phenobarbital	All forms of epilepsy except typical absence seizures	Enhance GABA transmission	Tablets Elixir Injection
Phenytoin	Tonic-clonic seizures Focal seizures	Sodium channel blocker	Tablets Chewable tablets Capsules Oral suspension Solution for injection
Prednisolone	Infantile spasms	Unknown mechanism of action	Tablets Soluble tablets Gastro-resistant tablets Oral solution Suspension for injection
Pregabalin	Focal seizures with or without secondary generalisation	Enhance GABA transmission	Capsules Oral solution
Primidone	All forms of epilepsy except typical absence seizures	Enhance GABA transmission	Tablets
Rufinamide	Lennox–Gastaut syndrome	Mixed receptors	Tablets Oral suspension
Sodium Valproate	All forms of epilepsy	Mixed receptors	Tablets Crushable tablets Gastro-resistant tablets Controlled-release tablets Modified-release granules Oral solution Solution for injection
Stiripentol	Dravet syndrome	Multiple mechanisms of action	Capsules Powder
Tiagabine	Focal seizures with or without secondary generalisation that are not satisfactorily controlled by other antiepileptics	Enhance GABA transmission	Tablets
Topiramate	Generalised tonic-clonic seizures Focal seizures with or without secondary generalisation Lennox–Gastaut syndrome	Mixed receptors	Tablets Sprinkle capsules Oral suspension
Vigabatrin	Focal seizures with or without secondary generalisation not satisfactorily controlled with other antiepileptics West syndrome	Enhance GABA transmission	Tablets Soluble tablets Granules for oral solution
Zonisamide	Focal seizures with or without secondary generalisation	Mixed receptors	Capsules Oral suspension

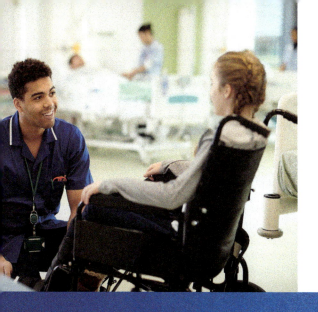

13

The Immune System and Immunisations

Sarah Greenshields

Aim

The aim of this chapter is to provide an understanding of the pharmacology associated with immunisation. This will include an overview of immunisations and their impact on the immune system, particularly in relation to children and young people. This will include the purpose, method and possible implications to practise.

Learning Outcomes

- To explore the pharmacology underpinning immunisations
- Identify the role, function and features for different types of immunisations
- Explain the impact of immunisations on the immune system
- Discuss the administration and possible side effects of immunisations
- Consider the challenges and the need for clear and accurate communication and documentation

Test Your Knowledge

Make some notes about your current knowledge regarding the following:

1. How would you define the term 'immunisation'?
2. How do immunisations work?
3. What diseases does the United Kingdom immunisation schedule cover?
4. What stages are included in the administration of a vaccine?
5. What is the 'green book' and what is its purpose?

Fundamentals of Pharmacology for Children's Nurses, First Edition. Edited by Ian Peate and Peter Dryden.
© 2022 John Wiley & Sons Ltd. Published 2022 by John Wiley & Sons Ltd.
Companion website: www.wiley.com/go/pharmacologyforCN

Introduction

The human body has three lines of defence to protect itself from pathogens (microorganism which can cause disease). The first is the skin and mucous membranes. When intact the membranes act as a non-specific physical barrier to stop or entrap invading pathogens. The cellular and chemical features of the skin also resist invasion. The dryness, acidity and temperature of the skin limit the growth of pathogens. The oily substance produced by glands in the skin as well as perspiration, cilia in the respiratory system and the shedding of dead skin cells remove potential pathogens from the skin.

If the pathogen is able to penetrate the first line of defence, the second non-specific line will usually destroy them. The second line of defence is a cellular and chemical response. This involve a complex combination of actions including; production of fever, creating interferons, inflammation, chemotaxis and phagocytosis. The third line of defence is the specific host defence, which is complex and multifaceted. Some of the basic fundamental third line immune responses are discussed within this chapter.

Within this chapter the drug group in focus will be immunisations. The rationale for choice is based in the interaction immunisations have with the immune system as well as the statistical relevance. A significant role of the immune system is to make a person resistant to specific illness and disease. One pharmacological approach to this is to vaccinate. The vast majority of children and young people in the United Kingdom (UK) will receive immunisations. For example, there is an expectation that the UK coverage for all routine childhood immunisations, evaluated up to five years of age, achieve 95% (NHS Digital, 2018). Although there has been some decline in vaccine uptake the number of children being immunised is significant and therefore it is a strong drug to analyse and understand.

The terms 'vaccination' and 'immunisation' are often used interchangeably. A vaccination is the administration of a harmless or less harmful form of a pathogen. This should cause the immune system to respond in order to protect an individual from a repeat exposure to the same pathogen (Kassianos, 2001). Immunisation refers to the process of both getting the vaccine and becoming immune to the disease following vaccination (Public Health England, 2018). The purpose of immunisation is threefold; to protect the individual, prevent disease in the community and to eradicate illness worldwide. In this chapter we will explore the role and actions of immunisations. First to fully understand this we need to consider the immune system.

Types of Immunity

The aim of the immune system is to recognise and destroy pathogens, protecting the health of the individual. As stated above, a pathogen is a microorganism which can cause disease. An antigen is a toxin or other foreign substance which initiates an immune response in the body, especially the production of antibodies. There are two main systems of immunity; innate (or natural) and acquired (or adaptive) (see Figure 13.1). The key difference is the recognition of antigens. The innate immune system is hard-wired and fixed. It generally recognises carbohydrates or lipids. The acquired immune system is not present at birth, it flexible and specific and tends to recognise proteins.

Vaccines provoke the recipient's immune system, causing it to produce a response. Vaccines cause the innate immune system to inflame whereas the acquired immune system has a specific response led by the white blood cells, specifically the T and B cell lymphocytes. Around 80% of the circulating human lymphocytes are T cells. These can be differentiated into four groups, shown in Table 13.1.

B cells are subdivided into two groups: plasma cells and NK (natural killer) cells. When stimulated, B cells can differentiate into plasma cells, which produce and release antibodies. The antibodies or memory cells formed in response to the vaccine then remain in the system ready to attack a specific pathogen if it re-enters the body at another time.

When considering acquired or adaptive immunity, you develop immunity to a specific antigen only when you are exposed to it or given the matching antibodies from a different source. Acquired immunity can be divided into two groups; active and passive acquired immunity. Active acquired immunity develops in response to antigen exposure. This can naturally occur due to contact in the environment or artificially take place after being administered a form of the antigen, via a vaccine or similar, to prevent disease. Passive acquired immunity occurs naturally when the transfer of maternal antibodies occurs across the placenta. It is artificially induced when antibodies are administered to combat infection.

Chapter 13 The Immune System and Immunisations

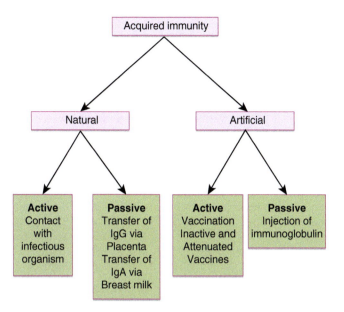

Figure 13.1 **Acquired (specific) immunity.** *Source:* Gormley-Fleming and Peate, 2019/John Wiley & Sons.

Table 13.1 **T cells.**

CYTOTOXIC T CELLS	HELPER T CELLS	SUPPRESSOR T CELLS	MEMORY T CELLS
Attack foreign cells or body cells which are identified as being infected with a virus	Stimulate the activation and function of both B and T cells	Inhibit the activation and function of T and B cells	Respond to a previously encountered antigen

Herd or population immunity is indirect protection of the population because a significant number of the group (usually around 85%, although it varies depending on the vaccine) are immunised. The primary goal with an immunisation schedule is to protect the recipient. However, those individuals are also less likely to be a source of infection to others. This means that individuals who cannot or choose not to be vaccinated will still benefit from the routine immunisation schedule.

How Immunisations Work

Immunisations aim to generate an acquired or adaptive immune response (World Health Organisation, 2019). This mirrors the response of the body when a natural infection occurs. Vaccines produce their protective effect by triggering active immunity and as a result forming immunological memory. This memory allows the immune system to spot natural infection and act rapidly to prevent infection. From birth humans are exposed to countless numbers of infectious agents. Responding to these helps the immune system to develop and mature. Compared with the challenge posed by the natural environment, vaccines provide specific exposure to a small number of antigens (Clinical Knowledge Summaries, 2018). Responding to these specific antigens uses only a tiny proportion of the capacity of an infant's immune system (Public Health England, 2018). Immunisations can on the whole be divided into two main types; live attenuated vaccines and inactivated vaccines.

Live Attenuated Vaccines

A pathogen, which may be a whole bacteria or virus, is grown in vitro so that it is weakened but can still reproduce. This causes an immune response but does not infect the individual with the disease. The live microorganism is attenuated but retains its immunogenic properties. Immunogenic is related to substances able to produce an immune response.

Chapter 13 The Immune System and Immunisations

Live attenuated vaccines tend to create a strong and lasting immune response although can be unstable. However, this type of vaccine is not suitable for people whose immune system is impaired, either due to drug treatment or underlying illness. Examples used in the UK immunisation schedule include the MMR and nasal flu vaccine.

Inactivated Vaccines

The vaccine contains either whole pathogens which have been inactivated by heat or chemical or a small part of the pathogen, which cannot cause disease. There are several different types of inactivated vaccine.

Inactivated vaccines do not contain any live bacteria or viruses and therefore cannot cause the diseases against which they protect, even in clients with a vulnerable immune system. The vaccine is more stable, but the response is not as strong and usually requires repeated doses and/or booster doses. Adjuvants, such as aluminium salts, are added to inactivated vaccines to help strengthen the response of the immune response through a variety of methods. As a result, local reactions (such as a red or swollen localised reaction) may be more evident and frequent with inactivated vaccines. For further information please see Table 13.2.

Table 13.3 highlights the properties of the three inactivated vaccines stated as examples above. The purpose of this is to support your knowledge of the featured of vaccines. Through the use of examples, it is hoped that your understanding of immunisation pharmacology is improved. To be able to explore the properties of further vaccines readers should refer to the 'Green Book' or the 'Electronic Medicines Compendium'.

Table 13.2 Examples of inactivated vaccines.

TYPE OF INACTIVATED VACCINE	DETAILS	EXAMPLE IN UK SCHEDULE
Whole inactivated	Contain whole inactivated viruses (no bacterial examples currently in schedule).	Polio vaccine (in the 6 in 1)
Sub-unit or acellular or polysaccharide	Do not contain any whole cells. May contain sugars or proteins from the surface of the pathogen so the body recognises them as antigens, or may contain inactivated versions of the toxins a bacteria releases.	Tetanus vaccine (in the 6 in 1)
Recombinant vaccines	Piece of DNA is taken from the virus or bacteria and inserted into other cells, such as yeast, to make them produce large quantities of active ingredient	Human Papillomavirus (HPV) vaccine

Source: The Green Book/Public Domain.

Table 13.3 The properties of three inactivated vaccines.

VACCINE	WHAT IS THE DISEASE?	PRODUCT NAMES	DOSE GIVEN
Polio vaccine (in the 6 in 1)	The virus replicates in the gut and has a high affinity for nervous tissue. Symptoms include headache, gastrointestinal signs, malaise and stiffness, with or without paralysis.	Infanrix-IPV Pediacil	A single dose of 0.5 ml should be administered
Tetanus vaccine (in the 6 in 1)	The disease is characterised by generalised rigidity and spasms of skeletal muscles. The case–fatality ratio ranges from 10 to 90%; it is highest in infants and the elderly	Infanrix-IPV Pediacil	A single dose of 0.5 ml should be administered
HPV vaccine	HPV is associated with genital warts and anogenital cancers in both men and women.	Gardasil Cervarix	A single dose of 0.5 ml should be administered

Source: The Green Book/Public Domain.

Conjugate Vaccines

The term 'conjugate' means 'connected' or 'joined'. Researchers found that polysaccharide vaccines were more effective if they were attached to another substance which creates a strong immune response. Commonly this involves joining a polysaccharide with one of the toxoid vaccines described in the Table 19.3. The immune system recognises the toxoids easily and this helps to generate a stronger immune response. In the UK immunisation schedule the Hib vaccine (in the 6-in-1) contains a polysaccharide joined to tetanus toxoid.

Immunisation and Public Health

Public Health is defined as 'the art and science of preventing disease, prolonging life and promoting health through the organized efforts of society' (Acheson, 1988). Immunisation is the most effective public health measure in preventing disease. An example of this was the worldwide eradication of small pox in 1980. The incidence of infectious disease has also been globally reduced, which can be referred to as containment. This can be seen through studying the epidemiology of diphtheria in the United Kingdom (UK) (see Figure 13.2). The vaccine was introduced in the UK in 1942. The rapid decline in reported cases and deaths can be viewed in this graph produced by Public Health England (2014).

Polio was a real threat until 50 years ago and caused significant ill health and permanent disability to individuals struck with the infection, but now in the UK it is completely eradicated. This is entirely due to a successful vaccination programme. However, eradicating infections is not just as simple as producing a new effective vaccination. It only works if the uptake of the new vaccination is high. Immunisation is the most effective public health measure in preventing disease. It can lead to eradication or containment of disease. It saves lives and provides opportunity to promote good health.

The Joint Committee on Vaccination and Immunisation (JCVI) is a significant partner in deciding which vaccines to include in the routine schedule. Rotavirus is the most common cause of vomiting and diarrhoea (gastroenteritis) in infants and young children. Prior to the vaccination programme, nearly every child will have had at least one episode of rotavirus gastroenteritis by five years of age. The rotavirus vaccination programme began on 1 July 2013 when children under four months were routinely vaccinated against this highly infectious illness using a droplet method (JCVI, 2013). The excellent news is that lab reports show there are 70% fewer cases of rotavirus during the same period when compared to the average over the last 10 seasons.

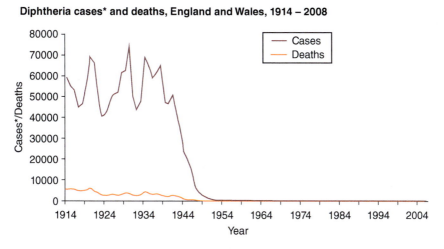

Figure 13.2 **Diphtheria cases and deaths, England and Wales, 1914–2008.** *Source:* Modified from Diphtheria: notifications and deaths, England and Wales.

Chapter 13 The Immune System and Immunisations

The immunisation programme in the United Kingdom is an expensive aspect of public health. It is funded and coordinated centrally by the Department of Health and NHS England. Records suggest that Department of Health is the largest purchaser of vaccinations in Europe. Most countries in the developed world tend to recommend the same kinds of vaccines for babies, children and adults. However, there is a variety between each countries programme because of epidemiology of the disease, differing approaches to deciding on vaccines and tradition. The Joint Committee on Vaccination and Immunisation considered evidence on the burden of disease, safety and how effective the vaccine is, and the financial impact (JCVI, 2013).

It is necessary to highlight that no vaccine can offer 100% protection and a small proportion of people can be infected despite immunisation. There are two main ways this occurs: primary or secondary vaccine failures (Public Health England, 2018). Primary failure occurs when a recipient of a vaccine does not have an initial immune response. An example would be the 5–10% of children who do not have a response to the first dose of the MMR vaccine. This is why a second dose of the vaccine is usually offered before starting school. Secondary failure is when a recipient has an initial response but this then reduces over time (Public Health England, 2018). An example given is the pertussis vaccine; again, a fourth (booster) dose is usually given to improve protection during the school years.

Immunisation Schedule

Each country will have a unique immunisation schedule. This will be formed in response to considerations regarding efficacy, safety and acceptability. The current schedule for children and young people the United Kingdom can be seen in Table 13.4. There are other vaccines to be considered as a result of the travel vaccination programme. When a family travels or migrates, they are exposed to a new climate, environment, culture and range of infections. Specialist travel vaccine clinics or the clients' general practice can offer advise and guidance on the best methods to programme immunisations (Kassianos, 2001).

If a client has an incomplete immunisation history, for example if they have moved from a country with a different schedule, their GP practice is responsible for assessing the immunisation history and providing advice and vaccinations to ensure the schedule is completed in a safe and timely manner. A useful resource is provided by The World Health Organisation, which highlights the immunisations provided in any country in the world (World Health Organisation, 2019).

Vaccine Uptake

Vaccine uptake could be influenced by a range of factors including personal, social cultural, religious and emotional factors (NHS Digital, 2018). Evidence suggest those at risk of lower uptake include those in deprived or mobile groups, those with chronic illness, children and young people in local authority care (NHS Digital, 2018). Parental attitudes are affected both by the extent of their knowledge of the disease and the vaccine (National Institute for Health and Care Excellence (NICE), 2009).

When immunising children and young people a practitioner will need to consider the anxiety of both client and their consenting adult. Depending on age the child or young person could be nervous or apprehensive about what to expect. This may be due to a previous negative experience or simply because of the anticipated pain. On occasion this can escalate and cause the child to present with very challenging behaviour or the young person to refuse the vaccination. Parents also report feeling an anxiety regarding their child being immunised, particularly as an infant. This can lead to avoidance or assertive assent.

It is a professional responsibility to keep up to date with policies and maintain awareness of parental concerns. Practitioners need to ensure there is time to prioritise being accessible so that children, young people and their family members feel able to ask questions and discuss concerns (Nursing and Midwifery Council, 2018). All health professionals should attempt to take opportunities to make every contact count to promote vaccination.

No vaccine is licensed for use in the United Kingdom until it has been extensively tested for efficacy, safety and acceptability. This includes careful assessment about any risks in balance with predicable benefits (JCVI, 2013). The aim is to protect the individual and prevent disease in the community. Even once a vaccine is licensed it continues to be monitored with surveillance in place for less common reactions or problems associated with immunisation.

Chapter 13 The Immune System and Immunisations

Table 13.4 Immunisation schedule.

AGE DUE	DISEASE PROTECTED AGAINST	VACCINE GIVEN	TRADE NAME	USUAL VACCINE SITE
Eight weeks old	Diphtheria, tetanus, pertussis (whooping cough), polio, Haemophilus influenzae type b (Hib) and hepatitis B	DTaP/IPV/Hib/HepB	Infanrix hexa	Thigh
	Pneumococcal (13 serotypes)	Pneumococcal conjugate vaccine (PCV)	Prevenar 13	Thigh
	Meningococcal group B (MenB)	MenB	Bexsero	Left thigh
	Rotavirus gastroenteritis	Rotavirus	Rotarix	By mouth
Twelve weeks old	Diphtheria, tetanus, pertussis, polio, Hib and hepatitis B	DTaP/IPV/Hib/HepB	Infanrix hexa	Thigh
	Rotavirus	Rotavirus	Rotarix	By mouth
Sixteen weeks old	Diphtheria, tetanus, pertussis, polio, Hib and hepatitis B	DTaP/IPV/Hib/HepB	Infanrix hexa	Thigh
	Pneumococcal (13 serotypes)	PCV	Prevenar 13	Thigh
	MenB	MenB	Bexsero	Left thigh
One year old (on or after the child's first birthday)	Hib and MenC	Hib/MenC	Menitorix	Upper arm/thigh
	Pneumococcal	PCV	Prevenar 13	Upper arm/thigh
	Measles, mumps and rubella (German measles)	MMR	MMR VaxPRO2 or Priorix	Upper arm/thigh
	MenB	MenB booster	Bexsero	Left thigh
Eligible paediatric age groups	Influenza (each year from September)	Live attenuated influenza vaccine	LAIV2, Fluenz Tetra	Both nostrils
Three years four months old or soon after	Diphtheria, tetanus, pertussis and polio	DTaP/IPV	Infanrix-IPV or Repevax	Upper arm
	Measles, mumps and rubella	MMR (check first dose given)	MMR VaxPRO2 or Priorix	Upper arm
Boys and girls aged twelve to thirteen years	Cancers caused by human papillomavirus (HPV) types 16 and 18 (and genital warts caused by types 6 and 11)	HPV (two doses 6–24 months apart)	Gardasil	Upper arm
Fourteen years old (school year 9)	Tetanus, diphtheria and polio	Td/IPV (check MMR status)	Revaxis	Upper arm
	Meningococcal groups A, C, W and Y disease	MenACWY	Nimenrix or Menveo	Upper arm

Source: Public Health England, 2019/Public Domain.

The 'Cold Chain'

Vaccines are biological products which lose potency with time. The change is irreversible and speeds up if proper storage is not ensured. The 'cold chain' is the process of storage and transporting vaccines within a safe temperature (Public Health England, 2018). The range is usually between 2 and 8 degrees Celsius. Maintaining the 'cold chain' is a professional responsibility to ensure maximum benefit to the client and reduction of vaccine waste. Stability does vary between vaccines, for example BCG vaccine is sensitive to heat and Hep B is sensitive to cold. Vaccines should also be stored within their original packaging until the point of administration as they may also be sensitive to light of different forms (Public Health England, 2018).

Clinical Considerations

The following is a list of commonly applied storage and transportation principles, although practitioners should review their local policies and procedures;

- Use a dedicated and calibrated fridge for storage
- Ensure there is a secondary supply of electricity in case of a failure
- Group vaccines in type and document amounts clearly
- Vaccines should be stored away from fridge sides
- Use of maximum and minimum thermometer, checking the temperature regularly
- Take action immediately if fault identified, vaccines which have not been stored in correct manner are no longer a licensed product
- Vaccines should be transported in approved cool boxes with insulation, so they do not directly come into contact with ice packs

Patient Specific Directions and Patient Group Directives

Immunisations can be prescribed however when part of the national schedule they are most commonly delivered with accordance with a Patient Group Direction or a Patient Specific Direction. Patient Group Directions (PGDs) allow some registered health professionals to administer specified medicines or products to a defined group of clients, without them being prescribed (NICE, 2017). They should be utilised in specific cases where it offers safe and effective access to care for clients. In the United Kingdom PGDs are frequently used by nursing staff to administer an immunisation programme.

A Patient Specific Direction (PSD) is a written instruction to administer a medicine or product to a list of individually named clients (NHS England, 2016). The clients are individually assessed by the prescriber who must evidence that the administration meets the needs of the client. PSDs are occasionally used as part of immunisation programmes such as the nasal flu vaccine.

Administration of Vaccines

Prior to vaccine administration there are a number of legal and professional requirements necessary to consider (Public Health England, 2018). They include;

- Up-to-date PGD if needed
- Expiry date, vaccine name and type clarified
- Ensuring valid and informed consent
- Suitability of vaccine type for the client, which incorporates a discussion regarding contraindications
- 'Cold chain' adherence
- Procedure needs to be explained clearly to the child or young person as well as their family member. This is commonly an injection, although it can be a nasal spray applicator.

However, there are also several environmental factors, for example, consideration of privacy and dignity and confirming an area for monitoring post vaccine, consent and vaccine preparation.

Consent must be obtained before the administration of all vaccines (Public Health England, 2018). Further legal developments may occur after this chapter has been written and health professionals should remember

Chapter 13 The Immune System and Immunisations

their duty to keep themselves informed of any such developments. There is no legal requirement for consent to immunisation to be in writing. The giving and obtaining of consent is viewed as a voluntary process, not a one-off event. The individual must be informed about the process, benefits and risks of immunisation and be able to communicate their decision. Consent remains valid unless the individual who gave it withdraws it.

For children a person with parental responsibility as outlined in the Children Act 1989 should provide consent. Those over the age of 16 are presumed by law to be able to consent for their own medical treatment. Those under 16 years of age are usually consented by a parent or legal guardian. If a young person is between 13 and 16 years old and deemed Gillick-competent, they will be able to consent for themselves. If a person aged 16 or 17 or a Gillick-competent child refuses treatment, that refusal should be accepted (Public Health England, 2018). Discussion regarding consent should always be supported by local and national policy and guidance. Confidentiality should also be explained and applied. Immunisations administered to young people in school are frequently an opportunity for the young person to share for themselves concerns about their health and well-being.

As part of preparation a practitioner may be required to reconstitute the vaccine as per product directions. However, there are numerous vaccines on the market which are ready to use when the packaging is opened. If the skin is clean, no further cleaning is necessary. Only visibly dirty skin needs to be washed with soap and water (Clinical knowledge summaries, 2018).

Injection technique will vary depending on the route required for the specific vaccine. Most commonly vaccines are administered by the intramuscular route (see skills in practice feature). The choice of needle length is usually 25mm blue needle as this is thought to be an appropriate length to reach the muscle tissue. The major injection sites include the thigh, upper arm and buttock (Public Health England, 2018). The aim is to avoid nerves and blood vessels. Selection of needle size and location of vaccine will be dependent on the age of the child young person as well as the route of injection required. Commonly vaccines in those over three years old are administered in the deltoid muscle. However, if a 1- to 2-year-old has good muscle mass, the deltoid may also be considered. The deltoid muscle is small, and the mass limits the volume of medication that can be injected – typically no more than 1 millilitre.

Consideration must be given to ensuring safe use of sharps. This includes disposing of vials, ampules, needles and syringes in the appropriate sharps bin. Record-keeping should include: vaccine name, batch number, expiry date, dose, site of administration, date and time, name, role and signature of practitioner. Immunisation should be recorded in all necessary locations; this may include a number of computer systems depending upon where you are completing the procedure (Public Health England and Royal College of Nursing, 2018).

Skills in Practice

How to Administer an Intramuscular Injection

This has been selected as this is the most common route of administration for vaccines in the United kingdom.

As with all nursing skills, the procedure will begin by ensuring that the practitioner is aware of the relevant associated policies, for example adhering to infection control policy. The practitioner will also need to be proficient in the skills required to complete the procedure safely. The drug will need to be checked according to the 5 Rs. The consent of the individual will need to be sought and appropriately respected and documented.

When supporting a child or young person to receive a vaccination the practitioner will be required to utilise necessary distraction techniques as well as demonstrating good communication to an appropriate level for the child's developmental stage. They may require additional support and reassurance to enable a successful administration. Always remember the strength of family-centred care, facilitating the parents or carers to offer support to the child or young person.

To locate this site, feel for the bone (acromion process) that is located at the top of the upper arm. The correct area to give the injection is two finger widths below the acromion process. At the bottom of the two fingers will be an upside-down triangle. The practitioner will need to give the injection in the centre of the triangle. Use a needle long enough to reach deep into the muscle. There is no requirement to clean the skin area. Research suggests stretching the skin and bunching the muscle helps with pain management and ensuring the vaccine reaches the muscle tissue.

Insert needle at a 90° angle to the skin with a quick thrust. In previous years nursing staff would aspirate prior to administration; however at the time of publication, this is no longer required as the specific recommended injection location does not have a major blood supply. If multiple injections need to be given in the same extremity, they should be separated by a minimum of 2cm, if possible. Remove the needle and dispose safely in a sharps box. Then apply gentle pressure with a soft dressing where required.

Clinical Considerations

Receiving an immunisation is on the whole a safe process Lang et al. (2014). However, there are contraindications specific to each vaccine administered. Practitioners should consider and assess supported by policy and The Green Book:

- Individuals with a history of a confirmed anaphylactic reaction to a previous dose of the vaccine
- Individuals with a history of a confirmed anaphylactic reaction to a component of the vaccine
- Individuals with current significant ill health, particularly with a fever
- Individuals with primary or acquired immunodeficiency
- Individuals on current or recent immunosuppressive or immunosuppressive biological therapy
- Infants born to a mother who received immunosuppressive biological therapy during pregnancy
- Those in contact with an individual with immunodeficiency, current recent immunosuppressive including biological therapy
- Pregnant women

Source: Public Health England, 2018/Public Domain.

Each assessment is specific to the person and the vaccine being given. In some instances, the benefit of that vaccination may outweigh the risk. In other instances, vaccination should be delayed rather than withheld, or alternative measures considered. For example, a child who is immunocompromised due to chemotherapy should not be immunised with a live vaccine. The most common contraindications are related to the body's ability to have an affective or safe immune response (Public Health England, 2018).

The circumstances for which the vaccine is licensed also require consideration. For example, some vaccines cannot be given to a client who is pregnant as they have not been confirmed as safe by testing in this group. Or there may be a contraindication to administering a type of vaccine when a client has recently received another vaccine (JCVI, 2013). It is important for practitioners to understand the need for maintaining contemporary knowledge and skills to complete a clear assessment prior to administration.

After administering a vaccine, a practitioner should observe for any immediate reactions. It is thought that around 15% of babies receiving a vaccination will experience mild symptoms, such as redness or swelling to the administration site (Royal College of Nursing, 2018). Adverse drug reactions in children should always be reported to the Committee of Safety of Medicines. This applies to serious reactions to established vaccines and every reaction for those drugs labelled with a black triangle. A black triangle is assigned to a newly licensed product.

Immunisation errors can occur due to vaccines with similar sounding names or similar looking packaging, expired vaccinations remaining in fridge, errors in reconstitution or issues with the cold chain (Lang et al., 2014). Practitioners may administer duplicate vaccines or administer them at the wrong time of the schedule as a result of records of child not being up to date, or have vaccination errors in vulnerable groups such as the looked after child due to lack of accurate patient information.

Common Reactions and Anaphylaxis

Practitioners will need to be open about any possible adverse reactions when completing the process to allow informed consent (Royal College of Nursing, 2018). However, the risks should be set in a context when compared to the risks of the disease. Common side effects vary depending on the vaccine type. However, common reactive symptoms include redness, swelling, hardening and pain at the site if injection. Some clients might suffer with temperatures, fatigue, headaches or joint pains (Public Health England, 2018).

Anaphylaxis can be defined as a severe, life-threatening and generalised reaction (Resuscitation Council UK, 2012). It is at the extreme end of the allergic spectrum and significant symptoms include rapidly developing life-threatening airway, breathing and/or circulation problems (Anaphylaxis Campaign, 2019). Frequently these symptoms are connected with skin and mucosal changes, urticaria, respiratory distress, wheeze, stridor, cough, profound hypotension, tachycardia, pallor or unresponsiveness. The presentation of signs and symptoms can vary greatly between individuals.

If a client started to display an anaphylactic reaction following administration of a vaccine, they will require immediate medical attention (Resuscitation Council UK, 2012). They should be consistently monitored and not left alone. They should be placed in the recovery position if safe and appropriate to do so. An intramuscular dose, calculated as per age, of adrenaline will need to be administered to the client. If available and required, a practitioner should administer oxygen via a face mask. They should be reviewed by medical staff in the Emergency Department or in the ward setting if this is where the vaccine was administered.

Chapter 13 The Immune System and Immunisations

A full history should be taken and recorded clearly as per local policy. Information should be shared and explained to parents/carers. In some circumstances, anaphylaxis may lead to a cardiac or respiratory arrest, which should be responded to with cardiopulmonary resuscitation as per emergency protocols.

Communication with the Child and Family

Various sources of information or experiences influence a client or their parents in the process of immunisation (NICE, 2009). Personal experience, beliefs, knowledge of the disease or its risks, support network, a healthcare professional's approach and the media all form understanding and beliefs. It tends to be that as the disease prevalence decreases, the perceived threat of it decreases and therefore the anxiety is focused on the threat of the vaccine. Practitioners need to be able to negotiate, be sensitive and respond to client or parental concerns. It may be helpful to focus on positives and emphasise the evidence of benefits; vaccines save lives and there is vast research base for this (NICE, 2009). It is a professional responsibility to provide the family with all the facts to ensure informed consent. Family members desire clarity, consistency, balanced information based on evidence, time and opportunity to discuss concerns.

When performing procedures, such as an immunisation, with children and young people communication is vital. The methods used to prepare the client for the injection will vary depending on age and capacity of the client (see Episode of Care to explore this further). The negative experiences associated with medical procedures can have a lifelong impact so it is imperative that any exposure to pain due to a medical intervention can be the best experience possible for the child (Martin et al., 1997). Practitioners should aim

Episode of Care

Administering Immunisations to Children and Young People Who Have a Learning Disability
Immunising can be viewed as a fundamental nursing skill. However, as with all intervention's nurses working with children and young people need to consider the holistic care of the client and their family. They also need to assess their approach in light of the age, stage and understanding of the client. There is a legal obligation to put reasonable adjustments in place to ensure equal access to healthcare services for people with disabilities (Equalities Act, 2010). These adjustments might be at a service level or at an individual level, for example offering a longer visit to someone who needs more time. Public Health England (2017) found that limited research studies have been completed to explore how individuals with a learning disability feel about needles. There was a dated qualitative study which found most participants liked seeing their doctor but 34% indicated a dislike of needles or had refused a blood test or vaccination (Martin et al., 1997). Another study found that almost a sixth of people with learning disabilities were described as having a significant fear of contact with medical professionals such that it might affect healthcare interventions. This included a fear of needles and it was recommended that such anxiety should be addressed by desensitisation work (Heslop et al., 2013).

To support the exploration of this episode of care a case study is presented alongside some questions for reflection:

Jasmin is a thirteen-year-old girl with global developmental delay. Her Mum has signed a consent form for Jasmin to be administered her human papilloma virus (HPV) vaccine in school. Mum is not present in school and Jasmin uses transport provided by the Local Authority to attend. The consent form indicates that Jasmin has a severe learning disability and epilepsy. Jasmin does not take any regular medications although is prescribed buccal midazolam for seizures lasting longer than five minutes. She does not have any allergies. Jasmin attends a specialist school and has a classroom support worker who she knows well. School staff share that Jasmin is only able to communicate through nonverbal methods, such as Makaton signs. She can become distressed with new people and tends to thrash her arms if frightened. Jasmin uses an electric wheel chair to mobilise. She likes music and the schools' 'sensory room'.

1. If Jasmin was to be immunised by you (under supervision), would there be any aspects where you would need more information?
2. Do you think you might have any concerns? How could you alleviate these concerns both for yourself and Jasmine?
3. What information from the case study would help you to assess, support and communicate effectively with Jasmin?
4. What have you learned that may help you to facilitate Jasmin safely receiving the immunisation?

Source: Based on Public Health England, 2017.

to minimise pain, distress and anxiety through explaining, calmly and honestly the process, administration and how it will feel. Sometimes this will require preparation and planning, for example discussing options for distraction or allowing time for questions

The Green Book

The Green Book has the latest information on vaccines and vaccination procedures, for vaccine preventable infectious diseases in the UK (Public Health, 2018). Part one of the book covers policies and practices and part two provides information about the specific diseases and vaccines. In practice settings The Green Book is an invaluable resource as it promotes and directs best evidenced-based practice. It is now available as an online resource and is updated regularly to reflect research and improvements.

Conclusion

This chapter has explored the pharmacology of vaccination and the body becoming immune to a disease. To fully understand this, it is important to recognise the features of the immune system and how different types of vaccine interact with it. Immunisation is a key part of public health provision although due to a complex range of factors vaccine uptake can vary in different groups and communities. Communication and documentation are vital skills in facilitating discussion with children and their families, ensuring informed consent and accurate record-keeping.

Glossary

Anaphylaxis: Severe, life-threatening and generalised reaction.
Acquired immunity: Immunity to a specific antigen only when you are exposed to it or given the matching antibodies from a different source. Acquired immunity can be divided into two groups; active and passive acquired immunity.
Cold Chain: The process of storage and transporting vaccines within a safe temperature.
Immunisation: The process of both getting the vaccine and becoming immune to the disease following vaccination.
Inactivated vaccine: A vaccine that contains either whole pathogens which have been inactivated by heat or chemical or a small part of the pathogen, which cannot cause disease. There are several different types of inactivated vaccine.
Innate immunity: Hard-wired and fixed immunity. It generally recognises carbohydrates or lipids.
Live attenuated vaccines: A pathogen, which may be a whole bacteria or virus, which is grown in vitro so that it is weakened but can still reproduce. This causes an immune response but does not infect the individual with the disease. The live microorganism is attenuated but retains its immunogenic properties.
Vaccination: The administration of a harmless or less harmful form of a pathogen. This should cause the immune system to respond in order to protect an individual from a repeat exposure to the same pathogen.

References

Acheson, D. (1988). Public Health in England: The Report of the Committee of Inquiry into the Future Development of the Public Health Function. London: HMSO.
Anaphylaxis Campaign (2019). Anaphylaxis: The Facts. www.anaphylaxis.org.uk/wp-content/uploads/2019/02/Anaphylaxis-The-Facts-2019.pdf (accessed 8 April 2019).
Children Act 2004, c. 31. www.legislation.gov.uk/ukpga/2004/31/contents (accessed 17 May 2019).

Clinical Knowledge Summaries (2018). *Immunizations: Childhood*. https://cks.nice.org.uk/immunizations-childhood (accessed 27 May 2019).

Equalities Act 2010. www.legislation.gov.uk/ukpga/2010/15/contents (accessed 3 June 2019).

Heslop, P., Blair, P., Fleming, P., Hoghton, M. et al. (2013). *Confidential Inquiry into Premature Deaths of People with Learning Disabilities (CIPOLD): Final report*. Bristol: Norah Fry Research Centre, University of Bristol. http://bristol.ac.uk/cipold/reports/ (accessed 23 May 2019).

Joint Committee on Vaccination and Immunisation (2013). *Code of Practice*. https://assets.publishing.service.gov.uk/government/uploads/system/uploads/attachment_data/file/224864/JCVI_Code_of_Practice_revision_2013_-_final.pdf (accessed 27 May 2019).

Kassianos, G.C. (2001). *Immunization; Childhood and Travel Health*. London: Blackwell Science.

Lang, S., Ford, K.J., John, T. et al. (2014). Immunisation errors reported to a vaccine advice service: intelligence to improve practice. *Quality Primary Care* 22(3): 139–146.

Martin, D.M., Roy, A., Wells, M.B., and Lewis, J. (1997). Health gain through screening -- users' and carers' perspectives of health care: developing primary health care services for people with an intellectual disability. *Journal of Intellectual and Developmental Disability* 22(4): 241–49.

Mayson-White, R. and Moreton, J. (1998). *Immunizing Children*. Oxford: Radcliffe Medical Press.

NHS Digital (2018). *Child Vaccination Coverage Statistics*. https://files.digital.nhs.uk/55/D9C4C2/child-vacc-stat-eng-2017-18-report.pdf (accessed 23 May 2019).

NHS England (2016). *Patient Specific Directions*. www.england.nhs.uk/south/wp-content/uploads/sites/6/2016/04/patient-specific-directions.pdf (accessed 23 May 2019).

National Institute for Health and Care Excellence (2009). *Immunisations: Reducing Differences in Uptake in Under 19s*. www.nice.org.uk/guidance/ph21 (accessed: 27 May 2019).

National Institute for Health and Care Excellence (2017). *Patient Group Directions*. www.nice.org.uk/guidance/mpg2 (accessed 23 May 2019).

Nursing and Midwifery Council (2018). *The Code: Professional Standards of Practice and Behaviour for Nurses, Midwives and Nursing Associates*. London: NMC.

Public Health England (2017). *Blood Tests for People with Learning Disabilities: Making Reasonable Adjustments*. https://assets.publishing.service.gov.uk/government/uploads/system/uploads/attachment_data/file/646489/Blood_tests_for_people_with_learning_disabilities.pdf (accessed 23 May 2019).

Public Health England (2018). *Immunisation Schedule*. https://assets.publishing.service.gov.uk/government/uploads/system/uploads/attachment_data/file/741543/Complete_immunisation_schedule_sept2018.pdf (accessed: 27 May 2019).

Public Health England (2018). *The Green Book*. www.gov.uk/government/collections/immunisation-against-infectious-disease-the-green-book (accessed 27 May 2019).

Public Health England and Royal College of Nursing (2018). *National Minimum Standards and Core Curriculum for Immunisation Training for Registered Healthcare Practitioners*. London: Public Health England.

Resuscitation Council (UK) (2012). *Emergency Treatment of Anaphylactic Reactions*. www.resus.org.uk/anaphylaxis/emergency-treatment-of-anaphylactic-reactions/ (accessed 8 April 2019).

Royal College of Nursing (2018). *Managing Childhood Immunisation Clinics*. www.rcn.org.uk/professional-development/publications/pub-007201 (accessed 27 May 2019).

World Health Organisation (2019). *Immunization*. www.who.int/topics/immunization/en/ (accessed 27 May 2019).

Further Resources

NHS Vaccination and Immunisation Schedule: www.nhs.uk/start4life/baby/vaccinations-and-immunisations-baby/

Gov. UK 'The Green Book': www.gov.uk/government/collections/immunisation-against-infectious-disease-the-green-book#the-green-book

e-Learning for Healthcare (Immunisation Programme): www.e-lfh.org.uk/programmes/immunisation/

Multiple Choice Questions

1. How do we define an immunisation?
- **(a)** Both the preparing and administering the vaccine
- **(b)** The process of both getting the vaccine and becoming immune to the disease following vaccination
- **(c)** The bodies response to the vaccine
- **(d)** Both the preparing, administering and recording of a vaccine

Chapter 13 The Immune System and Immunisations

2. What are the two types of immunity called?
   (a) Primary and secondary
   (b) Innate and natural
   (c) Innate (or natural) and acquired (or adaptive)
   (d) Acquired and adapted
3. What is a live attenuated vaccine?
   (a) A whole virus is injected to cause an immune response
   (b) The vaccine contains a small part of the virus or bacteria
   (c) The microorganism in the vaccine is heated to reduce its affect
   (d) The live microorganism is weakened but retains its immunogenic properties
4. What is the correct temperature for vaccine storage?
   (a) The normal range is between 2 and 8 degrees Celsius, however this can vary on vaccine type and brand
   (b) There is no correct temperature
   (c) The normal range is between 1 and 10degrees Celsius
   (d) Temperature standard completely depends on vaccine type
5. How should vaccines be transported?
   (a) Safely an according to risk assessments
   (b) In approved cool boxes with insulation, so they do not directly come into contact with ice packs
   (c) In approved insulated boxes
   (d) Dependent on trust or organisational policy
6. Can a child over the age of 16years consent for themselves?
   (a) Yes
   (b) No
   (c) Not if the parents disagree
   (d) Depends on the situation
7. What is a PGD (Patient Group Directive)?
   (a) The group of patient express a desire for a vaccine
   (b) Document allowing specific trained registered health professionals to administer specified medicines or products to a defined group of clients
   (c) a written instruction to administer a medicine or product to a list of individually named clients
   (d) A clear direction to a group a patient which suffer from one or more medical condition
8. What is a PSD (Patient Specific Directive)?
   (a) allow some registered health professionals to administer specified medicines or products to a defined group of clients, without them being prescribed
   (b) allows a patient to state which vaccine brand they consent to receiving
   (c) a written instruction to administer a medicine or product to a list of individually named clients
   (d) a vaccine which is specific to a patient group
9. Which of the following are possible contraindications to immunisation?
   (a) individuals with a history of a confirmed anaphylactic reaction to a previous dose of the vaccine
   (b) individuals with a history of a confirmed anaphylactic reaction to a component of the vaccine
   (c) Individuals with current significant ill health particularly with a fever
   (d) All of the above, as well as those specific to the vaccine and those clients who may be immuno-compromised or immunosuppressed
10. What factors will a practitioner need to consider prior to administration?
   (a) Consent, assessment of contraindications, vaccine preparation, client understanding and support
   (b) Consent, assessment of contraindications, client understanding and support
   (c) Assessment of contraindications, vaccine preparation, client understanding and support
   (d) Consent, assessment of contraindications, vaccine preparation
11. Which of the following are common side effects to a vaccination?
   (a) Redness and swelling
   (b) Hardening and pain at the site if injection
   (c) Some clients might suffer with temperatures, fatigue, headaches or joint pains
   (d) All of the above

12. What drug will a client experiencing anaphylaxis require?
- (a) Dexamethasone
- (b) Adrenaline
- (c) Salbutamol
- (d) Paracetamol

13. When is a vaccine a black triangle product?
- (a) A red triangle is assigned to a newly licensed product
- (b) A black triangle is assigned to a licensed product
- (c) A black triangle is assigned to a newly licensed product
- (d) A black triangle is assigned to a new product designed to address side effects

14. What should be recorded following a vaccination?
- (a) vaccine name, batch number and expiry date
- (b) dose and site of administration
- (c) date and time, name, role and signature of practitioner
- (d) All of the above

15. What is the site called you would commonly use to vaccinate a five-year-old?
- (a) Any muscle in the leg
- (b) Deltoid muscle, dependent on any specific patient need
- (c) Any major muscle
- (d) The biceps

Find Out More

The following is a list of conditions that are associated with the immune system. Take some time and write notes about each of the conditions. Think about the medications that may be used in order to treat these conditions and be specific about the pharmacokinetics and pharmacodynamics. Remember to include aspects of patient care. If you are making notes about people you have offered care and support to, you must ensure that you have adhered to the rules of confidentiality.

THE CONDITION	YOUR NOTES
Polio	
Diphtheria	
Hepatitis B	
Meningitis B	
Measles	

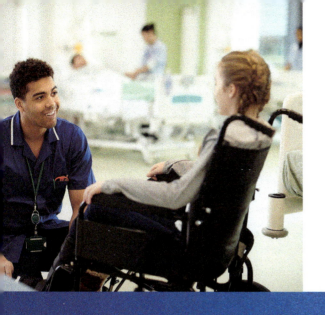

14

Medications and the Integumentary System

Sasha Ban and Peter Dryden

Aim
The aim of this chapter is to provide the reader with an introduction to common integumentary disease processes that may be encountered within clinical practice, and to explore the pharmacological therapies utilised in their management.

Learning Outcomes
After reading this chapter the reader will:
- Have gained an understanding of integumentary anatomy and physiology
- Have gained an understanding of concepts relating to the management of common integumentary disorders
- Understand key classes of integumentary medications and their pharmacology, and how understanding of such is crucial to the promotion of patient safety
- Understand the side effects of common integumentary pharmacotherapy and how this should be considered when counselling the patient and family to reach an informed decision regarding their care
- Have gained an understanding of the current evidence base behind the pharmacotherapy management of the common integumentary conditions reviewed in this chapter

Fundamentals of Pharmacology for Children's Nurses, First Edition. Edited by Ian Peate and Peter Dryden.
© 2022 John Wiley & Sons Ltd. Published 2022 by John Wiley & Sons Ltd.
Companion website: www.wiley.com/go/pharmacologyforCN

Chapter 14 Medications and the Integumentary System

Test Your Knowledge

1. Describe the principal functions of the integumentary system and its main components.
2. Name four common skin conditions.
3. Discuss the potential risks associated with steroid medication
4. List the common types of drugs used to treat skin conditions
5. Discuss the role and function of the National Institute of Health and Care Excellence in the management of skin disorders.

Introduction

The integumentary system, meaning 'covering', is one of the main protective systems of the body. It is the first line of defence against damage and is designed to prevent microorganisms entering the body (McLafferty, 2012). The integumentary system includes the skin, hair, nails, sensory nerve fibres and glands. The system has two layers: the epidermis layer and the dermis. The skin harbours many 'healthy' microbes. This system has a huge role to play in tactile perception, sensation, and prevention of damage to internal organs. It is a vulnerable system; as an external organ the skin and other parts of the system can be at risk of damage either from chemicals, irritants, ultraviolet light and/or microbes. Pharmacotherapy knowledge and understanding is essential in the safe medicines management and treatment of common disease processes, particularly in patients with skin conditions.

Anatomy and Physiology of the Integumentary System

The function of the skin is to provide protection, excretion and absorption, sensation, thermoregulation and synthesis of Vitamin D. It is a complex organ that can fulfill its function through its multiple layer structure.

- The skin provides protection as it is a continuous physical barrier surrounding internal organs. It has a water-resistant property. It provides a chemical barrier through an acid mantle of pH 5.5. Melanocytes produce the pigment melanin which creates a barrier against UV light and prevents damage to cells (McLafferty, 2012).
- The skin excretes water, sodium, urea, uric acid and ammonia in small amounts and absorbs carbon dioxide, heavy metals and topical medications (McLafferty, 2012).
- The skin can sense through neuroreceptors within its layers. Different receptors sense a range of sensations including touch, pressure and vibration (Peate, 2018).
- The skin regulates temperature by losing heat through convection, when the body's temperature regulates with the surrounding ambient temperature or when air passes over it. Heat loss occurs through conduction, either by touching something cooler or wearing wet cold clothes. Heat can be transferred through radiation and evaporation can cause heat loss, especially in infants and newborn due to insensible water loss (Peate and Nair, 2011).
- The skin synthesises vitamin D when exposed to UV radiation. In the presence of sunlight, a compound of vitamin D3, cholecalciferol, is synthesised from a derivative of the steroid cholesterol in the skin. The liver converts this to calcidiol, which is then converted in the kidneys to calcitriol (the active chemical form of the vitamin) (Peate and Nair, 2011).

The layers of the skin are divided into two: epidermis and dermis.

The Epidermis

The epidermis (or epithelial layer) is stratified squamous epithelia, composed of four to five layers (depending on body region) of epithelial cells and has no direct blood supply (Figure 14.1). Diffusion of nutrients and oxygen occurs through the multiple layers. The top layers of the epidermis are made up of keratinocytes, which are cells containing the protein keratin. These form the most superficial layer of the epidermis and are pushed upwards as new cells are produced below. By the time they have migrated to the surface they are dead cells. As keratinocytes move to the surface, they lose cytoplasm and become flattened, this results in compact

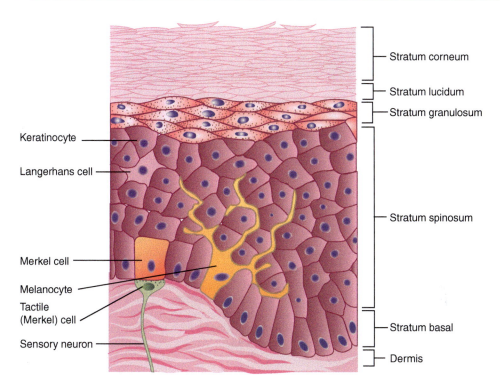

Figure 14.1 **Layers of the skin.**

layering in areas such as nails. The five layers of the epidermis are collectively known as strata (Figure 14.1). They have distinct names based on their function and appearance.

The Dermis

The dermis accounts for about 15–20% of the total weight of the body and varies in thickness. The structure of the dermis varies considerably from infants, children and adults. In the newborn, the skin is still developing and is approximately 60% of its adult thickness (Oranges et al., 2015). The epidermis and dermis layers are not securely attached at birth, these anchor within the first six months. The dermis layer has multiple functions, primarily to provide the epidermis with support and nutrients. These functions include vascular, neural, immunological, exocrine and muscular.

Common Skin Conditions

Having been introduced to the anatomy and physiology of the integumentary system, we will now introduce those skin conditions common in children and young people.

Impetigo

Impetigo is caused by a bacterial infection and it is the most common skin infection in children and occurs particularly in tropical or subtropical regions, or during the summer months in the northern hemisphere (Weller et al., 2015).

As a student or healthcare professional, you may become aware of two types mainly, bullous which is caused by the Staphylococcus aureus and additionally non-bullous which can be caused by β-haemolytic strains of streptococci.

Presentation

Impetigo presents mainly on the face, around the nose mouth and it usually starts as a small red itchy patch inflamed skin that quickly develops into vesicles that rupture and weep (Rutter, 2013: 300–301). The exudate from the wound dries into a brown, yellow sticky crust that can be highly contagious (Figure 14.2).

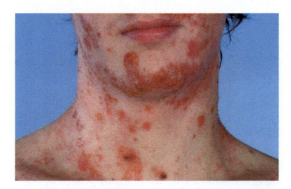

Figure 14.2 **Impetigo showing erosions, crusting and rupture blisters.** *Source*: Weller et al., (2015) Clinical Dermatology 5th edition, Wiley-Blackwell.

After the crusts dry out, they leave a red mark that usually fades without scarring. This can take from a few days to a few weeks.

As the condition does not cause any symptoms until 4 to 10 days after initial exposure to the bacteria, it is often easily spread especially with a family living in close quarters or close contact at nursery, school or college. It usually takes 1 to 3 days from the time of infection until symptoms show. The infection is spread by direct contact with lesions (wounds or sores) or nasal discharge from an infected person and scratching may also transmit the lesions further. The infection usually clears in time, even without treating with medication.

Treatment
Impetigo usually gets better by itself without any pharmaceutical interventions. However, because it is infectious and may cause CYP and their carers to miss out on education and employment, the condition is usually treated.

Hydrogen Peroxide
Hydrogen peroxide is a topical antiseptic used in wound cleaning which kills pathogens through oxidation burst and local oxygen production (Zhu et al., 2017) For initial treatment of non-bullous impetigo, hydrogen peroxide 1% cream should be considered (NICE, 2020a). Randomised controlled trials (RCTs) have shown that at this low dose, hydrogen peroxide cream is as effective as topical antibiotics for treating localised non-bullous impetigo (NICE, 2020a). The benefits for the CYP are that using topical hydrogen peroxide eliminates the risk of increasing antibiotic resistance when using topical or oral antibiotic cream.

At this low 1% concentration there are few side effects but it should be noted that the cream cannot be used around the eyes, it can cause skin irritation and it is incompatible with products containing iodine or potassium permanganate (BNFc, 2020).Currently, the cream only comes in one form (Crystacide 1% cream) which is licensed for use in children.

Treatment Course
The cream should be applied to the affected area 2–3 times a day for 5–7 days (NICE, 2020a). If a course of hydrogen peroxide is unsuccessful, offer:
- A short course of a topical antibiotic if impetigo remains localised or
- A short course of a topical or oral antibiotic if impetigo becomes widespread

Clinical Consideration

Topical and Oral Antibiotics
When the use of antibiotics is advised, the nurse practitioner/prescriber should consider the following:

- That both routes of administration are effective
- Any previous use of topical antibacterials that could have led to resistance
- The preferences of the patient and their family or carers (if appropriate), including the practicalities of administration (particularly to large areas).

Source: Based on NICE, 2020.

Chapter 14 Medications and the Integumentary System

If the CYP has an underlying health condition and could be at risk of becoming unwell quickly through complications of their condition and in all patients with bullous impetigo, an oral antibiotic should be prescribed.

Antibiotic Creams
Fusidic Acid
Fusidic acid and its salts are narrow-spectrum antibiotics used for staphylococcal infections and are derived from the fungus Fusidium coccineum and has been in continuous use since the 1960s. As with the hydrogen peroxide, fusidic acid should be applied to the affected area 3 times a day for 5–7 days. Caution should be taken to avoid contact with the patient's eyes and to avoid the development of resistance, fusidic acid should not be used for longer than 10 days. If a course of topical antibiotic is unsuccessful:

- Offer a short course of an oral antibiotic
- Consider sending a skin swab for microbiological testing

Oral Antibiotics
Although NICE (2020a) have produced guidelines to treat impetigo effectively, oral antibiotics should be prescribed on a patient by patient basis and acknowledge clinical considerations. Two of the commonly used antibiotics to treat impetigo are now discussed.

Flucloxacillin
Flucloxacillin is part of the penicillin group of drugs. They are bactericidal and act by interfering with bacterial cell wall synthesis (see Chapter 18). For those CYP who are not severely unwell, doses are advised in the BNFc online (2020) and can range from 25mg/kg twice daily for 7 days in neonates to 500 mg 4 times a day for 5–7 day, which highlights the need for extreme vigilance when prescribing in paediatrics.

Flucloxacillin is usually given four times a day, before breakfast, lunch, evening meal and bedtime so it is easier to remember to take them. Ideally, these times should be at least 3 hours apart and attention should be given to school-age children; for example, how the drug will be stored at school as liquid medicine needs to be refrigerated. Who will take responsibility to help the child administer when at school? The drug regimen may need to be altered to improve concordance alongside recognising the CYP's preference for tablets or liquid medicine.

As discussed in Chapter 18, it is important that the CYP completes the course of prescribed antibiotic. It can be difficult to persuade a CYP to continue to take oral antibiotics, especially when they start to feel better and see a difference with the impetigo. If they stop taking the antibiotic too soon, this could cause further infection in addition to decreasing future resistance. All this information should be given in an age-appropriate information leaflet for the CYP in addition to a separate one for the carers.

Side Effects of Flucloxacillin
Side effects with flucloxacillin are rare but safety-netting advice should be given around the potential for anaphylaxis and urgent attention and hospital admission especially if the child has never had a medicine from the penicillin family before. If the CYP gets a skin rash or itching, has problems breathing, seems short of breath or if their face, throat, lips or tongue start to swell, they need to call emergency services urgently. Other side effects which are more common but still rare include diarrhoea, abdominal pain and nausea/vomiting.

ADME of Flucloxacillin
Flucloxacillin can be administered orally or parenterally and absorption is more efficient when taken on an empty stomach. It diffuses well into most tissues and can be excreted in small quantities when breast-feeding. The drug is excreted really quickly by the kidney, with around 50% excreted within 6 hours of administration.

Clarithromycin
Clarithromycin is a semisynthetic macrolide antibiotic derived from erythromycin. Clarithromycin can be dispensed as tablets, liquid or granules, which is an important consideration in CYP for concordance and compliance with this medication regimen. For example, the use of granules for a young child when added to soft food such as yoghurt or even a small amount of fluid, may be an easier way for carers to administer the medication. One of the potential drawbacks with administering granules are that they should be swallowed

whole and not chewed as this would affect the absorption and distribution of the drug. A more measurable way to ensure that the appropriate dose has been taken is for carers to administer liquid medicine or tablets. For the treatment of impetigo, doses of clarithromycin can range from 7.5 mg/kg to a maximum dose of 500 mg in severe infections. Clarithromycin is usually given twice daily for 5–7 days.

Side Effects
Much like flucloxacillin, there are a few side effects to clarithromycin but the assessing nurse or student should ask if there are any allergies within the family or if the CYP has ever had a reaction to any medication, food or environment. As with flucloxacillin, some of the milder side effects of clarithromycin are diarrhoea, abdominal pains and nausea and vomiting. The same safety-netting advice and age-appropriate written information should be given to the CYP and their carers and the course of medication should always be completed.

Cellulitis
One of the complications of impetigo – cellulitis – occurs when the infection spreads to the lower dermis and subcutaneous tissue. It can cause the layers of the skin to become red and inflamed and may also be associated with pyrexia and pain. Provided the CYP is not acutely unwell and has no underlying health conditions, cellulitis can usually be treated with oral antibiotics, and painkillers such as paracetamol and ibuprofen can be used to relieve the pain.

Ringworm
This is a dermatophyte infection. Contrary to popular belief, ringworm is not caused by worms at all and is in fact caused by fungal skin infections known as tinea and is common in the CYP population. Ringworm usually presents as a red, itchy, circular rash with one or more rings with raised, bumpy, scaly borders with clearer skin in the middle (Figure 14.3).

Ringworm is caused by fungi called dermatophytes that live on skin hair nails and thrive in warm, moist areas. Three types of dermatophyte fungi cause tinea infections (ringworm).

- Trichophyton: skin, hair and nail infections
- Microsporum: skin and hair
- Epidermophyton: skin and nails

The infection can be contracted via:
- Human contact (anthropophilic spread from human to human)
- Animals (zoophilic spread cats, dogs and cattle)
- Soil (geophilic infections – quite rare)
- Indirect contact objects or materials which carry the infection, such as clothes, towels, or bedding)

Dermatophytes invade keratin and the inflammation they cause is due to metabolic products of the fungus or to delayed hypersensitivity.

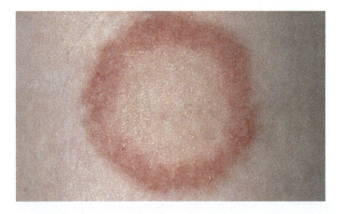

Figure 14.3 **Presentation of ringworm.** *Source:* image crown copyright@ https://www.nhs.uk/conditions/ringworm/

Presentation

The main symptom of ringworm is a red or silver rash which can appear anywhere on the body, including the scalp (tinea capitis) and groin. When first noticed, the rash may look dry and scaly and be accompanied by an itch or even look swollen.

Treating Ringworm

Ringworm is relatively easy to diagnose and treat by the nurse practitioner or paediatrician. Sometimes this can be done solely by visual assessment or if further clarity is needed, a small scraping of skin can be taken and sent to the microbiology labs for further clarification.

Topical Antifungals

NICE (2018) advise antifungals in the treatment of ringworm.

- Clotrimazole 1% cream
- Miconazole 2% cream
- Econazole 1% cream

Clotrimazole, miconazole and econazole are broad-spectrum antimycotic/antifungal medication and belong to a group of medicines called imidazoles that work by inhibiting the growth of fungal cells by altering the permeability of the fungal cell wall. The creams are usually applied 2–3 times daily for 4 weeks or 10 days after all skin lesions are healed. The CYP should avoid contact with the eyes and mucous membranes during use.

Side effects

Side effects with topical antifungals are uncommon and may include erythema, hypersensitivity reactions, itching, mild burning sensation, occasional local irritation (BNFc, 2020).

Drug Interactions

As clotrimazole is generally not significantly absorbed, drug interactions are not a major issue with its use (Crowley and Gallagher, 2017).

Possible complications of fungal infection of the body and groin include:

- Secondary bacterial infection – immunocompromised people are at increased risk.
- Fungal infection of the hand (tinea manuum) – this may develop as a result of scratching the affected area, and typically affects the dominant hand.

Clinical Consideration

Preventing Ringworm Spread

Do:
- Start treatment as soon as possible
- Wash towels and bedsheets regularly
- Keep your skin clean and wash your hands after touching animals or soil
- Regularly check your skin if you have been in contact with an infected person or animal
- Take your pet to the vet if they might have ringworm (for example, patches of missing fur)

Don't:
- Share towels, combs and bedsheets with someone who has ringworm
- Scratch a ringworm rash – this could spread it to other parts of your body

Source: www.nhs.uk/conditions/ringworm/ Public Domain.

Eczema

Eczema is particularly common in young children and infants, affecting 1 in 5 by the age of 2, approximately 15 million people in the UK (Cosh, 2016). Twenty-seven million prescriptions for topical agents used in the treatment of atopic dermatitis (eczema) at a cost of approximately £169 million were prescribed in 2015 (Health and Social Care Information Centre, 2016).

Chapter 14 Medications and the Integumentary System

Episode of Care Impetigo

Yolanda Green is a 14-year-old female with a learning disability who attends the walk-in centre with her father, alert and talkative after developing a red, itchy rash four days ago around her nose and mouth. Yolanda explains that the rash started small but the area affected has become larger and started to weep yesterday. Yolanda's medical notes indicate that she was prescribed fusidic acid had been applying it to the affected area but admits that she sometimes forgot to do this 3 times a day.

Yolanda's prescribed medications include:

- Fusidic acid cream applied to the affected area 3 times a day for 5–7 days
- Salbutamol 2–10 puffs, each puff is to be inhaled separately, repeat every 10–20 minutes or when required

Her allergies include penicillin.

On review of her medications it was agreed with Yolanda and her father that a course of oral antibiotics should be commenced and the fusidic acid (Fucidin) stopped. As Yolanda has an allergy to penicillin it was agreed to start clarithromycin 250 mg twice daily for 7 days.

There are opportunities here as a healthcare professional to provide Yolanda and her father with advice to prevent the spread of the impetigo to other members of the family.

Supported Self-Management

- It has been identified that Yolanda did not always use the fusidic acid as prescribed so she was given an information sheet on impetigo and her father will ensure that Yolanda takes the dose of clarithromycin twice daily
- Yolanda and her father were also given advice and written information on preventing the transmission to others including:
  - Keep sores, blisters and crusty patches clean and dry
  - Wash hands frequently
  - Wash sheets and towels at a high temperature after use and do not share with other family members
  - Do not prepare food for other people
  - Do not have close contact with CYP or adults with a weakened immune system (those receiving chemotherapy, for example)

Advice and Monitoring

In addition to the above, safety-netting advice given to Yolanda and her father on who to contact if the condition deteriorated or did not improve or Yolanda became unwell.

It is often referred to as atopic dermatitis, meaning allergy (atopic), skin (derma-) and inflammation (-itis). It is an allergic reaction that manifests as dry, itchy patches of skin that resemble rashes (Robinson, 2011). Within the dermal layers of the skin there are immune cells, and eczema is an immune response to an allergen. There is a breakdown of the skin barrier this can lead to exposure of allergens via the skin which may result in sensitisation (production of IgE antibodies) and the development of an allergy. In the initial stages of this response the allergen travels through the epidermis to the dermis where an immune cell, an antigen presenting cell starts the process of antibody formation, this process is referred to as sensitisation. Further exposure to the allergen following this initial response will result in an inflammatory response producing interleukins that communicate to cells in the body to produce histamine, leukotrienes and proteases (Iida et al., 2013). It is estimated that between 50–70% of children with eczema become sensitised to one or more allergens, often these are food allergies such as egg and nut and airborne allergens such as dust mite (Allergy UK, 2017).

The inflammatory response results in dry, inflamed, flaky, itchy skin, in severe cases and bleeding. These reactions are visible on the flexor surfaces and exposed parts of the skin. NICE (2007) guidance states that in Asian, black Caribbean and black African children atopic eczema can affect the extensor rather than flexures, and circular and hair follicle patterns may be more common. The first consideration is to prevent the permeability of the skin by ensuring that the skin is soft and well moisturised, avoidance to extremes of weather and chemical and environmental irritants. Symptoms of these conditions are usually managed with emollients and topically with corticosteroid or antihistamine creams that reduce the inflammatory immune response. In severe cases biologics can be used, see below.

Assessing and Diagnosing Atopic Eczema

Eczema has a wide spectrum from mild to severe (Table 14.1). Treatment and care are provided according to this and the age of the child. Many drugs are licensed by age, i.e. under 2 years of age, 2–12 years, over

Chapter 14 Medications and the Integumentary System

Table 14.1 Severity of eczema.

SKIN/ PHYSICAL SEVERITY	SIGNS AND SYMPTOMS	IMPACT ON QUALITY OF LIFE AND PSYCHOSOCIAL WELL-BEING	SIGNS AND SYMPTOMS	TREATMENT
Clear	Normal skin, no evidence of active atopic eczema	None	No impact on quality of life	None
Mild	Areas of dry skin, infrequent itching (with or without small areas of redness)	Mild	Limited impact on everyday activities, sleep and psychosocial well-being	Emollients and mild potency topical corticosteroids
Moderate	Areas of dry skin, frequent itching, redness (with, or without excoriation) and localised skin thickening	Moderate	Moderate impact on everyday activities and psychosocial well-being, frequently disturbed sleep	Emollients, moderate potency topical corticosteroids, topical calcineurin inhibitors and bandages
Severe	Widespread areas of dry skin, incessant itching, redness (with or without excoriation), extensive skin thickening, bleeding, oozing, cracking and alteration of pigmentation	Severe	Severe limitations of everyday activities and psychosocial functioning, nightly loss of sleep	Emollients, potent topical corticosteroids, topical calcineurin inhibitors, bandages, phototherapy, and systemic therapy

Source: Based on NICE, 2007.

12 years. At diagnosis, an assessment will include recording of their detailed clinical and treatment histories and identification of potential trigger factors (NICE, 2007).

Prevalence of atopic eczema is stated to be around 15–20% of school-age children are affected. The diagnosis primarily is concerned with pruritis plus three or more of the following (NICE, 2007):

- Visible dermatitis involving the skin creases, such as bends of knees and elbows (or visible dermatitis on the cheeks and/or extensor areas in children aged 18 months or under)
- Personal history of dermatitis in skin creases (or visible dermatitis on the cheeks and/or extensor areas in children aged 18 months or under)
- Personal history of dry skin in the last 12 months
- Onset of symptoms under the age of 2 years (do not use this criterion in children aged under 4 years)

Children and young people who have atopic eczema often have asthma, allergic rhinitis (hay fever) or food allergy. This order of progression is called the atopic march.

Topical Treatments

Emollients are prescribed on an individual basis suitable to the child's needs and preference. Emollients are used to hydrate and keep the skin smooth; they provide a protective layer for the skin. They can be left on the skin in large quantities (see Skills in Practice: Wet Wrapping). Emollient treatment should continue adjunct to all other treatment and can be used in the absence of symptoms too.

Topical corticosteroids are prescribed by potency levels depending on the severity and the area of the skin that is affected (see NICE, 2007). Application should only be once or twice daily for approximately 10–14 days following a 'flare-up'. The main side effect is skin atrophy (NICE, 2007), this is where the skin becomes thin and bruises easily. Prolonged use is contraindicated as it can cause long-term damage to the elasticity of the skin. Corticosteroids should be avoided where the skin is already thin, or the lowest potency used. The topical treatment with steroids suppresses the allergic reaction.

Topical calcineurin inhibitors are tacrolimus and pimecrolimus. These creams and ointments are used when other topical treatments have been tried and are not controlling the atopic eczema and there is a serious risk of damage to the skin if corticosteroids continue to be used. They have a non-steroidal anti-inflammatory effect on the allergic response, they inhibit the enzyme that triggers the T cell response. They are more expensive than corticosteroids and have side effects related to toxicity, hence the control of their usage. They can be used on children from 2 years of age with specialist support (NICE, 2017a)

Bandages and Dressings

Skills in Practice

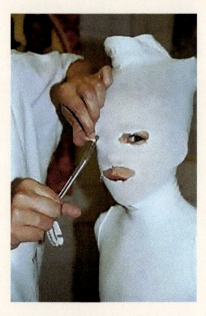

Figure 14.4 Eczema: wet wrapping. *Source:* NICE Guidance 2007, updated 2014.

Medicated dressings or dry bandages can be used for areas of chronic lichenification (localised skin thickening) either with emollients or emollients and topical corticosteroids. Whole-body (limbs and trunk) occlusive dressings (including wet wrap therapy) with topical corticosteroids should be used for 7–14 days only. Use can be continued with emollients alone until the atopic eczema is controlled.

Systemic Treatments

Narrow Band Ultraviolet (UV) Light Therapy/Psoralen and Long Wave Ultraviolet Light (PUVA)/Phototherapy

This treatment can be offered to children who are able to tolerate standing alone for 5-10 minutes. It is a regular treatment and patients need to be able to attend 2–3 times a week for 6–8 weeks to improve outcomes (National Eczema Society, 2018). It cannot be offered if a child is receiving any immunosuppressant medication. PUVA is ultraviolet treatment that is enhanced by taking psoralen before exposure; this increases the absorption of UV. Narrow band UV contains less of the burning rays and is becoming common place for treatment. UV light reduces the inflammation by dampening the activity of the immune system (National Eczema Society, 2018).

Immunosuppressive Drugs

Methotrexate (MTX) is thought to work by preventing cells of the immune system from dividing, but it is not entirely clear how it reduces the severity of eczema (Flohr and Irvine, 2013). It takes several weeks for MXT to accumulate inside cells (National Eczema Society, 2019). MTX and azathioprine (AZA) do not feature in NICE guidance for the treatment of eczema in CYP; however, studies have demonstrated positive outcomes for severe atopic eczema (Flohr and Irvine, 2013). MTX is used in children for the same conditions as in adults but is not licensed for any dermatological condition.

Biologic therapies are monoclonal antibodies (MAB) work by blocking the interleukin (IL) from binding to their cell receptors, this stops the immune system from overreacting. Dupilumab is designed to block two specific ILs, preventing the inflammatory response escalating in atopic eczema (NICE, 2020b). Adjunct therapies such as UV light and emollients are recommended to maintain clinical improvement. According to Smith et al. (2017) the drug is not yet routinely available for those aged less than 18 years, however some 12- to 17-year-olds are already being treated with dupilumab in the UK as part of an early access scheme. Research is ongoing for those under 12 years.

Psoriasis

Psoriasis is a systemic, immune-mediated, inflammatory skin disease which typically has a chronic relapsing-remitting course and may have nail and joint (psoriatic arthritis) involvement (Boehncke and Schon, 2015; NICE, 2017b). The prevalence of psoriasis is estimated to be around 1.3–2.2% in the UK (Parisi et al., 2011). Psoriasis can occur at any age, psoriasis is associated with joint disease in a significant proportion of patients (Ibrahim et al., 2009). It is an autoimmune disorder where too many skin cells are produced (Boehnke and Schon, 2015). In psoriasis, certain T cells are activated, and these produce tumour necrosis factor alpha (TNF-alpha) in excessive amounts. These cells act is if they are fighting an infection and this leads to rapid skin cell growth. There are a variety of types of psoriasis (Table 14.2). The most common is plaque psoriasis. Skin rapidly accumulates and looks silvery-white in appearance. Plaques from *plaque psoriasis* frequently occur on the skin of the elbows and knees, but can affect any area, including the scalp, palms of hands and soles of feet, and genitals (Young et al., 2017). Incidence in CYP has increased (Parisi, et al. 2013). Psoriasis varies in severity from minor localised patches to complete body coverage. The physical assessment of psoriasis includes recording the body surface area affected, any involvement of nails, high-impact and difficult-to-treat sites (for example, the face, scalp, palms, soles, flexures and genitals) and any systemic symptoms including fever and malaise. Fever and malaise are common in unstable forms of psoriasis, such as erythroderma or generalised pustular psoriasis (British Association of Dermatologists, 2020).

Assessment and Diagnosis

There are several validated assessment tools for adults with psoriasis and psoriatic arthritis, such as the Psoriasis Area and Severity Index (British Association of Dermatologists, 2020); however, these are not suitable for children.

Emollients/Topical Therapy

These are used as first line treatment in psoriasis in children and young people (NICE, 2017b). The purpose of an emollient is to remove the superficial scales. Once this top layer is removed it can enhance

Table 14.2 Types of psoriasis.

TYPE	SIGNS AND SYMPTOMS	AFFECTED AREAS	WHO
Plaque psoriasis	Raised, inflamed red skin covered with silvery-white scales	Anywhere but frequently elbows, knees, scalp and lower back	Most common. Both children and adults, mainly affects 30 years plus.
Guttate psoriasis (raindrop psoriasis)	Small pink-red spots	Scalp, upper arms, thighs and trunk	Starts in children and young people
Inverse psoriasis	Bright red, smooth skin but no scales	Skin folds and creases; armpits, groin, neck	Affects babies, may appear, and then not return, unlike psoriasis that starts in adults

the penetration of the topical treatments that are applied to the skin (Psoriasis and Psoriatic Arthritis Alliance, 2019) They also soften the plaques, this makes it more comfortable and flexible. Psoriasis can itch and emollients can give some pruritic relief. Emollients help to rehydrate the skin, they create a barrier, this prevents further water loss as well as protecting the skin from bacteria and irritants (NICE, 2017b).

Clinical Consideration

When the use of emollients is advised and topical medications are prescribed, the nurse practitioner/ prescriber should consider the following:

Emollient and Topical Medication Application
Topical medications do not reach their target site through the systemic circulation, they react directly to the area that they are applied to. Therefore, the action is rapid; however, small amounts of the medication may be absorbed through the skin into the circulation. It is imperative that topical medications are applied thinly and only for the prescribed duration (McGavock, 2017). For the same reason parents or practitioners who are applying the topical medication should wear gloves. Handwashing, post application, will reduce the risk of medication being transferred from hands to eyes and prevent any absorption into the nurse's/parent's hands. *Emollients* contain ingredients that can increase the risk of slipping, especially when used in the bath. They are designed to provide a barrier to the skin and care must be taken when moving and handling children.

Safe Storage and Ingestion
Parents/carers may often apply topical medications and emollients during a nappy change or at bath time, it may be convenient to have the products close by. These products need to be stored in a safe place away from small children. Ingestion can cause vomiting and diarrhoea (BNFc, 2020). Some medication may be affected by sunlight or damp conditions; ensure that safe storage is adhered to.

Expiry Dates
The therapeutic eff0ectiveness of medication reduces over time. Out-of-date topical medications and emollients should be disposed appropriately.

Disability Living Allowance
For many families there are additional costs to caring for a child or young person with a skin condition. The additional costs may include extra clothing, washing and time taken to apply and bandage affected areas. Practitioners should consider this and signpost families to apply for DLA where appropriate.

Source: BNFc, 2020; McGavock, 2017.

Corticosteroids

The risks for corticosteroids use are like those in eczema. Potency of corticosteroid creams is dependent on the need of the patient (NICE, 2017b). There can be systemic side effects if corticosteroids are used continuously to extensive areas of psoriasis; these can manifest as suppression of the hypothalamic-pituitary-adrenal axis, which could result in problems with growth and the development of Cushing's syndrome. Very potent corticosteroids in CYP are not recommended (BNF for Children (BNFc), 2020). Those CYP who are using corticosteroids for psoriasis should be reviewed at least annually to assess for the presence of steroid atrophy and other adverse effects (NICE, 2017b).

Vitamin D Preparations

Calcipotriol and tacalcitol are synthetic derivatives of vitamin D. They are antiproliferative, reducing the abnormal proliferation of keratinocytes that occurs in psoriasis, and they induce cell differentiation and cell death (Barrea, 2017). They are used as first line treatment for plaque psoriasis; calcipotriol applied once daily (only for children over 6 years of age) (BNFc, 2020). The vitamin D and analogues, calcipotriol, calcitriol, and tacalcitol are used for the management of plaque psoriasis. They should be avoided by those with calcium metabolism disorders and used with caution in generalised pustular or erythrodermic exfoliative psoriasis (enhanced risk of hypercalcaemia). Vitamin D and its analogues are effective and cosmetically acceptable alternatives to preparations containing coal tar or dithranol, they do not have an odour (NICE, 2017b).

Salicylic Acid

Salicylic acid is classified as a keratolytic, or peeling agent, and works by causing the outer layer of skin to shed (BNFc, 2020). It is a common and effective treatment for a wide variety of skin problems. As a psoriasis treatment, it acts as a scale lifter, helping to soften and remove psoriasis scales. Scalp psoriasis is usually scaly, and the scale may be thick and adherent. This requires softening with an emollient ointment, cream, or oil and usually combined with salicylic acid as a keratolytic. Some preparations for psoriasis affecting the scalp combine salicylic acid with coal tar or sulfur. The preparation should be applied generously and left on for at least an hour, often more conveniently overnight, before washing it off (BNFc, 2020).

Coal Tar Products

Coal tar is commonly used to treat psoriasis (BNFc, 2020). Tar can help slow the rapid growth of skin cells and restore the skin's appearance. It can help reduce the inflammation, itching and scaling of psoriasis. For chronic stable plaque psoriasis on extensor surfaces of the trunk and limbs preparations containing coal tar are moderately effective, but the odour is unacceptable to some children. Coal tar has anti-inflammatory properties that are useful in chronic plaque psoriasis; it also has antiscaling properties. Contact of coal tar products with normal skin is not normally harmful and preparations containing coal tar can be used for widespread small lesions; however, irritation, contact allergy and sterile folliculitis can occur. Leave-on preparations that remain in contact with the skin, such as creams or ointments, containing up to 6% coal tar may be used on children 1 month to 2 years; leave-on preparations containing coal tar 10% may be used on children over 2 years with more severe psoriasis.

Dithranol

Dithranol is an anthracene derivative that impairs DNA replication and decreases cell division and is effective for healing psoriatic plaques. Dithranol is used as a cream that is applied to the plaque for 30 minutes and then washed off. Treatment should be started with a low concentration such as dithranol 0.1%, and the strength increased gradually every few days up to 3%, according to tolerance (BNFc, 2020). Dithranol is an effective topical antipsoriatic agent but it irritates and stains the skin and it should be used only under specialist supervision. Adverse effects of dithranol are minimised by using a 'short-contact technique' and by starting with low concentration preparations. Dithranol is effective for chronic plaque psoriasis. Its major disadvantages are irritation (for which individual susceptibility varies) and staining of skin and of clothing. Dithranol is not generally suitable for widespread small lesions nor should it be used in the flexures or on the face. Proprietary preparations are more suitable for home use; they are usually washed off after 20–30 minutes ('short contact' technique). Specialist nurses may apply intensive treatment with dithranol paste which is covered by stockinette dressings and usually kept on overnight. Dithranol should be discontinued if even a low concentration causes acute inflammation; continued use can result in the psoriasis becoming unstable.

Phototherapy

The protocol for children is the same as for treatment of eczema. Phototherapy is available in specialist centres. Narrow band ultraviolet B (UVB) radiation is usually effective for chronic stable psoriasis and for guttate psoriasis. It can be considered for children with moderately severe psoriasis in whom topical treatment has failed, but it may irritate inflammatory psoriasis. The use of phototherapy and PUVA in children is limited by concerns over carcinogenicity and premature ageing (NICE, 2017b).

Systemic/Disease-Modifying Drugs

Ciclosporin, methotrexate and acitretin (NICE, 2017b) are systemic/disease-modifying drugs. Ciclosporin by mouth can be used for severe psoriasis and for severe eczema. Methotrexate can be used for severe resistant psoriasis; the dose is given once weekly and adjusted according to severity of the condition and haematological and biochemical measurements. Folic acid should be given to reduce the possibility of methotrexate toxicity. Folic acid can be given once weekly on a different day to the MXT; alternative regimens may be used in some settings. Acitretin, a metabolite of etretinate, is a retinoid (vitamin A derivative); it is prescribed by specialists. The main indication of acitretin is severe psoriasis resistant to other forms of therapy. It is also used in disorders of keratinisation such as severe Darier's disease (keratosis follicularis), and some forms of ichthyosis. Although a minority of cases of psoriasis respond well to acitre-

Chapter 14 Medications and the Integumentary System

tin alone, it is only moderately effective in many cases; adverse effects are a limiting factor. A therapeutic effect occurs after 2 to 4 weeks and the maximum benefit after 4 months. Consideration should be given to stopping acitretin if the response is inadequate after 4 months at the optimum dose. Continuous treatment for longer than 6 months is not usually necessary in psoriasis. However, some patients, particularly those with severe ichthyosis, may benefit from longer treatment, provided that the lowest effective dose is used, patients are monitored carefully for adverse effects, and the need for treatment is reviewed regularly. Topical preparations containing keratolytics should normally be stopped before administration of acitretin. Whilst using systemic medication the use of emollients should be encouraged, and topical corticosteroids can be continued if necessary.

Biologic Therapies

These are designed to block the condition in the immune system rather than treating the symptoms. Etanercept (a cytokine modulator) is licensed in children over 6 years of age for the treatment of severe plaque psoriasis that is inadequately controlled by other systemic treatments and photochemotherapy, or when these other treatments cannot be used because of intolerance or contraindications (NICE, 2017b). Adalimumab (a cytokine modulator) is licensed in children over 4 years for the treatment of severe chronic plaque psoriasis that is inadequately controlled by other topical treatments and phototherapies, or when these treatments are inappropriate (NICE, 2017b).

Episode of Care

Jennifer was 30 when she had her first child, Ben, now aged 12. She lives with her husband, Dan, they have daily support from Jennifer's parents as she finds some activities difficult and Dan works full time. Jen works from home; she was diagnosed with psoriatic arthritis 8 years ago.

Ben had severe cradle cap when he was a baby, they used several topical treatments to clear this up. It did not fully clear, Ben (now 12) still has scaling on his scalp. The GP diagnosed a fungal infection at the age of 2 years, Ben was treated with miconazole for six months. At the age of 4 years, several small red spots appeared around Ben's hair line and down his back and the GP prescribed topical corticosteroids for two weeks, this seemed to improve the spots. A month later a few red areas appeared on his lower limbs, these were treated with emollients and diagnosed as eczema. For the next few years Ben would be treated with intermittent steroid cream and emollients.

In Ben's first year at secondary school he developed small red spots on his arms. Within a month these had become itchy, inflamed, and started to shed white scales. He was referred to a dermatologist and diagnosed with psoriasis. He commenced topical creams, then PUVA and is currently on biologic therapy.

He has been referred to a psychologist following a clinic visit where he disclosed that he felt he wasn't coping, he could manage his medication and living with the fact that he might 'end up' like his mum, but he couldn't cope with the children at school calling him 'lizard man' and a 'freak'. The nurse practitioner is going into school to raise awareness of the condition. The school have been informed and are working with the bullies.

Conclusion

As a student healthcare practitioner, you will undoubtedly be involved in the care of patients with one or multiple types of skin conditions. These conditions can be complex and have the potential to have detrimental effects on a patient's activities of living. It is crucial that healthcare professionals involved in supporting this patient group to manage their acute and chronic disease processes have a sound understanding of the pathophysiological, pharmacological and evidence base that underpins the promotion of safe and effective care.

Glossary

Atrophy: A wasting away or diminution.

Carcinogen: A substance that causes cancer.

Cellulitis: A skin infection. It can be serious if it's not treated quickly.

Dermatophyte: Pathogenic fungus growing on skin, mucous membranes, hair, nails and other body surfaces.

Erythroderma: A severe and potentially life-threatening inflammation of most of the body's skin surface. It is also called generalised exfoliative dermatitis.

Excoriation: To wear off the skin (to abrade).

Hypersensitivity: Extreme physical sensitivity to particular substances or conditions.

Immunocompromised: A broad term that means a person's immune system is not working as well as it should be to protect the individual against infections.

integumentary: It comprises the skin and its appendages.

Lesion: A region in an organ or tissue that has experienced damage through injury or disease, such as a wound, ulcer, abscess, or tumour.

Pharmacotherapy: The treatment of disease with drugs.

Phototherapy: The use of light in the treatment of illness. Involves exposure to fluorescent light bulbs or other sources of light, such as, halogen lights, sunlight, and light emitting diodes (LEDs) to treat certain medical conditions.

Urticaria: Reddened, itchy welts that can be triggered by exposure to certain foods, medications or other substances (hives).

References

Allergy UK (2017). *Eczema: Are We Just Scratching the Surface?* www.allergyuk.org, (accessed 27 June 2020).

Barrea, L., Savanelli, M.C., Di Somma, C. et al. (2017). Vitamin D and its role in psoriasis: An overview of the dermatologist and nutritionist. *Reviews in Endocrine & Metabolic Disorders* 18(2), 195–205. doi: 10.1007/s11154-017-9411-6.

Boehnke, W-H. and Schon, M. (2015). Psoriasis. *The Lancet* 386(9997): 983–994. doi: 10.1016/S0140-6736(14)61909-7.

British Association of Dermatologists (2020). *Psoriasis Area and Severity Index* (PASI). www.bad.org.uk (accessed 25 July 2020).

BNF for Children (BNFc) (2020). British National Formulary for Children. www.bnfc.nice.org.uk (accessed 25 July 2020).

Cosh, J. (2016). Understanding the effects of eczema. *Nursing Children and Young People* 28(2): 9.

Crowley, P.D. and Gallagher, H.C. (2014). Clotrimazole as a pharmaceutical: past, present and future. *Journal of Applied Microbiology* 117(3): 611–617.

Flohr, C. and Irvine, A. (2013). Systemic therapies for severe atopic dermatitis in children and adults. *Journal of Allergy and Clinical Immunology* 132(3): 774e6.

Health and Social Care Information Centre (2016). *Prescription Cost Analysis, England*.

Ibrahim, G., Waxman, R., and Helliwell, P.S. (2009). The prevalence of psoriatic arthritis in people with psoriasis. *Arthritis and Rheumatism* 61: 1373–8.

Iida, H., Takai, T., Kamijo, S. et al. (2013). Protease allergen and barrier injury synergistically induce skin inflammation and antibody production. *Journal of Dermatological Science* 69(2), E6–E7.

McGavock, H. (2017). *How Drugs Work: Basic Pharmacology for Health Professionals*, 4e. London: CRC Press.

McLafferty, E. (2012). The integumentary system: anatomy, physiology and function of skin. *Nursing Standard* 27(3): 35–42.

NHS (2020). *Impetigo*. www.nhs.uk/conditions/Ringworm/ (accessed 7 July 2020).

NHS (2020). *Ringworm*. www.nhs.uk/conditions/Ringworm/ (accessed 7 July 2020).

National Eczema Society (2018). *Phototherapy*. https://eczema.org/wp-content/uploads/Phototherapy-Oct-18-1.pdf (accessed 25 July 2020).

Chapter 14 Medications and the Integumentary System

National Eczema Society (2019). *Methotrexate*. https://eczema.org/wp-content/uploads/Methotrexate-Oct-18-1.pdf (accessed 25 July 2020).

National Institute for Health and Care Excellence (2007). T*reatment of eczema in children and young people*. www.nice.org.uk/guidance/conditions-and-diseases/skin-conditions/eczema (accessed 25 July 2020).

National Institute for Health and Care Excellence (2017a). *Multiple Technology Appraisal of Adalimumab, Etanercept and Ustekinumab for Treating Plaque Psoriasis in Children and Young People [TA455]*. www.nice.org.uk/guidance/TA455 (accessed 25 July 2020).

National Institute for Health and Care Excellence (2017)b. *Psoriasis: Assessment and Management*. www.nice.org.uk/guidance/cg153 (accessed 25 July 2020).

National Institute for Health and Care Excellence (2020a). *Impetigo Antimicrobial Prescribing Guideline*. www.nice.org.uk/guidance/ng153/evidence/impetigo-antimicrobial-prescribing-guideline-pdf-7084856126 (accessed 21 July 2020).

National Institute for Health and Care Excellence (2020b). *Eczema – NICE Pathways*. https://pathways.nice.org.uk/pathways/eczema?UNLID=698701275202072693623 (accessed 21 July 2020).

Oranges, T., Dini, V., and Romanelli, M. (2015). Skin physiology of the neonate and infant: clinical implications. *Advances in Wound Care* 4(10): 587–595. doi: 10.1089/wound.2015.0642.

Paediatric Formulary Committee. *BNF for Children* (online) London: BMJ Group, Pharmaceutical Press, and RCPCH Publications. www.medicinescomplete.com (accessed 6 July 2020).

Parisi, R., Symmons, D.P.M., Griffiths, C.E.M., and Ashcroft, D.M. (2013). Global epidemiology of psoriasis: a systematic review of incidence and prevalence. *Journal of Investigative Dermatology* 133(2): 377–385.

Peate, I. (2018). *Fundamentals of Applied Pathophysiology: An Essential Guide for Nursing and Healthcare Students*, 3e, London, Wiley-Blackwell.

Peate, I. and Nair, M. (2011). *Anatomy and Physiology for Student Nurses*. London, Wiley.

Psoriasis and Psoriatic Arthritis Alliance (2019). *Emollients and Psoriasis*. www.papaa.org, accessed 28.6.20.

Robinson, J. (2011). Assessment and management of atopic eczema in children. *Nursing Standard* 26(1): 48–56.

Rutter, P. (2013). *Community Pharmacy: Symptoms, Diagnosis and Treatment*, 3e. Elsevier.

Smith, C., Jabbar-Lopez, Z., Yiu, Z. et al. (2017). British Association of Dermatologists guidelines for biologic therapy for psoriasis 2017. *Br J Dermatol* 177: 628–636. doi: 10.1111/bjd.15665.

Weller, R.B., Hunter, H., and Mann, M. (2015). *Clinical Dermatology*, 5e. Chichester: Wiley-Blackwell.

Young, M., Aldridge, L., and Parker, P. (2017). Psoriasis for the primary practitioner. *Journal of the American Association of Nurse Practitioners* 29(3). doi: 10.1002/2327-6924.12443.

Zhu, G., Wang, Q., Lu, S., and Niu, Y. (2017). Hydrogen peroxide: a potential wound therapeutic target? Medical principles and practice. *International Journal of the Kuwait University, Health Science Centre* 26(4), 301–308. doi: 10.1159/000475501.

Further Resources

NHS Conditions – Impetigo (online): www.nhs.uk/conditions/impetigo/

NHS Conditions – Ringworm (online): www.nhs.uk/conditions/Ringworm/

NICE NG153 – Impetigo antimicrobial prescribing (online): www.nice.org.uk/search?q=Impetigo%3a+antimicrobial+prescribing

NICE Eczema pathway or children under 12 years (online): https://pathways.nice.org.uk/pathways/eczema

Validated tools that assess the severity of skin disorders to decide treatment:

- Patient-Oriented Eczema Measure for severity (POEM)
- Children's Dermatology Life Quality Index (CDLQI)
- Infants' Dermatitis Quality of Life Index (IDQoL)
- Dermatitis Family Impact (DFI)

Multiple Choice Questions

1. What does integumentary mean?
   (a) Skin
   (b) Covering
   (c) Nail bed
   (d) Epidermis
2. As keratinocytes move to the skin surface, they lose what?
   (a) Oxygen
   (b) Nutrients

Chapter 14 Medications and the Integumentary System

(c) Vitamin D
(d) Cytoplasm
3. The dermis accounts for what percent of total body weight?
(a) 15–20%
(b) 25–30%
(c) 10–15%
(d) 35–40%
4. Which muscles contract in cold air or with heightened emotions?
(a) Pectoralis major
(b) Deltoid muscle
(c) Masseter and temporalis muscle
(d) Arrector pili
5. Approximately how many people are affected by eczema in the UK?
(a) 10 million
(b) 5 million
(c) 15 million
(d) 20 million
6. Methotrexate is thought to work by?
(a) Preventing cells of the immune system from dividing
(b) Preventing cells of the immune system from bursting
(c) Preventing cells of the immune system from dying
(d) Preventing cells of the immune system from being absorbed
7. In psoriasis, skin rapidly accumulates and looks _____ in appearance?
(a) Silvery-yellow
(b) Yellow-grey
(c) Grey-white
(d) Silvery-white
8. Children and young people who are using corticosteroids for psoriasis should be reviewed at least _____?
(a) 3 monthly
(b) 6 monthly
(c) 12 monthly
(d) Bi-annually
9. Impetigo is caused by a _____ infection?
(a) Viral
(b) Bacterial
(c) Fungal
(d) Yeast
10. How many days after initial exposure do impetigo symptoms present?
(a) 4–10 days
(b) 20–30 days
(c) 12–15 days
(d) 1–2 days
11. Hydrogen peroxide is a topical _____?
(a) Antibiotic
(b) Antifungal
(c) Antiviral
(d) Antiseptic
12. One of the drawbacks with administering clarithromycin granules are that they should not be?
(a) Swallowed
(b) Eaten with food
(c) Chewed
(d) Taken at night
13. Which of these are NOT dermatophyte fungi?
(a) Trichophyton:
(b) Microsporum:

(c) Epidermophyton
(d) Trichosporum
14. Dermatophytes invade _____?
    (a) Keratin
    (b) Epidermis
    (c) Dermis
    (d) d.Nose
15. Scarlet fever is caused by _____?
    (a) Streptococcus pyogenes
    (b) Streptococcus aureus
    (c) Epidermophyton
    (d) Zoophilic spread

Find Out More

The following is a list of common conditions that are associated with CYP who have skin conditions. Take some time and write notes about each of the conditions. Think about the medications that may be used in order to treat these conditions and be specific about the pharmacokinetics and pharmacodynamics. Remember to include aspects of patient care. If you are making notes about people you have offered care and support to, you must ensure that you have adhered to the rules of confidentiality.

THE CONDITION	YOUR NOTES
Herpes simplex (cold sores)	
Urticaria	
Scabies	
Fifth disease/parvovirus B19 (slapped cheek syndrome)	
Warts and verrucae	

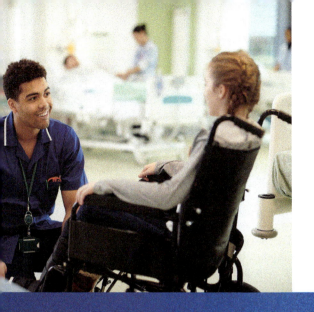

15

Medications Used in Children and Young People's Mental Health

Louise Lingwood, Edward Stephenson and Laura Stavert

Aim

This chapter provides the reader with an introduction to some of the mental health disorders (MHD) that may be encountered in clinical practice and supports a fundamental understanding of the common psychotropic medications used to treat common mental health conditions in children and young people (CYP). Psychopharmacology knowledge and understanding is essential to safe medicines management and the treatment of CYP who have a diagnosable MHD.

Learning Outcomes

- Gain an understanding of the pharmacokinetics and pharmacodynamics associated with each drug class.
- Categorise and evaluate the different groups of medications used to treat common mental health disorder in CYP.
- Gain an understanding of the risks associated with identified drug classes.
- Gain an understanding of the physical health monitoring necessary for identified drug classes and develop understanding of why this is necessary.

Fundamentals of Pharmacology for Children's Nurses, First Edition. Edited by Ian Peate and Peter Dryden.
© 2022 John Wiley & Sons Ltd. Published 2022 by John Wiley & Sons Ltd.
Companion website: www.wiley.com/go/pharmacologyforCN

Introduction

Mental health problems in CYP are estimated at 10–20% of the population worldwide (Kieling at al., 2011). One in eight 5–19-year-olds had at least one MHD when assessed in the United Kingdom (UK) in 2017 (NHS Digital, 2018). Half of lifetime mental health problems occur by the age of 14 and are often not recognised, leaving CYP struggling with their emotions, thoughts, the implications of behaviours and their relationships with peers and caregivers. A joint report published by Department of Health UK and Department for Education UK (2018) indicates that CYP wait too long for support and professional intervention (DH and DE, 2018). Medication use in this population has substantially increased in the last 15 years. It is often a difficult decision for parents and carers in partnership with psychiatric team members to consider medication as a way of managing the presentation of mental health problems and disorder and it should not be considered in isolation. It is important that MH problems are identified early to allow CYP to reach their full potential. CYP often will react differently to medication use and dose recalculations are often a part of the process in getting it right in individual cases. Drugs used are classed according to the ways that they function within the CYP's body. The drugs explored in this chapter are categorised by the effect that they have on the brain and behaviours. The categories explored in this chapter are stimulants and non-stimulants, hypnotics, antipsychotics, antidepressants, anxiolytics, mood stabilisers.

Skills for Practice 1

Remind yourself of the drug calculation used in CYP nursing

Basic Drug Calculations

What you want, over what you've got, times what it's in.

If you have a bottle of liquid medicine (500 mg in 5 ml) and your patient has been prescribed 120mg, it can appear to be a daunting calculation at first. Here's how it is done:

What you want (120mg) over *what you've got* (500mg) *times what it's in*
(5ml) 120/500 × 5 = 1.2ml to administer

What Is Psychopharmacology?

Pharmacology is the study of how drugs affect the body and *psychopharmacology* is the study of how drugs affect the brain and therefore behaviour. As discussed in Chapter 5, the two critical areas in understanding psychopharmacology are *pharmacokinetics* – this is related to how what the CYP's body does to the drugs as they are processed by the body and *pharmacodynamics* – this is related to understanding the mechanism of the actions of the drug or more simply how the drug causes an effect once it is distributed within the child or young person's body.

Most medications used in psychopharmacology act through neurotransmitters and have a direct effect on the brain. Serotonin, norepinephrine and dopamine are described as the main neurotransmitters. It is clear from comparison between the ways in which the drug causes effect in the adult body that there is a striking difference to the effect of the drug in children, due to the developing brain of the child. CYP have larger livers and kidneys in relation to their body mass than adults and therefore to simply reduce the medication dose and calculate it according to weight would not be safe and would place the CYP at risk of undertreatment (McVoy and Findling, 2017). In addition, severe side effects can result because of under or over dosage of medication.

Medications

Anxiety Disorders

The most prevalent disorders in CYP are anxiety disorders and they are often unrecognised and underdiagnosed (NICE, 2014). 7.2% of CYP aged 5–19 have experienced anxiety in some form (Vizard et al., 2017). 3.9% of 5- to 10-year-olds, 7.5% of 11–16-year-olds and 13.1% of 17–19-year-olds were diagnosed with

Chapter 15 Medications Used in Children and Young People's Mental Health

anxiety in 2017 (Vizard et al., 2017). The current ICD-10 (2019) states anxiety is characterised by anxious feelings or fear sometimes accompanied by physical symptoms, apprehension of danger, restlessness, tension, tachycardia and dyspnoea (shortness of breath) unattached to a clearly identifiable stimulus. There are two robust predictors (Creswell et al., 2020) of anxiety in CYP: first, if the CYP exhibits an inhibited temperament and, second, if the CYP's parent(s) have experienced an anxiety disorder. Comorbidity is commonplace among anxiety disorder in CYP and diagnostics can include observation, interview schedules and questionnaires (Creswell et al., 2020). In order to meet the threshold diagnosis of an anxiety disorder, a certain number of symptoms must be experienced beyond a minimum specified period and cause considerable personal distress, with an associated impairment in day-to-day functioning (Baldwin et al., 2014). Several different anxiety disorders exist, including Generalised Anxiety Disorder (GAD), Panic Disorder, Post-Traumatic Stress Disorder (PTSD) and Obsessive-Compulsive Disorder (OCD).

Reservations about drug treatment for anxiety disorders are common, not least due to the potential adverse effects which can be associated with these and the potential for dependence with drugs such as benzodiazepines. Nurses and Healthcare Assistants have a large role to play to ensure CYP, parents/carers understand the benefits associated with drug treatments and support them to balance these with the associated risks. Evidence-based psychological interventions are the first line of treatment in preference to pharmacological intervention (NICE, 2014).

Anxiolytics

Selective Serotonin Reuptake Inhibitors (SSRIs) are currently the second-line pharmacological treatment approach for most anxiety disorders as they appear to have a relatively quick onset of action but remain effective in the longer term and are generally well tolerated with few side effects (Baldwin et al., 2014). Where drug treatment has been effective, this should usually be continued for at least 12 months (Bazire, 2018).

Side effects of SSRIs can be seen in an escalation of anxiety rather than a decrease. There may be other indicators such as aggression and hostility and some CYP may develop suicidal thoughts (thinking about killing themselves or planning to do so). It is important to note any changes in appetite and changes to bowel movements. Some CYP state that they feel sick and report blurred vision and feeling dizzy.

Other Antidepressants Used in the Treatment of Anxiety
Sertraline

Sertraline acts to inhibit the reuptake of serotonin (5-hydroxytryptaline, 5-HT). It is used where the CYP has major depression but also is effective in the treatment of OCD and social anxiety and panic. There is little known about how this drug works. Sertraline is slowly absorbed and the estimated half-life ranges from 22–36 hours (De Vane et al., 2002).

Side effects include nausea, constipation, diarrhoea, vomiting, not being able to fall asleep or stay asleep, dry mouth, weight change, appetite changes and sweating. Some side effects can be very serious, including seizures, hallucinations and confusion, abnormal bleeding and bruising, hives, swelling and difficulty breathing. Sertraline can cause a decrease in appetite in CYP. It is therefore important to ensure that as nurses we spend time understanding what the CYP is feeling and be aware of medication changes and the possible side effects.

Benzodiazepines

Benzodiazepines are effective at managing symptoms of anxiety in the short term in adults. They are both anxiolytics and hypnotics and act at benzodiazepine receptors which are associated with gamma-aminobutyric acid (GABA) receptors. Examples include diazepam and lorazepam. They are not suitable for CYP except in cases of acute anxiety and insomnia (due to fear or sleepwalking), where diazepam may be used.

Diazepam

The main effect of diazepam is sedation, reduced anxiety and muscle relaxation. Diazepam should be a short-term treatment option and used with care. The CYP brain can become hypersensitive to the effects of diazepam and the effect can be reduced. The therapeutic effects of diazepam persist for a prolonged period following administration; it has a half-life of 1–2 days, but its metabolite is also pharmacologically active and has a half-life of 2–5 days (ABPI, 2019a). Promethazine is sometimes used as a sedative (BNF, 2020) sedative guidance.

Stimulants and Non-Stimulants

Common side effects of benzodiazepines include decreased alertness, confusion, dizziness, depression, gastrointestinal disorder, hypotension, respiratory depression, headaches, muscle weakness and balance issues and sleep disorder. A note of warning is that the CYP may experience thoughts of harming themselves or ending their lives. Uncommon side effects include agitation, although this is more likely in CYP than in adults. It is rare but again more common in CYP for their behaviour to become aggressive, making it essential for nurses to gain an understanding of what the CYP's behaviour is prior to medications being prescribed to enable robust clinical decision making in partnership with those who care for the child and where possible how the CYP feels.

Stimulants and Non-Stimulants

The most prevalent paediatric neuro-developmental disorder is Attention Deficit/Hyperactivity Disorder (ADHD), thought to be present in 2–5% of school-age children (Royal College of Psychiatrists, 2017). It is characterised by pervasive inattention and associated with impairments related to social, academic functioning in childhood with the addition of occupational impairment in adolescence and warrants holistic ongoing assessment (Nicholson, 2018). A diagnosis of ADHD can be made by a specialist healthcare professional with expertise in ADHD, for example, a specialist paediatrician or psychiatrist. The diagnosis should include an assessment of the CYP needs, level of impulsivity, coexisting conditions, social, familial and educational or occupational circumstances and physical health. For CYP, there should also be an assessment of their parents' or carers' mental health (NICE, 2019a). Nicholson (2018) reminds us that untreated ADHD can have a detrimental impact on a CYP's health and social outcomes. The risks of mismanagement of ADHD include substance abuse, self-harm and suicide, antisocial behaviours, educational attainment and future employment and life expectancy, highlighting the importance of continuous assessment.

There are two main categories of ADHD medication. These are known as stimulants and non-stimulants. Both act on the ways in which the neurons in the brain communicate with one another with the aim of increasing the ability to focus, improve memory and reduce restlessness and overactivity whilst increasing energy levels.

Stimulants

Stimulant drugs have been used for decades and have a strong evidence base relating to short-term use. They increase the activity of cells called neurons or nerve cells in the nervous system. Stimulant drugs are used to treat the symptoms of ADHD and are also used to treat narcolepsy (periods of deep sleep) in adults. Neurons are electrically excitable cells that receive sensory information from the outside world and send motor commands to the muscles in our bodies. The sensory information can be physical or chemical and correspond to our five senses – sight, touch, smell, hearing and taste.

A growth in concern has become apparent relating to a connection between stimulant medication and an exacerbation of risk relating to future substance misuse. A Swedish study examining the long-term effects of stimulant use in the treatment of ADHD disputed this and found no correlation and concluded that long-term use of stimulants decreased the risk of substance misuse (Chang et al., 2014). However, we must remain mindful that each CYP will present differently according to their chemical make-up.

Methylphenidate

Methylphenidate acts directly on the central nervous system (CNS) where it blocks the reuptake of norepinephrine and dopamine. Its mode of action is stimulation of the cerebral cortex and subcortical structures of the brain. It is used in the treatment of ADHD and Attention Deficit Disorder (ADD), fatigue (due to cancer) and depression. It is available in two forms an immediate release form and more recently in a variety of delivery systems for example a transdermal patch – 'Daytrana', enabling CYP not to be reliant on taking medications throughout the school day and it is also available as an oral liquid. The mode of action of methylphenidate is that it blocks the reuptake of the neurotransmitter dopamine.

Methylphenidate IR is commonly used as a medication which is administered orally for children, in children aged 4–6 years a dosage of 2.5mg daily up to 1.4mg. In children aged 6–17 years 5–60mg daily (unlicensed, the dosage above 90mg daily). The drug is targeted at those suffering from ADHD. Melatonin is not licensed for the treatment of narcolepsy in CYP.

Caution is advised in cases of agitation, alcohol dependence, anxiety, drug dependence, epilepsy, (discontinue if increased seizure frequency, family history of Tourette Syndrome, tics and susceptibility to angle-closure glaucoma).

Stimulant medications can cause side effects these can be categorised as common or very common, uncommon and very rare. Common side effects of stimulant medication include: alopecia; anxiety; appetite; arrhythmias; arthralgia; behaviour; cough; depression; diarrhoea; dizziness; drowsiness; dry mouth; fever; gastrointestinal discomfort; growth retardation; headaches; hypertension; laryngeal pain; mood altered; movement disorders; nasopharyngitis; nausea; palpitations; sleep disorders; vomiting; weight decreased. Uncommon side effects of stimulant medication include chest discomfort, constipation, dyspnoea, haematuria; hallucinations; muscle complaints; psychotic disorder; suicidal tendencies; tic; tremor and vision disorders. Some of the rare side effects of stimulant medication include anaemia, angina, cardiac death, Raynaud's, sexual disfunction and thrombocytopenia (NICE, 2021).

Non-Stimulant Medication

Whilst stimulant medications are often a first-choice treatment for ADHD in some cases there may be a requirement for non-stimulant medication. These alternative medications may be appropriate for CYP where there is a coexisting condition such as tic disorder as they in some cases are proven to treat both. In other cases where stimulant medication has not worked well or the side effects outweigh the benefits, there may also be a need to add a non-stimulant drug to already prescribed stimulant medication. However, those prescribing or supporting the CYP must remain mindful of the effects of polypharmacy on the developing child or young person and its long-term effects.

ADHD specific non-stimulants include atomoxetine (Strattera), which increases the amount of the neurotransmitter norepinephrine and is classified as an antidepressant medication. Non-stimulant medications do not have the risks associated with addiction (therefore not a controlled drug). They are not often related to side effects such as sleeplessness and agitation. Alternative non-stimulant drugs not routinely used include tricyclic antidepressants and Clonidine, a medication used to treat hypertension. NICE (2019a) currently indicates they should be avoided due to adverse side effects and efficacy of effect.

Hypnotic Medication

There is often a relationship between medical and mental health problems and sleep. CYP presenting for psychological and psychiatric assessment often report sleep problems (Mindell, 1999). The average individual will sleep a third of their lives and the Sleep Council recommendations (2020) for CYP are found in Figure 15.1. There are two broad groups that have been suggested as a type of hypnotic and appears to be effective for some patients with sleeping difficulties.

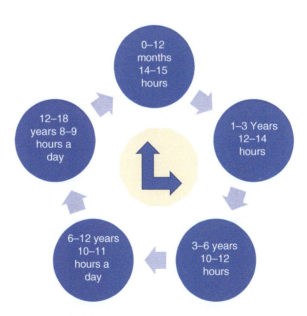

Figure 15.1 **Sleep hygiene recommendations.** *Source:* Adapted from Sleep Council UK, 2017.

Melatonin

Melatonin is a pineal hormone. It is unlicensed for use with CYP. As you will have discovered in earlier chapters, this does not prevent the use of medications in the care of CYP but the CYP and their carer must be told it is an unlicensed medication. Melatonin can be used in the treatment of CYP with autistic spectrum disorder (ASD) and for the management of sleep disturbance and ADHD. The mechanism by which melatonin improves sleep disturbance is unknown. Melatonin regulates the sleep waking cycle by chemically causing drowsiness and lowering the body temperature. Melatonin is also implicated in the regulation of mood, learning and memory, immune activity, dreaming, fertility and reproduction. Melatonin is also used for insomnia in patients with learning disabilities and is used for sleep onset insomnia and delayed sleep phase syndrome.

Manufacturers advise that modified-release tablets (not licensed) should be taken with or after food. Licensed immediate-release formulations should be taken on an empty stomach, two hours before or two hours after food – intake with carbohydrate-rich meals may impair blood glucose control (BNFc, 2020a). Instructions indicate initial 2–3mg/day for one-two weeks, then increase if necessary, to 4–6mg/day dose to be taken before bedtime; minimum 10 mg/day. The medication should be taken 30–60 minutes before bedtime. The manufacturer indicates that the medication should be avoided if hepatic impairment is present (BNFc, 2020a).

The evidence suggests that unlicensed melatonin products taken for ten days to four weeks may reduce sleep onset latency (the time it takes for a child to go to sleep) in children with sleep onset insomnia and ADHD by approximately 20 minutes. In addition, melatonin may improve average sleep duration by 15–20 minutes. These randomised control trials include stimulant and non-stimulant treated children aged 6–14 years with ADHD and suffering from sleep onset insomnia. The studies used daily doses of between 3 and 6mg of unlicensed melatonin described as 'fast release' or 'short-acting' administered shortly before bedtime.

Box 15.1 Sleep Hygiene Recommendations

- A warm (not hot) bath may help the CYP prepare for sleep
- Dimming the lights may support the CYP's body to produce the sleep hormone, melatonin
- Share a story time or encourage the CYP to read quietly or listen to some soothing music.
- Tablets, smartphones, TVs and other electronic gadgets can affect how easily children get to sleep
- Older children may also stay up late or even wake in the middle of the night to use social media
- Try to keep your child's bedroom a screen-free zone and get them to charge their phones in another room
- Encourage your child to stop using screens an hour before bedtime

Source: NHS/Crown copyright/Open Government Licence.

Associated improvement in ADHD related behaviour, cognition or quality of life was not robustly demonstrated. Unlicensed melatonin used in the randomised control trials appeared well tolerated in the short to medium term, with only transient mild to moderate adverse effects reported.

Non-pharmacological approaches should always be considered whether medication is considered to be appropriate or not. A sensible first step is to identify any potentially contributing factors such as pain and address these wherever possible. Although encouraging sleep hygiene may also be helpful, there is no evidence to suggest that such approaches are effective, though it is widely supported in current literature and guidance. Psychological therapies have also been shown to be effective in treating insomnia and should usually be considered as a first line approach before medication.

Antidepressants

Depression is an affective disorder which manifests in many ways but usually has depressed mood and/or loss of pleasure in most activities central to the presentation (NICE, 2009). Depression affects 1–3% of CYP across all ages, social backgrounds and ethnicity (Royal College of Psychiatrists, 2020). The use of antidepressant medication is controversial in the treatment of CYP and the current evidence base recommends that a stepped care approach is used to ensure the differing needs of CYP are met taking into consideration their social, personal and the characteristics of the depression experienced (NICE, 2019b).

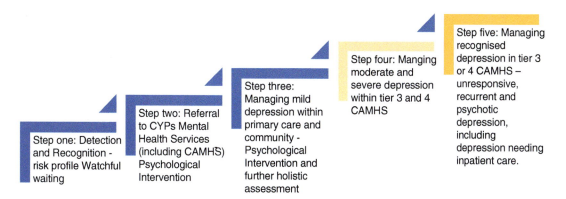

Figure 15.2 **Considerations for safe and high-quality practice.** *Source:* Adapted from NICE, 2019.

Evidence shows antidepressants are less effective in mild cases of depression (NICE, 2009). Psychological therapies should always be considered when treating depression in all the steps recommended in the latest NICE guidance beyond a period of watchful waiting in step one (NICE, 2019b) (Figure 15.2). For children that are under the age of 5 antidepressant medication is not recommended and should not be offered rather a need for parenting intervention is suggested. For children aged 5–11 and a young person aged between 12–18 antidepressant medication should only be offered in combination with a psychological therapy (NICE, 2019). Progress should be closely monitored with a focus on emergent adverse effects as may have an adverse drug reaction.

Moderate and Severe Depression in CYP
Selective Serotonin Reuptake Inhibitors (SSRIs)

The current evidence base recommends SSRIs as first line drug treatment due to their efficacy in treating low mood and their relatively good tolerability and side effect profile (NICE, 2009; Cleare et al., 2015; Joint Formulary Committee, 2019). Examples include fluoxetine, sertraline and citalopram. SSRIs act directly on the brain to block post-synaptic reuptake of the neurotransmitter *serotonin*5-hydroxytryptamine, 5-HT) and most also have minimal effect on other neurotransmitter systems including noradrenaline and dopamine (Smart et al., 2015).

Fluoxetine is the preferred antidepressant for use with CYP above the age of 5. Fluoxetine is advised for use in major depression for children aged 8–17 (BNFc, 2020b).

Most SSRIs are taken orally once daily and many are available in solid oral dosage forms (tablets and capsules) and some are commercially available in liquid form (e.g. liquid form of fluoxetine). For CYP fluoxetine can be taken orally with an initial dose of 10mg daily this is not available in a liquid form. The dose can be increased after one to two weeks of the initial dose up to 20mg (tablet or liquid form once at a dose of 20mg) as a daily or divided dose.

All SSRIs have contraindications. Those commonly associated with fluoxetine include use in poorly controlled epilepsy or should a patient enter a manic episode. It is important to be vigilant with regard to the monitoring of side effects. SSRIs are particularly associated with side effects that include headaches and Gastrointestinal (GI) disturbances (particularly nausea) and a number are associated with sexual dysfunction including reduced libido, though this varies within the drug class (Gartlehner et al., 2011).

Absorption
SSRIs are well absorbed from the GI tract following oral administration and are highly protein-bound. They are hepatically metabolised but notably fluoxetine has an active metabolite. Most SSRIs have half-lives of 24–36 hours. However, the half-life of Fluoxetine is significantly longer (4–5 days) (ABPI, 2018, 2019b, 2019c).

Side Effects of Fluoxetine
Common side effects include appetite changes, chills and gastrointestinal symptoms. CYP often complain about having a sore tummy and can experience nausea and diarrhoea. Some CYP experience cold sweats and

sleep disturbance. A small number of children become agitated and impulsive. More severe side effects include aggression, mania and panic. They may feel that their heart is racing, and this may present as risk-taking behaviour, increased suicidal thoughts are not common yet serious. The risk is at its greatest when the medication is first prescribed.

Tricyclic Antidepressants

Tricyclic antidepressants (TCA) are not recommended for use in children and are off licence.

Monoamine Oxidase Inhibitors (MAOI)

Monoamine oxidase (MAO) is an enzyme present throughout body tissues with particularly high concentrations in the gastrointestinal tract (GT) and the CNS. There are two subtypes:

- MAO-A which metabolises noradrenaline, serotonin, dopamine and tyramine
- MAO-B which metabolises tyramine, dopamine and phenylethylamine

Traditional MAOI antidepressants such as phenelzine, tranylcypromine and isocarboxazid irreversibly inhibit both MAO-A and MAO-B thereby inhibit reuptake of serotonin and noradrenaline. Common side effects include dizziness, drowsiness, peripheral oedema, GI disturbances (nausea, vomiting, dryness of the mouth, constipation), insomnia, blurred vision, tremor and postural hypotension. MAOIs are now only rarely used in the treatment of depression in adults, and rarely used in CYP partly due to dietary restrictions required whilst taking them as outlined in 'Clinical Considerations'.

Clinical Considerations

Dietary Restrictions – MAOIs

Whilst taking MAOIs adult patients must avoid foods rich in tyramine in order to avoid potentially fatal hypertensive crisis. Such foods include mature cheese, salami, pickled herring, meat or yeast extracts like Bovril® and Marmite® or fermented soya bean extract, and some beers, lagers or wines. Also to be avoided are foods containing dopamine (such as broad beans). These must be avoided for the duration of treatment with an MAOI and for 2 to 3 weeks after stopping.

Source: Modified from BNFc, 2020/NICE.

Other Antidepressants

Serotonin and Noradrenaline Reuptake Inhibitors (SNRIs)

Examples of drugs in this class are not used for CYP and include venlafaxine, duloxetine and reboxetine (inhibits noradrenaline reuptake only).

Considerations with Antidepressants

All antidepressant drugs are known to lower the seizure threshold and for this reason they need to be used with a degree of caution in patients with a known seizure disorder such as epilepsy. Patients treated with an antidepressant should begin to see an associated effect within two weeks of starting this and if no demonstrable response is noted by 3–4 weeks a dose increase or drug change should be considered by the healthcare provider.

Adverse Effects From Antidepressants

Suicidal behaviour

The use of antidepressants has been associated with an increased risk of suicidal thoughts and behaviour in adolescents under the age of 25 (National Health Service, 2009) and those with a history of suicidality (Joint Formulary Committee, 2019). Patients should be closely monitored for clinical worsening, suicidality and unusual changes in behaviour when commencing antidepressant treatment, following dose changes and where any risks are identified. As previously stated, suicidal behaviour may include attempted or completed suicide, preparatory acts for suicide and suicidal ideation (National Health Service, 2009).

Table 15.1 Symptoms associated with hyponatraemia.

1 Restlessness	2 Irritability
3 Drowsiness	4 Lack of energy
7 Confusion	8 Seizures

Source: Based on Meadows, 2019.

Table 15.2 Risk factors for developing antidepressant-related hyponatraemia.

• Female gender	• Heart failure
• Increasing age (likely related to higher rates of comorbidities and concurrent medicines)	• Liver cirrhosis
• Low BMI	• Malignancies
• History of hyponatraemia	• Reduced circulating volume
• Syndrome of inappropriate antidiuretic hormone secretion (SIADH)	• Urinary loss

Source: Modified from Taylor et al., 2019.

Hyponatraemia

Hyponatraemia is a rare state where a CYP has depleted plasma sodium levels. Sodium levels should usually be between 135–145mmol/L though this can vary between biochemistry laboratories so please check with individual local laboratories. It is an uncommon, but potentially severe side effect which is associated with SSRI and tricyclic antidepressants. Severe hyponatraemia is usually considered to be plasma level less than 125mmol/L however patients may be symptomatic even with sodium levels higher than this. Symptoms associated with hyponatraemia can be seen in Table 15:1 below.

Hyponatraemia is likely associated with most antidepressants, though not all drug classes have been investigated. The risk appears to be highest with Citalopram and lowest with Mirtazapine and Agomelatine. There are several other factors which can increase the risk of developing hyponatraemia outlined in Table 15.2.

Serotonin Syndrome

Serotonin syndrome is a physiological state where there is an excess of the neurotransmitter serotonin in the bloodstream, leading to adverse effects. It is relatively uncommon and is the result of using serotonergic drugs. Symptoms (summarised in Table 15.3) develop after starting, dose increase or overdose with a serotonergic drug and can arise after a few hours or even several days.

Symptoms can range from being mild in severity to life-threatening, and symptoms tend to be more severe in cases of overdose. Treatment of serotonin syndrome requires withdrawal of the causative agent(s) and any supportive therapy which may be required, according to presenting symptoms. The risk of developing serotonin syndrome increases where multiple drugs with serotonergic activity are used concurrently and although this may be appropriate in certain circumstances, patients should be made aware of this risk wherever necessary and advised of the symptoms to be vigilant for.

Table 15.3 Symptoms of serotonin syndrome.

AUTONOMIC DYSFUNCTION	NEUROMUSCULAR HYPERACTIVITY	ALTERED MENTAL STATE
• Increased heart rate	• Tremor	• Agitation
• Changes in blood pressure	• Hyperreflexia	• Confusion
• Hyperthermia	• Clonus	• Mania
• Shivering	• Rigidity	
• Diarrhoea		
• Sweating		

Source: Modified from Taylor et al., 2019.

Antidepressant Withdrawal

Antidepressant drugs should be withdrawn gradually to avoid precipitating acute discontinuation reactions unless a serious adverse event has occurred or there are serious risks associated with continuing. Current recommendations advise this should be done over at least a four-week period (NICE, 2019a). The onset of discontinuation effects can vary depending on the antidepressant used and so some patients may experience a degree of symptoms after only one missed dose, or if they do not take the full prescribed dose. Symptoms can vary in duration, type and severity and it is estimated that up to one third of patients will experience some degree of discontinuation symptoms (Taylor et al., 2019). There is some evidence to suggest fluoxetine discontinuation is well tolerated on account of its long elimination half-life (Taylor et al., 2019). Antidepressant discontinuation symptoms are outlined in Box 15.2 below.

Box 15.2 Antidepressant Discontinuation Symptoms

- Restlessness
- Problems sleeping
- Unsteadiness
- Sweating
- Abdominal symptoms
- Altered sensations (for example electric shock sensations in the head)
- Altered feelings (for example irritability, anxiety or confusion).

Source: Modified from BNFc, 2020/Pharmaceutical Press.

Antidepressant guidance can be located from the BNFc online site at https://bnfc.nice.org.uk/.

Antipsychotics

Psychosis often presents between 15 and 30 years of age (Van de Werf et al., 2014) and the age of onset is usually lower in males (Drake et al., 2016). Approximately 9.8% of CYP have experienced psychotic symptoms (Healy et al., 2019). The aim of antipsychotic treatment is to alleviate any distress the CYP experiences secondary to psychotic symptoms and to improve social and cognitive functioning. Antipsychotic medications are a range of medications that are used for some types of mental illness or disorder mainly schizophrenia, bipolar disorder (sometimes called manic depression). Of interest is that this group of drugs can also be used in the treatment of Alzheimer's disease. Other uses of antipsychotics include stabilising mood, reducing anxiety in anxiety disorders and reducing tics in Tourette Syndrome.

Clinical Consideration

Before determining that an antipsychotic medication is ineffective it is important to ascertain that patients have been adherent with their prescribed antipsychotic medication.

The common feature of most antipsychotic drugs is that they reduce dopaminergic neurotransmission, an action considered essential for their antipsychotic role. There are two types of antipsychotic medication and these are broadly referred to as first or second generation in terms of their properties and action. First generation antipsychotics' main property is the blocking of dopamine D2 receptors. Second-generation antipsychotics are a more heterogeneous group in terms of their pharmacological make-up and are more complex, acting upon multiple dopamine receptors, (D1, D2, D3, D4) and multiple serotonin (5-HT) receptors (5-HT2A, 5-HT2C, 5-HT1A and 5-HT1D, as well as others not identified) (Schneider et al., 2014).

Aripiprazole

Aripiprazole is recommended as an option for treating moderate to severe manic episodes in adolescents with bipolar I disorder, within its marketing authorisation (that is, up to 12 weeks of treatment for moderate to severe manic episodes in bipolar one disorder in adolescents aged 13 and older).

The drug works by partial antagonism at dopamine D2 and D3 receptors and has a reduced impact in terms of the extrapyramidal side effects that are present with other antipsychotic medication. The consequences of these extrapyramidal side effects can impact upon body movement and are generally considered to fall under the following four areas: Parkinsonism, dystonias, dyskinesias and akathisia.

Risperidone

Risperidone acts on the CNS to treat schizophrenia and other mental health conditions. It is a second-generation antipsychotic or atypical antipsychotic. It acts to balance dopamine and serotonin to improve thinking, mood and behaviour. Risperidone is a dopamine D2, 5-HT2A, alpha1-adrenoceptor and histamine-1 receptor antagonist. It is used in acute and chronic psychosis. It is not licensed for use in children for psychosis, mania or autism. It is, however, licensed for children and adolescents over five years of age for conduct disorders (serious problems with behaviours and emotions) but the licence only covers six weeks of use. Z-Track injection technique reminder is in Skills for Practice 15.2.

Risperidone is licensed to treat schizophrenia psychosis and mania as well as other conditions for defined short periods in terms of its license. It is used in CYP to target behaviour management problems, behaviours issues in terms of autistic spectrum disorder, and tics in Tourette Syndrome.

Olanzapine (Zyprexa®)

Olanzapine is an atypical antipsychotic used in the treatment for positive, negative and cognitive symptoms of schizophrenia and is helpful in the treatment of bipolar disorder. Due to the likelihood of weight gain and relationship with heart disease and its related problems, olanzapine is not often used with CYP. It is off licence and does not have a solid evidence base for use. The evidence in the adult population indicates that use is associated with insulin resistance, hyperglycaemia and type two diabetes. Its mode of action is that it blocks the D1, D2, 5-HT2A and 5-HT2C receptors, and mimics the 5-HT1A receptors. In schizophrenia it has a balance affect and counteracts an over or underactive dopamine system.

Mood Stabilisers

A mood stabiliser is used to treat disorders characterised by sustained and intense shifts in mood. An example of this is bipolar, which is a schizoaffective disorder. Bipolar disorder can be difficult to diagnose in CYP and diagnosis is much debated in the field of CYP psychiatry. It is thought to affect 1 in 100 people. It usually begins in late adolescence between the ages of 15 and 19. Symptoms can include extreme mood swings, manic episodes, high levels of activity and poor concentration. Low mood can occur characterised by disturbed sleep, thoughts of harming themselves and psychotic episodes (see Young Minds: https://youngminds.org.uk/find-help/conditions/bipolar-disorder/1).

Bipolar disorder often starts in adolescence and it can take as much as 6-years before an accurate diagnosis is formulated (Dagani et al., 2018). CYP can experience other problems clouding diagnosis including misuse of alcohol and illicit drugs. There may be a comorbidity with ADHD which may present as difficulties with focusing, for example, at school, maintaining positive relationships with peers and family members. It is also common for CYP with bipolar to experience an anxiety disorder. It is important to assess risk of harm as CYP may with extreme changes to behaviour and mood may express thoughts of suicide, engage in risk-taking behaviours or contemplate running away from home.

Common mood stabilisers include sodium valproate and lithium.

Sodium Valporate

The way sodium valporate works to stabilise mood is not well understood but it is thought to modify several biochemical pathways. Valproate is recommended for acute mania, acute bipolar depression (in combination with an antidepressant) and for prophylaxis of relapse (NICE, 2018). Valproate may commonly cause weight gain, diarrhoea; drowsiness, hallucinations headache; and hepatic disorders (Joint Formulary Committee, 2019; ABPI, 2018). It is important to note that 'Valproate medicines must no longer be used in women or girls of childbearing potential unless a Pregnancy Prevention Programme is in place' (Care Quality Commission, 2020).

Sodium valproate is rapidly and completely absorbed from the GI tract after oral administration, and it is thought the rate is delayed by food. There is a low proportion of protein binding and so therapeutic effects may not reflect free drug levels. Valproic acid, however, is highly protein-bound. Valproate undergoes extensive hepatic metabolism and in the form of sodium valproate has an elimination half-life of 13–19 hours (Buckingham, 2019; ABPI, 2018).

Skills for Practice 2

Z-Track Injection Technique (Figure 15.3)

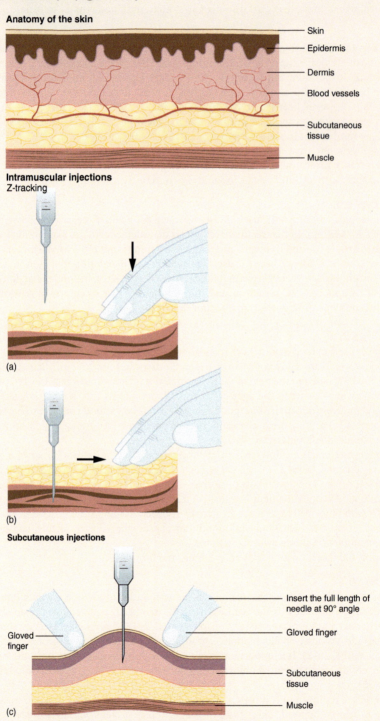

Figure 15.3 Z-track injection technique. *Source:* Bagness and Peate (2018).

Drug Interactions

Valproate is an *enzyme inhibitor*, meaning that it slows down some liver enzymes, causing certain medicines to be cleared from the body much more slowly than would be usual, with the potential for these to reach toxic levels. These medicines include clomipramine, warfarin, quetiapine and lamotrigine (Baxter and Preston, 2019).

Teratogenesis

Valproate carries a significant risk of birth defects and developmental disorders in children born to women who take Valproate during pregnancy. The current evidence base recommends that its use should be avoided in women under the age of 55 wherever possible for all indications (including epilepsy) but in cases where this is required that a robust pregnancy prevention plan is in place (MHRA, 2018b).

Lithium

Lithium is a naturally occurring element licensed to help get the mood changes experienced by the CYP under control. The exact mode of action by which it achieves mood stabilisation is poorly understood. It is principally used to treat affective disorders including bipolar affective disorder and depression (BPAD) and to prevent their recurrence. It may be less useful in the management of an acute manic episode due to the difficulty in quickly establishing the high doses which are often required.

Unfortunately, it is estimated that approximately 15% of patients with BPAD die of suicide. Treatment with lithium has been shown to reduce the risk of attempted and completed suicide in patients with BPAD by 80% (Taylor et al., 2019). Adverse reactions include fine tremor, polyuria, weight gain, cognitive impairment, drowsiness, metallic taste, poor coordination and gastrointestinal upset (e.g. nausea). These are often dose-dependent and may be alleviated to some extent with dose reduction where this is appropriate. Up to 1/5 of people who take lithium for over 10 years will develop some degree of renal impairment. Lithium is known to cause hypothyroidism in females, an effect that arises more commonly than in males (Psychiatric Times, 2002). Often treatment with levothyroxine is required. Hyperparathyroidism is also common with lithium treatment, and calcium monitoring is recommended during long-term treatment.

Toxicity (Taylor et al., 2019; Goodwin et al., 2016; MHRA, 2018a; NPIS, 2016)

Lithium is considered toxic when plasma levels are above 1.0mmol/L and toxic effects are reliably seen at levels of 1.5mmol/L and above. Signs of lithium toxicity can include vomiting and diarrhoea, cause tremor, blurred vision, polyuria, muscle weakness and confusion. Plasma levels above 2.0mmol/L are associated with increased disorientation and seizures which may lead to coma and ultimately can be fatal. If lithium toxicity is suspected, patients should have a hospital assessment as an emergency. There is no specific antidote; however, lithium treatment should be discontinued immediately, and supportive therapy provided including correction of electrolyte and fluid balance if indicated. In more serious cases dialysis may be required to minimise toxic effects.

Lithium blood levels are affected by fluid balance. This is of relevance should people taking lithium become physically unwell resulting in vomiting and/or diarrhoea. In these instances, total body water will reduce, leading lithium levels to increase. As such, any patient taking lithium who reports these symptoms should have a lithium level taken at the earliest opportunity. Any other situations leading to dehydration (e.g. excess sweating, reduced fluid intake) will have the same effect on lithium in the blood. Conversely, if patients dramatically increase their fluid intake this will likely lead to reduced lithium levels.

Baseline Monitoring (Taylor et al., 2019; Goodwin, 2016; NICE, 2018)

Lithium can have several adverse effects on thyroid, renal and cardiac function and baseline function must be checked before commencing lithium. This would usually include EGFR (estimated glomerular filtration rate) and thyroid and parathyroid function tests (e.g. TSH and calcium) would be expected as a minimum. An ECG is also recommended for those patients who are at increased risk of developing or have existing cardiac disease. Lithium commonly causes weight gain and so baseline measurement of this is helpful for assessing the severity of this side effect. Pregnancy should also be excluded as lithium may have teratogenic effects.

Ongoing Monitoring (Taylor et al., 2019; Goodwin, 2016)

Renal and thyroid monitoring should be checked at least every 6 months where this is found to be stable. Patients with a degree of impairment or additional concerns (e.g. chronic kidney disease, increasing age) may require more frequent monitoring.

Plasma monitoring of lithium levels should be closely monitored on initiation and once in therapeutic range every 3–6 months. Plasma monitoring may be helpful following dose changes however blood samples should not be taken until at least 5-days after dose changes to allow the new dose to reach steady state. Weight should be monitored due to the propensity for lithium to induce weight gain.

Discontinuation

Lithium treatment should be gradually reduced as abrupt discontinuation is associated with an increased risk of manic relapse in the first few months following this. Doses should be tapered and withdrawn over 4–8 weeks unless there are risks associated with doing so, such as in cases of overdose or toxicity where immediate withdrawal is necessary.

Conclusion

1–10 CYP experience mental health problems the prevalence of MHD in CYP is high. This chapter has explored what is meant by pharmacokinetics and dynamics and explored some of the medications that are prescribed within CYP mental health services. It provides an insight into the importance of holistic assessment, the presentation of the CYP, their history and their voice in clinical decision making and that of their families or carers. Before medications are considered and prescribed for CYP it is important that the relevant NICE guidance be taken into consideration and alternative therapies and approaches to treatment considered or offered in conjunction to medication. Many medications used to treat CYP are safe and effective. However, some are unlicensed, and side effects can differ between CYP and adults. It is important to remember that CYP metabolise medications faster than adults. Medications may need to be adjusted or changed as CYP grow and develop. It is essential that as nurses you have the clinical skills to monitor CYP physical health and it has been stressed that assessment should be a continuous process and be holistic in nature, capturing emotional well-being, social and spiritual elements of CYP's worlds as they experience it.

Episode of Care

Norman Gwynn is a 7-year-old male. His medical/nursing notes indicate that has ADHD.

Norman's prescribed medications include methylphenidate hydrochloride 30mg/day.

On review of his medications Tom has lost weight, is having difficulty sleeping and his parents report that he seems anxious.

This case presents many opportunities for improving the management of Norman's care. What additional pharmacological/social/nursing interventions could be considered and why?

Glossary

Akathisia: A movement disorder characterised by a subjective feeling of inner restlessness accompanied by mental distress and an inability to sit still.

Anti-psychotics: These medications work by altering brain chemistry to reduce psychotic symptoms, such as hallucinations, delusions and disordered thinking.

Anxiolytics: Medications used to relive anxiety.

Dyskinesia: Abnormal, uncontrollable, involuntary movements.

Dystonia: Uncontrolled and sometimes painful muscle movements (spasms).

Comorbidity: The simultaneous presence of two or more diseases or medical conditions in a patient.

Hypnotics: Medications used to help people fall asleep.

Metabolite: Any substance produced during metabolism (digestion or other bodily chemical processes). The term may also refer to the product that remains after a drug is broken down (metabolised) by the body.

Polyuria: The passing of large volumes of urine with an increase in urinary frequency.

Psychopharmacology: The scientific study of the effects of drugs on the mind and behaviour.

Psychotropic medications: Any medication capable of affecting the mind, emotions, and behaviour.

Tourette's Syndrome: A condition that causes a person to make involuntary sounds and movements called tics.

References

ABPI Medicines Compendium (2018) Summary of product characteristics for Paroxetine 10 mg Tablets. www.medicines.org.uk/emc/product/9582/smpc (accessed 21 June 2020).

ABPI Medicines Compendium (2019a) Summary of product characteristics for diazepam tablets BP 2mg. www.medicines.org.uk/emc/product/4523/smpc (accessed 21 June 2020).

ABPI Medicines Compendium (2019b). Summary of product characteristics for Lustral 50mg tablets. www.medicines.org.uk/emc/product/1070/smpc (accessed 24 June 2020).

ABPI Medicines Compendium (2019c) Summary of product characteristics for fluoxetine 20mg capsules. www.medicines.org.uk/emc/product/6013/smpc (accessed 21 June 2020).

Bagness, L. and Peate, I. (eds) (2018). *Midwifery Skills in Practice at a Glance*. Wiley-Blackwell.

Baldwin, D.S., et al. (2014). Evidence-based pharmacological treatment of anxiety disorders, post-traumatic stress disorder and obsessive-compulsive disorder: A revision of the 2005 guidelines from the British Association for Psychopharmacology. *Journal of Psychopharmacology* 1–37. DOI: 10.1177/0269881114525674.

Bazire, S. (2018). *Psychotropic Drug Directory 2018*. Dorsington: Lloyd-Reinhold Communications LLP.

Baxter, K. and Preston, C.L. (eds) (2019). *Stockley's Drug Interactions*, 12e. London: Pharmaceutical Press. www.new.medicinescomplete.com/ (accessed 21 June 2020).

BNF (2020). Sedative guidance. https://bnf.nice.org.uk/drug/promethazine-hydrochloride.html (accessed 25 June 2020).

BNFc (2020a). Melatonin. https://bnfc.nice.org.uk/drug/melatonin.html (accessed 2 June 2020).

BNFc (2020b). Fluoxetine. https://bnfc.nice.org.uk/drug/fluoxetine.html (accessed 20 May 2020).

Buckingham, R., (ed.) (2019). *Martindale: The Complete Drug Reference*. London: Pharmaceutical Press. www.new.medicinescomplete.com/ (accessed 21 June 2020).

Care Quality Commission (2020). High risk medicines: valproate. www.cqc.org.uk/guidance-providers/adult-social-care/high-risk-medicines-valproate (accessed 1 February 2020).

Chang, Z., Lichenstein, P., Halldner, L. et al. (2014). Stimulant medication and risk for substance abuse. *Journal of Child Psychology and Psychiatry*, 55(8): 878–885.

Cleare, A., Pariante, C.M., and Young, A.H. (2015). Evidence-based guidelines for treating depressive disorders with antidepressants: A revision of the 2008 British Association for Psychopharmacology guidelines. *Journal of Psychopharmacology* 2015, 29(5) 459–525. DOI: 10.1177/0269881115581093.

Creswell, C., Waite, P., and Hudson, J. (2020). Anxiety disorders in children and young people: assessment and treatment. *Journal of Child Psychology and Psychiatry* 61(6): 628–643.

Dagani, J., Baldessarini, R., Nielssen, O. et al. (2018). The age of onset of bipolar disorders. In: *The Age of Onset of Mental Disorder* (ed. De Girolamo, G., McGorry, P., and Sartorius, N.), 75–110. Switzerland: Springer International Publisher.

Department of Health and Social care and Department for Education (2018). Transforming children and young people's mental health provision: a green paper. www.gov.uk/government/consultations/transforming-children-and-young-peoples-mental-health-provision-a-green-paper (accessed 27 June 2020).

De Vane, L., Liston, H., and Markowitz, S. (2002). Clinical pharmacokinetics of sertraline. *Clinical Pharmacokinetics* 41(15): 1247–1266.

Drake, R.J., Addington, J., Viswanathan, A.C. et al. (2016). How age and gender predict illness course in a first-episode nonaffective psychosis cohort. *J Clin Psychiatry* 283–289.

Gartlehner, G., Hansen, R., Morgan, L. et al. (2011). Comparative benefits and harms of second generation antidepressants for treating major depressive disorder. *Annals of Internal Medicine* 155(11): 772–785.

Goodwin, G.M. et al. (2016). Evidence-based guidelines for treating bipolar disorder: Revised third edition recommendations from the British Association for Psychopharmacology. *Journal of Psychopharmacology*. 30(6): 495–553. DOI: 10.1177/0269881116636545.

Healy, C., Brannigan, R., Dooley, N. et al. (2019). Childhood and adolescent psychotic experiences and risk of mental disorder: A systematic review and meta-analysis. *Psychological Medicine* 49: 1589–1599.

International Statistical Classification of Diseases and Related Health Problems, 10th Revision (2019). https://icd.who.int/browse10/2019/en (accessed 03 June 2020).

Joint Formulary Committee (2019). *British National Formulary (BNF)* London: British Medical Journal (BMJ) Group and Pharmaceutical Press. www.medicinescomplete.com (accessed 24 May 2020).

Kieling, C., Baker-Henningham, H., and Belfer, M. (2011). Child and adolescent mental health worldwide: evidence for action. *The Lancet*, 378: 1515–1525.

Meadows, T. (2019). If antidepressant-induced hyponatremia has been diagnosed how should the depression be treated? www.sps.nhs.uk/articles/if-antidepressant-induced-hyponatremia-has-been-diagnosed-how-should-the-depression-be-treated-2.

Medicines Healthcare Regulatory Authority (MHRA) (2018a). Summary of product characteristics for Priadel 400mg prolonged release tablets. www.mhra.gov.uk/home/groups/spcpil/documents/spcpil/con1542949679637.pdf (accessed 21 June 2020).

Medicines Healthcare Regulatory Authority (MHRA) (2018b). Valproate use by women and girls. www.gov.uk/guidance/valproate-use-by-women-and-girls (accessed 25 May 2020).

Mindell, J.A. (1999). Empirically supported treatments in paediatric psychology: Bedtime refusal and night waking's in young children. *Journal of Paediatric Psychology* 24: 465–481.

McVoy, M. and Findling, R. (2017). *Clinical Manual of Child and Adolescent Psychopharmacology*, 3e. Arlington VA: American Psychiatric Association Publishing.

National Health Service (NHS) (2009). Antidepressants and suicide risk. www.nhs.uk/news/mental-health/antidepressants-and-suicide-risk/ (accessed 21 June 2020).

NHSDigital(2018).https://digital.nhs.uk/news-and-events/latest-news/one-in-eight-of-five-to-19-year-olds-had-a-mental-disorder-in-2017-major-new-survey-finds.

NICE (2009). *Depression in Adults: Recognition and Management. CG90.* www.nice.org.uk/guidance/CG90 (accessed 15 May 2020).

NICE (2014). Anxiety disorders. www.nice.org.uk/Guidance/QS53 (accessed 3 July 2020).

NICE (2018). *Bipolar disorder: assessment and management. CG185.* www.nice.org.uk/guidance/cg185 (accessed 21 June 2020).

NICE (2019a). Attention deficit hyperactivity disorder: diagnosis and management. www.nice.org.uk/guidance/NG87 (accessed 3 June 2020).

NICE (2019). Antidepressants. www.nice.org.uk/guidance/conditions-and-diseases/mental-health-and-behavioural-conditions/depression (accessed 3 June 2020).

NICE (2019). Depression in children and young people: identification and management www.nice.org.uk/guidance/NG134 (accessed 1 June 2020).

NICE (2021). Methylphenidate hydrochloride. https://bnfc.nice.org.uk/drug/methylphenidate-hydrochloride.html (accessed 20 April 2021).

Nicholson, T. (2018). Outcomes of untreated attention deficit hyperactivity disorder and the mental health nurse. *British Journal of Mental Health Nursing* 7(3): 113–118.

National Poisons Information Service (NPIS) (2016). Lithium. www.toxbase.org/Poisons-Index-A-Z/L-Products/Lithium/ (accessed 21 June 2020).

Royal College of Psychiatrists (2017). ADHD and hyperkinetic disorder. www.rcpsych.ac.uk/mental-health/parents-and-young-people/information-for-parents-and-carers/attention-deficit-hyperactivity-disorder-and-hyperkinetic-disorder-information-for-parents-carers-and-anyone-working-with-young-people?searchTerms=stimulants (accessed 22 June 2020).

Royal College of Psychiatrists (2020). Depression in young people. www.rcpsych.ac.uk/mental-health/parents-and-young-people/information-for-parents-and-carers/depression-in-young-people---helping-children-to-cope-for-parents-and-carers?searchTerms=depression%20children (accessed 3 June 2020).

Schneider, M., Debbane, M., Bassett, A. et al. (2014). Psychiatric disorders from childhood to adulthood in 22q11.2 Deletion Syndrome: Results from the International Consortium on Brain and Behaviour in 22q11.2 Deletion Syndrome. The American *Journal of Psychiatry* 171(6): 627–639.

Sleep Council (2020). Recommendations for sleep. https://sleepcouncil.org.uk/advice-support/sleep-hub/sleep-matters/how-much-sleep-do-we-need (accessed 22 June 2020).

Smart, C., Anderson, I.M., and McAllister-Williams, R.H. (2015). Monoamine hypothesis of depression. In: *Fundamentals of Clinical Psychopharmacology* (ed. Anderson, I.M. and McAllister-Williams, R.H.), 77. CRC Press.

Taylor, D.M., Barnes, T.R.E., and Young, A.H. (2019). *The Maudsley Prescribing Guidelines in Psychiatry*, 13e. Hoboken, NJ: Wiley Blackwell.

Van der Werf, M., Hanssen, M., Köhler, S. et al. (2014). Systematic review and collaborative recalculation of 133 693 incident cases of schizophrenia. *Psychol Med* 44(1): 9–16.

Vizard, T., Pearce, N., Davis, J. et al. (2018). Mental health of children and young people in England, 2017: Emotional disorders. https://digital.nhs.uk/data-and-information/publications/statistical/mental-health-of-children-and-young-people-in-england/2017/2017 (accessed 3 April 2021).

Further Resources

MIND Psychiatric medication A to Z: www.mind.org.uk/information-support/drugs-and-treatments/medication/drug-names-a-z/

National Institute of Mental Health 'Mental Health Medications': www.nimh.nih.gov/health/topics/mental-health-medications/index.shtml

Mental Health Foundation: www.mentalhealth.org.uk/a-to-z/d/drugs-and-mental-health

Multiple Choice Questions

1. Which of these drugs are not licensed for use in children for depression?
   (a) Diazepam
   (b) Methylphenidate
   (c) Amitriptyline
   (d) All of the above

2. Which is an example of a neurotransmitter?
   (a) Serotonin
   (b) Chloride
   (c) Sodium
   (d) Potassium

3. Clinicians should be aware of _____ steps in the management of depression?
   (a) 3
   (b) 7
   (c) 5
   (d) 8

4. Which of these drugs is a mood stabiliser?
   (a) Methylphenidate
   (b) Fluoxetine
   (c) Lithium
   (d) Atomoxetine

5. Which of these is a common side effect of SSRIs?
   (a) Chills
   (b) Growth retardation
   (c) Serum sickness
   (d) Vasculitis

6. Which of these drugs is used in sleep management?
   (a) Lithium
   (b) Pregabalin
   (c) Melatonin
   (d) Risperidone

7. Melatonin is a _____ hormone?
   (a) Thyroid
   (b) Pineal
   (c) Adrenal
   (d) Pituitary

8. What of these drugs are used in the treatment of anxiety in CYP?
   (a) Tricyclic antidepressants
   (b) MAOIs
   (c) SSRIs
   (d) Stimulant
   (e) Non-stimulant

9. What should be considered always in conjunction with pharmacological interventions in medication management for CYP?
   (a) CYP voice
   (b) Information
   (c) Psychological therapy
   (d) All of the above

10. Lithium requires monitoring of _____.
    (a) Cardiac function
    (b) Hyperparathyroidism
    (c) Weight
    (d) All of the above

Chapter 15 Medications Used in Children and Young People's Mental Health

11. What is the most common mental health in CYP?
    (a) Anxiety
    (b) Eating disorder
    (c) Schizophrenia
    (d) Bipolar
12. What is the age onset range for psychosis?
    (a) 10–20
    (b) 15–30
    (c) 6–12
    (d) 18–40
13. What is the name of a non-stimulant medication used to treat ADHD?
    (a) Atomoxetine
    (b) Fluoxetine
    (c) Methylphenidate
    (d) Concerta XL
14. Pharmacokinetics related to what?
    (a) Weight
    (b) What the CYP's body does to the drugs as they are processed by the body
    (c) The amount of the drug calculated
    (d) The ways the drugs are administered
15. How many hours sleep does a 7-year-old require?
    (a) 10–11
    (b) 12–14
    (c) 8
    (d) 9

Find Out More

The following is a list of common mental health conditions that are associated with CYP. Take some time and write notes about each of the conditions. Think about the medications that may be used in order to treat these conditions and be specific about the pharmacokinetics and pharmacodynamics. Remember to include aspects of nursing care. If you are making notes about CYP you have offered care and support to, you must ensure that you have adhered to the rules of confidentiality.

THE CONDITION	YOUR NOTES
Self-harm	
Obsessive-Compulsive Disorder	
Anorexia nervosa	
Generalised anxiety disorder	
Antisocial behaviour and conduct disorder	

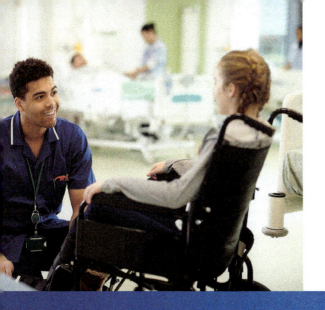

16

Medications Used in Children and Young People's cancer

Elaine Robinson and Leah Rosengarten

Aims

The aim of this chapter is to help the reader understand the pharmacology and pharmaceutical treatment options commonly used in Children and Young People's (CYP) cancer care.

Learning Outcomes

After reading this chapter, the reader will:

- Understand how cancer occurs in CYP in relation to the cell cycle
- Discuss the use of chemotherapies in the treatment of cancer for CYP
- Appreciate the role of immunotherapies in the management of CYP cancer
- Recognise how corticosteroids are used in CYP cancer care

Test Your Knowledge

1. What is the difference between normal cells and cancer cells?
2. What medicines are used in the treatment of cancer?
3. What considerations are relevant when prescribing and administering chemotherapy?
4. How is the immune system used in the treatment of cancer?
5. Why use corticosteroids in cancer care?

Fundamentals of Pharmacology for Children's Nurses, First Edition. Edited by Ian Peate and Peter Dryden.
© 2022 John Wiley & Sons Ltd. Published 2022 by John Wiley & Sons Ltd.
Companion website: www.wiley.com/go/pharmacologyforCN

Introduction

Over recent years, the NHS has seen a year on year increase in the number of cancer diagnoses but a year on year decrease in the number of people dying from cancer (Office for National Statistics (ONS), 2020). There are around 1900 new cases of cancer in children in the UK every year and it is estimated that around 1 in every 500 children in the UK will be diagnosed with cancer by the age of 14 (Cancer Research UK, 2020a). The most common cancers for children aged 0–14 years are leukaemia, brain, non-Hodgkin's lymphoma (males) and kidney (females). In young people, there are around 2,500 new cases of cancer diagnosed in the UK every day, with the most common cancers being lymphomas, carcinomas and germ cell tumours (Cancer Research UK, 2020b).

The average survival rate of young people diagnosed with cancer in the UK, who go on to live 5 years or more, is 84% (Cancer Research UK, 2020b): in children this figure is 82% (Cancer Research UK, 2020a). Both survival rates are much higher than those of adults in the UK, which sit at only 50% (Cancer Research UK, 2020c). Whilst it is not always clear why the survival rates of children and young people are much higher than adults, these are thought to include: CYPs get different types of cancers to adults which may respond better to treatment; CYPs often don't have other added health problems as well as cancer; and CYPs can often cope with more intense treatments. The latter will be discussed later in this chapter.

The goal of cancer treatment in the UK is to cure patients of their cancer through eradication of all cancer cells in their body (Cancer Research UK, 2017). In situations where a cure is not possible; treatments can be focused on prolonging life or improving the patients' quality of life through symptom management. Treatment options for cancer are not limited to drugs and may include surgery, radiotherapy, bone marrow or stem cell transplants and gene therapies among others. This chapter will consider the different drugs used in the treatment of cancer.

First, it is important that we develop a baseline understanding of what cancer is and the process of the normal cell cycle before we can appreciate the roles and mechanisms of drugs used in cancer.

Cancer

Cancer is a condition which occurs when cells in a certain part of the body grow and divide uncontrollably. When these cells grow abnormally, they can form a lump, which is called a tumour. Not all tumours are cancerous; tumours can be benign (not cancerous) or malignant (cancerous). The difference between these is that benign tumours will not spread to other areas of the body, but malignant tumours can spread to other tissues and organs.

Tumours that are benign will still continue to grow but typically only cause problems if they place pressure on nearby organs when they grow. Malignant or cancerous tumours in one part of the body can cast off cells which travel around the body and invade other organs. When these cells invade other organs they may start to grow and form a second tumour, which is called a metastasis. In blood cancer, cancerous cells behave in the same way as other cancer cells and build up in the blood or bone marrow but do not form tumours.

There are certain 'hallmarks' which are said to distinguish cancer cells from normal cells; these are displayed in Figure 16.1. Though it has been argued that not all cancers can be defined by the same six biological capabilities, appreciation of these common traits can lead to a greater understanding of the difference between cancer cells and normal cells and enhance the quality of care provided.

'Sustaining proliferative signalling' describes how a cancer cell ignores signalling to control growth. Where a normal cell's growth is carefully controlled through the production of growth-promoting signals, a cancer cell becomes self-sufficient in providing their own growth signals and do not require signalling from external cells to continue to grow. In addition to this, cancer cells also become resistant to anti-growth signals, which is the second hallmark, evading growth suppressors.

Activating tissue invasion and metastasis refers to the cancer cells' ability to invade and spread to surrounding tissues and organs rather than remaining in set boundaries as normal cells do. Additionally, cancer cells do not have a limit to how many times they can multiply and grow as a normal cell does; this is termed enabling replicative immortality.

The hallmark inducing angiogenesis identifies that the cancer cell can draw blood cells in to a tumour in order to feed it and ensure that it can continue to grow where a normal cell will attract blood vessels only

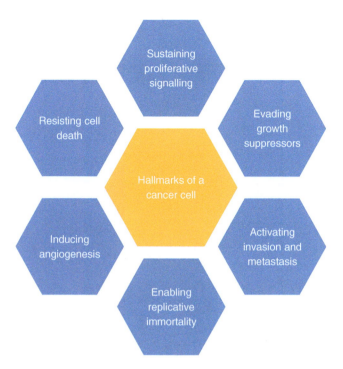

Figure 16.1 **Hallmarks of a cancer cell.** *Source:* Modified from Hanahan and Weinburg, 2011.

when they need to grow and feed. Lastly, the resisting cell death hallmark recognises that the cancer cell has an ability to ignore signals to die. Where a normal cell has a programme of self-destruction named apoptosis which is activated on occasions such as when DNA is damaged, a cancer cell can evade this process.

In short, a normal cell will: multiply and divide only when signalled to do so; stop multiplying and dividing when signalled to do so; perform one function that they were designed to perform; reproduce only a set number of times; attract blood vessels only when they need to grow; and self-destruct when necessary. A cancer cell will: multiply and divide uncontrollably; ignore signals to stop growing; invade other tissues and organs; continue to multiply and divide indefinitely; attract blood vessels to nourish itself constantly; and resist cell death.

Cell Cycle

The purpose of the cell cycle is for cells to reproduce themselves, to replace dead or injured cells and add new ones for tissue growth. The cell cycle is an ordered series of events which consists of two main periods: Interphase, when the cell is not dividing, and the Mitotic (M) phase, when the cell is dividing. The length of time that a cell takes to travel through its cycle varies depending on the type of cell but the times below serve as a guide. Figure 16.2 shows the cell cycle.

The interphase is a period of rapid growth during which the cell replicates its deoxyribonucleic acid (DNA). There are three phases within this period: G_1, S and G_2. The G phases are gaps or interruptions in DNA replication and the S phase involves the replication of DNA.

The G_1 phase is the gap between the mitotic stage and the S phase, during which the cell is preparing for DNA synthesis through genes directing the synthesis of ribonucleic acid (RNA) and proteins. This stage may last from 8 to 10 hours, though some cells remain in this phase for a longer time and are considered to be in the G_0 or resting phase. The S phase is between G_1 and G_2 and lasts approximately 8 hours, during which time all 46 chromosomes containing genetic DNA are copied, so both new cells that are formed will have matching DNA. Once a cell enters this phase it is committed to going through cell division. The G_2 phase is the gap between the S phase and mitosis, this phase may last for 4 to 6 hours, during which time cell growth continues and enzymes and other proteins are synthesised in preparation for cell division.

Chapter 16 Medications Used in Children and Young People's cancer

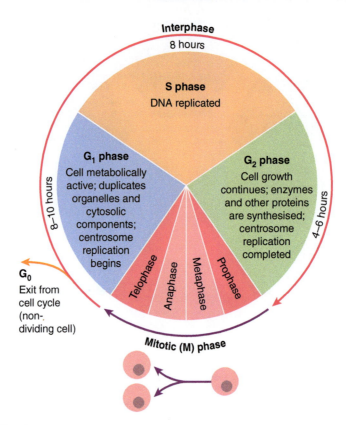

Figure 16.2 The cell cycle. *Source:* Ian Peate et al., 2018/John Wiley & Sons.

The M phase or mitosis is characterised by chromosomes passing through phases of change (cytokinesis) to form two genetically identical cells. Mitosis may be broken down into four distinct phases; prophase, where chromosomes form identical pairs, called chromotids; metaphase, where spindle fibres attach to chromosomes and chromotids begin to separate; anaphase, where two sets of new single-stranded chromosomes move to opposite ends of the cell; and telephase, where a nuclear membrane forms around each set of chromosomes, dividing the cell in two.

Children produce cells at a much quicker rate than adults because their cells are dividing faster in order to support their growth into an adult. Some infant cells can divide up to twice as fast as an adult's cell of the same type would, but this depends on the type of cell.

Understanding of the process of the cell cycle is important as certain drugs used in the treatment of cancer impact on specific points in the cell cycle. These drugs interrupt the process of the cell cycle in order to prevent the cancer from growing further or to kill the cancer cell completely.

Chemotherapies

Chemotherapy is the name given to the group of drugs which are cytotoxic, meaning that they are toxic to cells. Chemotherapy has been used in the treatment of cancer since the 1940s and today there are more than 100 different types of chemotherapy used in the UK. Childhood leukaemia was one of the first cancers to be effectively treated using chemotherapy.

Chemotherapy destroys cancer cells by interrupting the cell cycle and preventing the cells from multiplying further, though chemotherapy cannot distinguish between normal and abnormal cells so healthy cells can also be affected. The point at which a chemotherapy will interrupt the cell cycle differs depending on the type of chemotherapy.

Chemotherapy is used in both CYP and adult cancers, but CYPs can often tolerate higher doses of chemotherapy according to body weight than adults can. There are various reasons why this may be, but a key aspect is that children's cells divide much quicker than adults' cells, which means that they are able to recover quicker and more effectively after their chemotherapy.

Clinical Considerations

Types of chemotherapy are broken down into groups according to; their chemical structure, how they work and their relationships to other drugs. Some chemotherapies may belong to more than one group as they work in more than one way. Different chemotherapy agents are often given in combination with each other, to interrupt different points within the cell cycle.

Tables 15.1, 15.2, 15.3 and 15.4 display the commonly used chemotherapy agent for each group.

Preparations of Chemotherapy

Chemotherapy is most commonly given intravenously as either a bolus or infusion but can also be administered through the following routes:

- Orally – swallowed in pill, tablet, capsule or liquid form
- Subcutaneous – into the space between the skin and the muscle
- Intramuscular – into the muscle
- Intrathecal – into the spinal fluid
- Intraperitoneal – into the abdominal cavity
- Intravesicular – into the bladder
- Intrapleural – into the space between the lung and the lining of the lung
- Intra-arterial – into the artery that is supplying blood to the tumour
- Topical – onto the skin

Types of Chemotherapy

The British National Formulary (BNF) (Joint Formulary Committee, 2019) identifies four classes of chemotherapy;

1. Alkylating drugs
2. Antimetabolites
3. Anthracyclines and other antibiotics
4. Vinca alkaloids

Alkylating Drugs

Alkylating drugs or alkylating agents were the first chemotherapy drugs to be used to treat chemotherapy. The use of alkylating drugs to treat cancer were first discovered in the First World War, when sulfur mustards (mustard gas) were used as chemical weapons. As such, alkylating drugs are some of the most studied drugs used to treat cancer and still remain one of the most commonly used group of drugs for this purpose (Almeida et al., 2005).

Alkylating drugs are generally considered non-cell specific as their activity is not restricted to one specific point in the cell cycle (Pires et al., 2018). These drugs work through transferring alkyl carbon groups onto a wide range of biological molecules, prevent the proteins in the DNA from joining together as they should and eventually breaking the strands of DNA, stopping the cell from continuing to multiply and killing the cell (Fu et al., 2012).

As every aspect of the cell cycle is concerned with the replication of DNA, alkylating drugs can impact on every point in the cell cycle, but their biggest impact is thought to be within the S phase of the cell cycle where all 46 chromosomes are copied (Bignold, 2006). Table 16.1 identifies some of the commonly used alkylating drugs in CYP cancer care.

Antimetabolites

Antimetabolites structurally resemble normal biological molecules within a cell and work through interfering with the processes that require the use of that normal biological molecule (Gmeiner, 2002). As antimetabolites

Chapter 16 Medications Used in Children and Young People's cancer

Table 16.1 Commonly used alkylating drugs in CYP cancer.

DRUG	LICENSED FOR TREATMENT OF
Cyclophosphamide *oral or intravenous*	A wide range of malignancies including leukaemia, lymphomas and solid tumours
Ifosfamide (related to cyclophosphamide) *intravenous*	A wide range of malignancies including leukaemia, lymphomas and solid tumours
Melphalan *intravenous*	Neuroblastoma, multiple myeloma, polycythaemia vera, advanced ovarian adenocarcinoma
Lomustine *oral*	Hodgkin's disease resistant to conventional therapy, malignant melanoma and certain solid tumours
Carmustine *intravenous*	Multiple myeloma, non-Hodgkin's lymphoma and brain tumours

Source: Based on Joint Formulary Committee, 2019.

Table 16.2 Commonly used antimetabolites in CYP cancer care.

DRUG	LICENSED FOR USE IN
Methotrexate *intramuscular, subcutaneous, intravenous, oral and intrathecal*	Neoplastic diseases
6-mercaptopurine *oral*	Acute leukaemia's and chronic myeloid leukaemia
6-tioguanine *oral*	Acute leukaemia and chronic myeloid leukaemia
Fludarabine phosphate *oral or intravenous*	Advanced B cell chronic lymphocytic leukaemia (CLL)
Cladribine *subcutaneous, intravenous or oral*	Chronic lymphocytic leukaemia
Cytarabine *intravenous or subcutaneous*	Acute myeloid leukaemia
Gemcitabine *intravenous*	Solid malignancies

Source: Based on Joint Formulary Committee, 2019.

structurally resemble essential molecules, enzymes will mistake antimetabolites for other essential molecules and combine with them; this results in the exclusion of essential molecules from their normal role and creates a deficiency of that molecule (Woolley, 1959).

Antimetabolites attack cells at specific parts of the cell cycle, but the point at which this occurs in the cycle depends on which substance the antimetabolite interferes with. These drugs tend to be further classified according to which substance they inhibit, which can include; dihydrofolate reductase, tetrahydrofolate, purines and pyrimidines (Gmeiner, 2002). Table 16.2, identifies some of the commonly used Antimetabolites in CYP cancer care.

Anthracyclines and Other Antibiotics

Anthracyclines have been widely used in cancer treatment for over 50 years and are derived from antibiotics.

Though anthracyclines can induce many intracellular effects, their main mechanism of action is inhibition of topoisomerase II (Neilsen et al., 1996). Topoisomerase II is an enzyme which generates breaks in strands of DNA in order to regulate DNA processes (McClendon and Osheroff, 2007). Anthracyclines inhibit topoisomerase II through intercalating (inserting molecules) between base pairs of adjacent DNA, damaging the DNA and ultimately inducing apoptosis (Hortobágyi, 1997). Table 16.3, identifies some of the commonly used Anthracyclines and other Antibiotics in CYP cancer care.

Chapter 16 Medications Used in Children and Young People's cancer

Table 16.3 Commonly used anthracyclines and other antibiotics in CYP cancer care.

DRUG	LICENSED FOR TREATMENT OF
Daunorubicin *intravenous*	Acute myelogenous leukaemia and acute lymphocytic leukaemia
Doxorubicin hydrochloride *intravenous or intravesical*	Acute leukaemias, Hodgkin's and non-Hodgkin's lymphomas, paediatric malignancies and some solid tumours
Idarubicin hydrochloride *oral or intravenous*	Haematological malignancies
Mitoxantrone (structurally related to doxorubicin) *intravenous*	Non-Hodgkin's lymphoma
Pixantrone *intravenous*	Refractory or multiply relapsed aggressive non-Hodgkin's B cell lymphomas
Bleomycin *intramuscular, intravenous or intra-arterial*	Metastatic germ cell cancer and non-Hodgkin's lymphoma.
Dactinomycin *intravenous*	Various paediatric cancers

Source: Based on Joint Formulary Committee, 2019.

Table 16.4 Commonly used vinca alkaloids in CYP cancer.

DRUG	LICENSED FOR USE IN
Vinblastine sulfate *intravenous*	Variety of cancers including leukaemias, lymphomas and some solid tumours
Vincristine sulfate *intravenous*	Variety of cancers including leukaemias, lymphomas and some solid tumours
Vindesine sulfate *intravenous*	Variety of cancers including leukaemias, lymphomas and some solid tumours
Vinorelbine *oral or intravenous*	Usually relapsed or refractory solid tumours

Source: Based on Joint Formulary Committee, 2019.

Vinca Alkaloids

Vinca alkaloids are derived from certain types of plant and work through the inhibition of tubulin into microtubules (Zhou and Rahmani, 1992). Microtubules are needed to provide structure and shape to cells and when vinca alkaloids bind to tubulin, they prevent the tubulin from then being able to bind to microtubules (Moudi et al., 2013). This process ultimately blocks the ability of the cell to divide and causes apoptosis (Moudi et al., 2013). Table 16.4, identifies some of the commonly used Vinca alkaloids in CYP cancer care.

Side Effects of Chemotherapy

It has been noted that the effects of chemotherapy are not limited to only cancer cells but also impact on healthy cells. As chemotherapy affects the fastest dividing cells in the human body most, side effects of chemotherapy are more likely to occur in areas of the body where cells are fast dividing. Though individual chemotherapies will have differing side effects, common side effects are:

- Nausea and vomiting
- Alopecia
- Bone marrow suppression leading to
  - Anaemia (low red blood cell count)
  - Thrombocytopenia (low platelets)
  - Leukopenia (low white blood cell count)
- Mucositis
- Skin changes

As chemotherapy is usually given in cycles or set regimens, patients are clinically assessed before commencing every regimen to ensure that side effects are manageable. These assessments change depending on the point in treatment but frequently include blood tests and a full clinical exam. Healthcare professionals need to assess the patient to ensure that the impact of the patients' experienced side effects do not outweigh the benefit of the chemotherapy. Some side effects, such as nausea and vomiting, can be managed but others, such as mucositis, require the patient to be given time to recover before commencing more chemotherapy.

Clinical Considerations

According to the Control of Substances Hazardous to Health Regulations 2002 (COSHH), cytotoxic drugs are hazardous substances (HSE, online). Due to this, staff administering these drugs should: control their exposure to the substance, wear Personal Protective Equipment (PPE), monitor exposure in the workplace, use occupational health services to help identify risks if necessary, deal with spillages and contamination appropriately, dispose of waste correctly and report incidents as necessary according and in line with local policy and procedure (HSE, online).

Prescription and Administration of Chemotherapy

The National Chemotherapy Advisory Group (NCAG, 2009) give recommendations on the prescription of chemotherapy. They advise that the decision to initiate a programme of chemotherapy should be made by a consultant and that all patients must have a treatment plan in place for each cycle of chemotherapy they are given. NCAG (2009) direct that chemotherapy should only be prescribed by appropriately trained staff, according to predefined protocols and should be on pre-printed forms. Practice areas should keep an annually updated list of all staff who can prescribe chemotherapy and an oncology pharmacist should check all chemotherapy prescriptions. Exceptions may be made to the above in emergencies and extraordinary circumstances.

Drug Resistance

It is possible for cancer cells to be or become resistant to chemotherapy treatment. Occasions when cancer does not respond to chemotherapy treatment, may be termed 'refractory'. Some cancer cells may initially respond to chemotherapy, but later develop the ability to prevent chemotherapy drugs from entering the cell, or limit the amount of drug that enters the cell, to stop or minimise the amount of damage the drug can do.

Cyclophosphamide

Using the above categories, cyclophosphamide can be used as an example to gain a deeper insight into the use of a chemotherapy as an anticancer drug. Table 16.5 explains the properties of cyclophosphamide.

Episode of Care

Learning Disability

Jasmine was 16 years old when she presented to hospital with a seizure. On admission to hospital Jasmine also identified a month history of dizziness and vomiting. After initial testing, Jasmine was diagnosed with an ependymoma (a type of brain tumour), Jasmine is now 20 years old and has recently relapsed her ependymoma.

Jasmine has a moderate learning disability and lives in assisted living where she is visited regularly by her parents and older sister.

Jasmine is being treated with a combination of oral chemotherapies at home. Jasmine was prescribed $50mg/m^2$ of etoposide orally every day for a period of 3 weeks. She is now due to start taking 2.5mg/kg of cyclophosphamide orally every day.

Jasmine was given the correct number of tablets of etoposide to last for 3 weeks but on return to clinic to collect her cyclophosphamide tablets, Jasmine still has half of her tablets left in the bottle.

Jasmine was previously assessed as having capacity to manage her own medications, but she now seems confused by which medications she should take and when. Jasmine isn't able to remember which days she has taken her medications and which days she may have forgotten.

Before Jasmine can be discharged home, healthcare professionals need to reassess Jasmine's capacity to manage her own medications at home and develop a plan to ensure that she is compliant with her treatment regimen.

Table 16.5 Properties of cyclophosphamide.

Use	Can be used in the treatment of a wide range of malignancies, including some leukaemias, lymphomas and solid tumours (Joint Formulary Committee, 2019).
Dose	Must be individualised. The dose, duration of treatment and treatment intervals are adjusted according to the therapeutic indication of the patients scheme of chemotherapy (Electronic Medicines Compendium, EMC, 2017).
Administration	Can be given orally or intravenous (IV) as a bolus or an infusion.
Pharmacodynamics	An alkylating agent which affects the cell at the S or G2 phase of the cell cycle. It is not known whether cyclophosphamide works *only* through the alkylation of DNA but this is the drugs main known method of action (EMC, 2017).
Pharmacokinetics	Cyclophosphamide is inactive at administration but activated in the liver. Absorption – Quickly and almost completely absorbed parenterally and well absorbed orally. Distribution – Distributed widely around the body and can cross the blood–brain barrier, the placental barrier and is found in ascites. The parent compound binds poorly to plasma protein but the active metabolites are significantly protein bound. Metabolism – Activated in the liver. 2–4 hours after administration, the plasma concentrations of the active metabolites are maximal, after which plasma concentrations rapidly decrease. Excretion – The plasma half-life is about 4–8 hours in adults and children. Cyclophosphamide and its metabolites are primarily excreted by the kidneys (EMC, 2016, 2017).
Side effects (common or very common)	Bone marrow suppression and problems associated low blood counts, alopecia, physical weakness or lack of energy, cystitis, haemolytic uraemic syndrome, hepatic disorders, mucosal abnormalities, sperm abnormalities and progressive multifocal leukoencephalopathy (PML) (Joint Formulary Committee, 2019).

Immunotherapies in Treating Cancer

The Immune System

In immunotherapy, it is essential to understand the role of the immune system and how this line of therapy may influence cancer management plans.

The immune system plays a significant role in the development and progression of cancers (Coosemans et al., 2019; Hanahan and Weinberg, 2011). Natural antibodies within the immune system are proteins that fight infection when the body recognises something harmful, such as viruses and bacteria. In response to these harmful cells, signals are sent by the immune system, to interrupt growth and kill the invading cell (Figure 16.3).

Whilst some of the body's own malformed cells will be destroyed by the immune system responses, many cancers are able to avoid this process, as they act as part of the body's own structure rather than an invading cell. This allows the cancer cell to avoid attack and escape immune system pathways that are in place to block and reduce harm.

Though the immune system sometimes fails to destroy cancer cells initially, it can still be useful in the management and treatment of cancer. Immunotherapy uses substances that are naturally made by the body or made synthetically in a laboratory, to improve or restore the immune system in order to elicit or amplify an immune response.

Immunotherapy

Immunotherapy is a relatively new form of cancer therapy. Although first recognised by Dr William Coley in the 1800s, it was initially approved as part of cancer treatment in 1990. This was in the form of a cancer-based vaccine for tuberculosis (Cancer Research Institute, 2019) and since then advances in research and use of immunotherapy in cancer care have increased exponentially.

Chapter 16 Medications Used in Children and Young People's cancer

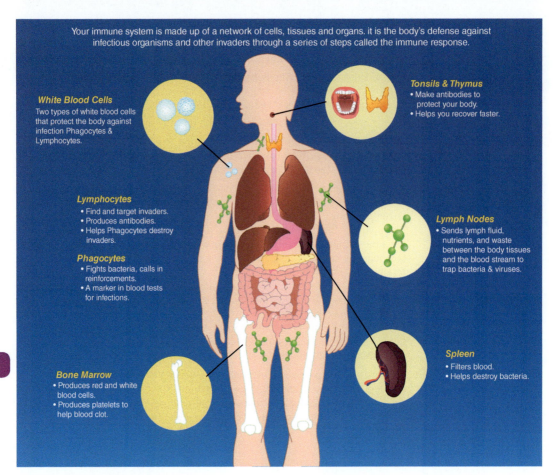

Figure 16.3 **The immune system.**

Immunotherapy is a form of treatment that can act to support the immune system in recognising specific cancer cells and either destroying them or stopping or slowing growth within the cancer cell (Schreiber and Smith 2011).

Immunotherapy can act to block the pathways that cancer cells often use to avoid immune responses and encourage the immune system to form memory cells against specific types of cancer. In certain cancers, it is thought that immunotherapy relaunches the immune system, allowing it to re-form and therefore producing cancer-specific antibodies that will be retained in immune memory and attack any returning cancer cells. Currently immunotherapy has been formulated to be suitable only for certain cancers due to cell composure within these cancer cells. Cancer immunotherapy is an artificial interaction with the immune system in an attempt to fight cancer.

The Use of Immunotherapy

Immunotherapy may be used independently or as part of a treatment regimen (with chemotherapy and or surgery), both in active and supportive pathways (see below). Using the body's own immune responses allows immunotherapy to respond to cancer only cells, preventing their growth and sparing healthy cells from this invasion, therefore reducing the severe side effects as commonly seen in chemotherapy.

- Active immunotherapy primes the immune system to recognise cancer cells as foreign, encouraging the production of antibodies or cytotoxic T cells to fight cancer, which aims to stop growth within the cancer cell (Yao et al., 2018).
- Supportive immunotherapy is non-specific strengthening of the innate immune system and acts as a secondary treatment line in slowing cancer growth (Vansteenkiste, 2012).

Immunotherapy is considered in addition to chemotherapy and radiotherapy for more resistant cancers, as part of an aggressive treatment plan and the effects of such treatment regimens remains under scrutiny (Coosemans et al., 2019).

Immunotherapy is used in a variety of treatment methods, including;
- Targeted antibodies
- Checkpoint inhibitors
- Bone marrow/stem cell transplant
- Adoptive cell transfer
- Cytokines

The role of each of the above are now discussed.

Targeted Antibodies

Advances in technology have allowed for the identification of proteins that are uniquely expressed within tumour cells. There are several types of targeted antibodies, each acting on different proteins. Monoclonal antibodies are manufactured antibodies that act by targeting specific proteins so the immune system can destroy these abnormal proteins. The purpose being to return cellular growth, differentiation and proliferation back to its healthy state. Monoclonal antibodies are made up of one protein type and bind to this particular epitope within the cell (Figure 16.4). Some monoclonal antibodies work by stimulating the immune system to respond and attack the cancer, rather than allowing natural immune regulation to see cancer proteins as part of the self and preventing continued antigen assault. Monoclonal antibodies target cancer cells by driving the immune system to release its brakes and remain active in the fight against harmful antigens (Saleh, 2019). Table 16.6 identifies some of the commonly used monoclonal antibodies in cancer care.

Checkpoint Inhibitors

Checkpoint inhibitors can also be considered a form of monoclonal antibodies. There are pathways in the immune system which are crucial in preventing cancer from being able to avoid immune responses and continue to grow. These pathways would normally contain a checkpoint to recognise and block invading organisms (such as cancer) and to allow immune responses to identify and destroy harmful cells.

Some cancers are able to fool the immune system and move through these pathways or checkpoints (PD-1/DD-L1, CTLA-4), which is where checkpoint inhibitor drugs may be useful. Checkpoint inhibitors are antibodies that act by stimulating the immune system to block these checkpoints, enticing immune recognition and response to occur, aiming to stop or slow growth of cancer cells (Johnson et al., 2019).

Figure 16.5 shows the action that occurs when checkpoint inhibitors such as Anti PD1 occur within the cell. Table 16.7 identifies some of the commonly used checkpoint inhibitors in cancer care.

See Table 16.8 for examples of checkpoint inhibitors.

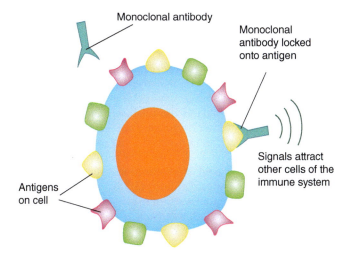

Figure 16.4 Mononuclear antibodies.

Chapter 16 Medications Used in Children and Young People's cancer

Table 16.6 Examples of monoclonal antibodies.

DRUG AND ROUTE	INDICATION	PHARMACODYNAMICS
Trastuzumab (Herceptin) intravenous infusion	Breast cancers that over express HER 2	Attach to HER2 cells to block growth signals
Rituximab intravenous infusion	Chronic lymphocytic leukaemia (CLL) Non-Hodgkin's lymphoma	Targets CD20 on B cells, immune responses then attach and kill CD20 (young cells in the bone marrow do not have CD20)

Source: Based on Joint Formulary Committee, 2019.

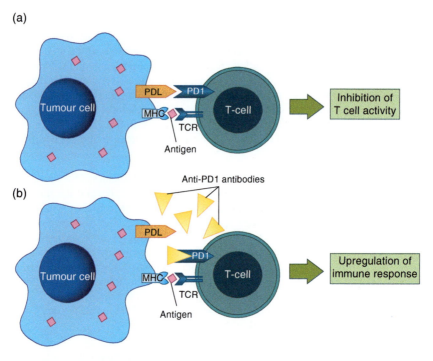

Figure 16.5 Cell activity with checkpoint inhibitor.

Bone Marrow and Stem Cell Transplant

Bone marrow transplants (BMT), also referred to as stem cell transplants, are used to replace diseased bone marrow with new healthy cells. This is a form of immunotherapy, as the transplanted marrow elicits the immune system to re-evaluate and re-launch, making it more able to respond to harmful cells following significant attack from diseases such as cancer. BMT is also used to replace cells within the immune system which have been permanently destroyed by cancer treatments (such as chemotherapy).

Bone marrow or stem cells can be donated from a matched donor or autologous, meaning they have been harvested, cleaned and stored and are later given back to the same person (Figure 16.6).

BMT and stem cell transplantation are used in conjunction with robust pharmaceutical regimens. Treatment to destroy the damaged immune system occurs pre BMT, alongside post BMT therapies which support the new cells to be established and minimise risk of rejection from the bodies original immune system. Table 16.9 identifies the indication for stem cell transplant or BMT bone in cancer care.

Adoptive Cell Transfer (ACT)

Adoptive cell transfer is the autologous use of genetically modified T cells to help activate T cell activity by stimulating T cells to recognise and target specific proteins on cancer cells. Before ACT can occur, depletion

Chapter 16 Medications Used in Children and Young People's cancer

Table 16.7 Properties of rituximab as a monoclonal antibody.

Treatment	Cancers such as: Follicular lymphoma, B cell non-Hodgkin's lymphoma, chronic lymphocytic leukaemia (CLL).
Dose	Adults 375mg/m^2 body surface. Child dose is strictly guided by individual protocols, weight of child and clinical presentation.
Administration	Always given as IV or subcutaneous infusion Patients must have close monitoring by a healthcare professional and be in an environment where full resuscitation facilities are available. Pre-medication of antipyretic and antihistamine is required alongside pre-hydration.
Pharmacodynamics	Rituximab is a monoclonal antibody that binds to transmembrane antigen CD20 on B cells. CD20 is present on normal and malignant B cells, but not on stem cells.
Pharmacokinetics	Absorption: Circulating B cells are depleted by rituximab within 3 weeks, effects can last up to 6 months. Distribution: Binding to B cells is seen on lymphoid cells in thymus, spleen, peripheral blood and lymph nodes. Excretion: Half-life varies depending on disease, with an average of 22 days. This is increased in patients with large tumour mass, in CLL can be up to 32 days. Serum concentrate after 4 doses can be detected after 3–6 months.
Common or very common side effects (a selection only listed)	Decreased appetite Bone marrow disorders Anxiety Myocardial infarction Conjunctivitis Insomnia Ear pain Dizziness Migraine Sepsis Multi-organ failure

Source: Joint Formulary Committee, 2019; Drugs.com, 2019.

Table 16.8 Other checkpoint inhibitors.

DRUG AND ROUTE	INDICATION	PHARMACODYNAMICS
Ipilimumab *intravenous infusion*	Melanoma	Stimulates T cell activation to destroy cancer cell
Avelumab *intravenous infusion*	Merkel cell carcinoma	Binds to PD1 (programmed death) receptor – at checkpoint to stimulate immune response

Source: Joint Formulary Committee, 2019; Kirkwood et al., 2001.

of lymphocytes is required, to support the immune system's ability to accept replaced T cells (Rosenberg et al., 2008). This is achieved through chemotherapy agents which destroy lymphocytes.

T cells without tumour activity are harvested via blood from the cancer patient (autologous), the T cell is separated from other components within the blood then genetically modified in vitro and allowed to multiply. A larger collection of stronger T cells now with tumour activity is infused back into the cancer patient. These engineered T cells have an enhanced ability to attack the proteins on the cancer cell (Restifo et al., 2012).

Table 16.10 identifies some of the commonly used ACT drugs in cancer care.

Chapter 16 Medications Used in Children and Young People's cancer

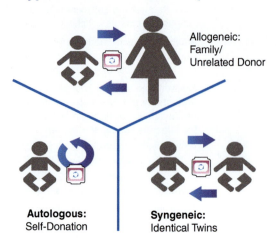

Figure 16.6 Types of bone marrow transplant.

Table 16.9 Indications for use of transplant.

ROUTE	INDICATION
Bone marrow/stem cells *intravenous infusion*	Leukaemia Lymphoma Multiple myeloma

Table 16.10 Examples of adoptive cell transfer drugs.

FORM OF ACT	INDICATION
Tisagenlecleucal	Acute lymphoblastic leukaemia in patients up to aged 25 years only
Axicabtagene	T cell lymphomas for patients who have failed conventional treatment twice

Source: National Institute for Health and Care Excellence (NICE), 2018a, 2018b.

Cytokines

Cytokines are memory bound proteins that act as a mediator of intercellular activity. Cytokines are responsible for signalling between cells and maintaining the balance of the Immune system. Cytokines act as messenger cells communicating and co ordinating responses to targeted antigens within the immune system (Lee and Margoln, 2011).

Engineered cytokine drugs stimulate the immune system to encourage T cell activity; they are able to interfere with the cancer cell by enticing the cancer cell to produce chemicals that are easily recognised as harmful within the immune system stimulating T cell attack. Cytokines also interfere with the way the cancer cell multiplies, attempting to reduce growth (Castro et al., 2018). Table 16.11 identifies some of the commonly used Cytokines in cancer care.

Side Effects of Immunotherapy

The side effects associated with immunotherapies vary between person to person and differ with each therapeutic agent. Table 16.12 details possible side effects from immunotherapy. The majority of side effects from immunotherapy are mild, due to the composition of immunotherapies in targeting cancer cells, thereby protecting healthy cells within the body. However, there are recorded incidences of severe and life-threatening effects from some patients. As immunotherapies stimulate the immune system, certain reactions should be expected (Kirkland et al., 2001, Joint Formulary Committee, 2018–19).

Chapter 16 Medications Used in Children and Young People's cancer

Table 16.11 Examples of cytokines.

DRUG AND ROUTE	INDICATION	PHARMACODYNAMICS
Interferon alpha *subcutaneous injection* *or intravenous injection*	Hairy cell leukaemia Non-Hodgkin's lymphoma Myeloma Liver or lymph metastasis of carcinoid tumour	Boosts immune systems response and reduce growth of cancer by interfering with action of proteins that affect growth
Interleukin 2/proleukin *subcutaneous injection* *or intravenous infusion*	Metastatic renal cancer	Aims to produce tumour shrinkage by inhibiting cell growth

Source: Based on Joint Formulary Committee, 2019.

Table 16.12 Side effects of immunotherapy.

MILD SIDE EFFECTS	SEVERE SIDE EFFECTS
Minor inflammation	Autoimmune response
Flu-like symptoms	Skin breakdown
Nausea	Mucositis
Headaches	Blood pressure irregularity
Body aches	Vomiting
Fatigue	Colitis
Itching (rash on less than 10% of body)	Paralysis
	Myocarditis
	Neurological disorders

Source: Haanen et al., 2017; Kirkwood et al., 2001; Joint National Formulary, 2019.

Immunotherapies (in particular checkpoint inhibitors) take the brakes off the regulation of the immune system, it is therefore crucial when administering immunotherapy that close monitoring of the patient occurs. This monitoring is needed because releasing the immune system control may entice attack from the immune system onto healthy functioning parts of the body. This could cause unpredictable, life-threatening side effects if early identification and treatment did not occur (Potter, 2014). Monitoring of the patient by healthcare professionals should seek to recognise any allergic responses or flu-like symptoms which may occur during or shortly after treatment.

Clinical Considerations

Immunotherapy treatments are rapidly becoming a popular choice in cancer care. They have expended treatment possibilities and are associated with less toxicity than traditional approaches. Guidelines for their use are differentiated by diagnosis, age and prognosis of each patient. Not all cancers and patients are responsive to immunotherapy. The risks and benefits of treatment as always is the priority in any consideration for immunotherapy (Haanen et al., 2017).

Source: Based on Haanen et al., 2017.

Episode of Care

Adult

Oluchi was 45 years old when she presented to her GP with a lump in her breast. Oluchi was the mother of three girls and lived in the city centre with her husband and children. After initial testing, Oluchi was diagnosed with breast cancer. Further testing showed that Oluchi's cancer staging was 2a and was HER2 positive.

Oluchi was initially given Trastuzumab (targeted antibody) to reduce the size of her tumour, before she had surgery to remove the tumour completely.

Throughout her treatment, Oluchi's experienced various side effects, including:

- Hot flushes and sweating
- Disinterest in sex
- Vaginal dryness
- Nausea and vomiting
- Pain in her joints
- Mood changes
- Fatigue

Oluchi will continue to receive oral Trastuzumab at 6mg/kg for at least 2 years after her surgery and will continue to see her specialist team in long-term follow-up clinic.

Healthcare professionals will need to offer ongoing psychological and physical support for Oluchi, monitoring her for side effects of treatment and to ensure that her cancer does not recur.

Corticosteroid Use in Cancer

Steroids

Steroids are hormones that are naturally produced within the body, these are produced in small amounts during physiological or emotional stress. Stress sends signals to the brain for the pituitary gland to release the adrenocorticotropic hormone (ACTH). ACTH acts by instructing the adrenal glands (located above the kidney) to release cortisol, the body's natural steroid. Cortisol once released it is picked up by cell receptors to respond to specific stress issues around the body (Ly and Wen, 2017).

Cortisol has several functions, it can help reduce inflammation, help control blood glucose, regulate the metabolism, control salt and water balance, maintain blood pressure and assist memory function. Cortisol receptors are present in a majority of body cells, each using the cortisol in a different way.

Although there is currently limited knowledge on the pharmacodynamics of steroids, it is reported that corticosteroids act in the body by altering transcription and protein synthesis within cellular activity (Wooldridge et al., 2001), thereby inhibiting the release of specific inflammatory mediators such as arachidonic acid.

Corticosteroids are manmade replicas of natural cortisol hormones (steroid). Corticosteroids are used as a means of supplying the body with an increased source of steroid, in order to encourage and produce the same effects within cells of the body that cortisol stimulates (Twycross, 1994). Corticosteroids act through genomic and non-genomic mechanisms. Genomic effects occur through gene translation or transcription. These include anti-inflammatory and immune suppression by excretion of anti-inflammatory cytokines and metabolic effects through suppression of the hypothalamic- pituitary-adrenal axis (Czock et al., 2005). Non-genomic effects occur through interaction with specific receptors such as glucocorticoids within cell membranes (Yu et al., 1981; Ly and Wen, 2017).

Using Corticosteroids to Treat Cancer

Corticosteroids act in a variety of ways. Primarily in cancer they are used for two principal functions, providing important components for modifying the fluid membrane and signalling molecules within the cell. These functions aim to reproduce responses within the immune system that are initiated by steroid activity, such as:

- Reduce inflammation
- Suppress immunity
- Reduce allergic reactions
- Stimulate appetite (metabolic effects)
- Control the balance of water and salt
- Regulate blood pressure
- Control mood and behaviour (Walsh et al., 2000, Zhou and Cidlowski, 2005)

The use of corticosteroids in cancer is part of well established treatment protocols. The type and stage of cancer often determines how corticosteroids will be used within pharmaceutical therapy plans (Table 16.13). Corticosteroids are used in cancer to achieve a variety of effects, such as reduce inflammation, suppress immune responses, treat the cancer (by attacking the cell), help alleviate sickness and improve appetite. Type and stage of cancer often indicates corticosteroid use within treatment or management plans. Corticosteroids

Chapter 16 Medications Used in Children and Young People's cancer

Table 16.13 **Examples of corticosteroid use in cancer.**

THERAPEUTIC PLAN	DESIRED EFFECT
In conjunction with chemotherapy	Inhibit inflammatory responses, reduce allergic reactions, help reduce sickness, increase appetite Maintain blood pressure Control balance of water and salt
Pre and post surgery	Reduce inflammatory responses
Post bone marrow transplant	Suppress immune system and reduce risk of rejection
Autonomously (advanced cancer)	Reduce inflammatory responses as part of symptom relief. Increase appetite

can be prescribed from diagnosis, throughout therapy or in palliative care (Ryken at al., 2010; Cancer Network, 2019). Anti-inflammatory and immune suppression are the main functions that signal use of corticosteroids in cancer patients. Reducing the inflammation around tumours, can help decrease the pressure on nerve endings, brain, spine or bone which are caused by the tumour. The corticosteroids ability to suppress the immune system by altering normal immune responses, although making the patient more susceptible to infection allows the immune system to be reprogrammed and other therapeutic agents to fight cancer cells. It is also thought that corticosteroids can induce programmed death within certain cells and help fight cancer (Joint Formulary Committee, 2019).

In cancer treatment there are four main corticosteroids in use. These are prednisolone, methylprednisolone, dexamethasone and hydrocortisone, as identified in Table 16.14.

Corticosteroids can be administered through oral, topical, intravenous and eye drops. Oral tablets or liquids and intravenous methods are the most common routes in cancer care. Each corticosteroid has its own half-life and intermediate-acting properties, defining differential indications for use (NICE, 2017).

Dexamethasone is one of the strongest corticosteroids. Dexamethasone holds 7.5 times greater effect opposed to prednisolone and hydrocortisone. The use of dexamethasone in cancer is a popular choice during initial treatment protocols. Long-term use is mainly restricted to palliative care (EMC, 2021). Table 16.15 outlines the properties of oral dexamethasone.

Side Effects of Corticosteroids

Corticosteroid use has several mild and severe associated side effects. It is well known that corticosteroids can mask the symptoms of infection and reduce immunity; therefore, stringent procedures should be in place to ensure safe use in cancer patients. Short-term use with low doses of corticosteroid have less complicated and

Table 16.14 **Examples of corticosteroid.**

ROUTE	EXAMPLE OF CORTICOSTEROID	INDICATION
Oral	Prednisolone Methylprednisolone Dexamethasone	Acute lymphoblastic leukaemia Chronic lymphocytic leukaemia Hodgkin's lymphoma Non-Hodgkin's lymphoma Mycosis lymphoma Aplastic anaemia
Intravenous	Hydrocortisone Methylprednisolone Dexamethasone	Brain tumours Spine tumours Cerebral oedema caused by tumours
Topical	Dexamethasone Hydrocortisone	Basal and squamous cell skin cancers
Eye drops	Dexamethasone	Prevent eye inflammation in leukaemia and lymphoma patients

Chapter 16 Medications Used in Children and Young People's cancer

Table 16.15 Dexamethasone.

Use	Dexamethasone is a corticosteroid that can be used for its anti-inflammatory, immune suppression and membrane stabilising properties within most cancers. It is also often used for the reduction of nausea and vomiting in patients undergoing chemotherapy (EMC, 2021).
Dose	Adult doses range from 0.5–10mg daily, depending on severity of disease. When used to treat nausea and vomiting, doses can range from 8–16mg/day (Joint Formulary Committee, 2018–19). Children's doses are calculated dependent on reason for use and stage of cancer, alongside the child's weight. Each individual child must be prescribed dose accordingly considering how they will manage the treatment.
Administration	Can be given as IV infusion, or oral in tablets and liquid form. Oral treatment should be taken as one dose each morning with or after food. Patients on high doses may be required to have doses more than once day (EMC, 2021; Joint Formulary Committee 2018–19).
Pharmacodynamics	Dexamethasone activates the transcription of corticosteroid sensitive genes. Effects of anti-inflammatory, immune suppression and cell anti-proliferation are caused by a decrease in the formation, release and activity of inflammatory mediators, inhibiting the specific function and migration of inflammatory cells.
Pharmacokinetics	Absorption: Oral dexamethasone is rapidly absorbed in the stomach and small intestine, creating a bioavailability of 80–90%. Distribution: It binds to plasma albumin; high doses give largest portion of drug that circulates within the blood. Metabolism: Partly metabolised by the kidneys. Half-life is up to 36 hours. Excretion: Metabolites are excreted as gluconates or sulfates and excreted by the kidneys (EMC, 2021).
Common or very common side effects	Adrenal suppression Anxiety Appetite increased Abnormal behaviour Cataract Cushing's syndrome Electrolyte imbalance Fluid retention, Headache Increased risk of infection Osteoporosis (Joint Formulary Committee, 2018–19)

more often immediate, short-term side effects. Long-term use with high doses of corticosteroids, which is more common in cancer patients, can present severe side effects that may take a prolonged time to resolve once treatment has ceased.

Clinical Considerations

High-dose and long-term use of corticosteroids requires healthcare practitioners to be alert to not only common side effects but also to the more uncommon and rare effects on an individual's physical and mental health, that can be attributed to this form of treatment. The elderly population are at increased risk of osteoporosis and children are more susceptible to retarded growth. Preterm infants may suffer extra complications such as cognitive impairment.

Source: Based on EMC, 2019.

Certain side effects may cause adverse reactions and irreversible damage (Yasir and Sonthalia. 2019). Table 16.16 details some of the more common side effects of long- and short-term use of corticosteroids; this list is not exhaustive. When administering corticosteroids, factors such as dose, duration and route alongside each patient's condition and health status need consideration for potential risk of side effects and adverse reactions.

Table 16.16 Side effects of corticosteroids.

SIDE EFFECTS IN SHORT-TERM USE (OFTEN LOWER DOSE)	SIDE EFFECTS IN LONG-TERM AND HIGH-DOSE USE
Insomnia	Weight gain
Gastrointestinal ulcers	Thinning of skin
Oral and vaginal candida	Cushingoid appearance
Anxiety	Osteoporosis *This may be permanent*
Glucose intolerance	Proximal myopathy
	Infection
	Impaired wound healing
	Gastrointestinal bleed
	Cardiac arrhythmias *This may be permanent*
	Cataracts *This may be permanent*
	Acne
	Increased risk of bone fracture
	Depression, suicidal thoughts
	Growth deceleration in children

Source: Yasir and Sonthalia, 2019; Sonauke et al., 2002.

Clinical Considerations

NICE (2017) stipulate that consideration for the use of corticosteroids should consider age of person (children and elderly being more susceptible to adverse side effects), certain conditions, (diabetes mellitus, hypertension and hepatic impairment require caution and close monitoring) in conjunction with the indication for use to ensure patient safety.

Source: Based on NICE, 2017.

Episode of Care

Child

Alex was 3 years old when he presented to hospital with a month history of flu-like symptoms and a recent development of a purpuric rash. After initial testing, Alex was diagnosed with Acute Lymphoblastic Leukaemia (ALL).

Alex lives at home on farm with his mother, father and one sister, aged 2 years. The family are struggling with income due to recent floods.

Alex was treated according to the UKALL 2011 trial guidelines which combines the use of corticosteroids and chemotherapy. As Alex's cancer was low risk, he was assigned to regimen A of the trial.

Alex was initially given a 4-week period of bi-daily, high-dose oral dexamethasone, alongside intravenous vincristine (weekly). Following this initial induction period (6 weeks), Alex was given a combination of intravenous and oral chemotherapy and oral corticosteroids over a period of 3 years to cure his leukaemia.

Throughout his treatment, Alex experience various side effects including;

- Initial weight gain
- Nausea and vomiting
- Alopecia
- Mucositis
- Weight loss (later in treatment)
- Decelerated growth

Prior to discharge, a nurse will need to ensure that Alex's family are educated and competent in recognising side effects of treatment and when to seek medical help.

Alex will continue to be followed up after his treatment by his specialist team in long-term follow-up. Healthcare professionals will need to offer ongoing psychological and physical support for Alex, monitoring him for side effects of treatment and to ensure that his cancer does not recur.

Conclusion

Treatment of cancer can occur using a number of different pharmaceutical options. Understanding of the difference between cancer cells and normal cells, allows for greater appreciation of the pharmacodynamics of each of these treatment options. When caring for patients with cancer, it is important that the nurse understands how each treatment regimen works and the side effects of these. The nurse also needs to be able to provide those receiving cancer treatment and if appropriate, their families with high-quality safe and effective care in a compassionate way. A holistic approach is advocated with the patient at the centre of all that is done

Different cancers have different properties and result in different abnormalities during the growth and multiplication of the cell. Not all treatments will be appropriate for all cancers, instead treatment must be tailored to the individual patient's cancer. Whilst one patient may have a single approach to treatment, other patients will require a combination of many different forms of treatment. Cancer care must be managed to ensure that the benefit of treatment outweighs the risk from adverse reactions or side effects.

This chapter has outlined some of the main pharmaceutical treatment options currently used for cancer in the UK. Advances in cancer research are continually developing and improving the care that can be offered to patients with cancer.

Glossary

Alopecia: The partial or complete loss of hair from areas of the body where it normally grows.
Antibodies: A blood protein produced in response to and counteracting a specific antigen. Antibodies combine chemically with substances which the body recognises as alien, such as bacteria, viruses and foreign substances in the blood.
Antigen: A toxin or other foreign substance which induces an immune response in the body, especially the production of antibodies.
Autoimmune: Relating to disease caused by antibodies or lymphocytes produced against substances naturally present in the body, producing the body's own autoimmune response.
Differentiation: The process by which cells, tissue and organs acquire specialised features, especially during embryonic development.
Epitope: The part of an antigen molecule to which an antibody attaches itself.
Molecule: A group of atoms bonded together, representing the smallest fundamental unit of a chemical compound that can take part in a chemical reaction.
Mucositis: Inflammation of a mucous membrane, especially that caused by cytotoxic therapy (radiation or chemotherapy).
Organism: An individual animal, plant, or single-celled life form.
Proliferation: Rapid reproduction of a cell, part, or organism.
Protein: Proteins are large molecules, composed of one or more chains of amino acids in a specific order, and are required for the structure, function, and regulation of the body's cells, tissues, and organs.
T cell: A lymphocyte of a type produced or processed by the thymus gland and actively participating in the immune response.
Toxic: Relating to or caused by poison.

References

Almeida, V.L., Leitão, A., Reina, L.C.B. et al. (2005). Cancer and nonspecific cycle-cell and nonspecific cycle-cell antineoplastic agents interacting with DNA: an introduction. *New Chemistry* 28(1): 118–129.
Bignold, L.P. (2006). Alkylating agents and DNA polymerases. *Anticancer Research* 26: 327–1336.
Cancer Research UK (2020a). Children cancer statistics. www.cancerresearchuk.org/health-professional/cancer-statistics/childrens-cancers (accessed April 2020).
Cancer Research UK (2020b). Young people's cancer statistics. www.cancerresearchuk.org/health-professional/cancer-statistics/statistics-by-cancer-type/young-peoples-cancers#heading-One (accessed April 2020).

Cancer Research UK (2020c). Cancer statistics for the UK. www.cancerresearchuk.org/health-professional/cancer-statistics-for-the-uk (accessed April 2020).

Cancer Research Institute (2019). https://www.cancerresearchuk.org (accessed August 2019).

Cancer Network (2019). https://www.cancernetwork/steroids.org (accessed August 2019).

Castro, F., Cardoso, A., Goncalves, R. et al. (2018). Interferon Gamma at the crossroads of tumour surveillance or evasion. *Frontiers in Immunology*. doi: 10.3389/fimmu.2018.00847.

Coosemans, A., Vankerckhoven, A., Baert, T. et al. (2019). Combining conventional therapy with immunotherapy: A risky business? *European Journal of Cancer*. 113: 41–44.

Czock, D., Keller, F., Rasche, F., and Haussler, U. (2005). Pharmacokinetics and pharmacodynamics of systemically administered glucocorticoids. doi: 10.2165/00003088-200544010-00003.

Drugs.com https://drugs.com/monograph/rituximab.html (accessed August 2019).

Electronic Medicines Compendium (EMC) (2016). Cyclophosphamide tablets 50mg. www.medicines.org.uk/emc/product/1813/smpc (accessed August 2019).

Electronic Medicines Compendium (EMC) (2017). Cyclophosphamide 1000mg powder for solution for injection or infusion. www.medicines.org.uk/emc/product/3525/smpc (accessed August 2019).

Electronic Medicines Compendium (EMC) (2020). Prednisolone 10mg tablets. www.medicines.org.uk/emc/product/7239/smpc#PRODUCTINFO (accessed 28 April 2021).

Electronic Medicines Compendium (EMC) (2021). Dexamethasone 1 mg tablets: Pharmacokinetic properties. www.medicines.org.uk/emc/product/12369/smpc#PHARMACOKINETIC_PROPS (accessed 28 April 2021).

Fu, D., Calvo, J.A., and Samson, L.D. (2012). Genomic instability in cancer: Balancing repair and tolerance of DNA damage caused by alkylating agents. *Nature Reviews Cancer* 12(2): 104–120.

Gmeiner, W.H. (2002). Antimetabolite incorporations into DNA: Structural and thermodynamic basis for anticancer activity. *Biopolymers* 65: 180–189.

Haanen, J., Carbonnel, C., Robert, C. et al. (2017). Management of toxicities from immunotherapy. doi: 10.1093/annoc/mdx225.

Hanahan, D. and Weinberg, R.A. (2011). The hallmarks of cancer: the next generation. doi: 10.1016/j.cell.2011.02.013.

Health and Safety Executive (HSE). Safe handling of cytotoxic drugs in the workplace. www.hse.gov.uk/healthservices/safe-use-cytotoxic-drugs.htm (accessed July 2019).

Hortobágyi, G.N. (1997). Anthracyclines in the treatment of cancer. *Drugs* 54(Supplement 4): 1–7.

Johnson, B., Manoucher, A., Haugh. A. et al. (2019). Neurological toxicity associated with immune checkpoint inhibitors: a pharmacovigilance study. *Journal for Immunotherapy of Cancer* 7: 134.

Joint Formulary Committee (2019). British National Formulary (BNF). Cytotoxic drugs. www.medicinescomplete.com/#/content/bnf/_979237904?hspl=chemotherapy#content%2Fbnf%2F_979237904%23section_979237904-0 (accessed April 2020).

Kirkwood, J., Lotze, M., and Yasko, J. (2001). *Current Cancer Therapeutics*, 4e. Philadelphia, PA: Port City Press.

Lee, S. and Margoln, K. (2011). Cytokines in cancer immunotherapy. *Journal of Cancer*. doi: 10.33901/cancers3043856.

Ly, K. and Wen, P. (2017). Clinical relevance of steroid use in neuro-oncology. *Current Neurology and Neuroscience Reports*. doi: 10.1007/s11910-017-0713-6.

McClendon, A.K., and Osheroff, N. (2007). DNA topoisomerase II, genotoxicity, and cancer. *Mutation Research* 623(1–2),: 83–97.

McEwen, B. (1991). Non genomic and genomic effects of steroids on neural activity. *Pharmacology* 12(4): 141–147.

Moudi, M., Rusea, G., Yien, C.Y.S., and Nazre, M. (2013). Vinca alkaloids. *International Journal of Preventative Medicine* 4(11): 1231–1235.

National Chemotherapy Advisory Group (NCAG) (2009). Chemotherapy services in England: Ensuring quality and safety. https://webarchive.nationalarchives.gov.uk/20130104173757/http://www.dh.gov.uk/en/Publicationsandstatistics/Publications/DH_104500 (accessed 20 April 20210).

Neilsen, D., Maare, C., and Skovsgaard, T. (1996). Cellular resistance to anthracyclines. *General Pharmacology: The Vascular System* 27(2): 251–255.

Office for National Statistics (ONS). (2020). Cancer registration statistics, England: 2017. www.ons.gov.uk/peoplepopulationandcommunity/healthandsocialcare/conditionsanddiseases/bulletins/cancerregistrationstatisticsengland/2017#cancer-registration-data (accessed April 2020).

Pires, J., Kreutz, O.C., Sayuri Suyenaga, E., and Perassolo, M.S. (2018). Pharmacological profile and structure-activity relationship of alkylating agents used in cancer treatment. *International Journal of Research in Pharmacy and Chemistry* 8(1): 6–17.

Restifo, N., Dudley, M., and Rosenberg, S. (2012). Adoptive immunotherapy for cancer: harnessing the T cell response. *Nature Reviews Immunology* 12: 269–281.

Rosenberg, S., Restifo, N., Yang, J. et al. (2008). Adoptive cell transfer: a clinical path to effective cancer immunotherapy. *Nature Reviews Cancer* 8: 299–308.

Ryken, T.C., McDermott, M., Robinson, P. et al. (2010). The role of steroids in management of brain metastases: A systemic review. *Journal of Neuro-Oncology*. doi: 10.1007/s11060-009-0057-4.

Saleh, N. (2019). Immunotherapy advances: 2019. *Oncology (Williston Park)* 33(10): 686508.

Schrieber, R.D. and Smyth, M.J. (2011). Cancer immunoediting: integrating immunity's role in cancer suppression and promotion. doi: 10.1126/science.1034864.

Twycross, R. (1994). Risks and benefits of corticosteroids in advanced cancer. *National Library of Medicine* 11(3): 163–168.

Vansteenkiste, J. (2012). Immunotherapy. doi: 10.1016/j.lungcan.2012.05.029.

Walsh, D., Doona, M., Molnar, M., and Lipnickey, V. (2000). Symptom control in advanced cancer: important drugs and routes of administration. *Oncology* 27(1): 69–83.

Wooldridge, J., Anderson, M., and Parry, M. (2001). Corticosteroids in advanced cancer. *Cancer Network* 15(2): 225–234.

Woolley, D. (1959). Antimetabolites. *Science* 129: 3349.

Yao, H., Wang, H., Li, C. et al. (2018). Cancer cell-intrinsic PD-1 and implications in combinatorial immunotherapy. doi: 10.3389/fimmu.2018.01774.

Yasir, M. and Sonthalia, S. (2019). Corticosteroids adverse effects. www.ncbi.nlm.nih.gov.

Yu, Z., Wrange, O., Baethius, J. et al. (1981). A study of glucocorticoid receptors in intracranial tumours. doi: 10.3171/jns.1981.55.5.0757.

Zhou, J. and Cidwlowski, J. (2005). The human glucocortoid receptor: one gene multiple proteins and diverse responses. doi: 10.1016/j.steroids.2005.02.006.

Zhou, X.J. and Rahmani, R. (1992). Preclinical and clinical pharmacology of vinca alkaloids. *Drugs.* 44(Supplement 4): 1–16.

Further Resources

National Cancer Peer Review-National Cancer Action Team: The NCAT have written a Manual for Cancer Services which supports the National Cancer Peer Review quality assurance programme for cancer services to enable quality improvement, in terms of both clinical and patient outcomes.

NICE guidelines: The National Institute for Health and Care Excellence (NICE) write evidence-based recommendations for healthcare in England. They provide a number of guidelines for the care and services suitable for most patients with certain types of cancer.

SIGN Guidelines: The Scottish Intercollegiate Guidelines Network (SIGN) develop and disseminate clinical guidelines for evidence-based healthcare practice in Scotland. They have developed a range of guidelines for use in cancer care.

Royal Pharmaceutical Society: The RPS provides pharmaceutical guidance for all healthcare practitioners in the UK. Information is available on current treatments for cancer.

Multiple Choice Questions

1. Over recent years, the UK has seen. . .
- **(a)** A decrease in the number of females diagnosed with cancer
- **(b)** An increase in the number of people dying from cancer
- **(c)** A decrease in the number of people dying from cancer
- **(d)** No change in the number of people diagnosed with cancer

2. Which of these is a 'hallmark of a cancer cell'?
- **(a)** Inducing angiogenesis
- **(b)** Apoptosis
- **(c)** Activating growth suppressors
- **(d)** Limited multiplication

3. At what stage in the cell cycle, does the cell completely divide?
- **(a)** M
- **(b)** G1
- **(c)** G2
- **(d)** S

Chapter 16 Medications Used in Children and Young People's cancer

4. What does cytotoxic mean?
   (a) Nourishes the cell
   (b) Stops the cell receiving messages
   (c) Stimulates the cell to grow
   (d) Poisonous to cells
5. Which of these is not a route that chemotherapy can be administrated?
   (a) Oral
   (b) Intravenous
   (c) Intrafollicular
   (d) Intrathecal
6. How does an antimetabolite work?
   (a) Inhibits topoisomerase II
   (b) Creates a deficiency of essential molecules
   (c) Transfers alkyl carbon molecules
   (d) Binds to tubulin
7. What are vinca alkaloids derived from?
   (a) Plants
   (b) Hormones
   (c) Horse urine
   (d) Synthetic compounds
8. Which of these is a common side effect of chemotherapy?
   (a) Changes to eye colour
   (b) Death
   (c) Hair loss
   (d) Perforated ear drum
9. What are the two main functions of the immune system?
   (a) Increase bone strength and fight infection
   (b) Fight infection and reduce inflammation
   (c) Stimulate growth and reduce inflammation
   (d) Control hair growth and support vision
10. Which one of the following is not part of the immune system?
    (a) White blood cells
    (b) Spleen
    (c) Lymph nodes
    (d) Liver
11. How does immunotherapy work?
    (a) Targets proteins on cancer only cells
    (b) Suppresses the immune system
    (c) Attracts cancer cells
    (d) Opens checkpoints in cancer cells
12. What is the role of supportive immunotherapy?
    (a) To prime the immune system
    (b) To stop growth within the cancer cell
    (c) To reduce growth in the cancer cell
    (d) To reduce inflammation
13. Who is the donor for an autologous bone marrow transplant?
    (a) Identical twin
    (b) Unrelated
    (c) Family
    (d) Self
14. Where are steroids naturally produced in the body?
    (a) The adrenal glands
    (b) Lymphocytes
    (c) The bone marrow
    (d) Testes

Chapter 16 Medications Used in Children and Young People's cancer

15. Why are corticosteroids used in the treatment of cancer?
- **(a)** To regulate heart and kidney function
- **(b)** Increase immunity and inflammatory responses
- **(c)** Reduce inflammation and allergic reactions
- **(d)** Support bone strength and growth

Find Out More

The following is a list of some of the cancers that are included in this chapter. Take some time and write notes about the treatment of each of the cancers and be specific about the pharmacodynamics and possible side effects of the medicines that would be used to treat this.

THE CONDITION	YOUR NOTES
Acute Lymphoblastic Leukaemia (ALL)	
Myeloma	
Hodgkin's lymphoma	
Breast cancer	
Melanoma	

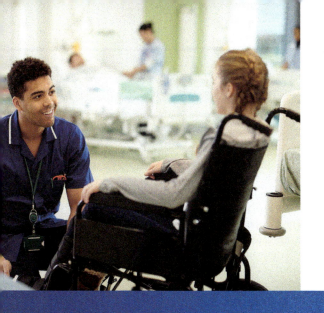

17

Analgesics

Claire Ford and Matthew Robertson

Aim
The aim of this chapter is to provide the reader with an introduction to some of the most common drugs used to manage pain in infants, children and young people (CYP). This chapter will also explore the concept of multimodal analgesic approaches, discuss the need for comprehensive individualised pain assessments, which are undertaken by healthcare providers in collaboration with CYP, parents and guardians and the importance of incorporating pharmacological and non-pharmacological strategies.

Learning Outcomes
After reading this chapter the reader will:

- Appreciate the importance of understanding the pharmacology associated with analgesic medications.
- Understand treatment optimisation in order to maintain therapeutic analgesic effects.
- Have a greater awareness of the importance of respecting individual choice, collaboration and utilising multimodal medication regimens for optimal delivery and satisfactory child-centred care.
- Recognise the importance of administering the right drug, in the right dose, via the right route, at the right time to manage pain.

Fundamentals of Pharmacology for Children's Nurses, First Edition. Edited by Ian Peate and Peter Dryden.
© 2022 John Wiley & Sons Ltd. Published 2022 by John Wiley & Sons Ltd.
Companion website: www.wiley.com/go/pharmacologyforCN

Chapter 17 Analgesics

Introduction

Pain is often experienced in early childhood ranging from minor scrapes and bumps, short periods of pain from the administration of a medical treatment e.g. immunisation, to long-standing pain which can be symptomatic of illness and disease (Mathews, 2011; Carter and Simons, 2014). While healthcare professionals are frequently faced with this clinical issue, pain can often be difficult to assess and manage as it is subjective, unique to each individual and activated by a variety of stimuli, including biological, physical and psychological (Boore et al., 2016). For individuals under the age of 19, pain management is further complicated due to considerable developmental, anatomical and physiological variation across the paediatric age range (Royal College of Anaesthetists (RCOA), 2020). When children and young people (CYP) state they are in pain, it is, therefore, every healthcare professional's duty to listen to what they say (Nursing and Midwifery Council (NMC), 2018); General Medical Council (GMC), 2019; Health and Care Professions Council (HCPC), 2019). Healthcare professionals must believe that pain is what the CYP says it is, observe for supporting information using appropriate and varied assessment approaches and act as soon as possible by utilising suitable management strategies. Unfortunately, pain is often not recognised in children, especially in those who are unable to self-report, such as neonates and treatment is frequently delayed and mismanaged (Petrack et al., 1997; Todd et al., 2002; Royal College of Nursing (RCN), 2009; Czarnecki et al., 2010; Mathews, 2011; Twycross and Finley, 2013). Pain left untreated (regardless of how it is manifested) can cause significant issues and negatively impact on physical health (e.g. recovery, sleep pattern, nutritional and hydration status) and emotional well-being (e.g. becoming socially withdrawn) (Vinall et al., 2012; Carter and Simons, 2014; Flasar and Perry, 2014; Twycross, 2017; Mears, 2018). Consequently, pain assessment, management and efficient pain alleviation should be a priority and episodes of pain should be anticipated in all neonates and CYP within the healthcare setting (RCN, 2009; Royal College of Emergency Medicine (RCEM), 2017).

Pain Pathways

The way in which pain is transmitted and modulated by the body and received and interpreted by the brain is extremely complex. This process is also associated with a variety of chemicals, neurons and electrical impulses and influenced by psychological and social elements (Ashelford et al., 2016). In order to understand the pharmacokinetics of analgesic drugs, it is important to examine these pain pathways in greater detail. Pain pathways are associated with ascending, descending and modulating processes, and while some medications are effective in interfering with the signals that are being sent to the brain, others could play a role in how the body responds to these signals after they are received and interpreted by the brain (see the illustration of a pain pathway in Figure 17.1).

The first part of the pathway is usually associated with the stimulation of sensory nerve endings 'nociceptors', by chemicals such as histamine and prostaglandins that are released when tissue injury or irritation occurs (Boyd, 2013). What needs to be noted here, is that despite some earlier beliefs that neonates' neurons are immature, nociceptive processes are present in early foetal development and the number of nociceptors in children are higher than in adults; thus pain signals are more easily initiated or more intense in this age range (Carter and Simons, 2014; Pancekauskaite and Jankauskaite, 2018). Once activated, these primary sensory neurons then carry impulses via afferent A-delta fibres (wide, myelinated, fast and associated with localised sharp pain) and C fibres (narrow, non-myelinated and slower) towards the central nervous system (CNS) (Todd, 2016). These terminate in the dorsal horn of the spinal cord and form synapses, where the action of neurotransmitters (i.e. glutamate and substance-P) continue to transfer the signals along relay neurons to the somatosensory cortex (Ashelford et al., 2016). In older children the junction within the spinal cord is fully functioning; however, in neonates these may not be fully operational, leading to signal disorganisation and confusion between tactile and nociceptive signals (Pancekauskaite and Jankauskaite, 2018). Neonates may, therefore, feel intense pain in response to a stimulus that is not usually associated with pain, such as touch.

The perception of the pain signals in the brain can also be influenced by a wide array of factors (depending on the level of development of the CYP) including psychological, physical and social and the response to the perceived pain signals could be in the form of emotional reactions and physiological responses, which activate the descending inhibitory efferent pathways (Smith and Muralidharan, 2014). Signals are transmitted

Chapter 17 Analgesics

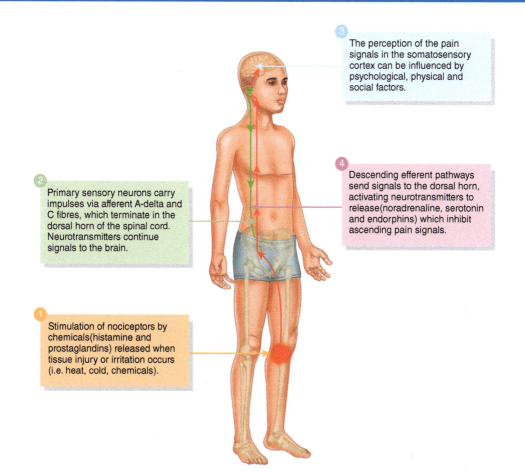

Figure 17.1 **Pain pathway.**

from the brain, back to the dorsal horn, where nerve endings are activated to release neurotransmitters (noradrenaline, serotonin and endorphins) which bind to the afferent pain fibres, inhibiting the synaptic transmission to the relay neurons. However, in neonates, this system may not be fully developed, and infants may have limited ability to respond in the same ways as an older child (Carter and Simons, 2014). It is in the descending pain pathway that opioids have been recognised as being the most effective medication, by inhibiting the synaptic transmission between the pain fibres. However, the way in which this occurs is different from the body's natural inhibitory mechanism. Opioid peptides, once bound to the appropriate receptors (mu – μ, kappa – κ and delta – δ) modulate pain input in two ways. By releasing a large number of calcium ions which block the presynaptic terminal and opening potassium channels which flood the synapse and hyperpolarises the neurons, preventing signals from passing across the synapse (Bannister, 2019).

Definitions and Categories of Pain

Before pain can be treated, it is necessary to understand and determine which type of pain the CYP is experiencing, as the choice of analgesic should be tailored to the type of pain and personal preferences of the child. See Figure 17.2 for the different types of pain. The first worldwide accepted definition of pain is from The International Association for the Study of Pain (IASP), which declares that pain is 'an unpleasant sensory and emotional experience associated with actual or potential tissue damage' (Merskey and Bogduk, 1994: 209). However, pain is not always directly linked to the amount of trauma as it can also be associated with

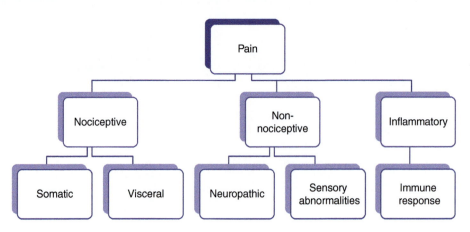

Figure 17.2 **Types of pain.** *Source: Adapted from Cunningham, 2017.*

psychological and emotional issues (Rodriguez, 2015). It is therefore multi-layered and the most commonly used classifications are separated by duration (acute or chronic), type (nociceptive, neuropathic and psychogenic) and site (somatic and visceral) (see Figure 17.2). Some overlap and CYP may present with one or more.

- **Acute:** serves a protective purpose, is of short duration (less than three months) and is reversible. It is predominantly nociceptive in nature, involves sensory processes and is treated very effectively with analgesics (Turk and Melzack, 2011; Kettyle, 2015).
- **Chronic:** serves no protective purpose and persists past the initial healing stage, usually more than three months. It is largely neuropathic, associated with an array of changes to the peripheral and central sensory pathways, typically connected with chronic disease and usually treated alongside psychological measures due to its extremely subjective nature (Tornsey and Fleetwood-Walker, 2012; Koneti and Perfitt, 2019).
- **Nociceptive:** is the most frequently experienced type of pain. It is a primitive sensation, protective in nature and involves the passing of information through primary afferent fibres to the cerebral cortex via pain receptors, referred to as 'nociceptors', which are stimulated and activated by tissue damage resulting from heat, cold, stretch, vibration or chemicals (Solaro and Uccelli, 2016; Mears, 2018).
- **Neuropathic:** is more degenerative in nature and usually occurs as a result of pain related to sensory abnormalities that can result from damage to the nerves (a nerve infection) or neurological dysfunction (a disease in the somatosensory nervous system). This type of pain may not be diagnosed immediately as it can manifest itself in various ways and can often be confused with acute persistent pain. Neuropathic pain is often managed with combined analgesic approaches (Colvin and Carty, 2012; Old et al., 2016).
- **Inflammation:** stimulation of nociceptive processes by chemicals released as part of the inflammatory process (Cunningham, 2017).
- **Somatic:** is a large part of the body's natural defence mechanism and is associated with nociceptive processes activated in skin, bones, joints, connective tissues and muscles (VanMeter and Hubert, 2014).
- **Visceral:** is a sensation and nociceptive process activated in the organs (e.g. stomach, kidneys, gallbladder) transmitted via the sympathetic fibres and linked to conditions such as irritable bowel syndrome and dysmenorrhoea (Boore et al., 2016).
- **Referred:** is pain that is felt in the skin that lies over an affected organ, or in an area some distance from the site of disease or injury (Patton and Thibodeau, 2016).

Importance of Individualised Pain Assessments

CYP react to pain in varying ways, depending on their level of development (Mathews, 2011). Therefore, in order to ensure an effective and child-centred holistic management plan is developed, it is important to understand how the pain is uniquely affecting the CYP from a biopsychosocial perspective (Twycross, 2017). In order to do this, healthcare professionals use a range of skills, such as the art of noticing, questioning techniques and active listening, which again will be aligned with the child's stage of development in order

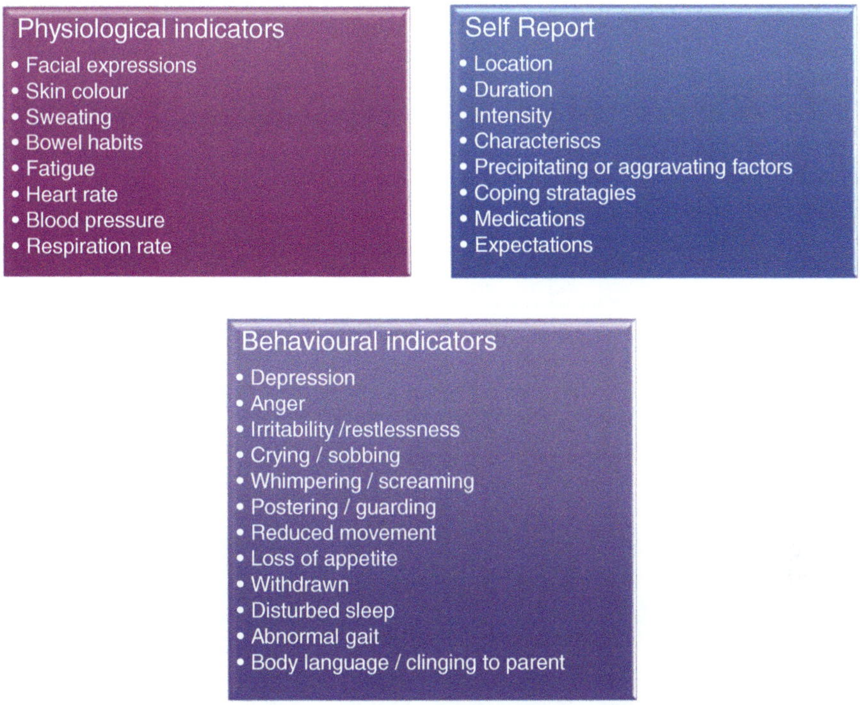

Chapter 17 Analgesics

Physiological indicators
- Facial expressions
- Skin colour
- Sweating
- Bowel habits
- Fatigue
- Heart rate
- Blood pressure
- Respiration rate

Self Report
- Location
- Duration
- Intensity
- Characteriscs
- Precipitating or aggravating factors
- Coping stratagies
- Medications
- Expectations

Behavioural indicators
- Depression
- Anger
- Irritability /restlessness
- Crying / sobbing
- Whimpering / screaming
- Postering / guarding
- Reduced movement
- Loss of appetite
- Withdrawn
- Disturbed sleep
- Abnormal gait
- Body language / clinging to parent

Figure 17.3 **Example of assessment approaches.** *Source:* Adapted from Kettyle, 2015; Cunningham, 2017; Twycross, 2017.

to assess what the child says (self-report) and how they behave (behavioural indicators) (see Figure 17.3 for more details on these assessment approaches). Another strategy often employed by healthcare professionals is the assessment and measurement of vital signs, as a correlation exists between how the body reacts (physiological indicators) and pain scores (e.g. respiratory rate, pulse and blood pressure (Bendall et al., 2011; RCN, 2017). This becomes even more relevant when attempting to take observations from CYP who are unable to self-report or verbalise, e.g. when a child is sedated (Association of Paediatric Anaesthetists of Great Britain and Ireland (APAGBI), 2012; Erden et al., 2018). It is important to remember that no one skill is superior, rather it is the culmination of information gathered via the various methods that enable a healthcare professional to determine if a CYP is in pain and understand how this pain is affecting them physically and emotionally (Cunningham, 2017; Twycross, 2017) Parents and guardians are invaluable during this process as they often witness how the pain is affecting their child first-hand (APAGBI, 2012; Carter and Simons, 2014).

Assessment Tools

Whilst vital observations may indicate that a child is in pain, questioning, measurement, interpretation skills and exploration of other contextual factors will assist with determining the intensity, severity, and effect of the pain on the child's well-being and quality of life (RCEM, 2017). This process can be aided with the use of specifically designed tools, which act as prompts for healthcare professionals and facilitate the assessment of one or more dimensions. The choice of tool will depend upon the age and development of the CYP, ability to self-report, the type of pain and the context of the healthcare setting (RCN, 2009) (see Figure 17.4). No one tool should be used in isolation but rather a multimodal approach needs to be adopted, which includes open communication between the child, parent and healthcare professional (see Clinical Consideration 1) (APAGBI, 2012).

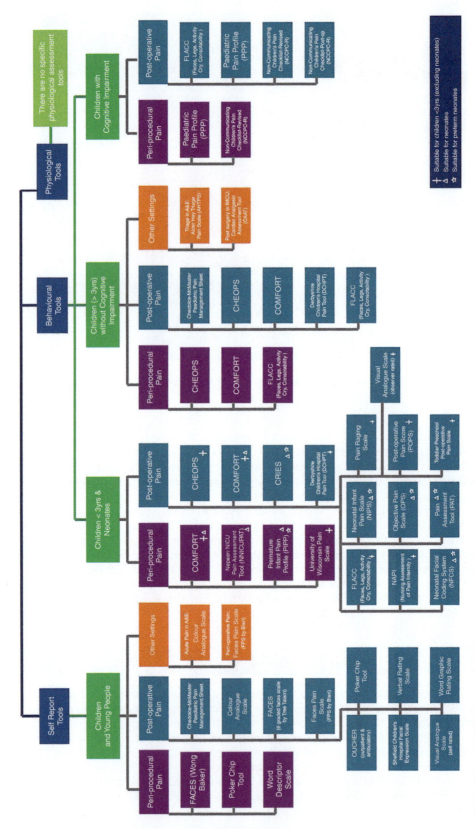

Figure 17.4 Algorithm for choice pain assessment tools. *Source:* Modified from Royal College of Nursing, 2009.

Clinical Consideration 1

A Child-centred and Tailored Approach
Regardless of which tool or mnemonic is used, as pain presentations are often unique, pain assessment will be unsuccessful if the healthcare professional fails to ascertain and interpret the signs and symptoms, uses assessment tools inappropriately and does not apply a child-centred approach to the overall assessment process, as the child's views should be paramount (RCN, 2009: RCEM, 2017; Intercollegiate Committee for Standards for Children and Young People in Emergency Care Settings, 2018).

Source: RCN, 2009; RCEM, 2017.

Multimodal Management Strategies

One of the primary goals is to pre-empt and prevent pain from occurring in the first instance; however, if pain cannot be avoided (as in the case of surgery) optimal analgesic management is vital. The word analgesia 'to be without the feeling of pain' is derived from the Greek language, and in terms of pain management relates to medication and alternative interventions (Laws and Rudall, 2013). Hence, pain management plans should incorporate a multi-modal approach using a range of pharmacological and non-pharmacological strategies (see Clinical Consideration 2), in order to successfully and holistically treat children' pain (APAGBI, 2012; Flasar and Perry, 2014). A combination approach is also recommended for pharmacological management, as several drugs have morphine sparing properties, which increases the effect of opioids; therefore, the use of adjuvants (e.g. opioids alongside NSAIDs and massage) is recommended (Boyd, 2013). Boore et al. (2016) state that this is an effective way to manage pain, but stress that the decisions about which management strategies to use, also need to take into consideration the context of the clinical situation, the CYP's level of acuity, the environment and physical space and the availability of resources. The clinical decisions associated with analgesic administration must also be made in line with Royal Pharmaceutical Society (RPS), (2019) recommendations, which state that any HCP administering medicines must possess a comprehensive

Clinical Consideration 2

Non-Pharmacological Strategies
Pharmacological treatments are not the only strategy at healthcare professionals' disposal, and true holistic management cannot be achieved without the incorporation of other non-pharmacological therapies. Some of these interventions are long-standing (Flasar and Perry, 2014) and when used correctly, can enhance a CYP's feelings of empowerment and involvement. However, due to limited resources, funding, space, time, knowledge of use, and personal beliefs, some therapies are not always fully utilised or embraced (Cullen and MacPherson, 2012). These can be placed into three main groups, (see Figure 17.5 below), and the choice of which to use will depend upon the child's preferences and development. The

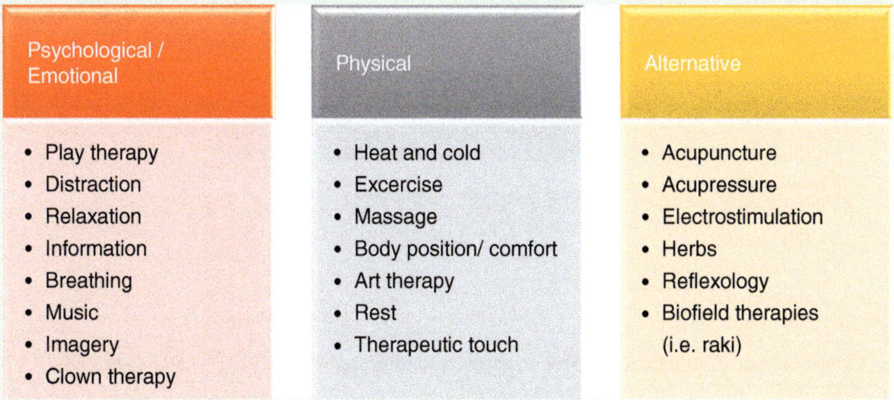

Psychological / Emotional	Physical	Alternative
• Play therapy	• Heat and cold	• Acupuncture
• Distraction	• Excercise	• Acupressure
• Relaxation	• Massage	• Electrostimulation
• Information	• Body position/ comfort	• Herbs
• Breathing	• Art therapy	• Reflexology
• Music	• Rest	• Biofield therapies
• Imagery	• Therapeutic touch	(i.e. raki)
• Clown therapy		

Figure 17.5 **Example of non-pharmacological management strategies.** *Source*: Adapted from Cunningham, 2017.

following strategies have been highlighted as they align with the fundamental core values of care and compassion and require very little in terms of resources or time.

- **Distraction:** This can take various forms, such as reading the child a story, using soap bubbles and clown therapy (Felluga et al., 2016; Longobardi et al., 2019). This basic skill often requires no equipment, can be done anywhere and is a useful way of taking the child's mind off their pain.
- **Play therapy:** This is a method of therapy where a variety of play and creative games/arts are used to help children discuss fears, this is particularly useful when children experience chronic and procedural pain (Scarponi and Pession, 2016).
- **Therapeutic touch (cuddles):** For centuries, the therapeutic placing of hands has proven to be a useful skill, and has beneficial physiological and psychological properties (Kettyle, 2015).
- **Environment:** Sound, lighting and the temperature of the child's immediate environment has also been shown to heighten or reduce perceptions of pain.

Source: Based on Healthcare Play Specialist Education Trust, 2015.

understanding of the drug itself, and an awareness of the potential risks and side effects. As well as the ability to accurately calculate precise doses for smaller children (RCOA, 2020).

Pharmacological Management

One very effective strategy that healthcare professionals have to treat pain is the use of pharmacological treatments, and the choice depends on whether the pain is nociceptive, non-nociceptive, inflammatory or of mixed origin. There are three main categories: opioids, non-opioids/non-steroidal anti-inflammatories and adjuvants/co-analgesics (see Figure 17.6). The most efficient pharmacological regime for moderate to severe pain often incorporates a combined approach, by administrating a specific drug in conjunction with adjuvants or co-analgesics (see Figure 17.7).

It is very important that the most appropriate drug is used to treat pain and the decision on which analgesic to choose should (whenever possible) be made in partnership with the child and parent (NMC, 2018; GMC, 2019; HCPC, 2019; RPS, 2019).

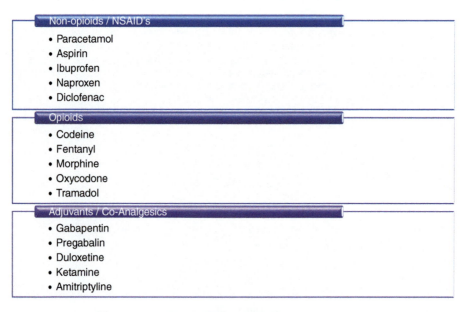

Figure 17.6 Classifications of pharmacological analgesics (examples). *Source:* Adapted from Smith and Muralidharan, 2014.

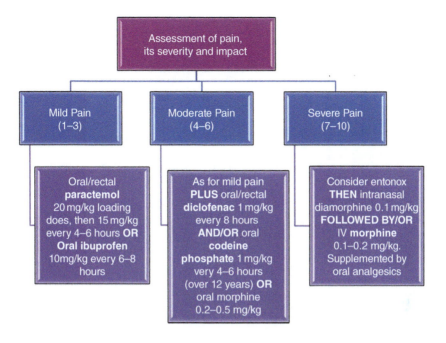

Figure 17.7 Algorithm for the pharmacological treatment of acute pain in the emergency department.
Source: Modified from RCEM, 2017.

Non-opioids

The most widely used and safest analgesic (when taken correctly) is acetaminophen, otherwise known as paracetamol, which can also be used as an antipyretic (Boyd, 2013). See Table 17.1 for further details of the pharmacokinetics, pharmacodynamics and common side effects of oral paracetamol. Whilst paracetamol is normally administered orally, depending on the age, weight and development of the CYP, Intravenous (IV) paracetamol is an effective way to bypass the absorption process, especially for drugs with a high degree of first-pass metabolism. IV paracetamol is therefore often used due to its ease of administration and rate of effectiveness as this route delivers the drug directly into the circulatory system (Neal, 2016). Rectal preparations are also available.

Pharmacodynamics and Pharmacokinetics
During the activation of nociceptors, prostaglandins which are converted from arachidonic acid by cyclooxygenases (COX) enzymes, binds to receptors and stimulates pain fibres to transmit signals more frequently, causing an increase in pain messages being sent to the brain. The exact mechanism of action is not fully understood (Young and Pitcher, 2016); however, it is believed that acetaminophen can hinder the production of prostaglandin centrally rather than peripherally. Following oral administration, paracetamol is rapidly absorbed from the gastrointestinal tract, its systemic bioavailability being dose-dependent and ranging from 70 to 90%. Its rate of oral absorption is predominantly dependent on the rate of gastric emptying, being delayed by food. It distributes rapidly and evenly throughout most tissues and fluids and has a volume of distribution of approximately 0.9L/kg. 10–20% of the drug is bound to red blood cells. Paracetamol is metabolised in the liver by conjugation with glucuronic and sulfuric acid and 85–95% is excreted in the urine within 24 hours.

Contraindications, Cautions and Side Effects
There are very few side effects associated with paracetamol; however, if taken in excess it can lead to serious hepatotoxicity (see Clinical Consideration 3) and death. When an overdose is suspected the antidote 'N-acetylcysteine' should be administered. Caution is advised for anyone with renal or hepatic impairment and heavy alcohol consumption can increase the risk of hepatotoxicity.

Table 17.1 Examples of non-opioids and non-steroidal anti-inflammatory drugs (NSAIDs) and the pharmacokinetics, pharmacodynamics and common side effects.

MEDICATION TYPE	ACETAMINOPHEN	SALICYLIC ACID DERIVATIVES	PROPIONIC ACID DERIVATIVES	SELECTIVE COX-2 INHIBITORS		OTHERS	
Medication name	Paracetamol	Aspirin	Ibuprofen	Celecoxib		Diclofenac	
Route of administration	Oral, rectal or intravenous infusion	Oral or rectal	Oral or topical	Oral		Oral, intramuscular injection, rectal, topical, intravenous infusion	
Dose (oral)	Dependent on age and weight – see BNFc	Neonate: 1–5mg/kg Child 1 month – 11 years: 1–5mg/kg Child 12–17 years: 75mg	Dependent on age and weight – see BNFc	Child 10–25kg: 50mg	Child over 25kg: 100mg	Child 9–13 (above 35kg) 2 mg/kg daily in 3 divided doses	Child 14–17: 75–100 mg daily in 2–3 divided doses
Frequency and timings (oral)	4–6 hours	Once daily	3–4 times a day	Twice daily		2–3 times a day	
Onset/duration	15–60 mins/6 hours	30–60 mins or 1–8 hours for coated tablets/12 hours	1–2 hours/5–10 hours	1 hour/8 hours		1 hour/12 hours	
Common side effects	No common side effects.	Bronchospasm	Fluid retention, gastrointestinal discomfort	Gastrointestinal discomfort, increase in the risk of a thrombotic event		Appetite decrease, gastrointestinal discomfort	
Absorption (A)	Rapidly absorbed from the gastrointestinal tract.	Rapidly by passive diffusion in the gastrointestinal tract.	Rapidly absorbed from the upper gastrointestinal tract.	Rapidly absorbed from the gastrointestinal tract.		Absorbed from the gastrointestinal tract but due to the first-pass metabolism, only 50% of the drug reaches systemic circulation unchanged.	
Distribution (D)	Distributes evenly throughout tissues and fluids – the volume of distribution is approximately 0.9L/kg.	Binds to albumin in the plasma and distributes rapidly into body fluid compartments. The volume of distribution is 10.5L/kg.	Binds to albumin in the plasma – the volume of distribution is 0.1L/kg.	Binds to albumin in the plasma – the volume of distribution is 400L.		Binds to albumin in the plasma – the volume of distribution is 1.4L/kg.	
Metabolism (M)	Predominately in the liver by conjugation with glucuronic and sulfuric acid.	Mainly in the liver by conjugation with glucuronic acid.	Ibuprofen is rapidly metabolised in the liver.	Mainly in the liver by conjugation with carboxylic and glucuronic acid		Predominately in the liver by conjugation with glucuronic and sulfuric acid.	
Excretion (E)	Excreted in the urine.	Excreted in the urine.	Excreted in the urine.	Predominantly excreted in the faeces and urine.		60–70% is eliminated in the urine and 30% is eliminated in the faeces.	

Source: BNFc, 2020/Pharmaceutical Press.

Chapter 17 Analgesics

Clinical Consideration 3

The Right Combination
Some medications such as paracetamol, are often found in combination medication (i.e. co-codamol) that can be purchased over the counter. Care must be taken, as they may contain drugs that the child or parent may be unaware of and this could lead to inadvertent overdose.

Non-Steroidal Anti-Inflammatory Drugs (NAIDs)

NSAID drugs are used not only for their anti-inflammatory actions but also for their analgesic and antipyretic properties. They are not effective for individuals experiencing visceral pain associated with the abdomen and chest but can be given as an adjuvant for children suffering from severe pain, due to their opioid-sparing effects. These are usually administered orally, however, these can also be administered via the rectal route or topically. There are a wide variety of NSAIDs, each with their own chemical composition; however, they are very similar in terms of the analgesic effect. One example of each type of NSAID and the pharmacokinetics, pharmacodynamics, common side effects and recommended corresponding dosages can be found in Table 17.1.

Pharmacodynamics and Pharmacokinetics

NSAIDs act on two enzymes: COX-1, which is expressed in the platelets, the gastrointestinal tract, the kidneys and always present in the body, and COX-2, which is found in the kidneys, the CNS and mainly induced in response to trauma (Smith and Muralidharan, 2014; Young and Pitcher, 2016). They restrict the synthesis of prostaglandin (which increases pain signals) both centrally and peripherally, but more effectively peripherally, at the site of the inflammation (Neal, 2016).

Contraindications, Cautions and Side Effects

Prostaglandin has beneficial effects in maintaining renal blood flow and preventing the lungs from collapse, therefore, care must be taken with individuals with asthma and poor renal function. Prostaglandin suppression can also result in gastrointestinal damage, nausea, gastritis, dyspepsia and in severe cases gastric bleeding, this is more common in neonates (BNFc, 2020; Boyd, 2013). Oral NSAIDs should, therefore, be taken with or after food and drugs may be enteric-coated. For NSAIDs which are COX-2 selective, gastrointestinal side effects can be reduced; however, inhibiting COX-2 can also increase cardiovascular risk and therefore they are not used routinely.

Opioid Agonists

Opioids are a class of drug that is naturally found within the opium poppy plant; however, some opioids can also be created synthetically and semi-synthetically. See Table 17.2 for further details of the pharmacokinetics, pharmacodynamics and common side effects of opioids. Stronger opioids (i.e. morphine) are indicated for the treatment of severe pain and weaker opioids (i.e. codeine) are often prescribed to manage mild to moderate pain. These will be discussed in greater detail later in this chapter.

Pharmacodynamics and Pharmacokinetics

Opioids bind to opioid receptors located within the CNS, the brain, the spinal cord and peripherally in the gastrointestinal tract. Once the opioids attach to the receptors, they block pain signals and release large amounts of dopamine throughout the body (Schumacher et al., 2015). There are four different types of opioid receptor (three of which have designated Greek letters (mu – μ, kappa – κ and delta – δ)) and different analgesics bind to these receptors in a variety of ways, which explains why there is a wide range of benefits and side effects associated with opioid use (Barber and Robertson, 2012). See Clinical Consideration 4 for additional information, which needs to be taken into consideration when in clinical practice and caring for children with a head injury.

Opioids are metabolised primarily by the liver, but this also takes place in the brain and the kidneys, and approximately 87% is excreted after 72 hours (MacKenzie et al., 2016). All opioids are able to cross the blood–

Table 17.2 Examples of opioids and the associated pharmacokinetics, pharmacodynamics and common side effects.

MEDICATION TYPE	OPIOIDS				
MEDICATION NAME	CODEINE	DIHYDROCODEINE	TRAMADOL	MORPHINE	FENTANYL
Route of administration	Oral, intramuscular injection	Oral, deep subcutaneous or intramuscular injection	Oral, intramuscular injection, intravenous injection or infusion	Oral, intramuscular, subcutaneous or intravenous injection or infusion, rectal	Intravenous injection or transdermal patches
Dose	Oral: 30–60mg Maximum 240mg daily (Child age 12–17)	Oral: 1–3 years old — 500mcg/kg; 4–11 years old — 0.5–1 mg/kg; 12–17 years old — 30mg	Oral: Child 12–17 50–100mg Maximum 400mg; IV: Child 12–17 Initially 100 mg, then 50–100 mg every 4–6 hours Usual maximum 400 mg/24 hours	Dependent on age and weight – see BNFc	Dependent on age and weight – see BNFc
Frequency and timings	4–6 hours orally	4–6 hours orally	4 hours orally	4 hours IV, slower with titration	4–6 hours IV
Onset/duration	30–60 mins/6 hours	30–60 mins/6 hours	Up to 60 mins/6 hours	6–30 minutes (depending on route)/4 hours	2–10 minutes/6 hours
Common side effects	Nausea and vomiting, constipation, cardiac arrhythmias (prolonged use)	Nausea and vomiting, constipation, paralytic ileus, abdominal pain	Seizures, serotonin syndrome	Nausea and vomiting, constipation, appetite decrease, dependence	Respiratory depression
Absorption (A)	Absorbed by the gastrointestinal tract, with a bioavailability of around 60%	Low bioavailability in the gastrointestinal tract, approximately 20% due to the first-pass metabolism	Rapidly absorbed in the gastrointestinal tract, bioavailability of 75%	Almost complete absorption in the upper intestine, approximately 95% bioavailability	Short distribution phase, high concentration of fentanyl found in well-perfused areas (lungs, brain, liver)

Distribution (D)	Extensively distributed into the tissues and plasma – the volume of distribution is 3–6L/kg	Distributed evenly into the tissues and plasma – the volume of distribution is 3–6L/kg	High affinity for tissue, distributed evenly – the volume of distribution is 2.6–2.9 L/kg	Low transfer for plasma, distributed most effectively in high alkaline areas e.g. upper intestine – the volume of distribution is 5.3L/kg	80% distributed in plasma – IV volume of distribution is 4L/kg
Metabolism (M)	70–80% of the oral dose is metabolised in the liver	Hepatic pre-systemic metabolism into active metabolite dihydromorphine	Extensive first-pass metabolism, from which there are 23 metabolites	Significant first-pass metabolism in the liver	Metabolised in the liver into a number of inactive metabolites
Excretion (E)	Renal elimination and urinary excretion – 90% after 6 hours	Renal elimination and urinary excretion	Hepatic elimination, metabolites excreted through urine (90%) and faeces (10%)	Renal elimination of morphine and metabolites, excreted through urine	Renal elimination of metabolites and urinary excretion

Source: BNFc, 2020/Pharmaceutical Press.

Chapter 17 Analgesics

brain barrier (BBB); however, those that can cross the BBB more easily (due to poor lipid solubility and protein binding) tend to be more potent (Schumacher et al., 2015).

Contraindications, Cautions and Side Effects

Caution should be taken when administering opioid analgesics, as there are several cautions and contraindications to be aware of. Firstly, it is of note that repeated opioid administration could result in opiate dependence. The National Institute for Health and Care Excellence (NICE) produced a document specifically focusing on opioid dependence, stating that signs of physical and psychological dependence can appear in as little as 2 to 10 days (NICE, 2019). It is also worth recognising that individuals may experience increased tolerance to the potency of an opiate with repeated usage, which may then develop into a dependence where pain cannot be managed with the medication prescribed (British National Formulary for Children (BNFc), 2020). However, the BNFc (2020) states that dependence is no deterrent for the control of severe pain.

Pain management is usually complex with adult patients with hepatic impairment due to the adverse reactions caused by the opioids. These reactions can result in sedation, constipation and sudden onset of hepatic encephalopathy (defined as a spectrum of neuropsychiatric abnormalities in patients with liver dysfunction). However, children have a large reserve of hepatic metabolic capacity, therefore it is suggested that the modification of types of drugs and dosages of opioids are often unnecessary (BNFc, 2020). The effect of opioid analgesics are prolonged and increased where renal impairment is present, and there may be an increase in cerebral activity. It is suggested that in these instances, opioid use should be avoided, or the dose reduced (BNFc, 2020).

One of the most serious side effects of opioid use is an increase in respiratory depression, which if not treated, could result in a significant brain injury, cardiac arrest or death (Lee et al., 2015). To treat respiratory depression, an opioid antagonist Naloxone, also known as an opiate reversal agent, should be administered (see Clinical Consideration 5). When injected intravenously, the effects of this agent occurs within 2 minutes of administration. The mode of action for Naloxone is not fully understood but it is thought to be a competitive opioid receptor antagonist, so it has a higher affinity to the receptor sites in the CNS, especially the mu receptor (Wang et al., 2016). Naloxone is primarily metabolised by the liver and its metabolites are excreted in the urine (Lynn and Galinkin, 2017).

Clinical Consideration 4

Opioids and Serious Head Injury

If a serious head injury has occurred, there may be a concern about intracranial pressure. In order to obtain accurate neurological observations healthcare professional will need to check the pupils of the individual are equal and reactive to light. In this instance, opioids should be avoided as they can have an impact on the individual's pupillary response (causing pinpoint pupils – see below) and therefore the healthcare professional would not be able to gain a true reading of the patient's neurological condition (Kosten et al., 2018). Pinpoint pupils are caused by opioid drugs as they stimulate the oculomotor nerves which shrink the diameter of the pupil. This phenomenon is still utilised as a vital diagnostic tool when testing for opioid overdose, as other causes of nonconsciousness tend to cause the pupils to dilate.

Source: Based on Kosten et al., 2018.

Clinical Consideration 5

Naloxone is very short-acting, with a half-life of approximately 30 to 80 minutes, which is shorter than the average half-life of some opiates. As a consequence, repeated administration may be necessary.

Other side effects such as nausea and vomiting, constipation, itching and drowsiness are generally proportionate to the type and strength of the opioid (Young and Pitcher, 2016). Specific types of opioids will now be explored in greater detail.

Chapter 17 Analgesics

Codeine Phosphate

Codeine phosphate is often referred to as a weak opioid as it is a less potent analgesic than some of its counterparts, such as morphine and fentanyl. As a weak opioid, it can be used to provide analgesia for mild to moderate pain. However, it is not to be administered to children under the age of 12 due to reports of morphine toxicity (MHRA, 2013). It is a naturally occurring opioid agonist with analgesic, antidiarrhoeal and antitussive properties (BNFc, 2020). If codeine is taken orally, 30–60mg every four hours is indicated with a maximum dosage of 240mg per day. Codeine can also be given by intramuscular injection; the same dosage applies.

Pharmacodynamics and Pharmacokinetics

Codeine will bind to many opioid receptor sites within the CNS and gastrointestinal system, causing a reduction in the release of neurotransmitters (Dubin and Patapoutian, 2010). Codeine has an advantage over morphine as it is well absorbed when administered orally, due to its bioavailability. However, the analgesic effect of this drug does not increase above a certain range, so higher quantities do not provide increased analgesia (Barber et al., 2012).

Contraindications, Cautions and Side Effects

Codeine is contraindicated for patients under the age of 12, due to the impact it can have on the respiratory system. Following this, there is a well-founded link between children who have recently had a tonsillectomy and adenoidectomy procedures and sleep apnoea when they have received codeine. For this reason, codeine is strictly contraindicated for these patients (MHRA, 2013). When administered over an extended period, codeine can also increase the risk of developing cardiac arrhythmias. In individuals at greater risk of these conditions, such children suffering from congenital heart disease, regular electrocardiograms (ECG) are recommended (Li and Ramos, 2017).

Dihydrocodeine

Dihydrocodeine is a semisynthetic opioid agonist which also possesses antitussive properties. This opioid is used to treat moderate to severe pain as well as severe dyspnoea. The recommended oral dose for a child ages 1–3 is 500mcg/kg every 4–6 hours; if the child is between 4–11 years old the dosage is 0.5–1mg every 4–6 hours and for an older child, ages 12–17, 30mg every 4–6 hours is the required dosage (BNFc, 2020). Like many of the other opioids, dihydrocodeine can be used in combination with other medications (i.e. co-dydramol contains dihydrocodeine and paracetamol) (Wiffen et al., 2016).

Pharmacodynamics and Pharmacokinetics

Once administered, dihydrocodeine is metabolised to dihydromorphine, a highly active metabolite with a high affinity for the mu-opioid receptor. The bioavailability of dihydrocodeine is relatively low (approximately 20%) if administered orally, this may be due to poor gastrointestinal absorption, this highlights the substantial role pre-systemic metabolism plays in reducing the bioavailability of this opioid (BNFc, 2020).

Contraindications, Cautions and Common Side Effects

Caution must be used when administering dihydrocodeine to a child with a history of pancreatitis as codeine-based medications have been linked with acute pancreatitis (Hastier et al., 2000). Additionally, when this drug is broken down into dihydromorphine a child can be placed at greater risk of the cardiovascular side effects of opioids such as arrhythmias and hypotension if they have severe right-sided heart failure (cor pulmonale) (BNFc, 2020).

Tramadol

Tramadol is a synthetic opiate analgesic indicated to treat moderate to moderately severe pain and has central analgesic properties similar to that of morphine (see below), although not as potent. In June 2014 tramadol was classified as a schedule three controlled drug (Stannard, 2019). For the treatment of acute pain, the initial

Chapter 17 Analgesics

oral dosage is 100mg followed by 50mg-100mg every 4–6 hours, the maximum daily dose is 400mg. If administered intravenously an initial loading dose of 100mg is recommended, followed by 50 mg every 10–20 minutes, up to total maximum 250 mg (including initial dose) in the first hour, after which 50–100 mg every 4–6 hours is recommended (BNFc, 2020).

Pharmacodynamics and Pharmacokinetics

Tramadol has a unique dual mode of action, acting both as a central opiate agonist and as a CNS reuptake inhibitor of norepinephrine and serotonin. It is therefore not surprising that due to tramadol's broad range of pain and inflammation targets it has been shown to be effective for a number of pain types such as neuropathic pain, postoperative pain, lower back pain, as well as pain associated with labour, osteoarthritis, fibromyalgia and cancer (Beyaz et al., 2016). Tramadol is primarily metabolised by the liver and the metabolites are excreted by the kidneys in urine.

Contraindications, Cautions and Side Effects

As tramadol may cause seizures, particularly if high doses of the drug are being used, it is contraindicated for children with poorly controlled or uncontrolled epilepsy (Beyaz et al., 2016). A secondary side effect of tramadol is serotonin syndrome, which is more commonly seen when taking antidepressants (SSRIs). However, a link has now been found between tramadol and serotonin syndrome due to tramadol's mode of action. Tramadol binds with the mu-opioid receptor in the CNS and inhibits the serotonin reuptake pathways, resulting in a build-up of serotonin in the CNS (Beakley et al., 2015). This has the potential to result in symptoms such as high body temperature, agitation, increased reflexes, tremor, sweating and dilated pupils (Hassamal et al., 2018).

Morphine

Morphine is a naturally occurring strong opioid that offers analgesia for severe pain as well as having the effect of euphoria and mental detachment. Due to morphine's potency, it has a duration of analgesia of approximately 4–6 hours compared to some of the weaker opiates that have a duration of 2–4 hours or less (BNFc, 2020). Morphine is often described as the 'prototypical opioid' creating a standard that other opioids are compared against (Barber and Robertson, 2012) (see Skills in Practice for details on how to insert a peripheral cannula for the administration of intravenous analgesic medications). The dosage must be adjusted to suit the child's age and weight to ensure they receive a safe amount of morphine, they should be closely monitored and the dosage should be adjusted according to individual response (BNFc, 2020).

Pharmacodynamics and Pharmacokinetics

Morphine predominantly binds to the mu and delta-opioid receptors found within the CNS, which in turn inhibits the voltage-gated channels needed for the pain signals to reach the brain.

Contraindications, Cautions and Side Effects

Nausea and vomiting are common side effects, therefore oral morphine should be administered after a meal or with food and it may be necessary to prescribe antiemetic (anti-sickness) medication (Smith and Laufer, 2014). Morphine has also been shown to have a noted effect on the gastrointestinal system as it slows the motility rate of the gastrointestinal tract, which often leads to constipation (BNFc, 2020). The reason for this is that there are also opioid receptors within the GI tract and when the agonists bind with them, it decreases gastric emptying and stimulates pyloric tone (Nelson and Camilleri, 2016). It is of note that any oral medication taken may take longer to absorb if they are being taken alongside morphine. To relieve the symptoms of opioid-induced constipation, high fibre foods, hydration and gentle exercise are recommended.

Fentanyl

Fentanyl is a strong synthetic opioid analgesic, which is approximately 100 times as potent as morphine. Consequently, fentanyl is only indicated for severe chronic pain and is mainly utilised within operating departments and critical care environments, as part of the general anaesthetic. Fentanyl can be administered via transdermal patches for chronic pain for older patients (16–17 years old), the patches release fentanyl at 12mcg or 25mcg per hour and these should be replaced every 72 hours, in a new location (BNFc, 2020). When assessing for the correct dosage of a transdermal patch, be mindful of the opioid requirement for the previous 24 hours. If fentanyl is being administered intravenously, only small amounts are required due to potency of the drug. For a child aged between 1 month and 11 years, the initial dosage is only 1–5mcg/kg (BNFc, 2020).

Pharmacodynamics and Pharmacokinetics

As a mu-opioid receptor agonist, fentanyl binds to these receptors 50 to 100 times more strongly than morphine; it also binds with the delta and kappa receptors but not as strongly (Brzakala and Leppert, 2019). Once fentanyl has successfully bound with the opioid receptors, it causes an influx of calcium ions (charged particles) into the cell, causing hyperpolarisation and the inhibition of nerve activity.

Contraindications, Cautions and Side Effects

Due to the potency of fentanyl, respiratory depression is a real concern; therefore, it is suggested that all opioids, especially fentanyl, should only be administered where an opioid antagonist is present, such as naloxone, and the individual's respiratory rate should also be closely monitored (Hill et al., 2019).

Adjuvants and Co-analgesics – Gabapentinoids

Gabapentinoids, such as pregabalin and gabapentin, are indicated for neuropathic pain and the treatment of focal seizures. For neuropathic pain, the recommended oral dose for 12- to 17-year-olds is the administration in increasing levels of day one, 300mg once; day two, 300mg twice; day three, 300mg three times throughout the day (BNFc, 2020). For younger children, the initial dosage is reduced depending on the age and weight of the child.

Pharmacodynamics and Pharmacokinetics

Gabapentin was developed to mimic the neurotransmitter GABA; however, it does not bind to the GABA receptors in the CNS. Instead, it has been found to bind to an auxiliary subunit ($\alpha 2\delta$-1) of voltage-gated calcium channels, which can be found at the synaptic terminals of 'excitable cells' such as muscle, neurons and glial cells (Kukkar et al., 2013). The gabapentin then inhibits calcium channels by reducing the number of available channels and preventing the neuropathic pain response from continuing to the brain (Fornasari, 2017).

Contraindications, Cautions and Side Effects

Caution needs to be applied to individuals who have a history of psychotic illness, as the listed potential side effects of gabapentin may aggravate their condition (BNFc, 2020). Caution should also be taken when administering high oral doses to young adults, as the levels of propylene glycol, acesulfame K and saccharin sodium may exceed the recommended WHO daily intake.

Inhalation Analgesics

Nitrous oxide (N_2O), commonly referred to as Entonox, is a well established anaesthetic and analgesic gas mixture for use with moderate pain with paediatric patients. The combination of 50% nitrous oxide and 50% oxygen is often found in paediatric emergency departments and trauma scenarios and is frequently used for the maintenance of anaesthesia (50–66% nitrous oxide for anaesthesia) (BNFc, 2020). When inhaled it provides pain relief as well as anaesthetic properties such as sedation.

Pharmacodynamics and Pharmacokinetics

The precise mechanism of action for the anaesthetic properties of nitrous oxide remains unknown; however, the most prevalent explanation is that the N_2O inhibits the pain receptors on the ascending pain pathway, blocking the neurons that carry the pain response via the afferent A-delta and C fibres. The analgesic mechanism of N_2O is better understood. The nitrous oxide forces the release of opioid peptides that bind to the

Chapter 17 Analgesics

opioid receptors in the brain and central nervous system. This results in the release of opioids in the brainstem blocking the pain signals on the descending pain pathway (Huang and Johnson, 2016). Nitrous oxide is absorbed via diffusion in the lungs and is eliminated and excreted by respiration with a duration of approximately 5 minutes (BNFc, 2020).

Contraindications, Cautions and Common Side Effects

Nitrous oxide may have a detrimental impact on patients, especially if those patients are experiencing entrapped air (i.e. pneumothorax, an underwater dive, intracranial air following head trauma or recent intraocular gas injection) (BNFc, 2020). The reason this should be avoided is due to the fact that administered nitrous oxide, has the potential to diffuse into these spaces, causing an increase in pressure which has the potential to be harmful and even fatal for the patient (i.e. in the case of pneumothorax, an increase in pressure would result in compromised respiration).

Local, Regional and Topical Analgesia

Local anaesthetics (LA) are used alone for specific regional analgesia as well as in combination with a general anaesthetic. The successful development of paediatric regional anaesthesia means it can be used to manage both acute and chronic pain, which makes it of vital importance when considering individuals with complex pain management needs (Lirk et al., 2014). The advances in ultrasound use for the administration of regional anaesthesia have made it a widespread intervention of paediatric pain management and is also frequently used within paediatric postoperative pain pathways (Shah and Suresh, 2013).

A topical analgesic is used to numb the surface of an area of the body. A common example of this is a eutectic mixture of local anaesthetics (EMLA); this is a combination of lidocaine 2.5% and prilocaine 2.5% (BNFc, 2020). EMLA comes in a cream form which can be applied to the skin to numb a localised area. For paediatric patients, it is usually administered when conducting small invasive procedures such as cannulation or venepuncture. The EMLA cream should be applied in a thick layer and covered with air and watertight dressing and left for a period of time before the procedure is carried out (see Table 17.3) (Maurice et al., 2002; BNFc, 2020).

Pharmacodynamics and Pharmacokinetics

Every local anaesthetic has different physicochemical properties, but they all share the same mode of action. They block the voltage-gated sodium channels in the axon of nerve cells, halting the transfer of electrons between the nerve cells and interrupting pain signals.

Toxicity

When injecting a local anaesthetic (LA) into the subcutaneous tissue, it is vital to aspirate and check position, as injecting the local anaesthetic into a blood vessel can result in complications from the toxic potential of this drug (see Clinical Consideration 6). Early symptoms of a mild LA toxicity include restlessness, tinnitus, slurred speech and a metallic taste in the mouth (Christie et al., 2015). In the most serious of cases, the local anaesthetic toxicity can enter the systemic circulation and cause a cardiac arrest through the inhibition of the

Table 17.3 **Dosages and administration time for EMLA cream.**

Neonates	Apply up to 1 g for a maximum of 1 hour before the procedure. Maximum 1 dose per day.
Child 1–2 months	Apply up to 1 g for a maximum 1 hour before the procedure, to be applied under occlusive dressing. Maximum 1 dose per day.
Child 3–11 months	Apply up to 2 g for maximum 1 hour before the procedure, to be applied under occlusive dressing. Maximum dosage of twice per day.
Child 1–11 years	Apply 1–5 hours before the procedure, a thick layer should be applied under occlusive dressing. Maximum dosage of twice per day.
Child 12–17 years	Apply 1–5 hours before procedure (2–5 hours before procedures on large areas e.g. split skin grafting), a thick layer should be applied under occlusive dressing.

Source: BNFc, 2020/Pharmaceutical Press.

calcium, potassium and sodium channels stopping the contraction of the heart. Initial signs include tachycardia and hypertension, followed by myocardial depression, vasodilation, hypotension and a multitude of cardiac arrhythmias such as sinus bradycardia, conduction blocks, ventricular tachyarrhythmia and eventually asystole. Local anaesthetic systemic toxicity (LAST) tends to have a delayed onset and so any unusual cardiovascular signs after LA administration should be recognised as local anaesthetic systemic toxicity (Christie et al., 2015). It has been identified that individuals who are at the extremes of ages are more susceptible to local anaesthetic systemic toxicity, so extra care and mindfulness should be adhered to when caring for these patients. However, with correct administration and following the guidelines, paediatric cases of LAST are low (Halim et al., et al., 2019).

Clinical Consideration 6

To treat LA toxicity the healthcare professional should assess airway, breathing and circulation in turn. If the child still has a strong cardiac output, 100% oxygen should be administered and the airway secured, followed by a 20% lipid emulsion intravenous infused, which absorbs toxins in the circulatory system, reducing the amount of toxin that is able to bind to the myocardium.

Source: Based on Ciechanowicz and Patil, 2012.

Skills in Practice

How to Insert a Peripheral Cannula for the Administration of Intravenous Analgesic Medications

Intravenous cannulation is a technique that involves the insertion of a fine flexible hollow tube, with an inner retractable needle, into a peripheral vein and worldwide, is the most commonly performed invasive procedure (Boyd, 2013). In order to carry out the procedure, additional equipment is required (see Figure 17.8), all of which should be checked prior to carrying out the procedure.

1. Communicate with the child and carer and provide them with relevant information in order for them to provide informed consent. This will also provide you with the opportunity to talk about previous experiences with cannulation, ascertain if the child has any allergies to dressings, assess for potential complications and physically prepare them and the environment prior to collecting the equipment. This could also be the prime opportunity to build rapport with the child and begin to use distraction techniques in order to reduce procedural anxiety. If a topical local anaesthetic is to be used, apply it to the chosen site and leave for 30–60 minutes prior to cannulation.
2. Depending upon the age of the child, ask the parent to hold them, encourage the mother to feed the infant, or employ multisensory stimulation before and during the procedure.
3. Decontaminate hands, and with the child's arm in a comfortable and appropriate position, apply the tourniquet above the chosen site. To encourage venous filling and vein distention, ask them to open

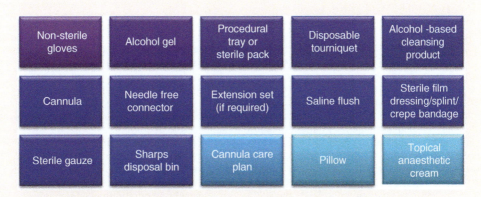

Figure 17.8 Equipment required for the insertion of a peripheral cannula for intravenous analgesic medications. *Source:* Adapted from Lister et al., 2020.

Chapter 17 Analgesics

and close their fist, use gravity by asking them to hang their arm down, apply a warm compress, or lightly stroke the vein in a downward motion (Phillips and Gorski, 2014).

4. With two fingers, palpate the vein in order to confirm suitability and release the tourniquet.
5. Decontaminate hands, clean the tray/receptacle and gather the equipment, ensuring that you check for damage and contamination. Place equipment into the clean receptacle or sterile pack using the aseptic non-touch technique (ANTT) (do not touch the key parts - the tip of the cannula and the end of the syringe for flushing).
6. Reapply the tourniquet; do not over tighten as this may obstruct arterial flow.
7. Clean the chosen site with the alcohol-based (2% chlorhexidine in 70% isopropyl alcohol) preparation equipment. Ensure that you abide by the manufactures application instructions and allow to dry for 30 seconds. Do not touch the skin or re-palpate the vein after application of the skin preparation.
8. While waiting for the skin preparation solution to dry, decontaminate hands and don gloves.
9. Prepare the cannula device by removing the needle guard and assessing the tip for damage.
10. Then with your non-dominant hand apply traction to the skin and stabilise the vein below the chosen site.
11. Insert the cannula at an angle of 20–30 degrees (depending on manufactures instructions) ensuring that the bevel is up and observe for the first flashback of blood into the cannula.
12. Lower the angle of insertion by dropping the cannula closer to the skin and advance the device slightly.
13. Then continue to advance the cannula and draw the stylet back noting the second flashback in the lumen of the cannula.
14. Slide the cannula over the needle, advancing further into the vein. Keeping traction on the skin will make this process easier.
15. Release the tourniquet, apply pressure beyond the cannula tip, loosen the cap at the end of the stylet and withdraw the needle, placing it immediately into the sharps waste container. In line with the Health and Safety Executive (2013) regulations, the cannula will have a safety device (active or passive) in place to prevent a sharps injury. Depending on the specific design, it may also have a passive safety feature that prevents the reinsertion of the needle back into the lumen of the cannula, reducing the risk of cannula tip damage. Reapply the cap before releasing pressure and fix the cannula in place with a semipermeable film dressing.
16. Flush with 0.9% sodium chloride (procedure for how this is undertaken will differ if using an extension set, or an integrated cannula), and ensure patient comfort.
17. Dispose of waste, remove PPE and decontaminate hands using the appropriate technique (Ford and Park, 2018, 2019).
18. Document your care (via paper-based or electronic platforms) according to local guidelines and protocols. This should include, as a minimum standard, your signature, date and designation, the time, cannula size, site of insertion, the number of insertion attempts, and any noted insertion complications. Further documentation such as the VIP score may also need to be completed, depending upon Trust requirements.

For the step-by-step guide please refer to the companion website.

Source: Adapted from Lister et al., 2020.

Episode of Care 1

Regional Block

Tom is a 7-year-old boy who was admitted to the emergency department by paramedics who had received a 999 referral after he fell from his bike and sustained a fracture of his lower leg. A pain assessment was undertaken at the scene, using self-report, behavioural and physiological approaches, and in agreement with Tom and his parents, nitrous oxide was administered whilst the leg was stabilised and during transportation to the hospital. On arrival Tom was seen by the Emergency Department nurse practitioner, who arranged diagnostic tests and an assessment by an orthopaedic registrar. They confirmed that he has fractured his tibia and discussed the need for surgery, to stabilise the fracture.

As part of the preoperative preparations, Tom was visited by an anaesthetic member of staff, who discussed perioperative analgesic requirements with him and his parents. A shared decision was made to utilise a left lower limb regional block as well as pharmacological strategies. These options were chosen as a regional blockade of the distal nerves of the lower limbs are usually well tolerated and have a low risk of systemic toxicity and neurological damage. This was administered prior to the general anaesthetic

Chapter 17 Analgesics

and involved an injection of a local anaesthetic around the nerves in the lower limb in order to achieve complete analgesia in the lower leg and foot. During this procedure, the operating department practitioner used distraction therapy, therapeutic touch and advanced communication skills in order to ensure that Tom's levels of anxiety and procedural pain were limited.

Following the procedure, Tom was transferred to the post-anaesthetic care unit where the specialist healthcare professionals closely monitored and assessed him for signs of pain and regional block functioning. As the effects of the blockade began to reduce, Tom was then encouraged to take pharmacological analgesics, which were necessary in order to pre-empt the onset of nociceptive pain. The choice of whether to administer non-opioids, NSAIDs and opioids were dependent on the assessment of the pain as well as Tom and his family's preferences.

Episode of Care 2

Chronic Pain

Samira is a 14-year-old girl who suffers from Juvenile Idiopathic Arthritis (JIA) and chronic pain. Samira has only recently been diagnosed with this condition, after experiencing unexplained joint pain for several months. She was initially started on a pain management pathway by her GP, which consisted of a combination treatment of paracetamol and ibuprofen to manage the inflammatory response and the pain.

After 10 weeks Samira and her mother returned to see her GP as she felt her management plan was not effective. Samira's self-reports of pain were investigated, and assessment tools were used to gain insight into the intensity and the impact on her well-being. She was then prescribed an additional opioid analgesic, tramadol, which was to be taken alongside the ibuprofen and the paracetamol prescription was stopped. The GP prescribed Samira 75mg of tramadol to be taken every 4–6 hours, up to a maximum daily dose of 400mg. The potential side effects were explained to Samira and her mum (nausea and vomiting, dry mouth, drowsiness, addiction and tolerance). The GP also discussed some non-pharmacological strategies including heat packs, massage and warm baths and the potential need for a referral to the paediatric rheumatologist or specialist pain team.

Conclusion

Pain management strategies are most successful when they incorporate multimodal approaches, which are chosen in partnership with the child and parent/carer (see Episodes of Care 1 and 2). This is not only to take advantage of the pharmacological benefits of a range of drugs but also to reduce potential side effects and adopt a holistic and child-centred approach to pain management. In order to achieve this safely and effectively, healthcare professionals must ensure that their knowledge and understanding of pharmacological management options are varied and up-to-date and if additional advice is required that they consult a prescriber or pharmacy professional (RPS, 2019).

Glossary

Acute: Generally refers to physical illnesses and conditions that are usually short-term
Analgesia: Absence of the sense of pain without loss of consciousness
Antitussive: A drug used to prevent or relieve a cough
Chronic: Conditions which in most cases cannot be cured, only controlled, often they are life-long and limiting in terms of quality of life.
Dyspepsia: Indigestion a persistent or recurrent pain or discomfort in the upper abdomen.
Enzymes: Biological molecules (usually proteins) that significantly speed up the rate of nearly all of the chemical reactions that take place within cells.
Hepatotoxicity: Relating to or causing injury to the liver.
Neuropathic pain: Describes the pain that develops when the nervous system is damaged or not working properly due to disease or injury.
Nociceptive pain: Describe the pain from physical damage or potential damage to the body.

Chapter 17 Analgesics

Opioids: A broad group of pain-relieving drugs that work by interacting with *opioid* receptors in the cells.
Pneumothorax: The presence of air or gas in the cavity between the lungs and the chest wall, causing collapse of the lung
Sleep apnoea: Occurs when breathing stops and starts whilst sleeping.
Somatic: Affecting or characteristic of the body as opposed to the mind or spirit
Synapse: The junction between two neurons (axon-to-dendrite) or between a neuron and a muscle

References

Ashelford, S., Raynsford, J., and Taylor, V. (2016). *Pathophysiology and Pharmacology for Nursing Students*. London: SAGE.

Association of Paediatric Anaesthetists of Great Britain and Ireland (APAGBI) (2012). Good practice in postoperative and procedural pain management. *Pediatric Anaesthesia* 22 (1): 1–79.

Bannister, K. (2019). Descending pain modulation: influence and impact. *Current Opinion in Physiology* 11(1): 62–66.

Barber, P. and Robertson, D. (2012). *Essentials of Pharmacology for Nurses*, 2e. New York: McGraw-Hill Education.

Barber, P., Parkes, J., and Blundell, D. (2012). *Further Essentials of Pharmacology for Nurses*, 1e. New York: McGraw-Hill Education.

Beakley, B., Kaye, A., and Kaye, A. (2015). Tramadol, pharmacology, side effects and serotonin syndrome: a review. *Pain Physician* 18(1): 195–400.

Bendall, J.C., Simpson, P.M., and Middleton, P.M. (2011). Prehospital vital signs can predict pain severity: analysis using ordinal logistic regression. *European Journal of Emergency Medicine* 8(6): 334–339.

Beyaz, S., Sonbahar, T., Bayar, F., and Erdem, A. (2016). Seizures associated with low-dose tramadol for chronic pain treatment. *Anaesthesia Essays and Researchers* 10(2): 376–378.

Boore, J., Cook, N., and Shepherd, A. (2016). *Essentials of Anatomy and Physiology for Nursing Practice*. Los Angeles, CA: Sage.

Boyd, C. (2013). *Clinical Skills for Nurses*. Chichester: Wiley.

British National Formulary for Children (BNFc) (2020). *BNFc – 79* (BNF). London: BMJ Group and Pharmaceutical Press.

British National Formulary for Children (BNFc) (2019). *BNFc – 78* (BNF). London: BMJ Group and Pharmaceutical Press.

Brzakala, J. and Leppert, W. (2019). The role of rapid onset fentanyl products in the management of breakthrough pain in cancer patients. *Pharmacological Reports* 71(3): 438–442.

Carter, B. and Simons, J. (2014). *Stories of Children's Pain: Linking Evidence to Practice*. London: SAGE.

Christie, L., Picard, J., and Weinberg, G. (2015). Local anaesthetic systemic toxicity. *British Journal of Anaesthesia* 15(3): 136–142.

Ciechanowicz, S., and Patil, V. (2012). Intravenous lipid emulsion – rescued at LAST. *Association of Anaesthetists of Great Britain and Ireland* 212(5): 237–241.

Colvin, L.A. and Carty, S. (2012). Neuropathic pain. In: *ABC of Pain* (ed. Colvin, L.A. and Fallon, M.), 25–30. Chichester: Wiley.

Cullen, M. and MacPherson, F. (2012). Complementary and alternative strategies. In: *ABC of Pain* (ed. Colvin, L.A. and Fallon, M.), 99–102. Chichester: Wiley.

Cunningham, S. (2017). Pain assessment and management. In: *Clinical Skills For Nursing Practice* (ed. Moore, T. and Cunningham, S.), 104–131. Oxford: Routledge.

Czarnecki, M.L., Simons, K., Thompson, J. et al. (2010). Barriers to paediatric pain management: a nursing perspective. *Pain Management Nursing* 11(1): 15–25.

Dubin, A. and Patapoutian, A. (2010). Nociceptors: the sensors of the pain pathway. *Journal of Clinical Investigations* 120(11): 3760–3772.

Erden, S., Demir, N., and Ugras, G. et al. (2018). Vital signs: Valid indicators to assess pain in intensive care unit patients? An observational, descriptive study. *Nursing and Health Sciences Journal* 20(4): 502–508.

Felluga, M., Rabach, I., Minute, M. et al. (2016). A quasi randomized-controlled trial to evaluate the effectiveness of clown therapy on children's anxiety and pain levels in emergency department. *European Journal of Pediatrics* 175(5): 645–650.

Flasar, C.E. and Perry, A. G. (2014). Pain assessment and basic comfort measures. In: *Clinical Nursing Skills and Techniques* (ed. Perry, A.G., Potter, P.A., and Ostendorf, W.R.), 345–374. London: Elsevier.

Ford, C. and Park, L.G. (2018). Hand hygiene and handwashing: key to preventing the transfer of pathogens. *British Journal of Nursing* 27(20): 1164–1166.

Ford, C. and Park, L.G. (2019). How to apply and remove medical gloves. *British Journal of Nursing* 28(1): 65–72.

Fornasari, D. (2017). Pharmacotherapy for neuropathic pain: a review. *Pain and Therapy* 6(1): 25–33.

General Medical Council (2019). *Good Medical Practice*. www.gmc-uk.org/ethical-guidance/ethical-guidance-for-doctors/good-medical-practice (accessed 14 June 2020).

Halim, NA., Christol, I., Tan, Z. et al. (2019). GP62 Lignocaine toxicity: a case report of the adverse effect of local anaesthesia Health and Safety Executive (2013). Sharp Instrument in community setting. *Archives of Disease in Childhood* 104(3): 54–55.

Health and Safety Executive (2013). *Healthcare Regulations 2013: Guidance for Employers and Employees*. Health and Safety Executive Publications.

Hassamal, S., Miotto, K., Dale, W., and Danovitch, I. (2018). Tramadol: understanding the risk of serotonin syndrome and seizures. *American Journal of Medicine* 131(11): 1382–1383.

Hastier, P., Buckley, MJ., Peten, EP., et al. (2000). A new source of drug-induced acute pancreatitis: codeine. *The American Journal of Gastroenterology* 95(11): 3295–3298.

Health and Care Professions Council (2019). *Standards of Conduct, Performance and Ethics*. www.hcpc-uk.org/standards/standards-of-conduct-performance-and-ethics/ (accessed 14 June 2020).

Healthcare Play Specialist Education Trust (2015). *Children Environments of Care Report May 2015*. www.hpset.org.uk/downloads/research_development/HPSET_CEC%20Report.pdf (accessed 21 July 2020).

Hill, R. et al. (2019). Fentanyl depression of respiration: comparison with heroin and morphine. *British Journal of Pharmacology* 14860: 1–12.

Huang, C. and Johnson, N. (2016). Nitrous oxide, from the operating room to the emergency department. *Current Emergency and Hospital Medicine Reports* 4(1): 11–18.

Intercollegiate Committee for Standards for Children and Young People in Emergency Care Settings (2018). *Facing the Future: Standards for Children in Emergency Care Settings*. London: Royal College of Paediatrics and Child Health.

Kettyle, A. (2015). Pain management. In: *Essentials of Nursing Practice* (ed. Delves-Yates, C.), 379–401. London: Sage.

Koneti, K. and Perfitt, J. (2019). Chronic pain management after surgery. *Surgery (Oxford)* 37(8): 467–471.

Kosten, T., Graham, D., and Nielsen, D. (2018). Neurobiology of opioid use disorder and comorbid traumatic brain injury. *JAMA Psychiatry* 75(6): 642–648.

Kukkar, A., Bali, A., Singh, N., and Jaggi, A. (2013). Implications and mechanism of action of gabapentin in neuropathic pain. *Archives of Pharmacal Research* 36(3): 237–251.

Laws, P. and Rudall, N. (2013). Assessment and monitoring of analgesia, sedation, delirium and neuromuscular blockade levels and care. In: *Critical Care Manual for Clinical Procedures and Competencies* (ed. Mallet, J., Albarran, J.W., and Richardson, A.), 340–354. Chichester: Wiley.

Lee, L.A., Caplan, R.A., and Stephens, L.S. et al. (2015). Postoperative opioid-induced respiratory depression – a closed claims analysis. *Journal of Pain Medicine* 122(1): 649–665.

Li, M. and Ramos, L. (2017). Drug-induced QT prolongation and torsades de pointes. *Pharmacy and Therapeutics* 42(7): 437–477.

Lirk, P., Picardi, S., and Hollmann, M. (2014). Local anaesthetics: 10 essentials. *European Journal of Anaesthesiology* 31(11): 575–585.

Lister S., Hofland, J and Grafton, H. (2020). *The Royal Marsden Hospital Manual of Clinical Nursing Procedures*, professional edn. Chichester: Wiley.

Longobardi, C., Prino, L.E., Fabris, M.A. et al. (2019). Soap bubbles as a distraction technique in the management of pain, anxiety, and fear in children at the paediatric emergency room: A pilot study. *Child Care Health Dev* 45: 300–305.

Lynn, R. and Galinkin, J. (2017). Naloxone dosage for opioid reversal: current evidence and clinical implications. *Therapeutic Advances in Drug Safety* 9(1): 63–88.

MacKenzie, M., Zed, P., and Ensom, M. (2016). Opioid pharmacokinetics-pharmacodynamics: clinical implications in acute pain management in trauma. *Annals of Pharmacotherapy* 50(3): 209–218.

Mathews, L. (2011). Pain in children: neglected, unaddressed and mismanaged. *Indian Journal of Palliative Care* 17(Suppl): S70–S73.

Maurice, S.C., O'Donnell, J.J., and Beattie, T.F. (2002). Emergency analgesia in the paediatric population. Part II Pharmacological methods of pain relief. *Emergency Medical Journal* 19(1): 101–105.

Mears, J. (2018). Pain management. In: *Acute and Critical Care Nursing at a Glance* (ed. Dutton, H. and Finch, J.), 10–11. Chichester: Wiley.

MHRA (2013). *Codeine for Analgesia: Restricted Use in Children because of Reports of Morphine Toxicity*. Medicines and Healthcare Products Regulatory Agency.

Merskey, H. and Bogduk, M. (1994). *Classifications of Chronic Pain*, 2e. Washington, DC: International Association for the Study of Pain Task Force on Taxonomy, IASP Press: 209–214.

Neal, M.J. (2016). *Medical Pharmacology at a Glance*, 8e. Chichester: Wiley.

Nelson, A. and Camilleri, M. (2016). Opioid-induced constipation: advances and clinical guidance. *Therapeutic Advances in Chronic Disease* 7(2): 121–134.

NICE (2019). *Opioid Dependence*. https://cks.nice.org.uk/opioid-dependence (accessed 29 September 2019).

Nursing and Midwifery Council (2018). *The Code: Professional Standards of Practice and Behaviour for Nurses, Midwives and Nursing Associates*. www.nmc.org.uk/standards/code/ (accessed 16 June 2020).

Old, E.A., Nicol, L.S.C., and Malcangio, M. (2016). Recent advances in neuroimmune interactions in neuropathic pain: The role of microglia. In: *An Introduction to Pain and its Relation to Nervous System Disorders* (ed. Battaglia, A.A.), 123–147. Chichester: Wiley-Blackwell.

Pancekauskaite, G. and Jankauskaite, L. (2018). Paediatric pain medicine: pain differences, recognition and coping acute procedural pain in paediatric emergency room. *Medicina* 54(94): 1–20.

Patton, K.T. and Thibodeau, G.A. (2016). *Structure and Function of the Body*, 15e. St Louis, MO: Elsevier.

Petrack, E.M., Christopher, N.C., and Kriwinsky, J. (1997). Pain management in the emergency department: patterns of analgesic utilization. *Paediatrics* 99(5): 711–714.

Phillips, L.D. and Gorski, L.A (2014). *Manual of I.V. Therapeutics: Evidence-Based Practice for Infusion Therapy*, 6e. Philadelphia, PA: F.A. Davis Company.

Rodriguez, L. (2015). Pathophysiology of pain: Implications for perioperative nursing. *AORN Journal* 101(3): 338–344.

Royal College of Anaesthetists (2020). *Guidelines for the Provision of Paediatric Anaesthesia Services 2020*. London: RCOA.

Royal College of Emergency Medicine (2017). *Management of Pain in Children*. London: The Royal College of Emergency Medicine.

Royal College of Nursing (2009). *The Recognition and Assessment of Acute Pain in Children*. London: RCN.

Royal College of Nursing (2017). *Standards for Assessing, Measuring and Monitoring Vital Signs in Infants, Children and Young People*. London: RCN.

Royal Pharmaceutical Society and Royal College of Nursing (2019). *Professional Guidance on the Administration of Medicines in Healthcare Settings*. London: Royal Pharmaceutical Society.

Scarponi, D. and Pession, A. (2016). Play therapy to control pain and suffering in pediatric oncology. *Front Pediatr* 4(132): 1–5.

Schumacher, M., Basbaum, A., and Naidu, R. (2015). Opioid agonists and antagonists. In: *Basic and Clinical Pharmacology* (ed. Katzung, B.), 553–574. New York: McGraw-Hill Education.

Shah, R.D. and Suresh, S. (2013). Applications of regional anaesthesia in paediatrics. *British Journal of Anaesthesia* 111(1): 114–124.

Smith, H. and Laufer, A. (2014). Opioid-induced nausea and vomiting. *European Journal of Pharmacology* 722(1): 67–78.

Smith, M.T. and Muralidharan, A. (2014). Pain pharmacology and the pharmacological management of pain. In: *Pain: A Textbook for Health Professionals*, 2e (ed. Van Griensven, H., Strong, J., and Unruh, A.M.), 159–180. London: Elsevier.

Solaro, C. and Uccelli, M. M. (2016). Pain in multiple sclerosis: from classification to treatment. In: *An Introduction to Pain and its Relation to Nervous System Disorders* (ed. Battaglia, A.A.), 345–360. Chichester: Wiley-Blackwell.

Stannard, C. (2019). Tramadol is not 'opioid-lite'. *BMJ* 365(1): 12095.

Todd, A.J. (2016). Anatomy of pain pathways. In: *An Introduction to Pain and its Relation to Nervous System Disorders* (ed. Battaglia, A.A.), 13–34. Chichester: Wiley.

Todd, K.H., Sloan, E.P., Chen, C., et al. (2002). Survey of pain aetiology, management practices and patient satisfaction in two urban emergency departments. *CJEM* 4(4): 252–256.

Tornsey, C. and Fleetwood-Walker, S. (2012). Pain mechanisms. In: *ABC of Pain* (ed. Colvin, L.A. and Fallon, M.), 5–10. Chichester: Wiley-Blackwell.

Turk, D.C. and Melzack, R. (2011). Prologue. In: *Handbook of Pain Assessment*, (ed. Turk, D. C. and Melzack, R.), 1–2. New York: Guilford Press.

Twycross, A. (2017). Guidelines, strategies and tools for pain assessment in children. *Nursing Times* 113(5): 18.

Twycross, A. and Finley, G.A. (2013). Children's and parents' perceptions of postoperative pain management: a mixed-methods study. *Journal of Clinical Nursing* 22(21–22): 3095–3108.

VanMeter, K.C. and Hubert, R.J. (2014). *Gould's Pathophysiology for the Health Professions*, 5e. St Louis, MO: Elsevier.

Vinall, J., Miller, S.P., Chau, V. et al. (2012). Neonatal pain in relation to postnatal growth in infants born very preterm. *Pain* 153: 1374–1381.

Wang, X., Zhang, Y., Peng, Y. et al. (2016). Pharmacological characterization of the opioid inactive isomers (+)-naltrexone and (+)-naloxone as antagonists of toll-like receptor 4. *British Journal of Pharmacology* 173(5): 856–869.

Wiffen, P.J., Knaggs, R., Derry, S. et al. (2016). Paracetamol (acetaminophen) with or without codeine or dihydrocodeine for neuropathic pain in adults. *Cochrane Database of Systematic Reviews* 12: 1465–1858.

Young, S. and Pitcher, B. (2016). *Medicines Management for Nurses at a Glance*. Chichester: Wiley.

Further Resources

National Institute for Health and Care Excellence (NICE): https://bnf.nice.org.uk/treatment-summary/pain-chronic.html

British Medical Association (BMA) 'Chronic pain: supporting safer prescribing of Analgesics: www.bma.org.uk/media/2100/analgesics-chronic-pain.pdf

Pain UK: https://painuk.org/

Chapter 17 Analgesics

Multiple Choice Questions

1. Which type of pain originates in the organs?
   - (a) Referred
   - (b) Somatic
   - (c) Visceral
   - (d) Nociceptive
2. Which pain assessment strategy is associated with the use of scales?
   - (a) Unidimensional tool
   - (b) Multidimensional tool
   - (c) Mnemonics
   - (d) The art of noticing
3. What classification of pharmacological analgesic is Aspirin?
   - (a) Opioid
   - (b) Non-opioid
   - (c) Non-steroidal anti-inflammatory
   - (d) Co-analgesic
4. NSAIDs are contraindicated in children who suffer from _____?
   - (a) Haemorrhoids
   - (b) Gastrointestinal ulceration
   - (c) Hyperthyroidism
   - (d) Hypotension
5. Which management strategy can be used alongside pharmacological approaches?
   - (a) Distraction
   - (b) Play therapy
   - (c) Touch
   - (d) All of the above
6. Which chemical is associated with the stimulation of nociceptors and is inhibited by NSAIDs?
   - (a) Prostaglandin
   - (b) Substance-P
   - (c) Histamine
   - (d) Bradykinin
7. What are A-delta fibres?
   - (a) Relay neurons
   - (b) Efferent pain fibres
   - (c) Afferent pain fibres
   - (d) Synapses
8. What is the name of the antagonist drug to reverse the effects of opioid-induced respiratory depression?
   - (a) Naproxen
   - (b) Naloxone
   - (c) Nefopam
   - (d) Nefazodone
9. How much EMLA cream should be used on a 6-month-old patient?
   - (a) 8g
   - (b) 3g
   - (c) 5g
   - (d) 2g
10. Which type of NSAIDs is Celecoxib?
    - (a) Acetaminophen
    - (b) Salicylic acid derivatives
    - (c) Propionic acid derivatives
    - (d) Selective COX-2 inhibitors

Chapter 17 Analgesics

11. How often should fentanyl transdermal patches be changed on a 16-year-old patient?
   (a) 36 hours
   (b) 24 hours
   (c) 72 hours
   (d) 48 hours
12. Which drug causes pinpoint pupils?
   (a) Paracetamol
   (b) Naproxen
   (c) Gabapentin
   (d) Morphine
13. Which route is not used for the administration of paracetamol?
   (a) Oral
   (b) Rectal
   (c) Intravenous infusion
   (d) Intramuscular
14. How many different types of opioid receptors are there?
   (a) 3
   (b) 4
   (c) 5
   (d) 6
15. What is the antidote for paracetamol overdose?
   (a) N-acetylcysteine
   (b) N-acetyl-para-aminophenol
   (c) Naloxone
   (d) Narcan

Find Out More

The following is a list of some of the conditions that are related to acute pain episodes or associated with children and young people who suffer from chronic pain. Take some time and write notes about each of the conditions. Think about the medications that may be used in order to treat these conditions and be specific about the pharmacokinetics and pharmacodynamics. Remember to include aspects of patient care. If you are making notes about children you have offered care and support to, you must ensure that you have adhered to the rules of confidentiality.

THE CONDITION	YOUR NOTES
Tonsillitis	
Sickle cell anaemia	
Migraine	
Urinary tract infection	
Arthritis	

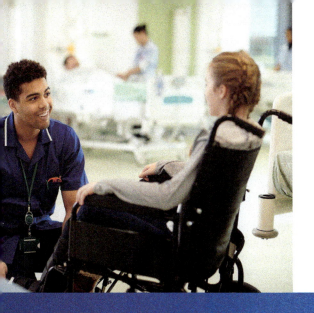

18

Antimicrobial Medications

Leah Rosengarten

Aims
The aim of this chapter is to help the reader understand the pharmacology and pharmaceutical treatment options commonly used for microbial organisms in Children and Young People (CYP).

Learning Outcomes
After reading this chapter, the reader will:
- Understand the different categories of microorganisms and how each can be harmful in CYP
- Discuss the risk of antimicrobial resistance and the role of antimicrobial stewardship
- Appreciate the use of antimicrobials in the treatment of infections
- Recognise the healthcare professional's role in antimicrobial prescribing

Test Your Knowledge
1. What is the difference between a bacteria and a virus?
2. What are the four main categories of antimicrobials?
3. How does antimicrobial resistance occur?
4. Why is a virus hard to treat?
5. What three key factors should a healthcare professional consider before prescribing an antimicrobial?

Fundamentals of Pharmacology for Children's Nurses, First Edition. Edited by Ian Peate and Peter Dryden.
© 2022 John Wiley & Sons Ltd. Published 2022 by John Wiley & Sons Ltd.
Companion website: www.wiley.com/go/pharmacologyforCN

Chapter 18 Antimicrobial Medications

Introduction

In everyday life, CYP are surrounded by incalculable numbers of microorganisms – in the air, on everything they touch and inside their own bodies. Microorganisms are organisms which are too small to be seen unaided by the human eye, which consist of a single cell. Most microorganisms are harmless, and some are even beneficial in our digestive and immune systems. However, others can be harmful. The most common illnesses in CYP (such as coughs and colds, chickenpox, earaches and tonsillitis) are all caused by microorganisms. Whilst some of these are rarely treated, as the child's own immune system can overcome the microorganism, others can be pharmacologically managed. This management may take the form of antimicrobials, which are drugs which kill or inhibit the growth of microorganisms.

In the UK we are privileged to have access to medications and high-quality healthcare, but it was only in 2005 that infectious conditions ceased to be the leading cause of death for 1- to 4-year-olds (ONS, 2017). Internationally, infectious conditions accounted for approximately 29% of deaths in children under 5 years in 2018 (UNICEF, 2020). This chapter will introduce the four classes of microorganisms and consider the pharmaceutical management of microorganisms in CYP. Another important feature within this chapter is an explanation of how microorganisms can develop resistance to antimicrobial drugs. Finally, the pharmacological mechanism of action of antimicrobial drugs will be discussed.

Microorganisms

Whilst most microorganisms live harmlessly inside the body and in the atmosphere, there are a small number which can be detrimental to our health. These harmful microorganisms can be categorised into four classes: Bacteria, Viruses, Fungi and Protozoa. The antimicrobial drugs which can be used to kill or inhibit the growth of these microorganisms derive simply from the name of the organism and are: antibacterial, antiviral, antifungal and antiprotozoal.

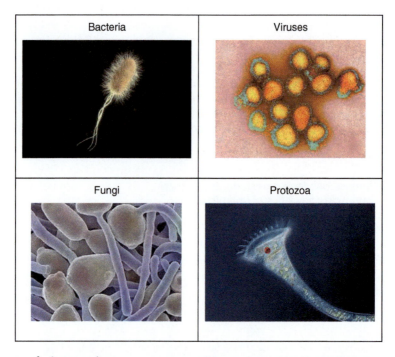

Figure 18.1 **Images of microorganisms** *Source:* (a) gaetan stoffel/Getty Images. (b) ©CDC/SCIENCE PHOTO LIBRARY/Getty Images. (c) Thomas Deerinck, NCMIR/Science Source. (d) FRANK FOX/Science Source.

Bacteria

There are about 10 times as many bacteria in the human body as there are human cells and many of these are not harmful. Bacteria can range in shape from spheres to rods to spirals. Bacteria can harm the human body through invading the immune system or through producing toxins, which damage body tissue. Bacteria are responsible for a range of diseases in humans including Streptococcus pneumoniae (pneumococcus), which can cause meningitis, and tuberculosis.

Viruses

Viruses are smaller than bacteria but also come in many different shapes. Viruses are not living organisms in the way that bacteria are; they are somewhere between an organism and a chemical. Viruses are made up of protein surrounding genetic material (either DNA or RNA). Viruses cause harm to humans as they take control of human cells and reproduce, eventually causing the host cell to die off. Common viruses which infect children are influenza and chickenpox.

Fungi

Fungi can live in the air, earth, water and in plants and due to this they often infect humans through their skins or lungs. Fungi usually will not cause infections in healthy CYP, but immune-compromised CYP are very susceptible. Less is known about how fungi causes harm in humans but it is thought to be in one of four ways;

- Fungal cells invade tissues and disrupt their function
- The fungus causes an immune response
- The fungus consumes energy and nutrients intended for the host
- The fungus excretes toxic metabolites

Common types of fungi which infect humans are Aspergillus and Candida (thrush).

Protozoa

Protozoa are single-celled organisms, similar to bacteria, which come in many different shapes and sizes. They differ from bacteria in that they are bigger and have a cell nucleus which makes them similar to other plant and human cells. Protozoa cause harm to humans when they feed off the host by surrounding the host's tissue with their cell membrane. This leads to tissue damage, which can be worsened if the host has an immune response to the protozoa or the protozoa produces toxic products. Common protozoa infections in humans are toxoplasmosis and malaria.

Antimicrobial Medications

Antimicrobials can be natural, synthetic or semisynthetic and their use varies according to the microorganism being treated and the host of the microorganism (the CYP requiring treatment). It is worth mentioning at this point that the terms 'antimicrobial', 'antibacterial' and 'antibiotic' are often used interchangeably. The term 'antibiotics', literally translated, means 'against life', which leads some authors to use it to describe all drugs which are effective against microorganisms, though the NHS (2020a) identifies that antibiotics are drugs which are used on bacterial infections. To minimise confusion throughout this chapter, antimicrobials will be referred to according to the class of microorganisms which they treat.

Alexander Fleming is credited with the development of the first antibacterial in 1928 and was awarded a Nobel Prize in 1945 for his work. Fleming discovered that mould created a substance which could kill bacteria, and named the substance penicillin. Following this discovery, many other scientists built on Fleming's work and, slowly, the assorted antibacterials that we use today in modern medicine were developed.

Antibacterial Medications

As was discussed earlier in this chapter, antibacterials are medications used to treat bacterial infection in CYP. There are hundreds of different types of antibacterials used in modern medicine, but they are usually classified in six groups: penicillins, cephalosporins, aminoglycosides, tetracyclines, macrolides and fluoroquinolones (NHS, 2020a).

Some antibacterial drugs may be effective against a varied range of bacteria, whilst others have very specific uses in only certain groups of bacteria. Different antibacterial drugs also work in different ways, some may kill the bacteria (bactericidal), whilst others inhibit the growth of the bacteria (bacteriostatic) (British Society for Antimicrobial Chemotherapy (BSAC), 2018). Bacteriostatic drugs are still beneficial in the treatment of harmful microorganisms as they allow the body's own immune system to more effectively target and kill the bacteria whilst inhibiting any further growth of the bacteria.

In order to understand the ways in which antibacterial drugs are effective against bacteria, it is first useful to understand a little about the structure of bacteria (Figure 18.2). Bacteria are prokaryotic cells, which means that they do not have a nucleus. Bacteria consist of the bacterial chromosome or nucleoid, ribosomes and cytoplasmic inclusions, and are surrounded by a cell membrane and cell wall. Bacteria are often encompassed by small, hair-like structures called pili and longer hair-like structures called flagellum which help the bacteria to move and attach to surfaces. Whilst some bacteria differ in the precise constituents, bacterial cells are largely consistent in their most important components and fundamental structure.

There are three main ways in which antimicrobial medications target bacteria; They target the cell wall or membranes that surround the bacterial cell, they target the systems that synthesise the nucleic acids DNA and RNA or they target the systems that synthesise proteins (the ribosome and associated proteins). As these three targets are either different or absent in the cells of humans, antibacterials are usually specific for bacteria and do not harm normal human cells (BSAC, 2018).

Bacteria can be classified in numerous different ways including by their shape and their oxygen demand, but one of the first ways in which an identified bacterium is classified, is the gram test. In 1882, Hans Christian Gram, a Danish bacteriologist, developed the Gram staining test, which is still used to identify bacteria today. It was identified that bacteria which retain a crystal violet dye when stained do this because of a thick layer of peptidoglycan on their cell wall, and these bacteria were named Gram-positive. Conversely, Gram-negative

Clinical Consideration

Mild stomach problems such as nausea, vomiting, diarrhoea, bloating and indigestion, abdominal pain and loss of appetite are common in the use of antibacterial medications (NHS, 2020a). CYP should be warned of the risk of these when prescribed antibiotics and advised when to report side effects or seek further help.

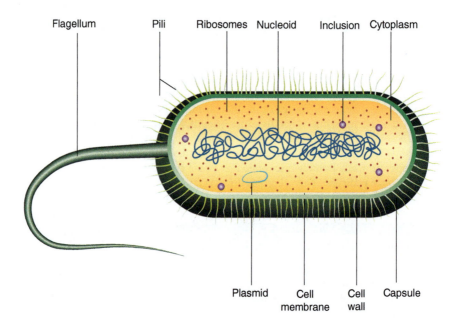

Figure 18.2 Basic cell structure.

bacteria do not retain the violet dye and are more resistant to treatment, because their cell wall is more difficult to penetrate.

Penicillins

Antibacterial drugs which belong to the Penicillin group are bactericidal as they interfere with the bacterial cell wall's ability to synthesise. These drugs bind to the penicillin binding proteins which are located on the inner membrane of the bacterial cell wall. Once bound to these proteins, penicillin inactivates them which results in weakening of the cell wall and rupture of the cell wall or membrane.

Penicillin are active against a number of gram-negative and gram-positive bacteria including but not limited to; Streptococci, Listeria, E.coli, Pneumococci and Salmonella. Table 18.1 lists the Penicillins commonly used in CYP and the conditions they are indicated to treat.

Clinical Consideration

Between 1–10% of patients who are exposed to penicillin may have an allergic reactions, with those who have a history of allergies such as asthma, hayfever and eczema being more at risk (Joint Formulary Committee, 2020a). It is important to note that patients who are allergic to penicillins are allergic to the basic structure of the drug, so they will be allergic to all drugs in this family.

Table 18.1 Commonly used penicillins in CYP.

DRUG	INDICATED FOR TREATMENT OF
Benzylpenicillin sodium *intravenous or intramuscular injection*	Mild to moderate susceptible infections (including throat infections and otitis media), pneumonia, cellulitis, endocarditis, meningitis and meningococcal disease
Phenoxymethylpenicillin (Penicillin V) *oral*	Oral infections, acute sore throat, otitis media and acute sinusitis
Flucloxacillin *oral or intravenous*	Infections due to beta-lactamase-producing staphylococci (including otitis externa), cellulitis, endocarditis, osteomyelitis, cerebral abscess, staphylococcal meningitis, staphylococcal lung infection in cystic fibrosis, erysipelas and as an adjunct in pneumonia and impetigo
Ampicillin *oral or intravenous*	Susceptible infections (including bronchitis, urinary tract infections, otitis media, sinusitis, uncomplicated community-acquired pneumonia, salmonellosis), group B streptococcal infection, enterococcal endocarditis and listeria meningitis
Amoxicillin *oral or intravenous*	Susceptible infections (including sinusitis, salmonellosis, oral infections), community-acquired pneumonia, acute exacerbation of bronchiectasis, acute cough (if systemically very unwell or at higher risk of complications), cystic fibrosis (treatment of asymptomatic haemophilus influenzae carriage or mild exacerbation), acute otitis media, lyme disease, listeria meningitis, anthrax and lower urinary tract infection
Piperacillin (only available in combination with the beta-lactamase inhibitor tazobactam) Piperacillin with tazobactam *intravenous*	Hospital-acquired pneumonia, septicaemia, complicated infections involving the urinary tract, skin or soft-tissues, complicated intra-abdominal infections, acute exacerbation of bronchiectasis and infections in neutropenic patients
Pivmecillinam hydrochloride *oral*	Acute uncomplicated cystitis, chronic or recurrent bacteriuria and urinary tract infections

Source: Data from Joint Formulary Committee, 2020b.

Cephalosporins

Cephalosporins are bactericidal and work in a similar way to penicillin antibacterial drugs. Cephalosporins attach to penicillin binding proteins to interrupt cell wall synthesis, leading to weakening of the cell wall and rupture of the cell wall or membrane. Since cephalosporins were first derived by fungus, and used clinically, specialists have been improving the structure of these drugs to make them effective against a wide range of bacteria. As such, each time the structure is changed, drugs of that structure are classified by generation. Cefalexin is the most widely used 'first generation' cephalosporin drug in CYP care.

Whilst Cephalosporins are active against a number of the same bacteria that penicillin is active against, they are used predominantly against Gram-positive bacteria such as Staphylococcus and Streptococcus. Table 18.2 demonstrates the commonly used cephalosporins in CYP care.

Aminoglycosides

Aminoglycosides are named as such due to the chemical structure of the compound; they are made up of amino groups which are attached to glycosides. Due to their chemical structure, aminoglycosides are effective against bacteria which attract aminoglycosides and possess the correct chemical characteristics to facilitate uptake of the drug in the cell. Once inside the bacteria, aminoglycosides bind to ribosomes and the cytoplasmic inclusions required for protein synthesis, which prevents them from working and causes cell death. Therefore, like penicillin and cephalosporins, aminoglycosides are bactericidal.

Aminoglycosides are active against a variety of Gram-positive and Gram-negative bacteria including Pseudomonas aeruginosa and Mycobacterium tuberculosis. Table 18.3 displays the commonly used aminoglycosides in the care of CYP.

Clinical Consideration

NICE (2017) guidance on sepsis advises that CYP with suspected sepsis give a broad-spectrum antimicrobial at the maximum recommended dose within 1 hour of identifying that they meet any high risk criteria in an acute hospital setting.

Though local guidelines on choice of broad-spectrum antimicrobials may differ, the guidance also states:

- If meningococcal disease is specifically suspected, give appropriate doses of parenteral benzyl penicillin in community settings and intravenous ceftriaxone in hospital settings
- For YP up to 17 years with suspected community-acquired sepsis of any cause, give ceftriaxone 80 mg/kg once a day with a maximum dose of 4 g daily at any age
- For children younger than 3 months, give an additional antibiotic active against listeria (for example, ampicillin or amoxicillin)
- Treat neonates presenting in hospital with suspected sepsis in their first 72 hours with intravenous benzylpenicillin and gentamicin

Toby is 16 years old, weighs 83kg and has suspected community-acquired sepsis. What antimicrobial might he be given and at what dose?

Tetracyclines

Tetracyclines are bacteriostatic as they interfere with a bacteria's ability to produce some necessary proteins which therefore inhibits their growth. Tetracyclines bind to ribosomes to prevent the transfer of RNA which then inhibits protein synthesis. This group of drugs can also be used to treat some virus and protozoal infections, due to its method of action.

Tetracyclines are effective against many bacteria including Propionibacterium acnes, brucella, borrelia burgdorferi, haemophilus influenzae and have a role in the management of methicillin-resistant *staphylococcus aureus* (MRSA) infections. Table 18.4 contains the commonly used tetracyclines in CYP care.

Macrolides

Macrolides can be both bacteriostatic and bactericidal depending on the concentration of the drug in the body, and the susceptibility of the bacteria. Their mode of action on the bacteria is that they bind to a subunit or ribosomes and inhibit the formation of proteins.

Chapter 18 Antimicrobial Medications

Table 18.2 Commonly used cephalosporins in CYP.

DRUG	INDICATED FOR TREATMENT OF
Cefotaxime *intravenous or* *intramuscular*	Uncomplicated gonorrhoea, severe exacerbations of *Haemophilus influenzae* infection in cystic fibrosis, congenital gonococcal conjunctivitis, infections due to sensitive gram-positive and gram-negative bacteria, surgical prophylaxis, haemophilus epiglottitis, meningitis
Ceftriaxone *intravenous or* *intramuscular*	Pneumonia, intra-abdominal infections, complicated urinary tract, skin and soft-tissue infections, infections of bones and joints, suspected bacterial infection in neutropenic patients, bacterial meningitis and bacterial endocarditis, surgical prophylaxis, uncomplicated gonorrhoea, pelvic inflammatory disease, syphilis, lyme disease, congenital gonococcal conjunctivitis and acute otitis media
Cefixime *oral*	Acute infections due to sensitive gram-positive and gram-negative bacteria and uncomplicated gonorrhoea
Ceftazidime *intravenous,* *intramuscular or* *inhalation*	Pseudomonal lung infection in cystic fibrosis, febrile neutropenia, meningitis, susceptible infections due to sensitive gram-positive and gram-negative bacteria, chronic *Burkholderia cepacia* infection in cystic fibrosis
Cefuroxime *intravenous,* *intramuscular or oral*	Susceptible infections due to gram-positive and gram-negative bacteria, cellulitis, erysipelas, lyme disease, surgical prophylaxis, urinary tract infection (lower), urinary tract infection, acute pyelonephritis

Source: Data from Joint Formulary Committee, 2020c.

Table 18.3 Commonly used aminoglycosides in CYP.

DRUG	INDICATED FOR TREATMENT OF
Amikacin *intravenous*	Serious gram-negative infections resistant to gentamicin, neonatal sepsis, pseudomonal lung infection in cystic fibrosis, acute pyelonephritis, urinary tract infection
Gentamicin *intravenous, intrathecal,* *intraventricular,* *intramuscular*	Bacterial eye infections, bacterial infection in otitis externa, septicaemia, meningitis and other CNS infections, biliary-tract infection, endocarditis, pneumonia in hospital patients, adjunct in listerial meningitis, neonatal sepsis, pseudomonal lung infection in cystic fibrosis, bacterial ventriculitis and CNS infection, acute pyelonephritis, urinary tract infection
Neomycin sulfate *topical*	Bacterial infection in otitis externa and bacterial skin infections
Streptomycin *intramuscular*	Tuberculosis, resistant to other treatment, in combination with other drugs, and as an adjunct to doxycycline in brucellosis
Tobramycin *topical, inhalation,* *intravenous*	Chronic *Pseudomonas aeruginosa* infection in patients with cystic fibrosis, pseudomonal lung infection in cystic fibrosis, septicaemia, meningitis and other CNS infections, biliary-tract infection, acute pyelonephritis, pneumonia in hospital patients, neonatal sepsis

Source: Data from Joint Formulary Committee, 2020d.

Macrolides are active against a range of bacteria similar to penicillin drugs and are therefore often seen as an alternative in CYP who have penicillin allergies. Macrolides are effective against a variety of Gram-positive bacteria including Streptococcus pneumoniae and some Gram-negative bacteria including Bordetella pertussis and Haemophilus influenzae. Table 18.5 identifies the commonly used macrolide antibacterial drugs in CYP care and the conditions they are licensed to treat.

Fluoroquinolones

Fluroquinolones are bactericidal as they inhibit both topoisomerase II and topoisomerase IV enzymes which are required for bacterial DNA replication, transcription, repair and recombination. Due to the interference with DNA replication, fluroquinolones carry a risk of adverse side effects for the CYP and their use is often

Chapter 18 Antimicrobial Medications

Table 18.4 Commonly used tetracyclines in CYP.

DRUG	INDICATED FOR TREATMENT OF
Doxycycline *oral*	Chlamydia, rickettsia and mycoplasma, acute sinusitis, acute cough [if systemically very unwell or at higher risk of complications], community-acquired pneumonia, acute exacerbation of bronchiectasis, acne, syphilis, uncomplicated genital chlamydia, non-gonococcal urethritis, pelvic inflammatory disease, Lyme disease, anthrax, periodontitis, Rocky Mountain spotted fever
Minocycline *oral*	Susceptible infections (e.g. chlamydia, rickettsia and mycoplasma) and acne
Rifampicin *oral or intravenous*	Brucellosis, legionnaires disease and serious staphylococcal infections in combination with other antibacterials, tuberculosis, pruritus due to cholestasis
Streptomycin *intramuscular*	Tuberculosis and as an adjunct to doxycycline in brucellosis

Source: Data from Joint Formulary Committee, 2020e.

Table 18.5 Commonly used macrolides in CYP.

DRUG	INDICATED FOR TREATMENT OF
Erythromycin *oral and intravenous*	Susceptible infections in patients with penicillin hypersensitivity (e.g. respiratory tract infections, legionella infection, skin and oral infections, and campylobacter enteritis), impetigo, cellulitis, erysipelas, acute cough (if systemically very unwell or at higher risk of complications), acute sore throat, acute otitis media, chlamydial ophthalmia, early syphilis, uncomplicated genital chlamydia, non-gonococcal urethritis, pelvic inflammatory disease, prevention and treatment of pertussis, acne, gastrointestinal stasis
Clarithromycin *oral and intravenous*	Cellulitis, erysipelas, impetigo, pneumonia, respiratory tract infections, mild to moderate skin and soft-tissue infections, acute exacerbation of bronchiectasis, acute cough (if systemically very unwell or at higher risk of complications), acute sore throat, acute otitis media, *Helicobacter pylori* eradication in combination with omeprazole, and amoxicillin or metronidazole, acute sinusitis
Azithromycin *oral and topical*	Prevention of secondary case of invasive group A streptococcal infection in patients who are allergic to penicillin, respiratory tract infections, otitis media, skin and soft-tissue infections, infection in cystic fibrosis, uncomplicated genital chlamydial infections, non-gonococcal urethritis, Lyme disease, mild to moderate typhoid due to multiple-antibacterial resistant organisms, trachomatous conjunctivitis caused by *Chlamydia trachomatis*, purulent bacterial conjunctivitis

Source: Data from Joint Formulary Committee, 2020f.

Table 18.6 Commonly used fluroquinolones in CYP.

DRUG	INDICATED FOR TREATMENT OF
Ciprofloxacin *topical, oral, intravenous*	Superficial bacterial eye infection, corneal ulcer, acute otitis externa, fistulating Crohn's disease, severe respiratory tract infections, gastrointestinal infection, acute exacerbation of bronchiectasis, pseudomonal lower respiratory tract infection in cystic fibrosis, complicated urinary tract infections, gonorrhoea, anthrax, acute pyelonephritis, urinary tract infection
Ofloxacin *topical*	Local treatment of eye infections

Source: Data from Joint Formulary Committee, 2020g.

limited. These drugs are related to the quinolone drug group, which are used in other countries, but only fluroquinolones are available in the UK (Joint Formulary Committee, 2020g).

Fluroquinolones have a wide spectrum of action, but current prescribing guidelines would tend to recommend the use of other antibacterial drugs for first line treatment in order to reserve the efficacy of this group of drugs. Fluroquinolones are effective against Enterobacteriaceae, Pseudomonas, Acinetobacter, Staphylococcus, Neisseria gonorrhoeae, Neisseria meningitidis, Haemophilus influenzae and Moraxella catarrhalis bacteria. Table 18.6 demonstrates the limited use of fluroquinolones in CYP care and the conditions the drugs are licensed to treat.

To exemplify the properties of just one antibacterial medication, Table 18.7 is included below.

Clinical Consideration

Hypersensitivity reaction to antimicrobial medications are not uncommon and healthcare professionals should be aware when to expect these to present.

NICE (2014) guide that anaphylaxis will usually present less than 1 hour after exposure, non-immediate reactions without systemic involvement will usually present 6–10 days after first exposure or within 3 days of the second exposure, and non-immediate reactions with systemic involvement can be expected anywhere from 3 days to 6 weeks after first drug exposure.

Antiviral Medications

As viruses are not living organisms in the same way that bacteria are, they are more difficult to pharmacologically manage as it is problematic to attempt to kill a virus, without also damaging the host that the virus has invaded. As such, antiviral drugs do not 'kill' the virus as such but work in a similar way to

Table 18.7 The properties of phenoxymethylpenicillin (Penicillin V).

Use	Oral infections, acute sore throat, otitis media and acute sinusitis (Joint Formulary Committee, 2020a).
Dose	Must be individualised according to the child's age and the severity of the infection.
Administration	Given orally in tablet or suspension form
Pharmacodynamics	Binds to penicillin binding proteins located on the inner membrane of the bacterial cell wall and inactivates these proteins resulting in weakening of the bacterial cell wall and lysis (EMC, 2017).
Pharmacokinetics	Absorption: Rapidly, but incompletely absorbed after oral administration and the absorption level is around 60%. Taking the medication with food slightly decreases the peak plasma concentration but does not affect the extent of absorption. Peak plasma concentrations are reached in about 45 minutes. The peak plasma concentration increases approximately in proportion with increased doses. Distribution: Widely distributed round the body tissues and fluids and more readily penetrates inflamed tissues. It also diffuses across the placenta into foetal circulation and small amounts appear in the milk of nursing mothers. Metabolism: Partially metabolised to inactive penicilloic acid by hydrolysis of the lactam ring. This metabolism occurs in the liver. Excretion: The plasma half-life of phenoxymethylpenicillin is about 45 minutes which may increase to four hours in renal failure. About 40% of the dose is eliminated in the urine either as under unchanged or as penicilloic acid in the first 10 hours after oral administration. Small excretion occurs in bile. Impaired absorption is seen in patients with coeliac disease (EMC, 2017).
Side effects (common or very common)	Diarrhoea, hypersensitivity, nausea, skin reactions, thrombocytopenia and vomiting are common or very common. Antibiotic associated colitis and leukopenia are uncommon and agranulocytosis, angioedema, haemolytic anaemia, hepatic disorders, nephritis tubulointerstitial, seizure and severe cutaneous adverse reactions (SCARs) are rare or very rare (Joint Formulary Committee, 2020b).

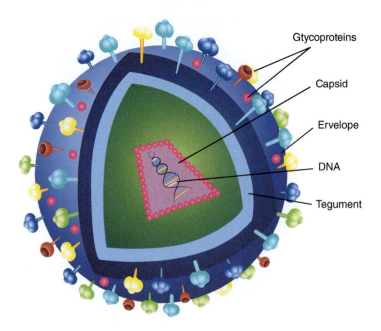

Figure 18.3 **Basic virus structure.**

bacteriostatic agents; they prevent the virus from replicating, in order to allow the body's own immune system to kill the virus.

The structure of a virus is quite simple in that is comprises of a nucleic acid core and is surrounded by a protein coat (Figure 18.3). The central nucleic acid of a virus is called the genome and consists of either DNA or RNA and viruses are labelled either a DNA virus or an RNA virus. The protein coat which surrounds the genome is called a capsid and, in some viruses, there is also an envelope of glycoprotein and phospholipid bilayer outside of the capsid. Additionally, some viruses may have additional proteins, such as enzymes, contained within them.

As well as being classified by DNA or RNA, viruses can also be classified into 4 groups based on their shape; filamentous, isometric, enveloped and head and tail. Filamentous viruses are long and cylindrical, isometric viruses are roughly spherical, enveloped viruses have surrounding capsids and head and tail viruses have spherical head and a filamentous tail and can infect bacteria.

Antiviral medications are not classified in the same way as other drugs may be but can be classified in accordance with the viruses they are active against; anti-herpes medications, anti-retrovirus medications, anti-influenza medications and non-selective antiviral drugs.

Anti-Herpes Medications

Herpes virus is a DNA virus which causes diseases such as chickenpox and genital herpes in CYP. As the herpes virus transfers DNA to the nucleus of the host cell, medications that are active against the herpes virus are drugs which interfere with DNA replication. Table 18.8 lists the commonly used anti-herpes medications in CYP.

Treatment of herpes simplex infections of the eye, mouth or genitals usually start at the initial onset of symptoms, with a topical antiviral drug, and lasts 5 days (Joint Formulary Committee, 2020h). Whilst varicella zoster infections (such as chickenpox) in a healthy child between 1 month and 12 years do not usually require treatment, neonates under 1 month and young people over the age of 12 often require pharmacological intervention to reduce the duration and severity of the infection.

Anti-Retrovirus Medications

A retrovirus is slightly different to other viruses; where a virus will insert their genetic material into a host cell and transcribe the cell to create 'daughter' virus cells, a retrovirus engages in a process called reverse transcription. All retroviruses carry RNA genetic material (not DNA), but once inside the host cell, the retrovirus can convert their RNA to DNA, which they integrate into the host cell and code in a process of reverse transcription. However, as retroviruses must engage in this process of reverse transcription quickly, the process is

Table 18.8 Commonly used anti-herpes medications in CYP.

DRUG	USE
Aciclovir *topical, oral, intravenous*	Usually first choice for systemic treatment of varicella zoster and systemic/topical treatment of herpes simplex
Foscarnet sodium *intravenous*	Mucocutaneous herpes simplex virus infections unresponsive to aciclovir in immunocompromised patients
Ganciclovir *intravenous*	More active against Cytomegalovirus (CMV) than aciclovir but also more toxic
Valaciclovir *oral*	Mild herpes zoster in immunocompromised CYP over 12 years and in CYP over 12 years for prevention of CMV following renal transplantation

Source: Data from Joint Formulary Committee, 2020h.

less accurate and causes offspring cells to be genetically different to the first retroviral cell. Human Immunodeficiency Virus (HIV) is an example of a retrovirus.

Whilst HIV is the most well known retrovirus, other retroviruses can have serious health implications and cause cancer. As such, treatment of retroviruses includes the aggressive use of antiviral medications. The antiviral medications most commonly used in CYP care are in the treatment of HIV and belong to one of six drug classes (Joint Formulary Committee, 2020i):

- Nucleoside reverse transcriptase inhibitors (or 'nucleoside analogue')
- Non-nucleoside reverse transcriptase inhibitors
- Protease inhibitors
- CCR5 antagonists
- Integrase inhibitors
- Fusion inhibitors

Each of the categories of antiretrovirals work in slightly different ways, and as such are given in combination. Fusion inhibitors and CCR5 antagonists work outside of the (CD4) cell which the HIV virus is intending to join to prevent the virus from being able to fuse with the cell. Nucleoside reverse transcriptase inhibitors inhibit the reverse transcriptase enzyme which HIV needs in order to be able to infect the cell and non-nucleoside reverse transcriptase inhibitors attach themselves to this same enzyme to prevent it from being able to convert RNA to DNA. Finally, protease inhibitors and integrase inhibitors inhibit the protease and integrase enzymes which HIV requires to reproduce itself. Initial treatment of HIV infection in CYP involves combination of two nucleoside reverse transcriptase inhibitors (NRTI) and one of either an integrase inhibitor, a non-nucleoside reverse transcriptase inhibitor, or a boosted protease inhibitor (Joint Formulary Committee, 2020i). Table 18.9 lists the drugs licensed for use in CYP's under each of these categories.

Table 18.9 Antiviral medications licensed for the treatment of HIV in CYP by drug class.

CLASS	DRUGS
Nucleoside reverse transcriptase inhibitors	Abacavir (ABC); Emtricitabine (FTC), Lamivudine (3TC); Stavudine (d4T), Tenofovir Alafenamide Fumarate (TAF), Tenofovir disoproxil fumarate (TDF), and Zidovudine (AZT)
Non-nucleoside reverse transcriptase inhibitors	Efavirenz (EFV), Etravirine (ETR), Nevirapine (NVP), and Rilpivirine (RPV)
Protease inhibitors	Atazanavir (ATZ), Darunavir (DRV), Fosamprenavir (FOS-APV), Lopinavir (LPV), Ritonavir (RTV), and Tipranavir (TPV)
CCR5 antagonist	Maraviroc (MVC)
Integrase inhibitors	Dolutegravir (DTG), Elvitegravir (EVG), and Raltegravir (RAL)
Fusion inhibitor	Enfuvirtide (T-20)

Source: Data from Joint Formulary Committee, 2020i.

Chapter 18 Antimicrobial Medications

Table 18.10 Commonly used influenze medications in CYP.

DRUG	USE
Oseltamivir *oral*	Prevention of influenza and for use in the first 48 hours of symptoms
Zanamivir *inhaled or intravenous*	Post-exposure prophylaxis of influenza, prevention of influenza during an epidemic and treatment for use in the first 36 hours of symptoms

Source: Data from Joint Formulary Committee, 2020j.

Anti-Influenza Medications

Influenza is caused by either influenza A, influenza B or influenza C viruses, all of which are RNA viruses. Whilst most strains of influenza are uncomplicated in the general population of CYP, some (usually associated with influenza A) may require treatment with antiviral medication (NICE, 2019).

Antiviral medications for influenzas are most effective if started immediately at the onset of symptoms and in CYP who are immunocompromised, they may be used for prophylaxis of influenza following exposure to the virus. Table 18.10 identifies the two antiviral drugs licensed for use in CYP care.

Non-Selective Antivirals

Some antiviral medications are non-selective in that they can be active against a variety of viruses instead of just one, but they are often less effective. An example group of drugs used as non-selective antivirals is interferons. Interferons are proteins which are produced by host cells in response to a viral invasion. Through administration of interferon drugs, the host's cells are stimulated to produce proteins which can prevent the synthesis of viral nucleic RNA or DNA.

In the COVID-19 global pandemic, which was first encountered in China in 2019, numerous selective and non-selective antivirals were trialled to assess if they could be used as treatment, though at the time of writing this chapter, none had been proved consistently effective (Izzi et al., 2020). Viruses continue to be difficult to treat because they are not living organisms which go through processes in the way of other microorganisms and because they hijack the body's own cells to reproduce.

To demonstrate the properties of just one antiviral medication, Table 18.11 is included.

Skills in Practice

Genevieve is a 6-week-old baby who requires aciclovir treatment for a herpes simplex infection. She weighs 4.2kg.

The BNFC (Joint Formulary Committee, 2020h) states that the dose of aciclovir is 20mg/kg every 8 hours, for 14 days, and that this should be given by intravenous infusion.

1. How much aciclovir does Genevieve need per dose?
2. How much aciclovir does Genevieve need in 24 hours?

Antifungal Medications

As was identified earlier in this chapter, fungi usually won't cause harm in healthy CYP, but immunocompromised children are at risk of complications arising from fungal infections. Treatment of fungal infections can be local or systemic, dependent on the location and severity of the fungal infection. Whilst antifungal resistance is not as much of a concern as antibacterial resistance, there are now an increasing number of fungi with resistance to antifungal medications which supports the need for principles of antimicrobial stewardship (discussed later in this chapter) to be applied to this group of drugs (BSAC, 2018).

As with bacteria, antifungal medications can either kill the fungus or prevent the growth of the cell and in order to appreciate the action of antifungal medications, understanding of the structure of fungal cells is useful. In contrast to bacteria and viruses, fungi can be either single-celled or complex, multicellular organisms. Fungal cells consist of a cell wall and cell membrane surrounding the nucleus and cytoplasm. Where the walls of bacteria and plant cells are made up of cellulose, fungi are made up of a compound called chitin. The

Table 18.11 The properties of Aciclovir.

Use	Usually first choice for systemic treatment of varicella zoster and systemic/topical treatment of herpes simplex (Joint Formulary Committee, 2020h)
Dose	Topically, dose is 5% cream applied 5 times per day. Oral and Intravenous doses must be individualised according to the child's age/weight and the severity of the infection.
Administration	Topical, oral or intravenously administered (Joint Formulary Committee, 2020h).
Pharmacodynamics	Aciclovir is a synthetic purine nucleoside analogue. Aciclovir triphosphate interferes with the viral DNA polymerase and inhibits viral DNA replication with resultant chain termination following its incorporation into the viral DNA (EMC, 2018).
Pharmacokinetics	As aciclovir plasma concentrations following topical application are below the limit of detection, no pharmacokinetic studies are available on topical aciclovir. For oral and intravenous administration; Absorption: Aciclovir is only partially absorbed from the gut. In fully grown CYPs and adults the terminal plasma half-life of aciclovir after administration of intravenous aciclovir is about 2.9 hours but this varies depending on a child's renal function. Distribution: Plasma protein binding is relatively low (9 to 33%) and drug interactions involving binding site displacement are not anticipated. Cerebrospinal fluid levels are approximately 50% of corresponding plasma levels Metabolism: Metabolised intracellularly in viral infected cells and is minimally metabolised by the liver. The terminal plasma half-life varies according to a child's age but in adults patients is 3.8 hours Excretion: Most of the drug is excreted unchanged by the kidney. Renal clearance of aciclovir is substantially greater than creatinine clearance, indicating that tubular secretion, in addition to glomerular filtration, contributes to the renal elimination of the drug. 9-carboxymethoxymethylguanine is the only significant metabolite of aciclovir and accounts for 10 to 15% of the dose excreted in the urine (EMC, 2018).
Side effects (common or very common)	When used by eye (topical): eye inflammation and eye pain are common or very common and skin reactions are uncommon. With oral use abdominal pain: diarrhoea, dizziness, fatigue, fever, headache, nausea, photosensitivity reaction, skin reactions and vomiting are common or very common. Agitation, anaemia, angioedema, ataxia, coma, confusion, drowsiness, dysarthria, dyspnoea, encephalopathy, hallucination, hepatic disorders, leukopenia, psychosis, renal impairment, renal pain, seizure, thrombocytopenia and tremor are rare or very rare. With intravenous use: nausea, photosensitivity reactions, skin reactions and vomiting are common or very common. Anaemia, leukopenia and thrombocytopenia are uncommon and abdominal pain, agitation, angioedema, ataxia, coma, confusion, diarrhoea, dizziness, drowsiness, dysarthria, dyspnoea, encephalopathy, fatigue, fever, hallucination, headache, hepatic disorders, inflammation localised, psychosis, renal impairment, renal pain, seizure and tremor are rare or very rare (Joint Formulary Committee, 2020h).

majority of the body of a fungus is made from very long, thin threads called hyphae which connect in a network of mycelium. Due to the long, thin shape of hyphae, they have a high surface area when compared to their volume, which allows them to absorb nutrients efficiently from their surrounding area (Figure 18.4).

Antifungal medications are often not as well tolerated as antibacterial medications and a number of antifungals also have significant drug-drug interactions with other medications (especially the azole drugs) which offer key considerations for the use of these medications (BSAC, 2018). Antifungal medications can be classified according to their mechanism of action and structure into azoles, polyenes and echinocandins (Ashbee et al., 2014). However, not all antifungal medications fit neatly into one of these categories, with flucytosine being an example of a miscellaneous antifungal. Flucytosine is licensed for the use of systemic yeast and fungal

Chapter 18 Antimicrobial Medications

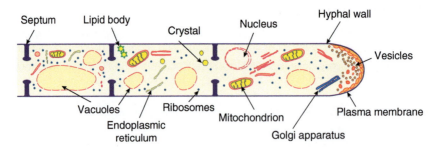

Figure 18.4 A fungal organism.

infections, and cryptococcal meningitis in CYP (Joint Formulary Committee, 2020k). Flucytosine works by preventing the fungal cell from producing the nucleic acids and proteins it needs to grow.

Azoles

Azole antifungal drugs make up most antifungal medications used in CYP care. Their method of action is to inhibit ergosterol, which is an important component of fungal cell membranes, through blocking the lanosterol 14 alpha demethylase enzyme required for synthesis. Table 18.12 displays the most commonly used azoles in CYP care.

Episode of Care

Learning Disability

Bao is 14 years old and lives at home with his parents and younger brother. Bao's family are originally from Vietnam and Mum speaks good English, but Dad requires a translator. Bao's father is his main care giver.

Bao has a moderate learning disability and has presented to his GP with a fungal nail infection on his left foot 3 times in the last 6 months. Today, Bao has presented again, with a fungal nail infection which is now also on his right foot and is red and sore.

Before Bao is given another prescription for an antifungal medication, healthcare professionals need to reassess Bao's and his father's understanding of the administration instructions for the previous medications he was prescribed. What else should healthcare professionals consider?

Table 18.12 Commonly used azole antifungal medications in CYP.

DRUG	USE
Clotrimazole *topical*	Fungal infection in otitis externa, fungal skin infections, superficial sites of infection in vaginal and vulval candidiasis, vaginal candidiasis
Econazole nitrate *topical*	Fungal skin infections, fungal nail infections, vaginal and vulval candidiasis
Fluconazole *oral or intravenous*	Candidal balanitis, vaginal candidiasis, vulvovaginal candidiasis, mucosal candidiasis, tinea capitis, tinea pedis, corporis, cruris, pityriasis versicolor, dermal candidiasis, invasive candidal infections, cryptococcal infections
Ketoconazole *oral or topical*	Endogenous Cushing's syndrome, seborrhoeic dermatitis and dandruff, pityriasis versicolor
Itraconazole *oral or intravenous*	Oropharyngeal candidiasis, pityriasis versicolor, tinea pedis, tinea manuum, tinea corporis, tinea cruris, tinea capitis, onychomycosis, histoplasmosis and systemic candidiasis, cryptococcosis and aspergillosis where other antifungal drugs inappropriate or ineffective
Miconazole *topical*	Fungal skin and nail infections, oral candidiasis, intestinal candidiasis
Tioconazole *topical*	Fungal nail infection
Voriconazole *oral or intravenous*	Invasive aspergillosis, Serious infections caused by s *cedosporium* spp., *f usarium* spp., or invasive fluconazole-resistant *c andida* spp. (including *C. krusei*).

Source: Data from Joint Formulary Committee, 2020l.

Table 18.13 Commonly used polyenes antifungal medications in CYP.

DRUG	USE
Amphotericin B *intravenous infusion*	Systemic fungal infections, suspected or proven infection in febrile neutropenic patients unresponsive to broad-spectrum antibacterials
Nystatin *oral*	Oral candidiasis, oral and perioral fungal infections

Source: Data from Joint Formulary Committee, 2020l.

Table 18.14 Commonly used echinocandin antifungal medications in CYP.

DRUG	USE
Caspofungin *intravenous*	Invasive aspergillosis, invasive candidiasis and empirical treatment of systemic fungal infections in patients with neutropenia
Micafungin *intravenous*	Invasive candidiasis, oesophageal candidiasis and prophylaxis of candidiasis in patients undergoing bone-marrow transplantation or who are expected to become neutropenic for over 10 days

Source: Data from Joint Formulary Committee, 2020l.

Polyenes

Polyene antifungal medications method of action lie in binding to ergosterol which is a type of steroid found in fungal cells membrane. Once bound, polyenes weaken the cell membrane which causes the cell to leak its contents and eventual cell death. Though there are fewer drugs belonging to this group, the two listed in Table 18.13 are commonly used in fungal infections in CYP.

Echinocandins

Echinocandin antifungal drugs are a relatively new class of antifungal drugs, having been first developed in the late 20th century. Their effect on fungal cells is to inhibit the enzyme glucan synthase which is an important competent of a fungal cell wall. Without the glucan synthase enzyme, the cell call becomes porous and the fungal cell dies. Table 18.14 identifies the two commonly used echinocandins in CYP.

To demonstrate the properties of just one antifungal medication, Table 18.15 is included.

Skills in Practice

Applying medication to the skin or mucous membrane is known as topical application. To apply medication in this way;

1. Wash hands and don PPE as appropriate
2. Gently smooth a thin layer of medication onto the skin in the direction the hair grows
3. Only apply the medication to the affected area
   Some topical medications will advise doses based on Finger Tip Units (FTU). This is the amount of medication which is dispensed from the tube onto an adult's fingertip. In a standard tube with a 5mm nozzles, this is approximately 0.5g of medication.
   CYP should be encouraged to administer their own topical medications as appropriate

Antiprotozoal Medications

Protozoa are single-celled organisms which have a cell membrane which binds the cell nucleus and organelles together. Like bacteria, protozoa have tiny hair-like structures called pseudopodia, flagella and cilia which aid movement of the organism. However, unlike bacteria, the cilia and flagella arising from the cell and sheathed inside the cell membrane, rather than external to it (Figure 18.5).

Much like antibacterial medications, antiprotozoal medications can either kill the protozoa or prevent their growth and ability to reproduce. As the protozoa for which most antiprotozoal medications are

Table 18.15 The properties of Fluconazole.

Use	Candidal balanitis, vaginal candidiasis, vulvovaginal candidiasis, mucosal candidiasis, tinea capitis, tinea pedis, corporis, cruris, pityriasis versicolor, dermal candidiasis, invasive candidal infections, cryptococcal infections (Joint Formulary Committee, 2020l).
Dose	Oral and Intravenous doses must be individualised according to the child's age/weight and the severity of the infection (Joint Formulary Committee, 2020l).
Administration	Oral or Intravenously administered (Joint Formulary Committee, 2020l).
Pharmacodynamics	Fluconazole is a potent and selective inhibitor of fungal enzymes necessary for the synthesis of ergosterol (EMC, 2019a).
Pharmacokinetics	Absorption: The pharmacokinetic properties of fluconazole are similar whether administered orally or by the intravenous route. After oral administration, fluconazole is well absorbed and plasma levels (and systemic bioavailability) are over 90% of the levels achieved after intravenous administration. Concomitant food intake does not affect oral absorption. Distribution: Fluconazole achieves good penetration in all body fluids studied. The levels of fluconazole in saliva and sputum are similar to plasma levels. In patients with fungal meningitis, fluconazole levels in the CSF are approximately 80% of the corresponding plasma levels. Metabolism: Minimally metabolised in the liver. Excretion: Excretion is mainly renal, with approximately 80% of the administered dose appearing in the urine as unchanged drug. Fluconazole clearance is proportional to creatinine clearance (EMC, 2019a).
Side effects (common or very common)	Diarrhoea, gastrointestinal discomfort, headache, nausea, skin reactions and vomiting are common or very common. Dizziness, flatulence, hepatic disorders, seizure, and altered taste are uncommon. Agranulocytosis, alopecia, dyslipidaemia, hypokalaemia, leukopenia, neutropenia, QT interval prolongation, severe cutaneous adverse reactions (SCARs), thrombocytopenia and torsade de pointes are rare or very rare (Joint Formulary Committee, 2020l).

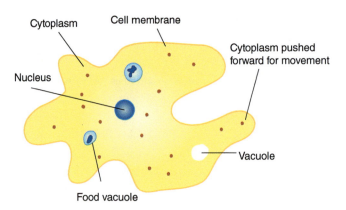

Figure 18.5 A protozoa organism.

formulated is malaria, these drugs are easily classified into one of two categories; antimalarials and other antiprotozoal medications.

Antimalarials

Whilst malaria is rare in the UK, it is not unheard of and children are at greater risk of becoming seriously unwell if exposed. Different antimalarial drugs treat different stages of the protozoal life cycle, and as such they are often used in combination with each other. Table 18.16 demonstrates the commonly used antimalarial medications in CYP.

Chapter 18 Antimicrobial Medications

Table 18.16 Commonly used antimalarials in CYP.

DRUG	USE
Artemether with lumefantrine *oral*	Treatment of acute uncomplicated falciparum malaria and chloroquine-resistant non-falciparum malaria
Artenimol with piperaquine *oral*	Treatment of uncomplicated falciparum malaria and non-falciparum malaria
Atovaquone with proguanil *oral*	Treatment of acute uncomplicated falciparum malaria and non-falciparum malaria
Chloroquine *oral*	Treatment of non-falciparum malaria
Doxycycline *oral*	Adjunct to quinine in treatment of plasmodium falciparum malaria in children over 12 years
Mefloquine *oral*	Treatment of malaria
Primaquine *oral*	Adjunct in the treatment of non-falciparum malaria caused by P.vivax infection and non-falciparum malaria caused by P.ovale infection

Source: Data from Joint Formulary Committee, 2020m.

Table 18.17 Commonly used antiprotozoal medications in CYP.

DRUG	USE
Metronidazole *topical, oral or intravenous*	Invasive intestinal amoebiasis, extra-intestinal amoebiasis, urogenital trichomoniasis, giardiasis
Tinidazole *oral*	Intestinal amoebiasis, amoebic involvement of liver, urogenital trichomoniasis, giardiasis
Mepacrine hydrochloride *intravenous*	Visceral leishmaniasis and cutaneous leishmaniasis
Sodium stibogluconate *intravenous or intramuscular*	Visceral leishmaniasis
Pentamidine isethionate *intramuscular*	Visceral leishmaniasis, cutaneous leishmaniasis, trypanosomiasis
Pyrimethamine *oral*	Congenital toxoplasmosis and toxoplasmosis in pregnancy
Sulfadiazine *oral*	Congenital toxoplasmosis and toxoplasmosis in pregnancy

Source: Data from Joint Formulary Committee, 2020n.

Other Antiprotozoal Medications

Protozoal infections are much less common than bacterial or viral infections in the UK, but they do still occur. One such example is toxoplasmosis, which is caused by the protozoa Toxoplasma gondii. Toxoplasmosis is contracted from CYP having contact with the faeces of infected animals (usually cats) or through eating infected meat (NHS, 2020b). Whilst the infection is usually harmless, it can cause problems in immunocompromised CYP and pregnant females (NHS, 2020b).

As with antimalarial protozoa, each antiprotozoal drug has a slightly different mechanism of action upon varied points of the protozoal cell cycle. Table 18.17 demonstrates the commonly used antiprotozoal medications in CYP.

To demonstrate the properties of just one antiprotozoal medication, Table 18.18 is included below.

Antimicrobial Resistance

There is currently a concern in the UK that with increasing use of antimicrobials, there is a rise in the development of antimicrobial resistant bacteria (Public Health England, 2015). To demonstrate how vast the use of antimicrobials is in the CYP population alone; globally 36% of inpatient CYP will receive at least one

Table 18.18 The properties of metronidazole.

Use	Invasive intestinal amoebiasis, extra-intestinal amoebiasis, urogenital trichomoniasis, giardiasis (Joint Formulary Committee, 2020n).
Dose	Doses must be individualised according to the child's age/weight and the severity of the infection (Joint Formulary Committee, 2020n).
Administration	Topical, oral or intravenous (Joint Formulary Committee, 2020n).
Pharmacodynamics	Precise mode of action is unknown but probably caused by interaction with DNS and different metabolites (EMC, 2019b)
Pharmacokinetics	Absorption: Metronidazole is rapidly and almost completely absorbed on administration of Flagyl tablets; peak plasma concentrations occur after 20 min to 3 hours. Distribution: The half-life of metronidazole is 8.5 ± 2.9 hours. Metabolism: Metronidazole is metabolised in the liver by hydroxylation, oxidation and glucuronidation. The major metabolites are a 2-hydroxy- and an acetic acid metabolite. Excretion: More than 50% of the administered dose is excreted in the urine, as unchanged metronidazole (approximately 20% of the dose) and its metabolites. About 20% of the dose is excreted with faeces. The plasma elimination half-life of metronidazole is approximately 8 hours, and of the 2-hydroxy-metabolite approximately 10 hours (EMC, 2019b).
Side effects (common or very common)	With intravenous use: dry mouth, myalgia, nausea, oral disorders, metallic taste and vomiting are common or very common. Asthenia, headache and leukopenia (with long-term or intensive therapy) are uncommon whilst agranulocytosis, angioedema, decreased appetite, ataxia, cerebellar syndrome, confusion, diarrhoea, dizziness, drowsiness, encephalopathy, epigastric pain, epileptiform seizure (with long-term or intensive therapy), flushing, hallucination, hepatic disorders, aseptic meningitis, mucositis, nerve disorders, neutropenia, pancreatitis, pancytopenia, peripheral neuropathy (with long-term or intensive therapy), psychotic disorder, seizure, severe cutaneous adverse reactions (SCARs), skin reactions, thrombocytopenia, dark urine and vision disorders are rare or very rare. With topical use skin reactions are common or very common. With vaginal use: pelvic discomfort, vulvovaginal candidiasis and vulvovaginal disorders are common and menstrual cycle irregularities and vaginal haemorrhage are uncommon. Agranulocytosis, ataxia, cerebellar syndrome, confusion, dizziness, drowsiness, encephalopathy, flushing, hallucination, headache, hepatic disorders, myalgia, neutropenia, pancreatitis, pancytopenia, psychotic disorder, seizure, skin reactions, thrombocytopenia, dark urine and vision disorders are rare or very rare (Joint Formulary Committee, 2020n).

antimicrobial during their admission (Versporten et al., 2016). Antimicrobial resistant infections are already estimated to be responsible for 700,000 deaths worldwide, each year (DH, 2019a). Unlike other drugs, the more that societies use antimicrobials, the less effective they become. Figure 18.6 displays how antimicrobial resistance occurs; whilst antimicrobials kill some bacteria in the body, resistant strains may remain and then multiply.

Whilst antimicrobial resistance can occur naturally through our continued use of antimicrobials, the incorrect use of these drugs compounds the problem. CYP who are prescribed antimicrobials when they are not needed or who take less than their prescribed doses of antimicrobials (through missing doses or stopping before the end of the course), can allow bacteria to develop resistance to the medication (DH, 2019b).

Antimicrobial Stewardship

Antimicrobial Stewardship is a relatively new term in healthcare, upon which the NHS is currently placing much focus (DH, 2019b). The goal of antimicrobial stewardship is to reduce unnecessary prescriptions of antimicrobials and educate healthcare professionals and service uses about correct use of these drugs.

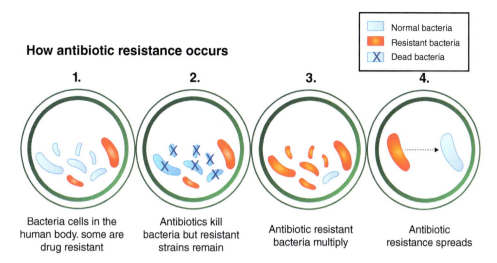

Figure 18.6 **How antibiotic resistance occurs.** *Source*: Public Health England, 2015/Public domain (OGL).

NICE guidance (2015: 8) defines antimicrobial stewardship as 'an organisational or healthcare-system-wide approach to promoting and monitoring judicious use of antimicrobials to preserve their future effectiveness'.

NICE (2015) provide clear guidance for prescribers of antimicrobials to ensure antimicrobial stewardship, but in short healthcare professionals must:

- Follow local and national guidelines to prescribe the shortest effective course, the most appropriate dose and the best route of administration of antimicrobials
- Consider the risk of antimicrobial resistance for individual patients and the population as a whole
- Consider taking microbiological samples before prescribing an antimicrobial and review the prescription when the results are available
- Document in the patient's records the reason for prescribing, or not prescribing, an antimicrobial and the plan of care as discussed with the patient, and their parent/carer
- Do not issue an immediate prescription for an antimicrobial to a patient who is likely to have a self-limiting condition
- Do not issue repeat prescriptions for antimicrobials unless needed for a particular clinical condition or indication

The CYP population is at increased risk of poor antimicrobial stewardship as healthcare professionals may be more likely to prescribe unnecessary antimicrobials in this population. Factors which influence healthcare professionals to prescribe antimicrobials in practice have been demonstrated to be (Cabral et al., 2015):

- The perceived vulnerability of children as a patient group
- Consulting and prescribing antibiotics were both perceived as the safer course of action
- Concern about disapproval of actions or missing something in a child
- The healthcare professional and parental experience on whether previous action had resulted in perceived increases or decreases in safety

Antimicrobial Education for Patients and Their Parents/Carers

Patient and parent/carer education is a key role for healthcare professionals when seeking to prevent antimicrobial resistance. Patients and their parents/carers need to be educated to take their full doses of antimicrobials, without missing any doses, stopping before the end of the course, or allowing anyone who is not prescribed the medication to take it (NICE, 2015).

Education for patients and their parents/carers when professionals decide to prescribe/not prescribe antimicrobials should incorporate: the likely nature of the condition; why prescribing an antimicrobial may not be the best option; alternative options to prescribing an antimicrobial; the patients' views on antimicrobials, taking into account their priorities or concerns for their current illness and whether they want or expect an

Chapter 18 Antimicrobial Medications

antimicrobial; the benefits and harms of immediate antimicrobial prescribing; what they should do if their condition deteriorates or they have problems as a result of treatment; and whether they need any written information about their medicines and any possible outcomes (NICE, 2015).

Episode of Care

Mental Health

Rhiann is 5 years old and lives at home with her mum, who is a single parent. Rhiann has no underlying healthcare conditions and is normally fit and well but her mum experiences severe health anxiety.

Rhiann recently started school and is enjoying being in reception and making new friends. She enjoys colouring and playing on her tablet.

Rhiann's mum is concerned as Rhiann has had three colds over the past few months, since starting school and she feels that Rhiann is barely getting over one cold before she gets another. Rhiann's mum has requested a prescription for 'antibiotics' to help Rhiann fight of this latest cold.

What factors should healthcare professionals include and consider when offering education to Rhiann's mum?

Prescribing Antimicrobials

The British National Formulary for Children (Joint Formulary Committee, 2020o) guides that clinicians must consider three key factors before choosing which antimicrobial to prescribe; the patient, the known or likely causative organism, and the risk of bacterial resistance with repeated courses.

The healthcare professional should consider the antibacterial sensitivity of the known or likely organism as well as the CYP's history of allergy, renal and hepatic function, immune status, ability to tolerate oral medications drugs, severity of illness, risk of complications, ethnic origin, age, whether taking other medication and, if female, whether pregnant, breast-feeding or taking an oral contraceptive (Joint Formulary Committee, 2020o). The Joint Formulary Committee (2020o) identify that CYP who may be at higher risk of treatment failure include those who have had repeated antibacterial courses, those who have had a previous or current culture with resistant bacteria and those at higher risk of developing complications.

Conclusion

Microorganisms which may be harmful to humans can be divided into four classes: bacteria, virus, fungi and protozoa. The medications used to treat these are known collectively as antimicrobials and are named after the microorganism they treat; antibacterial, antiviral, antifungal and antiprotozoal. Since Alexander Fleming first discovered penicillin in 1928, our understanding and use of antimicrobial medications has grown vastly.

Antibacterial medications are used in the management of bacteria and may be bactericidal (they kill the bacteria), or bacteriostatic (they inhibit the growth of the bacteria). Viruses are more difficult to pharmacologically manage than bacteria, as it is problematic to attempt to kill a virus without also damaging the host that the virus has invaded. These medications work by preventing the virus from replicating, whilst the body's own immune system destroys the virus.

Fungi can be either single-celled or complex, multicellular organisms whilst antifungal medications can either kill the fungus or prevent the growth of the fungus. Antifungal medications are often not as well tolerated as antibacterial medications and a number of antifungals also have significant drug-drug interactions with other medication. Finally, antiprotozoal medications are used to manage protozoa and can either kill the protozoa or prevent their growth and ability to reproduce.

Antimicrobial resistance occurs when antimicrobials kill some bacteria in the body, but resistant strains may remain and then multiply. The issue is compounded by the incorrect use of these drugs such as CYP who are prescribed antimicrobials when they are not needed or who take less than their prescribed doses of antimicrobials. To manage this, antimicrobial stewardship aims to reduce unnecessary prescriptions of antimicrobials and educate healthcare professionals and service uses about correct use of these drugs.

This chapter has outlined some of the main pharmaceutical treatment options currently used for microorganisms in CYP. The development of current medications and the search for new drugs is a continuous process in order to provide better outcomes for CYP.

Glossary

Aerobic: Relating to, involving, or requiring free oxygen.

Anaerobic: Relating to or requiring an absence of free oxygen.

Bactericidal: A substance which kills bacteria.

Bacteriostatic: A substance that prevents the multiplying of bacteria without destroying them.

Cytoplasm: The material or protoplasm within a living cell, excluding the nucleus.

Microorganism: Organisms which are too small to be seen unaided by the human eye, which consist of a single cell.

Organism: An individual animal, plant, or single-celled life form.

Pharmacological mechanism of action: The specific biochemical interaction through which a drug substance produces its pharmacological effect

Plasma membrane: A microscopic membrane of lipids and proteins which forms the external boundary of the cytoplasm of a cell or encloses a vacuole, and regulates the passage of molecules in and out of the cytoplasm.

Prokaryotic: A microscopic single-celled organism which has neither a distinct nucleus with a membrane nor other specialised organelles, including the bacteria and cyanobacteria

Ribosomes: A minute particle consisting of RNA and associated proteins found in large numbers in the cytoplasm of living cells

Sepsis: A potentially life-threatening condition caused by the body's response to an infection. The body normally releases chemicals into the bloodstream to fight an infection. Sepsis occurs when the body's response to these chemicals is out of balance, triggering changes that can damage multiple organ systems

Synthesise: The production of chemical compounds by reaction from simpler materials

Systemic: Relating to a full system, especially as opposed to a particular part.

References

Ashbee, H.M., Barnes, R.A., Johnson, E.M. et al. (2014). Therapeutic drug monitoring (TDM) of antifungal agents: guidelines from the British Society for Medical Mycology. *Journal of Antimicrobial Chemotherapy* 69(5): 1162–1176.

British Society for Antimicrobial Chemotherapy (BSAC). (2018). *Antimicrobial stewardship: from Principles to Practice.* www.bsac.org.uk/antimicrobialstewardshipebook/BSAC-AntimicrobialStewardship-FromPrinciplestoPractice-eBook.pdf (accessed June 2020).

Cabral, C., Lucas, P.J., Ingram, J. et al. (2015). 'It's safer to . . .': Parent consulting and clinician antibiotic prescribing decisions for children with respiratory tract infections: an analysis across four qualitative studies. *Social Science and Medicine* 136–137: 156–164.

Department of Health and Social Care (DH) (2019a). *Tackling Antimicrobial Resistance 2019–2024: The UK's Five-year National Action Plan.* https://assets.publishing.service.gov.uk/government/uploads/system/uploads/attachment_data/file/784894/UK_AMR_5_year_national_action_plan.pdf (accessed May 2020).

Department of Health and Social Care (DH) (2019b). *Contained and Controlled: The UK's 20-year Vision for Antimicrobial Resistance.* https://assets.publishing.service.gov.uk/government/uploads/system/uploads/attachment_data/file/773065/uk-20-year-vision-for-antimicrobial-resistance.pdf (accessed May 2020).

Electronic Medicines Compendium (EMC). (2017). Penicillin. www.medicines.org.uk/emc/product/1754/smpc (accessed June 2020).

Electronic Medicines Compendium (EMC). (2018). Aciclovir. www.medicines.org.uk/emc/product/11531/smpc (accessed June 2020).

Electronic Medicines Compendium (EMC). (2019a). Fluconazole. www.medicines.org.uk/emc/product/40/smpc#PHARMACOLOGICAL_PROPS (accessed June 2020).

Electronic Medicines Compendium (EMC). (2019b). Metronidazole. www.medicines.org.uk/emc/product/9238/smpc (accessed June 2020).

Health Education England (HEE). (2020). Antimicrobial resistance. www.hee.nhs.uk/our-work/antimicrobial-resistance (accessed June 2020).

Izzi, A., Messina, V., Rinaldi, L., Maggi, P. (2020). Editorial – Sofosbuvir/Velpatasvir as a combination with strong potential activity against SARS-CoV2 (COVID-19) infection: how to use direct-acting antivirals as broad-spectrum antiviral agents. *European Review for Medical and Pharmacological Sciences* 24(10): 5193–5194.

Chapter 18 Antimicrobial Medications

Joint Formulary Committee (2020a) British National Formulary (BNF). Penicillins. https://bnf.nice.org.uk/drug-class/penicillins-2.html (accessed June 2020).

Joint Formulary Committee (2020b) British National Formulary for Children (BNFC). Penicillins. https://bnfc.nice.org.uk/treatment-summary/penicillins.html (accessed June 2020).

Joint Formulary Committee (2020c) British National Formulary for Children (BNFC). Cephalosporins. https://bnfc.nice.org.uk/treatment-summary/cephalosporins.html (accessed June 2020).

Joint Formulary Committee (2020d) British National Formulary for Children (BNFC). Aminoglycosides. https://bnfc.nice.org.uk/treatment-summary/aminoglycosides.html (accessed June 2020).

Joint Formulary Committee (2020e) British National Formulary for Children (BNFC). Tetracyclines. https://bnfc.nice.org.uk/treatment-summary/tetracyclines.html (accessed June 2020).

Joint Formulary Committee (2020f) British National Formulary for Children (BNFC). Macrolides. https://bnfc.nice.org.uk/treatment-summary/macrolides.html (accessed June 2020).

Joint Formulary Committee (2020g) British National Formulary for Children (BNFC). Fluoroquinolones. https://bnfc.nice.org.uk/treatment-summary/quinolones.html (accessed June 2020).

Joint Formulary Committee (2020h) British National Formulary for Children (BNFC). Herpesvirus infections. https://bnfc.nice.org.uk/treatment-summary/herpesvirus-infections.html (accessed June 2020).

Joint Formulary Committee (2020i) British National Formulary for Children (BNFC). HIV infection. https://bnfc.nice.org.uk/treatment-summary/hiv-infection.html (accessed June 2020).

Joint Formulary Committee (2020j) British National Formulary for Children (BNFC). Influenza. https://bnfc.nice.org.uk/treatment-summary/influenza.html (accessed June 2020).

Joint Formulary Committee (2020k) British National Formulary for Children (BNFC). Flucytosine. https://bnfc.nice.org.uk/drug/flucytosine.html#indicationsAndDoses (accessed June 2020).

Joint Formulary Committee (2020l) British National Formulary for Children (BNFC). Antifungals, systemic use. https://bnfc.nice.org.uk/treatment-summary/antifungals-systemic-use.html (accessed June 2020).

Joint Formulary Committee (2020m) British National Formulary for Children (BNFC). Antimalarials. https://bnfc.nice.org.uk/treatment-summary/antimalarials.html (accessed June 2020).

Joint Formulary Committee (2020n) British National Formulary for Children (BNFC). Antiprotozoal drugs. https://bnfc.nice.org.uk/treatment-summary/antiprotozoal-drugs.html (accessed June 2020).

Joint Formulary Committee (2020o) British National Formulary for Children (BNFC). Antibacterials, principles of therapy. https://bnfc.nice.org.uk/treatment-summary/antibacterials-principles-of-therapy.html (accessed June 2020).

National Health Service (NHS). (2020a). Antibiotics. www.nhs.uk/conditions/antibiotics/ (accessed May 2020).

National Health Service (NHS). (2020b). Toxoplasmosis. www.nhs.uk/conditions/Toxoplasmosis/ (accessed June 2020).

National Institute of Health and Care Excellence (NICE). (2014). Drug allergy: diagnosis and management. www.nice.org.uk/guidance/cg183 (accessed June 2020).

National Institute of Health and Care Excellence (NICE). (2015).Antimicrobial stewardship: systems and processes for effective antimicrobial medicine use. www.nice.org.uk/guidance/ng15/resources/antimicrobial-stewardship-systems-and-processes-for-effective-antimicrobial-medicine-use-pdf-1837273110469 (accessed May 2020).

National Institute of Health and Care Excellence (NICE). (2017). Sepsis: recognition, diagnosis and early management. www.nice.org.uk/guidance/NG51/chapter/recommendations#managing-and-treating-suspected-sepsis-in-acute-hospital-settings (accessed June 2020).

National Institute of Health and Care Excellence (NICE). (2019). Influenza – seasonal. https://cks.nice.org.uk/influenza-seasonal#!backgroundSub (accessed June 2020).

Office for National Statistics (ONS). (2017).Causes of death over 100 years.www.ons.gov.uk/peoplepopulationandcommunity/birthsdeathsandmarriages/deaths/articles/causesofdeathover100years/2017-09-18 (accessed June 2020).

Public Health England (2015). Health matters: antimicrobial resistance. www.gov.uk/government/publications/health-matters-antimicrobial-resistance/health-matters-antimicrobial-resistance (accessed April 2020).

United Nations International Children's Emergency Fund (UNICEF). (2020). Childhood diseases. www.unicef.org/health/childhood-diseases (accessed April 2020).

Versporten, A., Bielicki, J., Drapier, N., Sharland, M., Goossens, H. (2016). The Worldwide Antibiotic Resistance and Prescribing in European Children (ARPEC) point prevalence survey: developing hospital-quality indicators of antibiotic prescribing for children. *Journal of Antimicrobial Chemotherapy* 71(4): 1106–1117.

Further Resources

FGDP guidelines: The Faculty of General Dental Practice offer guidelines for antimicrobial prescribing in dentistry.

Health Education England: Health Education England (HEE) have a number of resources, including an e-Learning resource, on antimicrobial resistance to help improve understanding for healthcare professionals.

Chapter 18 Antimicrobial Medications

NICE guidelines: The National Institute for Health and Care Excellence (NICE) write evidence-based recommendations for healthcare in England. They provide a number of guidelines for the prescription and administration of antimicrobials, including antimicrobial stewardship guidelines.

SIGN Guidelines: The Scottish Intercollegiate Guidelines Network (SIGN) develop and disseminate clinical guidelines for evidence-based healthcare practice in Scotland. They have developed a range of guidelines for prescription of antimicrobials for varying conditions.

Royal Pharmaceutical Society: The RPS provides pharmaceutical guidance for all healthcare practitioners in the UK. Information is available on the prescription of antimicrobials and includes antimicrobial stewardship guidance.

WHO: The World Health Organization take a proactive stance on reducing antimicrobial resistance and offer a series of publications with this focus. Guidance includes the use of antimicrobials in food producing animals as well as in healthcare.

Multiple Choice Questions

1. What would be the correct treatment for malaria?
   (a) Antibacterial
   (b) Antiviral
   (c) Antifungal
   (d) Antiprotozoal

2. What would be the correct treatment for genital herpes?
   (a) Antibacterial
   (b) Antiviral
   (c) Antifungal
   (d) Antiprotozoal

3. What does a bacteriostatic antibacterial drug do?
   (a) Kills bacteria
   (b) Stops bacteria from growing
   (c) Encourages bacterial growth
   (d) Changes a bacteria to a fungus

4. What is the function of pili on bacterial cells?
   (a) To keep them warm
   (b) To fight off attacking medications
   (c) Movement within the body
   (d) To allow cell division

5. What does it mean if a bacterium is stained violet in the Gram test?
   (a) The bacteria are Gram-positive
   (b) The bacteria are Gram-negative
   (c) The bacteria are part of the staphylococcus family
   (d) The bacteria are not part of the staphylococcus family

6. How do antiviral medications work?
   (a) They kill viruses
   (b) They inhibit virus's growth
   (c) They make the body temperature rise
   (d) They make the body temperature lower

7. What shape is a filamentous virus?
   (a) Roughly spherical
   (b) Head- and tail-shaped
   (c) Envelope-shaped
   (d) Long and cylindrical

8. How common are photosensitivity reactions with intravenous aciclovir administration?
   (a) Common or very common
   (b) Uncommon
   (c) Rare or very rare
   (d) Unheard of

Chapter 18 Antimicrobial Medications

9. What group are most at risk from complications arising from antifungal infections?
   (a) Children under 12
   (b) Young people
   (c) Immunocompromised CYP
   (d) CYP who have had their flu vaccine
10. What is the cause of a toxoplasmosis infection?
   (a) Bacteria
   (b) Virus
   (c) Fungus
   (d) Protozoa
11. Where is metronidazole metabolised?
   (a) The kidneys
   (b) The lower intestines
   (c) The liver
   (d) The stomach
12. What does antimicrobial stewardship involve?
   (a) Reducing unnecessary prescriptions of antimicrobials
   (b) Educating CYP and their parents/carers on the correct use of antimicrobials
   (c) Educating healthcare professionals on the correct use of antimicrobials
   (d) All of the above
13. Is antimicrobial resistance a problem in the current healthcare climate?
   (a) No, microorganisms are easily killed as long as we use the right antimicrobial
   (b) There are only a few resistant microorganisms in existing so this is not yet a problem for our current healthcare agenda
   (c) Yes, antimicrobial resistant infections are responsible for thousands of deaths each year and the problem is set to continue rising.
14. Which of the following could increase antimicrobial resistance?
   (a) A CYP taking antimicrobials which were not prescribed for them.
   (b) A CYP taking a prescribed antiviral to treat chickenpox.
   (c) A CYP completing the full course of their antimicrobial medication even after they start to feel better.
   (d) A CYP who takes paracetamol for their common cold virus.
15. Which of the following should the healthcare professional consider before prescribing an antibacterial medication?
   (a) The antibacterial sensitivity of the known organism
   (b) The CYP's ability to tolerate oral drugs
   (c) The CYP's renal function
   (d) All of the above

Find Out More

Below is a list of conditions addressed in this chapter. Take some time and write some notes about the treatment of each condition and be specific about the pharmacodynamics and possible side effects of the medicines that would be used to treat this.

THE CONDITION	YOUR NOTES
Bacterial meningitis	
Influenza A	
Thrush	
Toxoplasmosis	
Human immunodeficiency virus (HIV)	

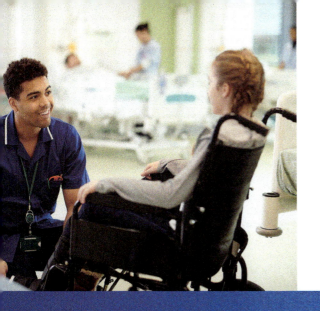

19

Adverse Drug Reactions

Claire Pryor and Carol Wills

Aim

This chapter will discuss what is meant by the term 'adverse drug reaction' (ADR), the mechanisms underpinning ADRs, and your role and responsibility in caring for children and young people (CYP) who may experience ADRs. This will be linked to your professional and regulatory codes of practice.

Learning Outcomes

By the end of this chapter, you will be able to:

- Understand what is meant by the term 'adverse drug reaction'
- Recognise how ADRs may present in children
- Demonstrate how to respond to ADRs appropriately for your scope of practice
- Understand some of the common pharmacological mechanisms underpinning ADRs

Test Your Knowledge

1. Are ADRs to immunisations always unexpected?
2. Is a ADR is also a type of adverse event?
3. What are two features of a type A ADR?
4. What are two features of a type B ADR?
5. What colour is the UK card system used to report adverse drug reactions?

Fundamentals of Pharmacology for Children's Nurses, First Edition. Edited by Ian Peate and Peter Dryden.
© 2022 John Wiley & Sons Ltd. Published 2022 by John Wiley & Sons Ltd.
Companion website: www.wiley.com/go/pharmacologyforCN

Introduction

Within all fields of healthcare, medication and medication administration form part of treatment plans and care optimisation. Medicines are given with the intention of having a beneficial effect. Unfortunately, medications can also produce unwanted or unexpected effects and reactions.

Each medication may have a range of potential adverse reactions, side effects or cause adverse events. The terminology can be confusing, and some phrases are often interchanged. As a healthcare professional, it is important that events, effects or actions are described, detailed and documented clearly to support effective communication and individualised care planning for the patient.

Additionally, it is also important that the healthcare professional has an awareness of what adverse drug reactions may look like, the required immediate care, but also follow-up care for both the CYP and also their family or carers.

Adverse reactions in CYP may not present in the same way as adults and the reactions may be different or not so well known. This can be due to differences in the drug's pharmacokinetics and less testing of drugs in CYP. Drugs being used which are not specifically licensed for paediatric use or the intended use for the child or young person's condition. 'Off-label' means a drug is being used for a condition or purpose not specified in its licence, at different doses to the licence, or in an age range not indicated in the licence; 'unlicensed use' is when a drug is not available with a licence for the intended use in this country but does elsewhere and is imported.

The term 'adverse drug reaction' (ADR) has had multiple definitions over the years, and inclusions of different components. These are often interchanged without explanation. Put simply, an ADR can mean a range of harm occurring from the use of medication (Rieder, 2017). That said, it is important to understand the different occurrences that may fall into the ADR bracket.

The World Health Organisation (WHO) defines an adverse reaction as:

a response to a medicine which is noxious and unintended, and which occurs at doses normally used in man

World Health Organisation, 2000

The European Medicines Agency further supports this definition, defining an adverse drug reaction as:

a response to a medicine which is noxious and unintended, and which occurs at doses normally used in man for the prophylaxis, diagnosis or treatment of disease or the modification of physiological function

European Medicines Agency, 2001

These definitions express clear relationships between the medication and the unwanted reaction to that medication.

In practice, this terminology can often be confused with adverse events.

Clinical Considerations

There are accepted risk factors for ADRs are common across the life span from birth to older age and some specifically shown to increase risk in children.

1. Previous reactions to other medicines
2. Polypharmacy (multiple medications in use)
3. Female gender
4. Extremities of age (i.e. very young or very old)
5. Reduced capacity of organs function impacting on medication excretion (renal and hepatic systems)
6. Drug doses used (larger)
7. Some genetic polymorphisms
8. General anaesthetic use
9. Off-label drug use

Source: Adapted from Rieder, 2012, 2017.

Adverse reactions are commonly termed adverse drug reactions (ADRs). The differentiation between the two terms is seen in the causal relationships and the dose indication. ADRs are noted to be directly linked to and caused by a specific medication when used at the intended dose. Adverse events happen during a treatment period. However, they may or may not be caused by medication (just happen in the same timeframe as a medication is being used). In addition, they may be caused by inappropriate dose schedule or other factors that do not relate to the pharmacology of the drug being given. As such, ADRs are classed as a type of adverse event (Schatz and Weber, 2015)

Adverse Events

An adverse event is defined as:

> any untoward medical occurrence that may appear during treatment with a pharmaceutical product but which does not necessarily have a causal relationship with the treatment
> **(World Health Organisation, 2002)**

The term 'adverse event' is a broad term that encompasses sensitivities, allergic reactions, outcomes from contraindicated medication being administered and adverse drug reactions.

Side Effects

Side effects are actions of the drug, often unwanted, but are known about, predictable, and patient education can be given to the patient and carers or patent prior to therapy commencement. Some medications are chosen specifically for their perceived beneficial side effect actions. An adverse drug reaction may happen immediately or evolve over a long period of time (Ferner and McGettin, 2018). It could simply be described as an unpleasant effect, or it could equally be life-threatening and require an urgent response to save the person's life. Patients may not associate their symptoms with a medication (Ferner and McGettin, 2018). As such, healthcare professionals must have an understanding of both the medication's desired effect, but also potential adverse effects and how to manage these within the scope of their practice. Side effects, contraindications and cautions for medicines can all be found using the British National Formulary for Children (BNFC) (print or online), the Electronic Medicines Compendium (EMC online) as well as accessing both patient information leaflets (PILs) or the summary of product characteristics (SmPCs). PILs are the leaflets that are included in the medication packets for patient use. This information is written specifically to increase patients' understanding of the medication they are taking. SmPCs are written specifically for healthcare professionals and details how the medication acts and how it is to be used. For more information about how to use such prescribing formularies and resources, please see Chapter 2.

Your professional body will determine your required and expected competence regarding medication administration and associated care.

- For nursing associates, this is Annex B, section 10 of the Standards of proficiency for nursing associates (Nursing and Midwifery Council, 2018b) which details procedural competencies required for administering medication safely. In applying knowledge of recognising and responding to adverse effects of medications, you will practice within: Platform 1 'Being an accountable professional', Platform 3 'Provide and monitor care', Platform 5 'Improving safety and quality of care' and specifically Annexe B 'Procedures to be undertaken by the nursing associate'
- Nurses must pay attention to accountability and safety in medicines administration and line with Annexe B section 11 of the standards of proficiency for registered nurses (Nursing and Midwifery Council, 2018a)
- Health and Care Professions Council (HCPC) registered professionals need to have a clear and current awareness of their profession's medicines entitlement (Health and Care Professions Council, 2020)

Clinical Consideration

An adverse drug reaction is harmful, occurs with a normal therapeutic dose and is not the response which was intended – it is directly linked to a medicine being used.

Chapter 19 Adverse Drug Reactions

Table 19.1 Classification of adverse drug reactions.

TYPE OF ADR	TITLE	FEATURES	EXAMPLE
A	Augmented	Reaction occurs at normal therapeutic drug dose Usually dose-dependent Can be an exaggeration of the drugs normal actions	Respiratory depression with opioids
B	Bizarre	Unexpected/novel reactions Not expected by the drug action Often allergic Medication induced disease	Rash with antibiotics Anaphylaxis
C	Continuing	Sometimes named 'chronic' Persists for a long duration	Potential for osteonecrosis of the jaw due to bisphosphonates
D	Delayed	Do not present initially Occur sometime after medication use Some are time-critical	Leucopenia presenting up to six weeks post lomustine (a chemotherapy drug) administration
E	End-of-use	Present after the drug has been stopped/withdrawn	Insomnia following benzodiazepine discontinuation

Source: Modified from Medicines and Healthcare Products Regulatory Agency, 2018.

ADRs can present with varied severity inclusive of minor, moderate, severe and fatal reactions. ADRs are categorised from A–E depending on both the nature of the reaction and the timescale. Table 19.1 details the full ADR classification system and gives examples using the guidance determined by the Medicines and Healthcare Products Regulatory Agency (Medicines and Healthcare Products Regulatory Agency, 2018). Most commonly, ADRs are categorised as type A or type B.

Type A reactions (augmented) are seen when a medication is given at the usual therapeutic dose, but the action of the drug is exaggerated. It is important to note that not only the desired action of the drug should be recognised, but also any known undesired actions. Augmented Reactions (Type A ADRs) are the most common type of reaction; in other words, they can be expected from what we know about the pharmacology of the drug and how it works. It is an exaggerated response which occurs with the normal therapeutic dose of the product. An example of this would be a person taking anti-coagulants to treat or prevent blood clots. Blood clots can be life-threatening and can cause a stroke so people susceptible to this may be prescribed an anticoagulant e.g. warfarin (warfarin sodium). These drugs work by making the blood take longer to clot (some call this thinning the blood) so the person would have frequent blood tests to ensure that the time the blood takes to clot are within safe and therapeutic limits. Expected side effects may include bruising from a relatively minor knock or upset stomach. A Type A reaction, however, would be sudden or severe internal bleeding as a result of taking a normal dose of the drug e.g. vomiting blood or passing blood in faeces. Some Type A adverse reactions can be minimised by reducing the dose of the drug (National Institute for Health and Care Excellence, 2017) so a referral back to the prescriber or health professional managing their care is indicated if this is suspected so that they may assess the nature and severity of the reaction and subsequent care.

Type B reactions ('bizarre') are reactions that are unexpected and not predicable in relation to the normal action of the drug ('novel'). These types of reactions are rare in comparison to Type A reactions, but they are life-threatening and need fast responses to prevent death. A Type B Reaction requires immediate recognition and treatment. These often present as allergic reactions such as skin rashes or anaphylaxis.

Preventing ADRs

Prevention of ADRS is paramount and involves all members of the CYP clinical team and parents/carers depending on their role. The principles of preventing ADRs include only using medication for which there us a good intention or need, ask about previous reactions to drugs and drug formulations, prescribe as few medications as possible and give clear instructions, use familiar medications and be alert for ADRS with new drugs, consider if additives (or excipients such as colouring agents) are appropriate or causing ADRs – consider alternative formulations, review medication history including over the counter drugs used, appreciate age-related hepatic (liver) or renal (kidney) disease, or development genetic considerations, and the effect on drug metabolism and excretion. Finally, always communicate with the child or young person, parent or carer if serious ADRs could occur (Paediatric Formulary Committee, 2020a)

Recognising ADRs

Practising in accordance with your regulatory body standards, healthcare professionals must be able to recognise the effects of medication as well as recognise allergies, drug sensitivity, side effects, contraindications, and adverse reactions.

A practical approach to ADRS is demonstrated in Table 19.2 and offers a practical approach to potential ADRs.

Primarily, Rieder's approach takes a measured and methodical process. Starting this process, clinicians need to be open to the idea that patient presentation could be underpinned by and ADR. Following this willingness to consider medication induced events, the clinician must perform a comprehensive history and assessment to gain a full picture of preceding events and action. Children or young people may not be able to clearly express their symptoms or understand what is happening, and therefore parental/guardian opinion may be required (Paediatric Formulary Committee, 2020b). With this information, the clinician then needs to analyse the information in line with up-to-date and reputable pharmaceutical information (see Chapter 2). The British National Formulary *for children* (BNFc), medication information sheets or online resources (such and TOXBASE or the electronic medicines compendium) will help in determining the likelihood of an ADR taking place.

If an ADR is determined, actions move to providing assistive and targeted care in keeping with the specific ADR and patient presentation. Concluding the approach is the aftermath. This is frequently overlooked (Rieder, 2012) but it is vital for safe and effective care of both the specific patient and also other medication users. Aftermath steps should include careful, clear contemporaneous documentation in patient records and appropriate communication with the wider team (General Practitioner for example), use of identification strategies (allergy wrist bands or alerts, for example), and discussions with the child, parents, or guardian. Education where appropriate, and appropriate reporting to regulatory bodies following local and national protocol (internal incident reporting and reporting to the Medicines and Healthcare products Regulatory Agency (MHRA)).

Clinical Consideration

ADRs can occur in any health or social care setting. As well hospital or clinic based care, you may be involved in caring for people in the wider community or social care setting: For example in patients' own homes following commencement of a new mediation by the General Practitioner, or reactions to vaccinations in clinic or in their own home. Community nursing teams who administer specific medications in people's own homes or community settings may carry emergency medication to treat severe reactions (such as anaphylaxis).

Table 19.2 The Five As of drug-induced adverse events.

Appreciation	*Could this be an ADR?*
Assessment	*What is the history of the event? What clinical tests or features are key? Timing and strength of medications.*
Analysis	*Differential diagnosis: drug/medication vs disease? (Is this actually an ADR?)*
Assistance	*Symptom relief, treatment, or considerations for the diagnosis. Interventions.*
Aftermath	*How does this effect future treatment? What is required now?*

Source: Adapted from Rieder, 2012, 2018.

No matter what area of care you are involved in, it is paramount that you consider this setting and are aware of the local policy and process for requesting support or emergency care.

Recognising ADRs may appear complex; however, a good understanding of the patient's condition, history and the pharmacokinetic and pharmacodynamic properties of the medicines they take will support timely recognition and appropriate action. As shown in Table 19.1 ADRs may not always present on first administration of medication, subsequent administrations may produce an ADR, or they may present after a considerable amount of time taking the medication. Vigilance in recognising signs or symptoms of potential ADRs is vital. It could be a change in skin colour, shortness of breath, a new skin rash, confusion or a report from a parent of the child or young person being non-specifically unwell, or an exaggeration of the desired effect that gives the first cue that an ADR may be present. Patients or parents may offer information to you during your interactions with them, and appropriate questioning and careful listening may glean important clues and details.

The history of taking specific medications, first dose or long-term treatment may assist in categorisation of ADR, additional medications including herbal, supplements or over the counter medications is essential as these too may produce ADRs and contribute to potential medication interactions for example.

Previous drug reactions are documented in the patient's notes and medication charts. This should be matched by a patient wristband (if clinical policy) that clearly identifies what medication has caused the reaction. It is vital that this information is checked and updated when a new reaction is identified.

Clinical Consideration

ADRs do not only occur in prescribed medication (prescription-only medicine or POM). They may be caused by medications bought from shops without any health professional guidance e.g. at a supermarket (known as General Sales List product or GSL) or following the guidance of a pharmacist (Pharmacist-only medication or P). Additionally, recreational drugs may cause ADRs, and more recently special attention has been placed on vape devices and e-cigarettes.

With the range of routes of administration available, it is essential that consideration is given to how adverse reactions could present. All healthcare professionals are accountable for their knowledge base and clinical competence, and as such should understand that both the mechanism of administration and the pharmaceutical properties of the medicine itself may cause adverse reactions.

Adverse reactions may present in a number of different ways: local presentations such as inflammation or irritation of the site of administration, systemic reactions due to the action of the medication, or more unspecified presentations which may not be easily identified as being due to the medication such delirium (a new change in awareness or attention: often called acute confusion) in an acutely unwell person, and following the commencement of a new medication.

Clinical Consideration

Adverse reactions may occur due to:

1. The action of the medication
2. The route of administration

Healthcare professionals must have an awareness of both to ensure safe and effective care.

ADRs and Immunisations

Immunisations may cause predictable ADRs and those delivering vaccine and immunisation care (see Chapter 13) must be aware of these, and the potential for unpredictable reactions as with any drug. These are classified as Adverse Events Following Immunisation (AEFIs) and have four categories: programme-related, vaccine-induced, coincidental and unknown (Public Health England, 2013). Common AEFIs include local reactions such as swelling or pain at injection site with systemic reactions including fever malaise and myalgia (to name a few) (Public Health England, 2013). It is paramount that healthcare professionals involved in any aspect of immunisation or vaccine care are aware of the specifics of the vaccines being used, understand the child or young person's overall health or medical conditions, and have appropriate training for their role and expectations in care provision. Following immunisations or vaccines patients should be observed for immediately presenting ARDs (Public Health England, 2013).

Whilst most AEFIs are mild and manageable, anaphylactic reactions may occur and have the potential to be fatal. Anaphylaxis is discussed later in this chapter.

Episode of Care

Daisy was an eight-year-old child with long-term underlying health conditions. She attended her GP practice for her annual Flu vaccine with her father. Daisy had received the vaccine every year previously for several years without complication. On attending the clinic, she was reviewed by the practice nurse and with her father's consent the vaccinations was administered.

Whilst sitting in the clinic post vaccination Daisy complained of increased pain at the injection site and an unusual hot sensation. The GP reviewed Daisy and found an unexpected skin reaction appeared to be present extending past the usual injection site. The GP, nurse, Daisy and her father agreed an appropriate course of care and management of the reaction and the practice nurse completed the MHRA Yellow Card report online using https://yellowcard.mhra.gov.uk/ this could have been completed via post using the cards in the BNFc.

To complete the form the nurse registered herself with the system before creating a report. The nurse ensured that this was sent to the GP using the MHRA system and updated Daisy's records indicating a suspected ADR had occurred. The GP and nurse talked with Daisy and her father to explain the reaction and gave advise about home care and subsequent vaccinations. Daisey was observed in the clinic for a time period before being reviewed again by the GP and allowed home in her father's care.

Allergic Reactions

Allergic reactions have both patient- and drug-related risk factors. Having an awareness of medication sensitivities and allergic reactions is vital when providing patient care. Allergies or hypersensitivity occurs due to the body recognising a usually harmless antigen (such as a drug or pollen) and harmful. The immune system over produces antibodies to the antigen in an attempt to protect the body (Carne and Owen, 2019). A severe allergic reaction is caused by a person being exposed to a drug for a second time and which their body has already produced antibodies against. The second exposure triggers an immediate response by the antibodies and mast cells which flood a range of chemicals including histamine, into the bloodstream and tissues (Carne and Owen, 2019). This can occur with any medicine (or indeed non-medicine e.g. food allergy or bee-sting) and so it is extremely important to check for allergies and ensure that any allergies are recorded in the patient notes.

An allergic reaction may be immediate, or it may take hours. In an anaphylactic reaction this can be within 5 to 60 minutes of the allergen being taken (depending on the route).

Anaphylaxis

Anaphylaxis is a type of allergic reaction. The Resuscitation Council defines Anaphylaxis as:

A severe, life-threatening, generalised or systemic hypersensitivity reaction

(Resuscitation Council UK, 2008)

An anaphylactic reaction can result as a hypersensitivity or a severe allergic reaction and is a medical emergency.

A diagnosis of anaphylactic reaction is likely if a patient who is exposed to a trigger (allergen) unexpectedly develops a sudden illness (usually within minutes of exposure) with rapidly progressing skin changes and life-threatening airway and/or breathing and/or circulation problems (Resuscitation Council UK, 2008: 13). The

CYP will feel and look unwell and can become very anxious. Rapid in onset, anaphylaxis may present with (Resuscitation Council UK, 2008; National Institute for Health and Care Excellence, 2011):

- Airway compromise and/or
- Difficulty in breathing (bronchospasm with tachypnoea) and/or
- Skin and mucosal changes and/or
- Problems with the circulatory processes (hypotension and/or tachycardia)

However, a definitive list of all features, always present is not feasible as the reaction may vary.

Drugs such as non-steroidal anti-inflammatory drugs (NSAIDs) and antibiotics are common causes of anaphylaxis in children (Cardinale et al., 2019). Other common causes of anaphylactic reactions include environmental agents such as stings from insects, contact with latex or hair dye, food and nut allergies (Pumphreys, 2004).

To reiterate, anaphylactic reactions present suddenly and have a rapid progression over several minutes. The patient may visibly appear unwell or report feeling unwell and be anxious. The Resuscitation Council UK (2008) stipulate that three criteria indicate that an anaphylactic reaction is present:

1. Sudden onset with rapid progression
2. Life-threatening compromise of airway, and/or breathing, and/or circulation
3. Finally skin or mucosal changes

and advocate an ABCDE approach to recognition and management (Resuscitation Council UK, 2008).

The airway, breathing and circulation (ABC) compromise may present as difficulty in breathing due to airway swelling (throat or tongue oedema) or stridor (a high-pitched noise heard on inspiration). Importantly, the CYP may self-report feeling as if their throat is closing, or have a hoarse voice (Resuscitation Council UK, 2008). Compromised breathing may be signalled by shortness of breath, wheeze or increased respiratory rate (tachypnoea) and may resemble life-threatening asthma in children. The shortness of breath and an increased respiratory rate may result in tiredness and ultimately lead to cyanosis and respiratory arrest.

Circulatory issues may present as pale clammy skin (indicating shock), hypotension (low blood pressure) and tachycardia (increased pule rate). The patient may have a change in consciousness or lose consciousness due to circulatory compromise; and ultimately a slowing of the pulse leading to cardiac arrest.

As noted previously, both respiratory or cardiac arrest may occur (Resuscitation Council UK, 2008) due to a compromised airway (A), breathing (B) and circulation (C). Disability (D) may relate to an altered neurological state (confusion, agitation, loss of consciousness and so on) due to decreased brain perfusion or gastrointestinal issues such as pain, vomiting or incontinence. Through exposure (E) skin and mucosal changes may be evident, and often are the first indication of a reaction occurring.

Skin and mucosal changes can be subtle or dramatic such as flushing of the skin, itchy hives or welts (urticaria) or a deeper reaction causing swelling of the tissues commonly eyelids, lips and mouth or throat (angiooedema) and a patchy or red rash (erythema), important criteria to support the diagnosis. Such skin and mucosal signals are present in over 80% of anaphylactic reactions and often the first notable feature. It is important to remember, however, that skin reactions without the life-threatening ABC problems do not signify an anaphylactic reaction.

The Resuscitation Council (UK) anaphylaxis algorithm is presented in Figure 19.1. Offering a clear process for emergency management, healthcare professionals must ensure that they work within their scope of practice, confidence, and competence at all times.

Clinical Consideration

Anaphylaxis is a serious and life-threatening allergic reaction. It is rapid in onset and presents with compromise to airway, breathing and circulation. In addition, mucosal and skin changes are often present. All patients irrespective of clinical setting should expect:

- Recognition that they are severely unwell
- A prompt and early request for assistance
- Assessment and treatment following the ABCDE process
- Adrenaline therapy if indicated (adrenaline is also known as epinephrine)
- Referral and follow-up by an allergy specialist

Source: Modified from Resuscitation Council UK, 2008.

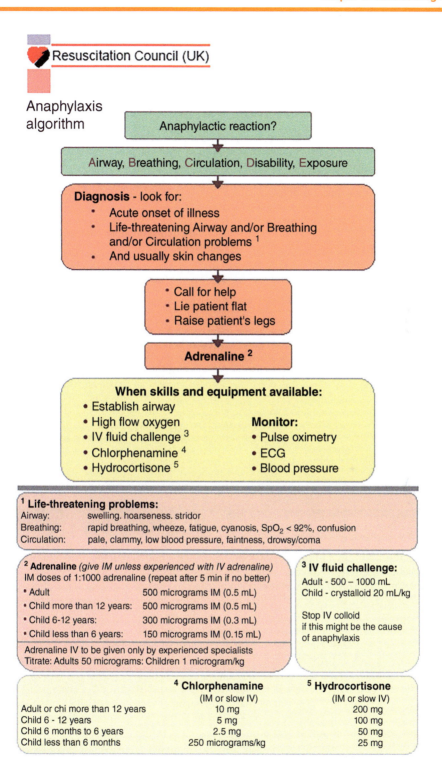

Figure 19.1 **Anaphylaxis algorithm.** Resuscitation Council UK, 2008/Elsevier.

Chapter 19 Adverse Drug Reactions

As Figure 19.1 shows, the management of anaphylaxis for children, young people and adults is the same in principle and practice, with changes occurring only in drug dosing and fluid administration. It is paramount that the clinical team pay attention to these variations.

Clinical Consideration

Anaphylaxis is a serious and life-threatening allergic reaction. The person or parent/carer of someone who has had an anaphylaxis reaction may experience anxiety because of fear of subsequent reactions. Important factors for supporting someone with a history of anaphylaxis include:

1. Information about what anaphylaxis is
2. Information on what the trigger allergen is
3. Appropriate management strategy education for anaphylaxis
4. Appropriate referral to allergy specialists
5. Follow-up provision of support and guidance. This should be tailored to the individual and always follow the advice of the medical or specialist clinical teams.

Episode of Care

Jacob is a 17-year-old admitted to the surgical unit for planned day surgery. The admitting nurse welcomed him and confirmed his name, date of birth and the reason for his admission. During Jacob's admission process the nurse asked him about his past medical history, medication he took (including prescribed, over the counter, herbal/supplements and recreational drugs). Jacob reported having an allergic reaction to penicillin when he was a small child. This presented with a skin rash and vomiting. The nurse checked the Trust policy regarding patient identification bands as he was aware different Trusts had different systems. Following the policy, the nurse ensured that he gave Jacob an identity band that included his demographic details, and an additional red allergy band that detailed the type of drug Jacob was allergic to. The nurse then ensured that the medical and nursing notes were updated with this information and ensured that the team was aware of this information.

Medicines Safety and Reporting ADRs

Prior to being authorised with a product licence (or marketing authorising), the product must have undergone clinical trials to demonstrate its effectiveness and safety profile. The safety profile will detail the types of reactions, contraindications and cautions identified within the clinical trial data. This offers practitioners information about what is to be expected from the product. A limitation of this, however, is that clinical trials are undertaken on a very select group of people, e.g. a specific age range or people with a specific condition. It is not until there is more widespread use of the product that we then begin to find out how some people may react to the product or how it may interact with other drugs or new reactions etc that may not have been identified. These new products (or sometimes old products with a new use or ingredient) are assigned a black triangle (see the BNFc) to warn health professionals that the product is new and that all suspected adverse reactions must be reported to the MHRA. This information is then used to build the safety profile further and identify any risks associated with the product (pharmacovigilance) and consider whether they are common, rare, serious etc. The MHRA will consider the potential risks to the patient if not treated with the medication and the risk associated with the side effects of the medication. Health professionals are then alerted to any identified risks through safety alert systems, drug leaflets and medicine formularies such as the BNFc. The MHRA work collaboratively with the European Medicines Agency and the World Health Organisation so that all drug safety data is monitored and shared.

The MHRA is responsible for ensuring that quality and efficiency is maintained, and also providing education and up-to-date information for healthcare professionals and the public on the safety of medicine and devices. The MHRA collects information and reports regarding ADRs to influence regulatory frameworks, ensuring any risk associated with a medicine or device is proportionate and effective.

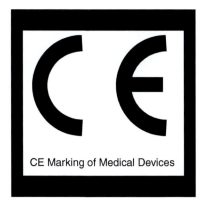

Figure 19.2 CE mark of approved devices.

The MHRA accepts reports from all healthcare professionals and self-reports from patients or consumers of products. Information collected relates to side effects (or ADRs), medical device adverse incidents, defective medicines, counterfeit or fake medication or devices and from 2016 the MHRA started collecting information on ADRs in relation to e-cigarettes (Medicines and Healthcare Products Regulatory Agency, 2019). The MHRA also collect information about devices such as thermometers, instructions for use, wheelchairs and condoms. Medical approved devises carry CE mark (Figure 19.2) to show it has reached the approved requirements as outlined by the MHRA (Medicines and Healthcare Products Regulatory Agency, 2015a).

Episode of Care

Kevin is a 13-year-old boy who has attended Accident and Emergency with his foster carer after having a suspected anaphylactic reaction in a restaurant. Kevin has not had a previous anaphylaxis and no known allergies. His foster carer called an ambulance and he was treated initially in the restaurant. This treatment included the administration of adrenaline before being transferred to hospital.

Following emergency care and treatment, the medical team referred Kevin to a specialist allergy service. This was to ensure that the correct treatment plan could be made for Kevin in partnership with his foster carer and also to support and educate them about anaphylaxis. Before Kevin was discharged from Accident and Emergency, he was prescribed an adrenaline auto-injector pen and both himself and his carer were given training in its use. This included information about what anaphylaxis is, signs and symptoms of anaphylaxis, being shown how to use the injector pen, practising using a training injector pen and being provided with information about how and when to use it. This allowed Kevin and his carer to feel able to manage any potential reactions whilst awaiting specialist assessment.

Full and contemporaneous documentation was made, and all relevant health professionals informed of this occurrence (including his GP).

Reporting ADRs via The Yellow Card System

All healthcare professionals have a responsibility for reporting suspected ADRs, be able to recognise and respond to adverse or abnormal reactions to medications within their scope of practice. As such you need to know when and how to escalate any concerns around ADRs and how to take appropriate action. Reporting ADRs may include both professional and organisational systems (such as employer internal systems following employer policy as well as using the yellow card system). The Yellow Card Scheme is the medicines safety monitoring system in the UK and is operated by the Medicines and Healthcare products Regulatory Agency (MHRA), who govern the licensing of medicines and medical devices in the UK.

Chapter 19 Adverse Drug Reactions

Clinical Consideration

- The *yellow card system* is the UK medicines safety monitoring system.
- This is different to the British Paediatric Surveillance Unit *orange card scheme*
- **Even if a suspected ADR has been reported to the BPSU it should still be reported using to the MHRA using the yellow card system.**

It is considered good practice for healthcare professionals to report any suspected ADRs or incidents to the MHRA using the yellow card scheme. This facilitates accurate reporting and recognition of ADRs both known and new in relation to medicines, interactions between medicines and medical devices. Reporting can take place using hard copies of the yellow cards found at the back of print version of the BNFC, online via https://yellowcard.mhra.gov.uk/ or through the yellow card mobile app.

Reporting ADRs in children and neonates is vitally important as (as discussed previously) pharmacolites of a drug may differ in children to adults, drugs may have not been tested extensively in children, 'off-label' use or licensing complexity may be present, some drugs may effect a child's growth or development (consider delayed ADRs which are not present in adults) and there is dose/formulation and illness presentation complexity (Paediatric Formulary Committee, 2020a)

The yellow card has four distinct sections which are critical for accurate reporting. It is asked that as much information as possible is provided. The MHRA request information (if known) in relation to:

1. The suspect drug
   - Administration route
   - Dose information, including frequency and daily dose
   - Date/dates of administration
   - Brand and batch number if the ADR relates to a vaccine
2. The suspect reaction
   - When the suspect reaction happened
   - The severity of reaction
   - Treatment administered
   - Reaction outcome
3. Patient information
   - Sex of patient
   - Age when reaction occurred
   - Weight
   - Patient initials and identification number.

      The MHRA requests at least one piece of information from section 3 and note that requesting the patient's initials and identification number does not breach any confidentiality agreement between the patient ad healthcare provider (Medicines and Healthcare Products Regulatory Agency, 2015b).

4. Details of the reporting individual
   - Name and address should be provided for receipt of the report, future contact or follow-up

In addition to these four criteria, additional information may be provided including any medicines taken in the past three months including prescription medicines and those bought over the counter, medical history and known allergies, any pertinent test results, drugs taken during pregnancy (if applicable) and any congenital abnormalities and date of last menstrual period (if applicable) and any re-challenge of the medicine (Medicines and Healthcare Products Regulatory Agency, 2015b)

A medicine de-challenge and re-challenge test (re-exposure test) is when a practitioner reintroduces a medicine that has previously caused a reaction in a patient (Meyboom, 2013). Or it may be that medications are removed (de-challenge) and are not reintroduced. The aim of these tests is to establish causality (i.e. is it the drug causing the reaction (ADR) or has a reaction occurred during treatment, but not caused by the drug (Marante, 2018)) or to obtain information knowledge that may benefit future patients or to establish patient tolerance at a lower dose (Meyboom, 2013).

It is paramount to note here that such challenges may pose significant and life-threatening danger to patients and should only be conducted by appropriately trained practitioners under strict regulation and guidance.

In addition, if it is unclear whether someone else has reported the ADR it is advisable to send an additional yellow card, or if new information is available. The MHRA will collate the reports and omit any duplication of information (Medicines and Healthcare Products Regulatory Agency, 2015b). It is recommended that a copy of the completed yellow card should be included in the patent's notes to ensure accurate documentation and future reference.

Clinical Consideration

All healthcare professionals have a part to play in recognising, responding to and reporting adverse drug reactions and any concerns relating to drugs or medical devises. This must be in line with the employer's policy, role and responsibilities. The MHRA yellow card scheme supports reporting and investigation of concerns and suspected issues or incidents. These are inclusive of

1. ADRs
2. Incidents where a medical device was involved
3. Medicines of poor quality (defective)
4. Fake medication or devices
5. Safety information or concern regarding e-cigarettes and refill devices

   Modes of reporting can be through

1. Hard copy yellow cards as found in the print version of the BNF
2. Online via https://yellowcard.mhra.gov.uk/
3. Using the yellow card mobile app

Conclusion

This chapter has introduced and defined what adverse drug reactions are, how they can be prevented, their presentation and your role in suspecting, treating and reporting of ADRS. Specific focus has been placed on children and young people and how ARDs can be the same or differ to adults. As a healthcare professional, your practice needs to align to your professional regulations and your job requirements.

References

Cardinale, F., Amato, D., Felicia, M., et al. (2019). Drug-induced anaphylaxis in children, *Acta Biomedica* 30–35.

Carne, E. and Owen, N. (2019). Care of the adult with an immunological condition. In: *Essentials of Nursing Adults* (ed. Elcock, K., Wright, W., Newcombe, P., and Everett, F). London: Sage.

European Medicines Agency (2001). Directive 2001/83/EC of the European Parliament and of the Council of November 2001 On the Community Code Relating to Medicinal Products for Human Use. *Official Journal L* 311 28/11/2001: 67–128.

Ferner, R. and McGettin, P. (2018). Adverse drug reactions. *The British Medical Journal*, 363.

Health and Care Professions Council (2020). *Sale, Supply and Administration of Medicines*: Health and Care Professions Council. www.hcpc-uk.org/about-us/what-we-do/medicine-entitlements/sale-supply-and-administration-of-medicines/ (accessed 13 July 2020).

Marante, K. (2018). The challenges or adverse drug reaction evaluation. *Journal of Pharmacovigilance* 6(3).

Medicines and Healthcare Products Regulatory Agency (2015a) *Medicinal Devices: Conformity Assessment and the CE Mark*: Medicines and Healthcare Products Regulatory Agency. www.gov.uk/guidance/medical-devices-conformity-assessment-and-the-ce-mark (accessed 15 July 2020).

Medicines and Healthcare Products Regulatory Agency (2015b) *What to include in your yellow card of an adverse drug reaction*. https://assets.publishing.service.gov.uk/government/uploads/system/uploads/attachment_data/file/404416/What_to_include_in_your_Yellow_Card_of_an_adverse_drug_reaction.pdf (accessed 12 October 2019).

Medicines and Healthcare Products Regulatory Agency (2018). *Guidance on adverse drug reactions: classification of adverse drug reactions*: Medications and Healthcare products Regulatory Agency. https://assets.publishing.service.gov.uk/government/uploads/system/uploads/attachment_data/file/752688/Guidance_on_adverse_drug_reactions.pdf (accessed 12 October 2019).

Medicines and Healthcare Products Regulatory Agency (2019). *Yellow Card: about yellow card*. https://yellowcard.mhra.gov.uk/the-yellow-card-scheme/ (accessed 15 October 2019).

Meyboom, R. (2013). Intentional rechallenge and the clinical management of drug-related problems. *Drug Safety* 36(3): 163–165.

National Institute for Health and Care Excellence (2011). *Anaphylaxis: Assessment and Referral after Emergency Treatment*. National Institute for Health and Care Excellence.

National Institute for Health and Care Excellence (2017). *Adverse drug reactions*. https://cks.nice.org.uk/adverse-drug-reactions (accessed 16 October 2019).

Nursing and Midwifery Council (2018a) *Future Nurse: Standards of Proficiency for Registered Nurses*, London: Nursing and Midwifery Council.

Nursing and Midwifery Council (2018b) *Standards of proficiency for nursing associates*: Nursing and Midwifery Council. www.nmc.org.uk/standards/code/ (accessed 20 September 2019).

Paediatric Formulary Committee (2020a) *British National Formulary for Children Adverse Reactions to Drugs* London: BMJ Group, Pharmaceutical Press, and RCPCH Publications. https://bnfc.nice.org.uk/guidance/adverse-reactions-to-drugs.html (accessed 14 July 2020).

Paediatric Formulary Committee (2020b) *British National Formulary for Children Adverse Reactions to Drugs: Special Problems*: London: BMJ Group, Pharmaceutical Press, and RCPCH Publications. https://bnf.nice.org.uk/about/frequently-asked-questions-for-the-bnf-and-bnf-for-children-bnfcgeneral.html (accessed 2 June 2020).

Public Health England (2013). *Immunisation Against Infectious Disease*. London: Public Health England.

Pumphreys, R. (2004). Fatal anaphylaxis in the UK: 1992–2001. *Novartis Foundation Symposia* 257(257): 116–128.

Resuscitation Council UK (2008). Emergency treatment of anaphylactic reactions: Guidance for healthcare providers.

Rieder, M. (2012). Novel approaches to adverse drug reactions in children, *Pediatric Clinics of North America* 59: 1001–1004.

Rieder, M. (2017). Adverse drug reactions in children: pediatric pharmacy and drug safety. *Journal of Pediatric Pharmacology and Therapeutics* 1: 4–9.

Rieder, M. (2018) Adverse drug reactions across the age continuum: epidemiology, diagnostic challenges, prevention and treatments. *The Journal of Clinical Pharmacology* 58: S36–S47.

Schatz, S. and Weber, R. (2015). Adverse drug reactions. *American Collage of Clinical Pharmacology* Pharmacology Self Assessment Program (PSAP): 5–26.

World Health Organisation (2000). *Safety Monitoring of Medicinal Products. Guidelines for Setting Up and Running a Pharmacovigilance Centre*. London: World Health Organisation.

World Health Organisation (2002). *The Importance of Pharmacovigilance: Safety Monitoring of Medicinal Products*. Geneva: World Health Organisation.

Further Resources

The Green Book Public Health England (2013) *Immunisation Against Infectious Disease*. London: Public Health England. Available at: www.gov.uk/government/collections/immunisation-against-infectious-disease-the-green-book

National Institute for Health and Care Excellence (2017) *Adverse drug reactions*. Available at: https://cks.nice.org.uk/adverse-drug-reactions

National Institute for Health and Care Excellence (2016) Anaphylaxis Quality standard [QS119] Available at: www.nice.org.uk/guidance/qs119

Resuscitation Council UK (2008). Emergency treatment of anaphylactic reactions: Guidance for healthcare providers. Resuscitation Council UK.

Multiple Choice Questions

1. What is a type C ADR?
 (a) Caution
 (b) Continuing
 (c) Critical
 (d) Common

2. Adverse reactions may occur due to:
   (a) The action of the medication
   (b) The route of administration
   (c) Both
3. What differentiates an adverse drug reaction from an adverse event?
   (a) The reaction happens during therapy with medication but may not be caused by the medication
   (b) The reaction is caused by the medication
4. ADRs can be
   (a) Mild or moderate
   (b) Moderate or severe
   (c) Severe
   (d) Mild, moderate or severe
5. What is a type D ADR?
   (a) Detrimental
   (b) Delayed
   (c) Damaging
   (d) Deferred
6. ADRs always occur on first administration of the drug. True or false?
   (a) True
   (b) False
7. ADRs only occur in prescription-only medicines. True or false?
   (a) True
   (b) False
8. Risk factors for allergic reactions relate to
   (a) Patient risk factors
   (b) Patient and drug risk factors
   (c) Drug risk factors
9. How many key features does anaphylaxis have?
   (a) 3
   (b) 4
   (c) 2
10. The yellow card scheme supports reporting via which systems?
    (a) Online
    (b) Paper
    (c) Mobile application
    (d) All of the above
11. Only paper copies of yellow cards are available for ADR reporting. True or false?
    (a) True
    (b) False
12. The yellow and orange card schemes are the same. True or false?
    (a) True
    (b) False
13. Following the approach outlined by Rieder – how many As are there when considering ADRs?
    (a) 4
    (b) 6
    (c) 5
    (d) 7
14. One of these As is anaphylaxis. True or false?
    (a) True
    (b) False
15. Anyone can report ADRs using the yellow cards. True or false?
    (a) True
    (b) False

Answers

Chapter 1

1. c; **2.** d; **3.** b; **4.** c; **5.** b; **6** c; **7.** b; **8.** a; **9.** a; **10.** b; **11.** c; **12.** d; **13.** c; **14.** d; **15.** b

Chapter 2

1. c; **2.** a; **3.** a; **4.** b; **5.** c; **6.** b; **7.** d; **8.** c; **9.** b; **10.** a; **11.** c; **12.** c; **13.** c; **14.** b; **15.** c

Chapter 3

1. b; **2.** c; **3.** c; **4.** a; **5.** d; **6.** d; **7.** a; **8.** c; **9.** c; **10.** a; **11.** b; **12.** d; **13.** d; **14.** d; **15.** d

Chapter 4

1. a; **2.** b; **3.** b; **4.** a; **5.** e; **6.** d; **7.** d; **8.** b; **9.** a; **10.** f; **11.** b; **12.** d; **13.** b; **14.** a; **15.** a

Chapter 5

1. a; **2.** a; **3.** e; **4.** b; **5.** a; **6.** d; **7.** b; **8.** d; **9.** a; **10.** a; **11.** c; **12.** a; **13.** c; **14.** a; **15.** b

Chapter 6

1. c; **2.** d; **3.** c; **4.** a; **5.** b; **6.** d; **7.** d; **8.** c; **9.** a; **10.** a; **11.** c; **12.** b; **13.** b; **14.** d; **15.** a

Chapter 7

1. a; **2.** c; **3.** b; **4.** d; **5.** a; **6.** a; **7.** b; **8.** c; **9.** a; **10.** c; **11.** b; **12.** d; **13.** a; **14.** b; **15.** b

Fundamentals of Pharmacology for Children's Nurses, First Edition. Edited by Ian Peate and Peter Dryden.
© 2022 John Wiley & Sons Ltd. Published 2022 by John Wiley & Sons Ltd.
Companion website: www.wiley.com/go/pharmacologyforCN

Chapter 8

1. c; **2.** b; **3.** a; **4.** c; **5.** a; **6.** d; **7.** a; **8.** c; **9.** a; **10.** b; **11.** b; **12.** b; **13.** a; **14.** b; **15.** c

Chapter 9

1. c; **2.** c; **3.** c; **4.** a; **5.** b; **6.** c; **7.** b; **8.** a; **9.** a; **10.** b; **11.** a; **12.** b; **13.** a; **14.** a; **15.** a, c

Chapter 10

1. a, c, d; **2.** b; **3.** d; **4.** b; **5.** c; **6.** b; **7.** b; **8.** e; **9.** c; **10.** b; **11.** b, c, d; **12.** c; **13.** c; **14.** a; **15.** c

Chapter 11

1. c; **2.** b; **3.** c; **4.** a; **5.** b; **6.** a; **7.** c; **8.** d; **9.** b; **10.** a; **11.** b; **12.** c; **13.** b; **14.** a; **15.** a

Chapter 12

1. c; **2.** b; **3.** b; **4.** d; **5.** a; **6.** c; **7.** a; **8.** d; **9.** c; **10.** b; **11.** a; **12.** a; **13.** c; **14.** b; **15.** c

Chapter 13

1. b; **2.** c; **3.** d; **4.** a; **5.** b; **6.** a; **7.** b; **8.** c; **9.** d; **10.** a; **11.** d; **12.** b; **13.** c; **14.** d; **15.** b

Chapter 14

1. b; **2.** d; **3.** a; **4.** d; **5.** c; **6.** a; **7.** d; **8.** c; **9.** b; **10.** a; **11.** d; **12.** c; **13.** d; **14.** a; **15.** a

Chapter 15

1. d; **2.** a; **3.** c; **4.** c; **5.** a; **6.** c; **7.** b; **8.** c; **9.** d; **10.** d; **11.** a; **12.** b; **13.** a; **14.** b; **15.** a

Chapter 16

1. c; **2.** a; **3.** a; **4.** d; **5.** c; **6.** b; **7.** a; **8.** c; **9.** b; **10.** d; **11.** a; **12.** c; **13.** d; **14.** a; **15.** c

Chapter 17

1. c; **2.** a; **3.** c; **4.** b; **5.** d; **6.** a; **7.** c; **8.** b; **9.** d; **10.** d; **11.** c; **12.** d; **13.** d; **14.** a; **15.** a

Chapter 18

1. d; **2.** b; **3.** b; **4.** c; **5.** a; **6.** b; **7.** d; **8.** a; **9.** c; **10.** d; **11.** c; **12.** d; **13.** c; **14.** a; **15.** d

Chapter 19

1. a; **2.** c; **3.** b; **4.** d; **5.** b; **6.** b; **7.** b; **8.** b; **9.** a; **10.** d; **11.** b; **12.** b; **13.** c; **14.** b; **15.** a

Index

absorption, 281
  cell membrane, drug crossing, 72–73
  defined, 71
  factors affecting, 75
absorption, distribution, metabolism and excretion
  (ADME) of drugs, 70, 79–80
  flucloxacillin, 261
  warfarin *versus* aspirin, 113
Academic Education Institutions (AEIs), 51
acetylcysteine, 188
Aciclovir, 355
acid-base balance, 138
acitretin, 269–270
acquired immunity, 242, 243
activating tissue invasion, 294
active acquired immunity, 242
active immunotherapy, 302
active transport, 73
Act of Parliament *see* Statute Law
acute asthma, management of, 176
acute inflammatory demyelinating
  polyradiculoneuropathy (AIDP), 228
acute kidney injury (AKI), 130
acute pain, 320
adjuvants, 244, 333
adolescents, 9–10
adoptive cell transfer (ACT), 304–306
ADR *see* adverse drug reaction (ADR)
adrenal glands disorders, medication in, 162–165
adrenaline (epinephrine), 119–121
adrenoceptor agonists, 182
adverse drug reaction (ADR), 368
  adverse events, 369
  allergic reactions, 373
  anaphylaxis, 373–376
  CE mark of approved devices, 377
  classification of, 370
  and immunisations, 372–373
  medicines safety and reporting, 376–377
  preventing, 370–371
  recognising, 371–372
  side effects, 369–370
  Type A reactions, 370
  Type B reactions, 370

Yellow Card Scheme, 377–379
adverse events, 369
Adverse Events Following Immunisation (AEFIs), 372
air pressure needle free devices, 157
airway, breathing and circulation (ABC), 374
alkylating drugs, 297, 298
allergic reactions, 373
allergic rhinitis, 185
alpha-adrenergic blockers, 114
alpha blockers (AB), 114
Alport syndrome, 136
aminoglycosides, 348, 349
aminophylline, 84, 185, 186
aminosalicylates, 213
amiodarone, 116–117
amitriptyline hydrochloride, 232
amoxicillin, 100, 178
analgesics *see* pain
anaphylaxis, 250–251, 373–376
angiogenesis, 294
angiotensin converting enzyme (ACE) inhibitors, 113, 143, 144
angiotensin II, 143
Angiotensin II Receptor Antagonists (A2RA), 114
antagonists, 83
anthracyclines, 298–299
anti-androgenic drugs, 161
antibacterial medications, 345–351
antibiotics
  for cystic fibrosis, 179
  impetigo, 261
  for respiratory disorders, 187–188
anticoagulant medications, 112–113
  aspirin, 112, 113
  warfarin, 112–113
antidepressant discontinuation symptoms, 284
antidepressant-related hyponatraemia, 283
antidepressants, 232–233, 280–284
  adverse effects from, 282–284
  antidepressant withdrawal, 284
  considerations with, 282
  hyponatraemia, 283
  serotonin and noradrenaline reuptake inhibitors
    (SNRIs), 282
  serotonin syndrome, 283

Fundamentals of Pharmacology for Children's Nurses, First Edition. Edited by Ian Peate and Peter Dryden.
© 2022 John Wiley & Sons Ltd. Published 2022 by John Wiley & Sons Ltd.
Companion website: www.wiley.com/go/pharmacologyforCN

388 Index

antidepressant withdrawal, 284
antidiuretic effect, 123
antidiuretic hormone (ADH), 123
antidysrhythmic drugs, 114–117
  amiodarone, 116–117
  atenolol, 116
  diltiazem, 117
  labetalol, 116
  lidocaine, 115
  metoprolol, 116
  propafenone, 115
  quinidine, 115
  sotalol hydrochloride, 116–117
  verapamil, 117
antiemetic, 231
antiepileptic drugs (AEDs), 222–223
  for epilepsy, 222–223, 238–240
  for migraine, 232
antifungal medications, 354–357
  azoles, 356
  echinocandins, 357
  polyenes, 357
anti-herpes medications, 352, 353
anti-influenza medications, 354
antimalarials, 358, 359
antimetabolites, 297–298
antimicrobial medications
  antibacterial medications, 345–351
  antifungal medications, 354–357
  antimicrobial education, for patients and their parents/
    carers, 361–362
  antimicrobial resistance, 359–361
  antimicrobial stewardship, 360–362
  antiprotozoal medications, 357–359
  antiviral medications, 351–354
  microorganisms, 344–345
  prescribing, 362
antimicrobial resistance, 359–361
antimicrobial stewardship, 360–362
antimuscarinic bronchodilators, 182
antiprotozoal medications, 357–359
antipsychotics, 284–285
anti-retrovirus medications, 352–353
anti TFN-a antibody treatment, 213
antiviral medications, 351–354
  anti-herpes medications, 352, 353
  anti-influenza medications, 354
  anti-retrovirus medications, 352–353
  non-selective antivirals, 354
anxiety, 108
  antidepressants for, 277–278
  anxiolytics, 277
  medication for, 276–278
anxiolytics, 277
aripiprazole, 284–285
aromatase inhibitors, 161
arrythmia, 115
aspirin, 112, 113
asthma, 175–177, 185
  acute asthma, management of, 176

  caused by, 175
  classes of medication, 175
  inhalers for, 175
  self-management education, 175
atenolol, 23, 116
atopic dermatitis *see* eczema
atopic eczema, 264–265
atorvastatin, 111
atropine sulfate, 121
Attention Deficit Disorder (ADD), 278
Attention Deficit/Hyperactivity Disorder (ADHD)
  non-stimulant medication, 279
  stimulant medications, 278
augmented reactions, 370
autistic spectrum disorder (ASD), 280
autonomy, 39, 40
Aveeno Cream for dermatitis, 22
azathioprine, 55
azithromycin, 187
azoles, 356

babies, considerations for, 7
bacteria, 345, 346
B cells, 242
BCG vaccine, 248
behavioural adverse events (BAEs), 224
beneficence, 38
benign intracranial hypertension (BIH), 156
benzodiazepines, 226, 227, 277
beta-adrenergic receptors, 116
beta agonists, 83, 184
beta blockers (BB), 116, 122
  contraindications of, 116
  for migraine, 231
  sub-classifications of, 117
bicarbonate supplements, 139, 142–143
bioavailability, 78, 231
biologic therapies, 270
biotransformation, 76–78
bipolar disorder, 285
blood–brain barrier (BBB), 75
blood pressure monitoring, 145
Bolam test, 35–36
bone marrow transplants (BMT), 304, 306
botulinum toxin, 233
branded and generic drugs, 223
breast milk, 75–76
British Heart Foundation (BHF), 108
British National Formulary (BNF), 19, 76, 77
British National Formulary for Children (BNFc), 18, 59
  back matter of, 22
  borderline substances, 22
  cautionary and advisory labels for dispensed
    medication, 23
  chapters, 20
  conversions and abbreviations, 23
  emergency care protocols, 23
  front matter, 20
  interactions, 22
  online and mobile application, 23–24

text format and information purpose, 20
units, 23
British Society for Paediatric Endocrinology and
    Diabetes (BSPED), 159
brivaracetam (BRV), 224
bronchiolitis, 178
bronchodilation, 119
bronchodilators, 175, 182, 184–185
    adrenoceptor agonists, 182
    antimuscarinic bronchodilators, 182
    leukotrienes, 182, 185
    xanthines, 185–186
buccal formulations, 93
buccal lorazepam, 226, 227
buccal midazolam, 226
Buccolam (midazolam), 93

caecum, 199
calcineurin inhibitors, 136–138
calcipotriol, 268
calcium, 137
calcium channel blockers (CCB), 117, 231–232
calcium mobilisers, 117
calcium supplements, 138
cancer, medication used in, 294
    cell cycle, 295–296
    chemotherapies, 296–300
    corticosteroid, 308–311
    cyclophosphamide, 300–301
    drug resistance, 300
    hallmarks of, cell, 295
    immunotherapies for, 301–308
    malignant/cancerous tumours, 294
candesartan, 114
cannabidiol, 225
captopril, 113, 144
carbamazepine, 84
carbimazole, 152
cardiac output, 121
cardiovascular system, medication used in
    actions of, 115
    for acute clinical scenarios, 114
    affecting chronic conditions, 110–112
    alpha blockers (AB), 114
    angiotensin converting enzyme (ACE) inhibitors, 113
    Angiotensin II Receptor Antagonists (A2RA), 114
    anticoagulant medications, 112–113
    with chronotropic effect, 121–123
    electrophysiological system, 114–117
    with inotropic effect, 117–120
cardiovascular system (CVS) pharmacology, 108–109
care coordination, 63–64
carrier protein, 73
Case Law *see* Common Law
catecholamines, 116
cell membrane
    drug crossing, 72–73
    layers, 72
cell structure, 346
cellulitis, 262

CE mark of approved devices, 377
cephalosporins, 348, 349
CFTR modulators, 189
channel protein, 73
checkpoint inhibitors, 303–305
chemotherapies, for cancer, 296–301
    preparations of, 297
    prescription and administration of, 300
    side effects of, 299–300
    types of, 297–299
child and adult airway, 174
Children Act 1989, 249
Children Act 2004, 36, 43
    principles of, 36
children and young people (CYP)
    ACE inhibitors for, 144
    antiepileptic drugs for, 223
    appropriate medicine for, 90
    cancer *see* cancer, medication used in
    competence in, 42
    considerations for, 7
    ethical research, 40
    furosemide dosage for, 135
    Gillick and Fraser guidance, 42
    liquid rectal formulations in, 94
    mental health *see* mental health, medication for
chronic constipation, 211
chronic kidney disease (CKD), 130
chronic pain, 320, 337
chronotropic drugs, 114
chronotropic effect, cardiovascular drugs with, 121–123
chyme, 197
ciclosporin, 136, 137, 269
Civil Law, 35
clarithromycin, 261–262
    side effects of, 262
class monograph, 20
    contraindication and, 24
clotrimazole, 263
coal tar products, 269
codeine phosphate, 331
Code of Conduct, 2
Coeliac disease, 22
cognitive behavioural therapy (CBT), 233
cold chain, 248
colomycin, 188
Common Law, 34
community-acquired pneumonia (CAP), 178–179
competitive antagonist, 83
complementary and alternative medicines (CAM), 58
comprehensive assessment, 55
confidentiality, 53
congenital adrenal hyperplasia (CAH), 161, 163
congenital anomalies, 136
congenital hypothyroidism, 152
conjugate vaccines, 245
consequentialism theory, 38
constipation, 208–211
    causes of, 208
    osmotic laxatives, 210, 211

390 Index

constipation (*cont'd*)
  pharmacokinetics, 211
  stimulant laxatives, 210–211
  suppositories, 209–210
containment, 245
continuity of care, 63
controlled drugs, 6
convulsive status epilepticus (CSE), 226, 227
coordination of care, 63–64
corticosteroids, 134, 163, 164, 166
  for cancer, 308–311
  for Crohn's disease, 212
  for eczema, 265
  psoriasis, 268
  for respiratory disorders, 186–187
co-trimoxazole, 187
COVID-19 global pandemic, 354
Creutzfeldt–Jacob disease (CJD), 154
Criminal Law, 34
Crohn's disease (CD), 211–214
  pharmacological treatment for, 212–214
  treatment of, 212
  types, 212
croup, 177–178
Crown Prosecution Service (CPS), 34
Cushing's syndrome, 268
cyclophosphamide, 136, 137, 300–301
cystic fibrosis (CF), 179–180
  non-pharmaceutical management for, 179
  pharmaceutical management, 179
cytokines, 306, 307

Darier's disease, 269
Data Protection Act, 39
decision-making process, 9
deflazacort, 83
deontology, 39
depression, 280
dermis, 259
Desitrend® granules, 224
DesmoMelt (desmopressin), 93
dexamethasone, 164, 186, 187, 310
diabetes management, medication in, 163, 167–168
diazepam, 277–278
digitalis, 122
digoxin, 84, 122
dihydrocodeine, 331
dihydrotestosterone (DHT), 159
diltiazem, 117
diltiazem hydrochloride, 122
diphtheria, 245
direct hormone replacements, 159
displacement values, 100–101
disposable pen devices, 157
distraction techniques, 10–11, 95
distributive justice, 41
dithranol, 269
diuretics, 123
dobutamine hydrochloride, 119–120
dopamine hydrochloride, 119, 120, 122

dornase alfa, 188
Dravet syndrome (DS), 225
drug, defined, 2
drug calculations, 276
drug-drug interactions, 355
drug formulations
  displacement values, 100–101
  enteral feeding tubes, 97–99
  excipients, 96–97
  inhalation administration, 95
  intravenous route, 95–96
  licensing of paediatric medicines, 90–91
  mucous membranes, administration via, 93–94
  oral route of administration, 91–93
  parenteral administration, 95
  rectal administration, 93
  topical administration, 94
  types of, 91–96
drug history (DH), 70
drug monograph, 20–21, 23
drug resistance, 300
Drug Tariff, 26–27
Duchenne Muscular Dystrophy (DMD), 83
duodenum, 198
dupilumab, 267
dyslipidaemias, 111

echinocandins, 357
econazole, 263
eczema, 263–267
  assessment and diagnosis, 264–265
  bandages and dressings, 266
  severity of, 265
  systemic treatments, 266–267
  topical treatments, 265–266
electroconvulsive therapy (ECT), 35
electrolyte disorders, treatment of, 138–145
  bicarbonate supplements, 139, 142–143
  calcium supplements, 138
  phosphate binders, 138, 139, 141
  potassium binders and supplements, 138–139, 142
  vitamin D supplements, 138, 140
electronic medicines compendium, 26
electrophysiological system, 114–117
emergency medications, 226–228
EMLA cream, 334
emollients, 265, 267–268
enalapril, 113, 144
endocardium, 110
endocrine disorders, medication used in
  of adrenal glands, 162–165
  in diabetes management, 163, 167–168
  drugs for blocking puberty/action of sex steroids,
    160–161
  mecasermin (Increlex®), 156–158
  medications, affecting growth, 154–157
  of puberty, 154–156
  reduce action of sex steroids, drugs for, 161–162
  somatropin, 154–156, 158
endocrine function, of pancreas, 199

endocrine glands
  and hormones, 154
  location of, 153
endocrine system, 152–154
  endocrine glands location, 153
  endocrines glands and hormones, 154
  negative feedback system, 153
  positive feedback loop, 153
  terminology used in, 155
endogenous pathway, 111
end-stage renal disease (ESRD), 130
end-stage renal failure (ESRF), 133
enteral feeding tubes, 97–99, 204–208
  on CYP and their family, 207
  legal aspects of medication administration via, 207
  risks associated with medication administration via, 206
  sites of, 205
enteral medicines, 73–74
enteral tube feeding, 202
enteric-coated tablets, 9
enzyme inhibitor, 287
epicardium, 110
epidermis, 258–259
Epidyolex, 225
epilepsy
  antiepileptic drugs, 222–223
  cannabidiol, 225
  defined, 221
  emergency medications, 226–228
  lamotrigine, 223–224
  levetiracetam, 224
  seizure types, 222
  sodium valproate, 223
epinephrine, 119, 121
ergonomics, 63
European Medicines Agency (EMA), 89
evolocumab, 112
excipient-related toxicity, 96–97
excipients, 96–97
excretion, 78
exocrine function, of pancreas, 199
exogenous pathway, 111
ezetimibe, 112

facilitated diffusion, 73
familial hypercholesterolaemia, 110
family-centred care approach, 5
Family Law Reform Act, 41
fentanyl, 332–333
fidelity, 39
first-order elimination, 77
first-pass effect, 77
five As of drug-induced adverse events, 371
  5 Moments of Medication Safety, 53, 54, 60
Fleming, Alexander, 345
flucloxacillin, 8, 179, 261
  ADME of, 261
  side effects of, 261
fluconazole, 358

fluid balance, 136
flunarizine, 231
fluoxetine, 77, 281
  side effects, 281–282
fluroquinolones, 349–351
flutamide, 161
focal seizures, 222
focused assessment, 55
folic acid, 269
follicle-stimulating hormone (FSH), 160
formoterol, 184
frequently relapsing nephrotic syndrome (FRNS), 136
fungi, 345
furosemide, 135–136
fusidic acid, 261

gabapentin, 229, 333
gabapentinoids, 333
gallbladder, 199
gastroenterology
  constipation, 208–211
  Crohn's disease (CD), 211–214
  enteral feeding tubes, 204–208
  gallbladder, 199
  gastrointestinal system, anatomy and physiology of, 196–197
  gastro-oesophageal reflux disease, 200–204
  large intestine, 199–200
  liver, 199
  medication administration, 204–208
  pancreas, 199
  small intestines, 198–199
  stomach, 197
gastrointestinal system (GI), anatomy and physiology of, 196–197
gastro-oesophageal reflux (GOR), 200
  clinical manifestations, 201
  management of, 202
gastro-oesophageal reflux disease (GORD)
  clinical manifestations, 201
  management of, 202
  pharmacological treatment for, 202
  Proton Pump Inhibitors (PPIs), 202–204
Gaviscon˜, 202
generalised seizures, 222
generalised tonic-clonic seizures (GTCS), 225
General Medical Council (GMC), 37
general sales list, 6
gentamicin, 84
Gillick and Fraser guidance, 42
glucagon, 163, 168
glucocorticoids, 134, 186, 187
glutamate and gamma-aminobutyric acid (GABA), 222
gonadotrophin-releasing hormone analogues (GnRha), 160–161
Good Clinical Practice (GCP) principles, 40
growth hormone (GH), 154, 156
Guillain–Barre Syndrome (GBS), 228
  acute inflammatory demyelinating polyradiculoneuropathy, 228

392 Index

Guillain–Barre Syndrome (GBS) (*cont'd*)
  infections, 228
  intravenous immunoglobulin for, 228
  mortality rate in, 228
  plasmapheresis/therapeutic plasma exchange for, 228
  symptoms, 228

haemodynamic effectors, 123
half-life of medication, 81
head and neck, regions of, 233
HEADSS for Adolescents tool, 55–57
Health and Care Professions Council (HCPC), 37
Health and Safety Executive (HSE), 37
healthcare, 37
  duty of care and, 37
  regulation of, 37
health promotion, 52
heart
  anatomy and blood flow of, 109
  function, 109–110
  layers of, 109, 110
  left side of, 110
  right side of, 110
  structure of, 109
  valves, 109
heart valves, 109
hepatic first pass metabolism, 77, 78
hepatic impairment, 111
herpes virus, 352
Hib vaccine, 245
high-efficacy agonist, 82
history of presenting complaint (HPC), 70
holistic assessment, 52–53
hormone replacement therapy (HRT), 159
human chorionic gonadotrophin (HCG), 159
human factors approach, 63
Human Immunodeficiency Virus (HIV), 353
human immunoglobulin, 228
human normal immunoglobulin (HNIG), 228
Human Rights Act, 39
Human Tissue Act, 39
hydrochloric acid (HCl), 197, 198
hydrocortisone, 164, 186
hydrogen peroxide, 260
hyoscine hydrobromide patches, 94
hyperkalaemia, 137
hypersensitivity reaction, 351
hypertension, 141
hypertonic saline inhalation, 188
hypnotic medication, 279
hypocalcaemia, 138
hypogonadotrophic hypogonadism, 160
hypokalaemia, 137
hyponatraemia, 283
hypothyroidism, 111, 162
hypovolaemia, 133

ibuprofen, 80, 230
ideas, concerns and expectations (ICE), 70
ileum, 198–199

immune system, 301, 302
immunisation, 242
  adverse drug reaction and, 372–373
  cold chain, 248
  common reactions and anaphylaxis, 250–251
  communication with child and family, 251–252
  conjugate vaccines, 245
  inactivated vaccines, 244
  and law, 38
  live attenuated vaccines, 243–244
  Patient Group Directives, 248
  Patient Specific Directions, 248
  and public health, 245–246
  schedule, 246, 247
  vaccine administration, 248–250
  vaccine uptake, 246
immunity types, 242–243
immunosuppressant medication, 213, 267
immunotherapies, for cancer, 301–308
  active immunotherapy, 302
  adoptive cell transfer, 304–305
  bone marrow transplants, 304, 306
  checkpoint inhibitors, 303–305
  cytokines, 306, 307
  side effects of, 306–308
  supportive immunotherapy, 302
  targeted antibodies, 303
impetigo, 259–262, 264
  antibiotic creams, 261
  cellulitis, 262
  clarithromycin, 261–262
  flucloxacillin, 261
  fusidic acid, 261
  hydrogen peroxide, 260
  oral antibiotics, 261
  presentation, 259–260
  treatment, 260
  treatment course, 260–261
inactivated vaccines, 244
Increlex*, 156–157
infancy, 7–8
infections, 228
inflammation, 320
inflammatory bowel disease (IBD), 43, 211
infliximab, 213, 214
  action of, 213
influenza, 354
informed consent, 39–41
inhalation administration, 95
inhalation analgesics, 333–334
inhaled antibiotics, 179
inhalers, 182
  for asthma, 175
inotropic drugs, 114
inotropic effect, cardiovascular drugs with, 117–120
insulin-like growth factor 1 (IGF-1), 154, 157
insulins, 163, 167
  absorption rates and length of action of, 169
  syringe, 157
integumentary system, medication and

anatomy and physiology of, 258
   dermis, 259
   eczema, 263–267
   epidermis, 258–259
   impetigo, 259–262
   psoriasis, 267–270
   ringworm, 262–263
International Study of Kidney Disease in Children
   (ISKDC) regimen, 134
intramuscular injection, 249
intravenous analgesic medications, 335–336
intravenous antibiotics, 179
intravenous immunoglobulin (IVIG), 228–229
intravenous route of administration, 95–96
intrinsic activity, 82
ipratropium, 182, 185
isoniazid, 91

jejunum, 198
Joint Committee on Vaccination and Immunisation
   (JCVI), 245
Joint Royal Colleges Ambulance Liaison Committee
   Clinical (JRCALC) Guidelines, 27
justice, 39, 41

Kaftrio, 189
Kalydeco, 189
kidney structure, 131
KidzMed project, 44–45

labetalol, 116
lamotrigine (LTG), 223–224
large intestine, 199–200
large volume spacer, 177
laryngotracheobronchitis, 177–178
law
   Civil Law, 35
   Common Law, 34
   Criminal Law, 34
   and immunisations, 38
   Statute Law, 34
   Tort Law, 35
legal and ethical issues
   Bolam test, 35–36
   Children Act 2004, 36
   Civil Law, 35
   Common Law, 34
   competence, assessing and promoting, 42
   Criminal Law, 34
   duty of care and healthcare, 37
   ethical principles and theories, 38–39
   medication adherence and administration, 43–44
   parental responsibility, 43
   research, 39–42
   Statute Law, 34
   Tort Law, 35
Lennox–Gastaut Syndrome (LGS), 224, 225
letrozole, 161
leukotrienes, 182, 185
levamisole, 136

levetiracetam (LEV), 224, 227
levodopa, 77
levothyroxine, 162
licensing of paediatric medicines, 90–91
lidocaine, 115
lipid profile, 110
lisinopril, 113, 144
lithium, 84, 287
   baseline monitoring, 287
   discontinuation, 288
   plasma monitoring, 288
   renal and thyroid monitoring, 287
   toxicity, 287
live attenuated vaccines, 243–244
liver, 199
local anaesthetics (LA), 334–335
local anaesthetic systemic toxicity (LAST), 335
long-acting beta$_2$ agonists (LABA), 182
loop diuretics, 123, 135
lorazepam, 277
Losartan Potassium, 114
low cardiac output syndrome (LCOS), 117

macrolides, 179, 348–350
mecasermin (Increlex˙), 156–157
Medical Protection Society (MPS), 35
medication categories, 21
medicinal forms, 20–21, 23
medicinal product, 26, 27
medicine
   administration, 3
   controlled drugs, 6
   defined, 2
   general sales list, 6
   within healthcare, 3
   pharmacy medications, 6
   prescription-only medicines, 6
   types, 6
medicine management, 6–7, 50
   assessment, 53–55
   checking, 59
   complementary and alternative medicines (CAM), 58
   coordination of care, 63–64
   employer and colleagues, 51–52
   evaluation, 59–60
   health promotion, 52
   holistic assessment, 52–53
   ill health prevention, 52
   leading and managing nursing care and working in
     teams, 60–61
   planning, 58
   providing and evaluating care, 58–59
   safety and quality improvement, 62–63
   self-medication, 55, 58
Medicines and Healthcare products Regulatory Agency
   (MHRA), 24, 26, 223, 376
Medicines for Human Use (Clinical Trials) Regulations, 39
medicines optimisation, 5
Medicines Safety Improvement Programme, 62
melatonin, 232, 280

menotrophin, 160
Mental Capacity Act (MCA) 2005, 41, 42
mental health, medication for, 276
  antidepressants, 282–284
  antipsychotics, 284–285
  anxiety disorders, 276–278
  moderate and severe depression in, 281–282
  monoamine oxidase inhibitors, 282
  mood stabilisers, 285–288
  selective serotonin reuptake inhibitors, 281
  tricyclic antidepressants, 282
mesangiocapillary glomerulonephritis (MCGN), 133
metabolism, 76–78
  defined, 76
  first-pass metabolism, 77
  phases of, 76
  rate, 77
metastasis, 294
Metformin, 163, 168
methotrexate (MTX), 43, 213, 267, 269
methylphenidate, 278–279
metoprolol, 116
metred dose inhalers (MDIs), 175
metronidazole, 360
miconazole, 263
microorganisms, 344–345
microtubules, 299
Mid-Staffordshire Health trust, 41
migraine, 230–233
  antidepressant drugs, 232–233
  antiepileptic drugs, 232
  beta blockers, 231
  calcium channel blockers, 231–232
  melatonin, 232
  neurotoxins, 233
  preventative treatments, 231–233
  rescue treatment, 230–231
  serotonin modulators, 232
milrinone, 117, 119, 120
mineralocorticoids, 163, 165
mini assessment, 55
minimal change disease (MCD), 133
minimal change nephrotic syndrome (MCNS), treatment
    of, 134–138
  calcineurin inhibitors, 136–138
  contraindications, 134–135
  furosemide, 135–136
  prednisolone, 134
  SRNS, recommendations for management of, 134
monoamine oxidase (MAO), 282
monoamine oxidase inhibitors (MAOI), 282
monoclonal antibodies (MAB), 188–189, 267, 303, 304
Montelukast, 185
Monthly Index of Medical Specialities (MIMS), 24–26
mood stabilisers, 285–288
morphine, 332
mucolytics, 179, 188
mucous membranes, administration via, 93–94
Mycophenolate mofetil (MMF), 136, 137
myocardium, 110

naloxone, 330
Narrow Band Ultraviolet (UV) Light Therapy, 266
Narrow Therapeutic Index (NTI), 84
nasogastric tube (NGT), 74, 97, 205
National Institute for Health and Care Excellence
    (NICE), 23, 29
National Patient Safety Agency (NPSA), 3
natural killer (NK) cells, 242
nebuliser device, 180
negative chronotropes
  beta blockers (BB), 122
  digitalis, 122
  digoxin, 122
  diltiazem hydrochloride, 122
negative feedback system, 153
nephron structure, 131
nephrotic syndrome (NS), 130, 132–133
nervous system, medication used in, 220
  epilepsy see epilepsy
  Guillain–Barre Syndrome (GBS), 228–230
  migraine, 230–233
  Status Migrainosus (SM), 234
nervous system, parts of, 220
neuron, 221
neuropathic pain, 320
neurotoxins, 233
NHS Litigation Authority (NHS LA), 35
NHS prescription, 26–27
nociceptive pain, 320
non-competitive antagonist, 83
non-enteric-coated tablets, 10
non-maleficence, 39
non-opioids, 325–327
non-opioids and non-steroidal anti-inflammatory drugs
    (NSAIDs), 326, 327
non-selective antivirals, 354
non-steroidal anti-inflammatory drugs (NSAIDs), 230,
    326, 327
non-stimulant medication, 279
noradrenaline, 120, 122–123
norepinephrine, 120
Nursing and Midwifery Council (NMC), 2, 18, 37,
    51, 70

Octagam', 228, 229
oedema of airways, 174
oestrogen, 159
off-label medication, 78
Olanzapine (Zyprexa'), 285
omalizumab, 188
OnabotulinumtoxinA (botulinum toxin), 233
ondansetron, 231
ongoing assessment, 55
opioids, 319
  agonists, 327–330
  by receptor binding, 83
oral route of administration, 91–93
  advantages, 91
  disadvantages, 91
  flexible dosing with tablet formulations, 93

liquid formulations for, 91–92
solid dosage formulations for, 92
Orkambi, 189
orogastric tube (OGT), 74
osmotic laxatives, 210, 211
over the counter (OTC), 55
oxygen-haemoglobin dissociation curve, 181
oxygen therapy, 181–182
in children, 183
oxygen-haemoglobin dissociation curve, 181

Package Leaflets (PLs), 26
Paediatric Formulary Committee (PFC), 19
pain, 318
assessment tools, 321–322
child-centred and tailored approach, 323
codeine phosphate, 331
definitions and categories of, 319–320
dihydrocodeine, 331
fentanyl, 332–333
gabapentinoids, 333
individualised pain assessments, 320–321
inhalation analgesics, 333–334
local anaesthetics (LA), 334–335
morphine, 332
multimodal management strategies, 323–324
non-opioids, 325–327
non-pharmacological strategies, 323
non-steroidal anti-inflammatory drugs, 326, 327
opioid agonists, 327–330
pathways, 318–319
pharmacological management, 324–325
regional analgesia, 334–335
topical analgesic, 334–335
tramadol, 331–332
palivizumab, 188
palliative care, 20
pancreas, 199
paracetamol, 5, 25, 325
for migraine, 230
pharmacokinetics of, 80–81
sales, 22
paraldehyde, 227
parasympathetic innervation, 117, 118
parental responsibility, 43
parenteral administration, 95
parenteral medicines, 74
Parkinson disease, levodopa for, 77
passive acquired immunity, 242
passive diffusion, 72
passive transport, 72–73
past medical history (PMH), 70
Patient Group Directions (PGDs), 248
Patient Information Leaflets (PILs), 26
patient safety, 62
Patient Specific Direction (PSD), 248
penicillins, 347–351
Penicillin V, 351
percutaneous endoscopic gastrostomy (PEG) tube, 97, 201, 205

percutaneous endoscopic jejunostomy (PEJ), 74
peripheral alpha antagonist, 114
peritonitis, 134
pharmaceutical and prescribing reference guides
British National Formulary for Children (BNFc), 18
Drug Tariff, 26–27
electronic medicines compendium, 26
Joint Royal Colleges Ambulance Liaison Committee Clinical (JRCALC) Guidelines, 27
local and national prescribing guidelines, 29
NHS prescription, 26–28
NICE prescribing guidance, 29
Scottish Intercollegiate Guidelines Network (SIGN), 29
pharmacodynamics, 2, 81, 276
adverse effects, 85
agonist, 82–83
antagonists, 83
codeine phosphate, 331
dihydrocodeine, 331
fentanyl, 332–333
inhalation analgesics, 333–334
local, regional and topical analgesia, 334
morphine, 332
non-opioids, 325
non-opioids and non-steroidal anti-inflammatory drugs, 326, 327
opioid agonists, 327–329
of Proton Pump Inhibitors, 203–204
therapeutic index, 84
tramadol, 332
pharmacokinetics, 2, 276
absorption, 71–74
codeine phosphate, 331
constipation, 211
dihydrocodeine, 331
distribution, 74–76
elimination, 78–79
fentanyl, 332–333
inhalation analgesics, 333–334
local, regional and topical analgesia, 334
of loop diuretics, 135
metabolism, 76–78
morphine, 332
non-opioids, 325
non-opioids and non-steroidal anti-inflammatory drugs, 326, 327
opioid agonists, 327–329
paediatric, 79–80
of paracetamol, 80–81
principles, 70–71
of Proton Pump Inhibitors, 202–203
of statins, 111
tramadol, 332
pharmacology
adolescents, 9–10
babies, considerations for, 7
children and young people, considerations for, 7
defined, 2
distraction techniques, 10–11
infancy, 7–8

pharmacology (*cont'd*)
  medicine administration, 3
  medicines optimisation, 5
  medicine within healthcare, 3
  preservation of safety, 3
  rights of medication administration, 7
  safety within paediatric care, 5
  social prescribing, 4
  tablets, 10
  therapeutic, 3–4
pharmacy medications, 6
phenoxymethylpenicillin, 351
phenytoin, 84
phosphate, 137
phosphate binders, 138, 139, 141
phototherapy, 266, 269
pimecrolimus, 266
pitressin, 123
pizotifen, 232
placenta, 75–76
plaque psoriasis, 267
plasma cells, 242
pneumonia, 178–179
polio, 245
polycystic kidney disease, 136
polyenes, 357
positive chronotropes
  adrenaline (epinephrine), 121
  atropine sulfate, 121
  dopamine hydrochloride, 122
positive feedback loop, 153
positive inotropes, 117
  adrenaline, 119, 120
  dobutamine hydrochloride, 119–120
  dopamine hydrochloride, 119, 120
  milrinone, 117, 119, 120
  noradrenaline (norepinephrine), 120
potassium, 137
potassium binders, 138–139, 142
potassium homeostasis, 138
potassium-sparing diuretics, 123
potassium supplements, 138–139, 142
prednisolone, 134, 164, 186, 187
prescription-only medicines, 6
presenting complaint (PC), 70
pre-systemic metabolism, 77
preventer medications, 187
primary active transport, 73
prochlorperazine, 231
pro-drugs, 77
product information, 26
progesterone, 159
promethazine, 277
propafenone, 115
propranolol, 231
prophylactic penicillin, 134
protein binding, 74–75
Proton Pump Inhibitors (PPIs)
  pharmacodynamics of, 203–204
  pharmacokinetic properties of, 202–203

side effects of, 203
transportation of, 203
protozoa, 345
Psoralen and Long Wave Ultraviolet Light (PUVA), 266
psoriasis, 267–270
  assessment and diagnosis, 267
  biologic therapies, 270
  coal tar products, 269
  corticosteroids, 268
  dithranol, 269
  emollients/topical therapy, 267–268
  phototherapy, 269
  salicylic acid, 269
  systemic/disease-modifying drugs, 269–270
  types of, 267
  vitamin D preparations, 268
Psoriasis Area and Severity Index, 267
psychopharmacology, 276
psychosis, 284
psychotropic drug, 4
puberty, endocrine disorders of
  defined, 158
  dihydrotestosterone, 159
  direct hormone replacements, 159
  human chorionic gonadotrophin, 159
  menotrophin, 160
  oestrogen, 159
  progesterone, 159
  testosterone, 159
public health, immunisation and, 245
Public Prosecution Service (PPS), 34
pyridoxine (vitamin B6), 224

quinidine, 115

reagent strip procedure, 132
receptor-mediated ion channel, 82
recombinant insulin-like growth factor 1 (IGF-1), 156
rectal administration, 93
rectal diazepam, 226
rectal paraldehyde, 226, 227
referred pain, 320
regional analgesia, 334–335
Registered Nurses, 51, 58
relapse, defined, 133
renal impairment, 111
renal sodium reabsorption, 113
renal system, anatomy and physiology of, 130–132
renal system, medication in
  common renal conditions, 132
  minimal change nephrotic syndrome, treatment of, 134–138
  nephrotic syndrome (NS), 132–133
  to treat electrolyte disorders, 138–145
renal tubular acidosis, 137, 139
renal tubulointerstitial disease, 137
renin angiotensin aldosterone system (RAAS), 143
rescue medication, 226
Research Ethics Committees (RECs), 40
respiratory medicines, 180

antibiotics, 187–188
bronchodilators, 182, 184–185
CFTR modulators, 189
corticosteroids, 186–187
monoclonal antibodies, 188–189
mucolytics, 188
oxygen therapy, 181–182
respiratory system, medications in
asthma, 175–177
bronchiolitis, 178
child and adult airway, 174
croup, 177–178
cystic fibrosis (CF), 179–180
pneumonia, 178–179
reusable pen devices, 157
rights of medication administration, 7
ringworm, 262–263
drug interactions, 263
presentation of, 262–263
tinea infections, 262
topical antifungals, 263
treatment for, 263
Risk Minimisation Materials (RMMs), 26
risperidone, 285
rituxamab, 136, 137
rituximab, 305
rizatriptan, 231
rotavirus, 245
Royal Pharmaceutical Society (RPS), 70

safety alerts, 26
salbutamol, 83, 184
salbutamol inhaler, 10
salicylic acid, 269
salmeterol, 184
scalp psoriasis, 269
Scottish Intercollegiate Guidelines Network (SIGN), 24, 29
secondary active transport, 73
second messenger system, 82
seizure types, 222
Selective Serotonin 5-HT1-Receptor Agonists, 230
selective serotonin reuptake inhibitors (SSRIs), 231, 277, 281
absorption, 281
self-medication, 55, 58
sensitisation, 264
serotonin and noradrenaline reuptake inhibitors (SNRIs), 282
serotonin modulators, 232
serotonin syndrome, 283
sertraline, 277
short-acting beta$_2$ agonists (SABA), 182
signal transduction, 72
simvastatin, 111
Situation, Background, Assessment and Recommendation (SBAR) communication tool, 60, 61
skin layers, 259
sleep hygiene recommendations, 279, 280
slipped upper capital femoral epiphysis (SUFE), 156

small intestines, 198–199
social history (SH), 70
social prescribing, 4
sodium bicarbonate supplement, 141
sodium chloride, 165
sodium valproate, 223, 232, 285, 287
somatic pain, 320
somatropin, 154–156, 158
sotalol hydrochloride, 116–117
statins, 110–111
atorvastatin, 111
cautions/considerations for, 111
pharmacokinetics of, 111
side effects, 112
simvastatin, 111
Status Migrainosus (SM), 234
Statute Law, 34
steady state (SS), 81
stem cell transplants *see* bone marrow transplants (BMT)
stenosis, 109
steroid-resistant nephrotic syndrome (SRNS), 133, 134, 136
steroids, 60, 152, 186, 187, 308
steroid sensitive nephrotic syndrome (SSNS), 133
steroid sparing agents, 136
stimulant laxatives, 210–211
stimulant medications, 278
stomach, 197
subcutaneous injections, injection devices for, 157
sublingual formulations, 93
suicidal behaviour, 282
sumatriptan, 231
Summaries of Product Characteristics (SPCs/SmPCs), 26
supportive immunotherapy, 302
suppositories, 209–210
sustaining proliferative signalling, 294
Symkevi, 189
sympathetic innervation, 117, 118
synapses, 221
systemic/disease-modifying drugs, 269–270

tacalcitol, 268
tacrolimus, 137, 266
targeted antibodies, 303
T cells, 242, 243, 305
teicoplanin, 84
teratogenesis, 287
terbutaline, 184
termination of action, 81
testosterone, 159
tetracyclines, 348, 350
theophylline, 84, 185, 186
therapeutic drug monitoring, 85
therapeutic index, 84
Therapeutic pharmacology, 3–4
therapeutic plasma exchange (TPE), 228, 229
therapeutic range, 81
thiazide diuretics, 123
tiotropium, 182
tobramycin, 188

398 Index

topical administration, 94
topical analgesic, 334–335
topical antifungals, 263
topical calcineurin inhibitors, 266
topical medication, 74
topical medications, 267–268
topiramate, 232
Topoisomerase II, 298
Tort Law, 35
toxoplasmosis, 359
tramadol, 331–332
tricyclic antidepressants (TCA), 282
triptans, 230, 231
tuberculin syringe, 157
tumour, 294

urinalysis, 132, 133
utilitarian theory, 38

vaccines
  administration of, 248–250
  conjugate vaccines, 245
  Green Book, 252
  inactivated vaccines, 244
  live attenuated vaccines, 243–244
  uptake, 246
Valsartan, 114
vancomycin, 84

vasoactive drugs, 114
  noradrenaline, 122–123
  vasopressin, 123
vasopressin, 123
Vaughan-Williams classification, 115
veracity, 39
verapamil, 117
vinca alkaloids, 299
viruses, 345
  structure, 352
visceral pain, 320
visual infusion phlebitis (VIP) score, 122
vitamin D, 130, 137
  deficiency, 137
  preparations, 268
  supplements, 138, 140

warfarin, 112–113
White coat syndrome, 108
World Health Organization (WHO), 89, 368

xanthines, 185–186

Yellow Card Scheme, 24, 377–379

zolmitriptan, 231
Z-track injection technique, 286
Zyprexa*, 285